Geriatrics: Clinical Diagnosis and

Geriatrics: Clinical Diagnosis and Treatment

Edited by Benjamin Thornberg

hayle medical

New York

Hayle Medical,
750 Third Avenue, 9th Floor,
New York, NY 10017, USA

Visit us on the World Wide Web at:
www.haylemedical.com

ISBN: 978-1-63241-550-9

Cataloging-in-Publication Data

Geriatrics : clinical diagnosis and treatment / edited by Benjamin Thornberg.
    p. cm.
Includes bibliographical references and index.
ISBN 978-1-63241-550-9
1. Geriatrics. 2. Aging. 3. Gerontology. 4. Older people--Diseases--Treatment.
5. Clinical medicine. 6. Older people--Health and hygiene. I. Thornberg, Benjamin.
RC952 .G47 2019
618.97--dc23

Table of Contents

Preface

An aged human body differs from a younger body in physiology, particularly due to the gradual decline of the different organ systems with age. This decline is significantly influenced by past medical history and lifestyle choices. Some of the major impairments in the elderly include incontinence, immobility, instability and impaired memory/intellect. Elderly people may suffer from multiple complications and hence need special focus on medications. Geriatrics or geriatric medicine is a specialization in healthcare medicine, which is concerned with the treatment and prevention of diseases and disabilities in the elderly. Some of the geriatric-related services or specializations in geriatric medicine include cardiogeriatrics, geriatric nephrology, geriatric oncology, psychogeriatrics, etc. A geriatrician aims to achieve independence, continued functional abilities and quality of life in their patients. This book contains some path-breaking studies in the field of geriatrics. Also included herein is a detailed explanation of the clinical diagnosis and treatment techniques of geriatric medicine. It is appropriate for students seeking detailed information in this area as well as for experts.

The information shared in this book is based on empirical researches made by veterans in this field of study. The elaborative information provided in this book will help the readers further their scope of knowledge leading to advancements in this field.

Finally, I would like to thank my fellow researchers who gave constructive feedback and my family members who supported me at every step of my research.

Editor

Montreal cognitive assessment reflects cognitive reserve

Jae Myeong Kang[1†], Young-Sung Cho[2,3†], Soowon Park[4], Byung Ho Lee[5], Bo Kyung Sohn[2], Chi Hyun Choi[3], Jeong-Seok Choi[2,3], Hee Yeon Jeong[2,3], Seong-Jin Cho[1], Jae-Hong Lee[6] and Jun-Young Lee[2,3*]

Abstract

Background: The Montreal Cognitive Assessment (MoCA) is known to have discriminative power for patients with Mild Cognitive Impairment (MCI). Recently Cognitive Reserve (CR) has been introduced as a factor that compensates cognitive decline. We aimed to assess whether the MoCA reflects CR. Furthermore, we assessed whether there were any differences in the efficacy between the MoCA and the Mini-Mental State Examination (MMSE) in reflecting CR.

Methods: MoCA, MMSE, and the Cognitive Reserve Index questionnaire (CRIq) were administered to 221 healthy participants. Normative data and associated factors of the MoCA were identified. Correlation and regression analyses of the MoCA, MMSE and CRIq scores were performed, and the MoCA score was compared with the MMSE score to evaluate the degree to which the MoCA reflected CR.

Results: The MoCA reflected total CRIq score (CRI; $B = 0.076$, $P < 0.001$), CRI-Education ($B = 0.066$, $P < 0.001$), and CRI-Working activity ($B = 0.025$, $P = 0.042$), while MMSE reflected total CRI ($B = 0.044$, $P < 0.001$) and CRI-Education ($B = 0.049$, $P < 0.001$) only. The MoCA differed from the MMSE in the reflection of total CRI ($Z = 2.30$).

Conclusion: In this study, we show that the MoCA score reflects CR more sensitively than the MMSE score. Therefore, we suggest that MoCA can be used to assess CR and early cognitive decline.

Keywords: MoCA, Cognition, Cognitive reserve, Dementia, Mild cognitive impairment

Background

In recent years, the number of patients with dementia has increased worldwide. This increase emphasizes the importance of early detection and treatment of dementia. Therefore, the development and standardization of effective screening tools are required. The Montreal Cognitive Assessment (MoCA) is known to distinguish patients with Mild Cognitive Impairment (MCI) from the normal population [1]. MoCA has shown higher sensitivity in detecting cognitive decline than the Mini-Mental State Examination (MMSE) [2], another common clinical screening tool for Alzheimer's disease (AD). Previous studies have indicated that the MoCA exhibits high sensitivity and specificity in other languages as well. Moreover, MoCA is not only highly sensitive in identifying patients with AD, but also non-AD patients who demonstrate behavioral variants of frontotemporal dementia [3], dementia associated with Parkinson's disease [4], and vascular dementia [5].

Cognitive Reserve (CR) is a concept based on the plasticity of the brain. CR is believed to counter the effects of aging or brain damage. It has been suggested that environmental factors play an important role in the onset of AD. Moreover, a meta-analysis reported that higher CR lowers the risk for incidence of dementia to 54% [6]. CR is associated with diverse factors of life experience such as higher intellectual quotient (IQ), education, occupational complexity and duration, and lifestyle [7]. Several measures have been developed to assess CR using these variables. The Cognitive Reserve Index questionnaire (CRIq), which has been developed by Nucci et al. [8], has advantages over other measures assessing comprehensive CR; CRIq measures 3 subdomains, i.e.,

* Correspondence: benji@snu.ac.kr
†Jae Myeong Kang and Young-Sung Cho contributed equally to this work.
2Department of Psychiatry, SMG-SNU Boramae Medical Center, Boramae-Ro 5-Gil, Shindaebang-dong, Dongjak-gu, Seoul, Republic of Korea
3Department of Psychiatry and Behavioral Science, Seoul National University College of Medicine, Boramae-Ro 5-Gil, Shindaebang-dong, Dongjak-gu, Seoul, Republic of Korea
Full list of author information is available at the end of the article

education, occupation, and leisure activities, which are the most used proxies of CR [9]. Unlike other measurements, which only evaluate current activities of 1 or 2 domains, CRIq considers activities from all 3 subdomains throughout adulthood, including the frequency of the activities.

As the MoCA exhibits higher sensitivity than the MMSE in cognitive decline in the early stages of AD, the MoCA might be more sensitive to factors such as age, sex, and CR than MMSE. Recently, a study reported that educational domain in CR can affect MoCA and MMSE scores in patients with MCI [10]. However, to the best of our knowledge, no prior studies have assessed the degree to which MoCA reflects CR. Moreover, comparisons of the level at which MoCA and MMSE reflect CR are lacking. In the present study, we examined the associations of demographic factors (sex, age, and education) and CR with MoCA and compared the level of reflection of CR in MoCA and MMSE using CRIq as a comprehensive measure of CR.

Methods

Subjects

Subjects were recruited from a community-based center from March 2013 to June 2016 through recruitment announcements. Assessments of their physical and neuropsychiatric disorders were performed by 2 community dementia center consultant psychiatrists with 6 years and 15 years of experience, respectively.

Subjects with dementia or any mental or physical disease that may affect cognitive functioning, such as alcohol or other substance abuse, history of infarction, any evidence of central nervous system disorders or brain damage were excluded. Patients with severe major depressive disorders, altered state of consciousness like delirium, severe loss of hearing or sight, or language disorders were also excluded. However, patients with general medical problems, well-controlled diabetes, essential hypertension, or mild impairment of vision or hearing due to aging were not excluded if the impairment did not restrict their ability to perform the tests. Exclusion criteria were determined by psychiatrists on the basis of diagnostic criteria in the Diagnostic and Statistical Manual of Mental Disorders, fourth Edition (DSM-IV) [11].

A total of 221 subjects participated in this study and the age of subjects ranged from 60 to 90 years. Informed consent was obtained from all participants and the study was approved by the institutional review board of SMG-SNU Boramae Medical Center.

Data collection

Clinical neuropsychological tests (MoCA and MMSE) were administered to all subjects by mental health center specialists and professional dementia researchers (nurses,

clinical psychologists) who had experience with the tests for an average of 10 years. CR was assessed using the self-reported CRIq completed by the subjects and interviews with the subjects' close family members.

Measurements

Korean version of Montreal cognitive assessment (MoCA-K)

MoCA is a screening instrument to detect MCI developed by Nasreddine et al. Administration of MoCA takes about 10 to 15 min. Higher scores indicate better cognition; the maximum score is 30 [2]. There are 12 items for cognitive domains; memory is tested by a short-term memory recall task (5 points); visuospatial ability is tested using a clock-drawing test (CDT; 3 points) and a 3-dimensional cube copy (1 point); executive function is tested using a trail-making test, part B (TMT-B; 1 point), a phonemic fluency task (1 point), and a 2-item verbal abstraction task (2 points); attention, concentration, and working memory is tested using a sustained attention task (1 point), a serial subtraction task (3 points), and digits forward and backward tasks (1 point each); language is tested using a 3-item confrontation naming task with low-familiarity animals (lion, camel, rhinoceros; 3 points) and repetition of 2 syntactically complex sentences (2 points); orientation in time and place was also tested (6 points). MoCA-K was standardized for Koreans. It should be taken into consideration that the words for the short-term memory recall task and the TMT-B were replaced by Korean words and the semantic fluency task was replaced by a phonemic fluency task. One point was added for subjects with 6 years or less of education in MoCA-K to account for the large illiteracy in elderly Koreans [12]. In the current study, however, we did not add the correction point, to investigate normative data of MoCA-K without any adjustment.

Mini-mental state examination-dementia screening (MMSE-DS)

MMSE is the most commonly used dementia screening tool that can be performed in the relatively short time of 5 to 10 min. The MMSE consists of 30 questions with a maximum score of 30. Higher scores indicate better cognition. The MMSE tests the following 7 cognitive domains: orientation in time and place, memory registration and recall, attention and calculation, and language. In Korea, there are several standardized forms of the MMSE, such as MMSE-K [13], K-MMSE [14], MMSE-KC [15]. However, the present study was conducted using MMSE-DS [16]. MMSE-DS has been developed to reflect the specific characteristics of the Korean elderly population and add cultural sensitivity. Normative data and test accuracy were validated for the Korean elderly population using age, sex, and years of education. Scores under 25 indicate cognitive impairment [16].

Korean version of cognitive reserve index questionnaire (K-CRIq)
The CRIq has been developed by Nucci et al. It consists
of 20 questions collecting demographic information, the
number of years of education, and occupational and leisure activities throughout adulthood [8]. Regarding the
years of education (CRI-Education), both formal and
non-formal education and training years were included.
The working activity (CRI-WorkingActivity) value is divided into 5 levels depending on the cognitive load involved. The leisure activity area (CRI-LeisureTime) is
measured by evaluating cognitive activity, except for
education and occupation activity, using 17 questions to
evaluate the type and frequency of cognitive activity.
Considering the effect of aging, scores for each category
are obtained using age as an independent variable. The
scores of 3 domains are calculated again to an average of
100 and a standard deviation of 15 to obtain the total
CRIq score (CRI). Choi et al. reported a Korean version
of CRIq normalized to age and sex [17].

Statistical analyses
Descriptive statistics were used to obtain the mean score
and standard deviation for demographic characteristics
and scores for MMSE, MoCA, and CRIq. Independent
t-tests were used to compare the scores of different
groups divided by sex. To measure correlations between
the demographic variables and MoCA scores, Pearson
correlation, and multivariate linear regression analyses
(independent variable: age, sex, and years of education)
were used. The interactions between age and years of
education in MoCA were analyzed by multivariate regression analysis using interaction terms.

Univariate and multivariate linear regression analyses,
using a stepwise method, were used to evaluate the correlation between CR and the MoCA and MMSE scores.
To avoid multicollinearity, the total CRI score was analyzed separately from subdomains of CRIq. In order to
compare the degree to which the MoCA and MMSE
scores reflect CR, correlation coefficients were compared
using Fisher's *r*-to-*z* transformation, and regression coefficients were compared using *z* transformation. All statistical analyses were performed using Statistical Package
for the Social Sciences (SPSS) version 23.0 (SPSS, Inc.,
Chicago IL) and statistical significance was defined as
$P < 0.05$ (2-tailed).

Results
Demographics and clinical characteristics
Table 1 shows the demographic and clinical results of
the subjects that participated in this study. CRIq is presented
as the total score (CRI) and the 3 subdomains, i.e.,
CRI-Education, CRI-WorkingActivity, and CRI-LeisureTime.
When the results of the male and female subjects were compared, male subjects showed significantly higher scores of

CRI, CRI-Education, and CRI-WorkingActivity ($P < 0.001$)
than female subjects; female subjects exhibited a significantly higher CRI-LeisureTime score than male
subjects ($P < 0.001$).

Relationships between demographical variables and MoCA
Table 2 shows descriptive data of MoCA scores using
age, sex, and educational level. MoCA scores were associated with all 3 demographic variables, showing higher
scores for subjects with longer educational times (correlation analysis: $r = 0.446$, $P < 0.001$), younger age (correlation analysis: $r = -0.347$, $P < 0.001$), and male subjects
(independent *t*-test: $t = 2.903$, $P = 0.004$).

When the demographic variables were analyzed using
multivariate linear regression analysis, education level
showed moderating effect on the influence of age on
MoCA score. The higher the education level was, the
lower the degree of MoCA score decreased with age
($B = 0.017$, $P = 0.023$, Additional file 1: Table A1).

Correlations of MoCA, MMSE, and CR
Pearson correlation was performed between MoCA,
MMSE and CRIq scores (Table 3).

Correlation of MoCA score with total CRI was $r =
0.383$, $P < 0.001$; with CRI-Education $r = 0.356$, $P
< 0.001$; CRI-WorkingActivity $r = 0.246$, $P < 0.001$, and
CRI-LeisureTime $r = 0.224$, $P = 0.001$). Semi-partial correlation analysis adjusting sex was performed in order to
find relation between MoCA, MMSE, and CRIq scores
adjusting the effect of sex because age and years of education were already adjusted in CRIq and it showed
comparable results (Additional file 1: Table A2).

Linear regression analyses were performed to investigate the effect of CRIq on the MoCA and MMSE
scores (Table 4).

We conducted univariate linear regression analyses for
total and each subdomain score of CRIq, and multivariate linear regression analyses using a stepwise method
based on the 3 subdomains of CRIq. Total CRI and the
3 subdomains of CRIq were analyzed separately to avoid
multicollinearity. The results showed a significant association of the total CRI and MoCA scores ($B = 0.076$,
$P < 0.001$), with an explanatory power of 15% ($R^2 =
0.147$, $F = 37.723$, $P < 0.001$). In the final model of
multivariate regression analysis using stepwise
method ($F = 18.245$, $P < 0.001$), CRI-Education and
CRI-WorkingActivity also showed correlations with the
MoCA score (CRI-Education: $B = 0.066$, $P < 0.001$;
CRI-WorkingActivity: $B = 0.025$, $P = 0.042$), with an explanatory power of 14% ($R^2 = 0.143$). CRI-LeisureTime
was not included in the final regression model. For the
MMSE score, univariate linear regression analysis ($F =
35.416$, $P < 0.001$) indicated that the total CRI was signifi-
cantly correlated with the MMSE score ($B = 0.044$, $P = 0.042$)

Table 1 Demographic and clinical characteristics

	Male (n = 95)	Female (n = 126)	Total (n = 221)	P value
Age (year)	74.60 ± 5.54	73.39 ± 5.79	73.91 ± 5.70	0.118
60–74	50 (52.6%)	74 (58.7%)	124 (56.1%)	
75–90	45 (47.4%)	52 (41.3%)	97 (43.9%)	
Education (year)	10.65 ± 4.61	8.83 ± 4.81	9.61 ± 4.80	0.005
0–6	29 (30.5%)	56 (44.4%)	85 (38.5%)	
7–12	35 (36.8%)	38 (30.2%)	73 (33.0%)	
13-	31 (32.6%)	32 (25.4%)	63 (28.5%)	
MMSE	27.47 ± 1.83	26.94 ± 2.23	27.17 ± 2.08	0.041
MoCA	23.40 ± 3.21	22.03 ± 3.65	22.62 ± 3.53	0.004
CRIq				
CRI	107.32 ± 18.46	99.28 ± 16.10	102.74 ± 17.57	0.001
CRI-Education	106.11 ± 15.63	99.30 ± 16.04	102.23 ± 16.19	0.002
CRI-WorkingActivity	114.50 ± 20.70	92.32 ± 11.55	101.86 ± 19.49	< 0.001
CRI-LeisureTime	95.44 ± 16.32	106.80 ± 19.13	101.92 ± 18.80	< 0.001

Data are shown in mean ± standard deviation or number (%)
MMSE Mini-mental Status Examination, *MoCA* Montreal Cognitive Assessment, *CRIq* Cognitive Reserve Index questionnaire

and the explanatory power was 14% (R^2 = 0.139). When all 3 domains of CRIq were treated as independent variables in the multivariate linear regression analysis (F = 36.655, P < 0.001), only CRI-Education was included in the final model with significant effects (B = 0.049, P < 0.001). The explanatory power was 14% (R^2 = 0.143).

Table 2 Mean, standard deviation, and selected percentiles of the MoCA-K by age, educational level, and sex in the normal Korean elderly

Educational level (year)	Male (n = 95)			Female (n = 126)		
	0–6	7–12	13-	0–6	7–12	13-
Age (year)						
60~ 74						
N	16	19	15	33	24	17
Mean	23.44	24.05	25.33	21.88	23.54	25.12
Standard deviation	2.80	3.47	1.92	3.55	2.89	2.37
Lower quartile	21.25	22.0	24.0	19.0	21.0	23.0
Median	23.0	25.0	26.0	23.0	23.50	26.0
Upper quartile	25.50	27.0	27.0	24.50	26.0	26.0
75~ 90						
N	13	16	16	23	14	15
Mean	19.69	22.50	24.69	18.87	19.71	23.47
Standard deviation	2.29	3.25	2.27	3.08	2.76	2.95
Lower quartile	18.50	19.25	23.0	15.0	18.0	21.0
Median	19.0	23.0	25.0	20.0	19.0	24.0
Upper quartile	21.0	24.75	26.0	21.0	22.0	26.0

MoCA-K Montreal Cognitive Assessment

Comparison between MoCA and MMSE on reflection of CRIq

Correlations of MoCA and MMSE scores with CRIq are shown in a scatter plot (Fig. 1). The zero-order correlation coefficients shown in Table 3 were compared using Fisher's r-to-z transformation. We observed no significant difference in total CRI (r for MoCA = 0.383, r for MMSE = 0.373) and CRI-Education (r for MoCA = 0.356, r for MMSE = 0.379). In addition, we compared the multivariate regression coefficient B shown in Table 4, which represents the correlation slope between the CRIq score and MoCA or MMSE scores; MoCA scores tended to show a larger slope than MMSE scores. We observed a significant difference in total CRI (B for MoCA = 0.076, B for MMSE = 0.044, Z = 2.30) but not in CRI-Education (B for MoCA = 0.066, B for MMSE = 0.049, Z = 1.06).

Discussion

In this study, the MoCA was associated with years of education, age, and sex. In addition, MoCA was also significantly associated with CR. Furthermore, we compared

Table 3 Correlation analyses between CRIq score and MMSE or MoCA scores

	CRI	CRI-Education	CRI-WorkingActivity	CRI-LeisureTime
MoCA	r = 0.383	r = 0.356	r = 0.246	r = 0.224
	P < 0.001	P < 0.001	P < 0.001	P = 0.001
MMSE	r = 0.373	r = 0.379	r = 0.165	r = 0.268
	P < 0.001	P < 0.001	P = 0.014	P < 0.001

CRIq Cognitive Reserve Index questionnaire, *MMSE* Mini-mental State Examination, *MoCA* Montreal Cognitive Assessment

Table 4 Univariate and multivariate regression analyses between CRIq score and MoCA and MMSE scores

Dependent variable	Independent variable	B	Standard Error	t	P value
Univariate regression analyses					
MoCA	CRI	0.076	0.012	6.14	< 0.001
	CRI-Education	0.077	0.014	5.64	< 0.001
	CRI-WorkingActivity	0.044	0.012	3.76	< 0.001
	CRI-LeisureTime	0.042	0.012	3.39	0.001
MMSE	CRI	0.044	0.007	5.95	< 0.001
	CRI-Education	0.049	0.008	6.05	< 0.001
	CRI-WorkingActivity	0.018	0.007	0.01	0.014
	CRI-LeisureTime	0.030	0.007	4.11	< 0.001
Multivariate regression analyses[a]					
MoCA	CRI-Education	0.066	0.014	4.59	< 0.001
	CRI-WorkingActivity	0.025	0.012	2.05	0.042
MMSE	CRI-Education	0.049	0.008	6.05	< 0.001

[a]Multivariate linear regression: independent variables are CRI-Education, CRI-WorkingActivity, and CRI-LeisureTime. The variables included in the final models of multivariate regression analyses using stepwise method are presented

CRIq Cognitive Reserve Index questionnaire, *MoCA* Montreal Cognitive Assessment, *MMSE* Mini-mental State Examination

the degree to which CR was reflected in the MoCA and MMSE. Our results showed that the MoCA score reflected CR better than the MMSE score.

The first findings of our study are the MoCA scores. MoCA scores tended to be higher for the patients with more years of education and of younger age. These results are similar to results from previous normative studies [18, 19]. Additionally, aging had a larger effect on MoCA scores in a population with lower education than in a population with higher education. This result indicates

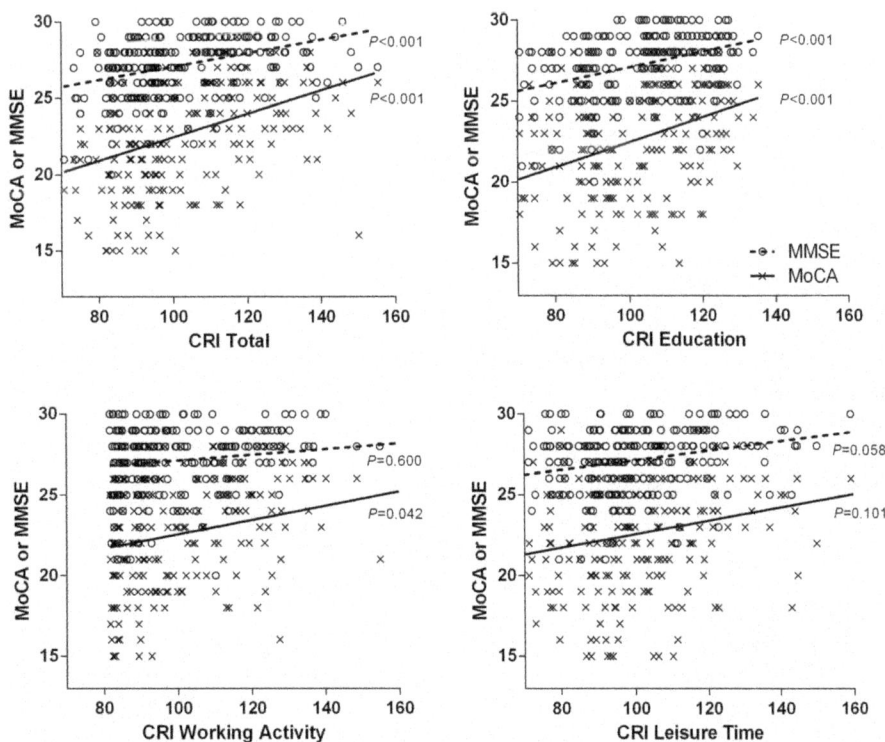

Fig. 1 Correlation between MoCA or MMSE and CRIq. *P* values for the subdomains of CRIq are obtained from the multivariate regression analyses using stepwise method (dependent variable: MoCA or MMSE, independent variables: CRI-Education, CRI-WorkingActivity, CRI-LeisureTime). *MoCA* Montreal Cognitive Assessment, *MMSE* Mini-Mental State Examination, *CRIq* Cognitive reserve index questionnaire

that the effect of education overcomes the effect of aging. This is in line with previous studies suggesting that education is a major factor in CR [20, 21]. Regarding this significant effect of education, Nasreddine et al. have included one correction point in the MoCA for individuals with education of 12 years and below. In Korea, Lee et al. set a similar correction point in the MoCA-K for individuals with 6 years or less of education, considering the low level of education in Korea [12]. However, in this study, the correction point was not applied to determine the association between normative scores of MoCA-K and CR or demographic variables. MoCA scores were higher in male subjects than in female subjects, which is in line with the results of the Chinese MoCA study [22] and an MMSE normative study performed on Koreans [23]. This sexual discrepancy in normative data is considered to reflect a tendency of elderly men to have more intellectual, social, and physical opportunities than women due to gender role differences.

Our results demonstrated that both MoCA and MMSE correlate with CR, although MoCA score reflects CR more sensitively than MMSE score. In regression analyses with total and subdomain scores of CRIq, the MoCA score reflected total CRI, CRI-Education, and CRI-WorkingActivity, while the MMSE score only reflected total CRI and CRI-Education. In addition, the correlation slope between the total CRI and MoCA scores was significantly higher than that between the total CRI and MMSE scores. We suggest that this discrepancy was due to differences in the tools of assessment employed by the MoCA and MMSE; MoCA contains various assessment tools for frontal lobe function (TMT-B, copy of a cube, CDT, letter A tap, letter fluency), which are not included in MMSE, making it sensitive to and reflective of CR in various cognitive subdomains [24]. It is known from previous studies that connectivity in the frontal lobe plays an important role in CR [25, 26]. This can be more prominent in the elderly. Compared to young individuals, old individuals use different brain networks [27]. Scarmeas et al. investigated the brain regions related to CR and found that the inferior frontal region is related to CR only in old subjects [28]. The increase in activity and connectivity in the prefrontal area of patients with AD, compared with normal controls, has been interpreted to reflect the recruitment of cognitive resources [9, 29]. Increased activity in the prefrontal cortex has also been associated with tasks such as episodic, retrieval, and recognition memory, which are the most basic memory functions and are frequently affected by cognitive decline [25].

In particular, our study suggests that only the MoCA scores can sensitively reflect CRI-WorkingActivity among the subdomains of CRIq. This association between MoCA and the vocational ability is attributed to the assessment of frontal lobe function by MoCA. The effect of vocational ability on CR can be explained by the motivation to participate in cognitively stimulating daily activities, neuronal plasticity, and executive functions, making it a favorable domain to examine CR [30, 31]. Many studies have shown that vocational abilities are dependent on frontal lobe function in patients with traumatic brain injuries and vascular degenerative changes. Since the frontal lobe is involved in language, arithmetic processing, attention, planning and strategy application, and willful action, it can be a good indicator of vocational ability [32–34]. Proxies such as educational or occupational achievements, and IQ have been used to characterize CR previously [7, 31]. In conjunction with our results, it appears that it would be clinically beneficial to use MoCA as a brief cognitive screening tool for the assessment of both cognitive function and reserve.

Recently, interest in CR has increased because of its importance in identifying and managing patients with preclinical and prodromal AD. Lacking a current disease-modifying treatment, CR can be another interesting candidate for the prevention and treatment of AD. Accordingly, the number of studies investigating treatments using cognitive stimulation is sharply increasing [35]. CR consists of these lifetime experiences. High levels of CR have been reported to be capable of lowering the risk of incidents of dementia, its clinical symptoms, and its pathologic changes, as shown by neuroimaging studies [6, 10, 36–38].

Our study shows that MoCA score correlates with CR, especially in terms of education and working activity, which corresponds to executive function. Therefore, MoCA can be a useful tool to evaluate CR and to screen the subtle changes in cognition. However, our present study has limitations that should be taken into account when evaluating the results. For example, our study only included a small number of participants, and the participants in this study had fewer years of education than those in studies from other countries. Future larger studies supported by more validating methods and biological assays are required to overcome these limitations.

Conclusion

This study confirms that MoCA reflects CR, and that CR is reflected more sensitively by the MoCA score than the MMSE score. The clinical use of the MoCA is expected to increase markedly, because it provides an easy way to evaluate cognitive function and CR, without any additional tests or large-scale batteries. This study may provide valuable insight for future, large community-based studies of early cognitive decline and CR.

Abbreviations

CDT: Clock-Drawing Test; CR: Cognitive Reserve; CRIq: Cognitive Reserve Index questionnaire; DSM-IV: Diagnostic and Statistical Manual of Mental Disorders, fourth Edition; IQ: Intellectual Quotient; MCI: Mild Cognitive Impairment; MMSE: Mini-Mental State Examination; MoCA: Montreal Cognitive Assessment; TMT-B: Trail-Making Test, Part B

Acknowledgements

Not applicable.

Funding

This study was conducted without financial support. All authors are independent from the funding sources.

Author's contributions

All authors listed above contributed significantly to this study. JYL: study concept and design, critical review and approval for final manuscript; JMK, YSC: data acquisition, data analyses, writing and editing manuscript; SP: data analyses and interpretation; BHL: data analyses, critical review, and editing manuscript; JHL, BKS, JSC, HYJ, SJC: critical review; CHC: data acquisition, critical review, and editing manuscript. All authors have read and approved the final version of the manuscript.

Competing interests

The authors declare that they have no competing interests.

Author details

[1]Department of Psychiatry, Gil Medical Center, Gachon University College of Medicine, Incheon, Republic of Korea. [2]Department of Psychiatry, SMG-SNU Boramae Medical Center, Boramae-Ro 5-Gil, Shindaebang-dong, Dongjak-gu, Seoul, Republic of Korea. [3]Department of Psychiatry and Behavioral Science, Seoul National University College of Medicine, Boramae-Ro 5-Gil, Shindaebang-dong, Dongjak-gu, Seoul, Republic of Korea. [4]Department of Education, Sejong University, Seoul, Republic of Korea. [5]Department of Psychology, Salisbury University, Salisbury, Maryland, USA. [6]Department of Neurology, Asan Medical Center, University of Ulsan College of Medicine, Seoul, Republic of Korea.

References

1. Petersen RC, Smith GE, Waring SC, Ivnik RJ, Tangalos EG, Kokmen E. Mild cognitive impairment: clinical characterization and outcome. Arch Neurol. 1999;56(3):303–8.
2. Nasreddine ZS, Phillips NA, Bédirian V, Charbonneau S, Whitehead V, Collin I, Cummings JL, Chertkow H. The Montreal cognitive assessment, MoCA: a brief screening tool for mild cognitive impairment. J Am Geriatr Soc. 2005;53(4):695–9.
3. Freitas S, Simões MR, Alves L, Duro D, Santana I. Montreal cognitive assessment (MoCA): validation study for frontotemporal dementia. J Geriatr Psychiatry Neurol. 2012;25(3):146–54.
4. Hoops S, Nazem S, Siderowf A, Duda J, Xie S, Stern M, Weintraub D. Validity of the MoCA and MMSE in the detection of MCI and dementia in Parkinson disease. Neurology. 2009;73(21):1738–45.
5. Freitas S, Simoes MR, Alves L, Vicente M, Santana I. Montreal cognitive assessment (MoCA): validation study for vascular dementia. J Int Neuropsychol Soc. 2012;18(06):1031–40.
6. Valenzuela MJ, Sachdev P. Brain reserve and dementia: a systematic review. Psychol Med. 2006;36(04):441–54.
7. Stern Y. Cognitive reserve in ageing and Alzheimer's disease. Lancet Neurol. 2012;11(11):1006–12.
8. Nucci M, Mapelli D, Mondini S. Cognitive reserve index questionnaire (CRIq): a new instrument for measuring cognitive reserve. Aging Clin Exp Res. 2012; 24(3):218–26.
9. Horwitz B, McIntosh AR, Haxby JV, Furey M, Salerno JA, Schapiro MB, Rapoport SI, Grady CL. Network analysis of PET-mapped visual pathways in Alzheimer type dementia. Neuroreport. 1995;6(17):2287–92.
10. Liu Y, Cai Z-L, Xue S, Zhou X, Wu F. Proxies of cognitive reserve and their effects on neuropsychological performance in patients with mild cognitive impairment. J Clin Neurosci. 2013;20(4):548–53.
11. American Psychiatric Association: Diagnostic and statistical manual of mental disorders DSM-IV-TR fourth edition (text revision). 2000.
12. Lee J-Y, Lee DW, Cho S-J, Na DL, Jeon HJ, Kim S-K, Lee YR, Youn J-H, Kwon M, Lee J-H. Brief screening for mild cognitive impairment in elderly outpatient clinic: validation of the Korean version of the Montreal cognitive assessment. J Geriatr Psychiatry Neurol. 2008;21(2):104–10.
13. Park JH, Kwon YC. Modification of the mini-mental state examination for use in the elderly in a non-western society. Part 1. Development of korean version of mini-mental state examination. Int J Geriatr Psychiatry. 1990;5(6): 381–7.
14. Kang Y, Na DL, Hahn S. A validity study on the Korean mini-mental state examination (K-MMSE) in dementia patients. J Korean Neurol Assoc. 1997; 15(2):300–8.
15. Lee JH, Lee KU, Lee DY, Kim KW, Jhoo JH, Kim JH, Lee KH, Kim SY, Han SH, Woo JI. Development of the Korean version of the consortium to establish a registry for Alzheimer's disease assessment packet (CERAD-K) clinical and neuropsychological assessment batteries. J Gerontol B Psychol Sci Soc Sci. 2002;57(1):P47–53.
16. Kim TH, Jhoo JH, Park JH, Kim JL, Ryu SH, Moon SW, Choo IH, Lee DW, Yoon JC, Do YJ. Korean version of mini mental status examination for dementia screening and its' short form. Psychiatry investig. 2010;7(2):102–8.
17. Petersen RC, Roberts RO, Knopman DS, Boeve BF, Geda YE, Ivnik RJ, Smith GE, Jack CR. Mild cognitive impairment: ten years later. Arch Neurol. 2009; 66(12):1447–55.
18. Rossetti HC, Lacritz LH, Cullum CM, Weiner MF. Normative data for the Montreal cognitive assessment (MoCA) in a population-based sample. Neurology. 2011;77(13):1272–5.
19. Freitas S, Simões MR, Alves L, Santana I. Montreal cognitive assessment (MoCA): normative study for the Portuguese population. J Clin Exp Neuropsychol. 2011;33(9):989–96.
20. Roe CM, Xiong C, Miller JP, Morris JC. Education and Alzheimer disease without dementia support for the cognitive reserve hypothesis. Neurology. 2007;68(3):223–8.
21. Kemppainen NM, Aalto S, Karrasch M, Någren K, Savisto N, Oikonen V, Viitanen M, Parkkola R, Rinne JO. Cognitive reserve hypothesis: Pittsburgh compound B and fluorodeoxyglucose positron emission tomography in relation to education in mild Alzheimer's disease. Ann Neurol. 2008; 63(1):112–8.
22. Wen H, Zhang Z, Niu F, Li L. The application of Montreal cognitive assessment in urban Chinese residents of Beijing. Zhonghua Nei Ke Za Zhi. 2008;47(1):36–9.
23. Lee DY, Lee KU, Lee JH, Kim KW, Jhoo JH, Youn JC, Kim SY, Woo SI, Woo JI. A normative study of the mini-mental state examination in the Korean elderly. J Korean Neuropsychiatr Assoc. 2002;41(3):508–25.
24. Julayanont P, Phillips N, Chertkow H, Nasreddine ZS. Montreal cognitive assessment (MoCA): concept and clinical review. In: Cognitive screening instruments. London: Springer; 2013. p. 111–51.
25. Grady CL, McIntosh AR, Beig S, Keightley ML, Burian H, Black SE. Evidence from functional neuroimaging of a compensatory prefrontal network in Alzheimer's disease. J Neurosci. 2003;23(3):986–93.
26. Supekar K, Menon V, Rubin D, Musen M, Greicius MD. Network analysis of intrinsic functional brain connectivity in Alzheimer's disease. PLoS Comput Biol. 2008;4(6):e1000100.
27. Stern Y, Habeck C, Moeller J, Scarmeas N, Anderson KE, Hilton HJ, Flynn J, Sackeim H, van Heertum R. Brain networks associated with cognitive reserve in healthy young and old adults. Cereb Cortex. 2005;15(4):394–402.
28. Scarmeas N, Zarahn E, Anderson KE, Hilton J, Flynn J, Van Heertum RL, Sackeim HA, Stern Y. Cognitive reserve modulates functional brain responses during memory tasks: a PET study in healthy young and elderly subjects. Neuroimage. 2003;19(3):1215–27.
29. Jagust WJ, Friedland RP, Budinger TF, Koss E, Ober B. Longitudinal studies of regional cerebral metabolism in Alzheimer's disease. Neurology. 1988;38(6): 909–12.
30. Buchman AS, Bennett DA. Loss of motor function in preclinical Alzheimer's disease. Expert Rev Neurother. 2011;11(5):665–76.
31. Scarmeas N, Stern Y. Cognitive reserve: implications for diagnosis and prevention of Alzheimer's disease. Curr Neurol Neurosci Rep. 2004;4(5): 374–80.
32. Menon V, Rivera S, White C, Glover G, Reiss A. Dissociating prefrontal and

parietal cortex activation during arithmetic processing. Neuroimage. 2000; 12(4):357–65.

33. Baldo JV, Shimamura AP, Delis DC, Kramer J, Kaplan E. Verbal and design fluency in patients with frontal lobe lesions. J Int Neuropsychol Soc. 2001; 7(05):586–96.

34. Frith CD, Friston K, Liddle PF, Frackowiak RS. Willed action and the prefrontal cortex in man: a study with PET. Proc Biol Sci. 1991;244(1311):241–6.

35. Winblad B, Palmer K, Kivipelto M, Jelic V, Fratiglioni L, Wahlund LO, Nordberg A, Bäckman L, Albert M, Almkvist O. Mild cognitive impairment– beyond controversies, towards a consensus: report of the international working group on mild cognitive impairment. J Intern Med. 2004;256(3):240–6.

36. Scarmeas N, Zarahn E, Anderson KE, Habeck CG, Hilton J, Flynn J, Marder KS, Bell KL, Sackeim HA, Van Heertum RL. Association of life activities with cerebral blood flow in Alzheimer disease: implications for the cognitive reserve hypothesis. Arch Neurol. 2003;60(3):359–65.

37. Perneczky R, Drzezga A, Diehl-Schmid J, Schmid G, Wohlschläger A, Kars S, Grimmer T, Wagenpfeil S, Monsch A, Kurz A. Schooling mediates brain reserve in Alzheimer's disease: findings of fluoro-deoxy-glucose-positron emission tomography. J Neurol Neurosurg Psychiatry. 2006;77(9):1060–3.

38. Bennett DA, Wilson R, Schneider J, Evans D, De Leon CM, Arnold S, Barnes L, Bienias J. Education modifies the relation of AD pathology to level of cognitive function in older persons. Neurology. 2003;60(12):1909–15.

2

Adherence to driving cessation advice given to patients with cognitive impairment and consequences for mobility

Dafne Piersma[1][*] (iD), Anselm B. M. Fuermaier[1], Dick De Waard[1], Ragnhild J. Davidse[2], Jolieke De Groot[2], Michelle J. A. Doumen[1], Rudolf W. H. M. Ponds[3], Peter P. De Deyn[4], Wiebo H. Brouwer[1,4] and Oliver Tucha[1]

Abstract

Background: Driving is related to social participation; therefore older drivers may be reluctant to cease driving. Continuation of driving has also been reported in a large proportion of patients with cognitive impairment. The aim of this study is to investigate whether patients with cognitive impairment adhere to driving cessation advice after a fitness-to-drive assessment and what the consequences are with regard to mobility.

Methods: Patients with cognitive impairment ($n = 172$) participated in a fitness-to-drive assessment study, including an on-road driving assessment. Afterwards, patients were advised to either continue driving, to follow driving lessons, or to cease driving. Approximately seven months thereafter, patients were asked in a follow-up interview about their adherence to the driving recommendation. Factors influencing driving cessation were identified using a binary logistic regression analysis. Use of alternative transportation was also evaluated.

Results: Respectively 92 and 79% of the patients adhered to the recommendation to continue or cease driving. Female gender, a higher Clinical Dementia Rating-score, perceived health decline, and driving cessation advice facilitated driving cessation. Patients who ceased driving made use of less alternative modes of transportation than patients who still drove. Nonetheless, around 40% of the patients who ceased driving increased their frequency of cycling and/or public transport use.

Conclusions: Adherence to the recommendations given after the fitness-to-drive assessments was high. Female patients were in general more likely to cease driving. However, a minority of patients did not adhere to driving cessation advice. These drivers with dementia should be made aware of the progression of their cognitive impairment and general health decline to facilitate driving cessation. There are large differences in mobility between patients with cognitive impairment. Physicians should discuss options for alternative transportation in order to promote sustained safe mobility of patients with cognitive impairment.

Keywords: Dementia, Driving cessation, Adherence to driving cessation advice, Alternative transportation, Mobility

Background

Continuation of driving after being diagnosed with dementia has been found repeatedly [1–10]. Nevertheless, with the progression of the disease, cognitive abilities needed for safe driving gradually decrease and driving cessation is likely to become inevitable [11, 12]. It is difficult to define when a patient with dementia is no longer fit to drive [13] because of large individual differences in the patterns of dysfunctions, related to the different aetiologies of dementia [14, 15]. Therefore, the most appropriate moment to cease driving needs to be assessed on a case-by-case basis [16].

The decision to cease driving is not easily made as driving is associated with social participation, independence, and well-being [17, 18]. Some patients with dementia cease driving suddenly, e.g. from one day to another, or as a result of an accident, diagnosis, or other critical event, while others cease driving gradually [19]. These patients

* Correspondence: d.piersma@rug.nl
[1]Department of Clinical and Developmental Neuropsychology, University of Groningen, Groningen, The Netherlands
Full list of author information is available at the end of the article

may drive less kilometres (i.e. driving reduction) or avoid difficult driving situations (i.e. driving restriction) before ceasing driving entirely [19]. However, a proportion of patients with dementia continues to drive despite evidence of a decreased fitness to drive [20]. Some of these patients did not recall their fitness-to-drive assessment, others were not aware of their own cognitive impairment (due to decreased insight associated with dementia) or believed that their cognitive impairment did not affect driving safety [13, 16, 21–25]. According to the last group, the assessment process was 'not fair' and did not accurately reflect their fitness to drive [13, 16, 21]. These findings suggest that fitness-to-drive assessments should be comprehensive, comprising several types of tasks and sources of information, and that guidance for patients with dementia in interpreting a recommendation about driving is essential [25–28].

The process of driving cessation is affected by intrapersonal, interpersonal, and environmental factors [29]. Intrapersonal factors are factors related to the driver, interpersonal factors are derived from relationships with others involved in decisions about driving, and environmental factors are external influences not associated to the driver or the relationship with others.

Intrapersonal factors include, among others, age, gender, the presence and awareness of decline in physical, visual, and cognitive abilities as well as an opinion regarding the importance of driving and one's own driving safety. With increasing age, driving cessation becomes more likely [30], especially females are more likely to cease driving than men, even prematurely [31, 32]. An important reason for driving cessation among older drivers is perceived health decline, in particular in vision and cognition [10, 22, 30, 31, 33–38]. Cognitive impairment is strongly associated with various aetiologies of dementia that are characterized by distinct symptoms and impairments, therefore driving cessation might be more likely in one or the other aetiology of dementia. Seiler and colleagues [9] reported that as many as 90.9% of the patients with dementia with Lewy bodies (DLB) ceased driving whereas only about 55–65% of the patients with Alzheimer's disease (AD), vascular dementia (VaD) and frontotemporal dementia (FTD) ceased driving. Furthermore, older people reported other reasons for driving cessation such as no need to drive anymore (e.g. because of retirement), decreased confidence while driving or lack of enjoyment during driving, and costs of fuel and upkeep of the car [18, 34, 39–41].

Interpersonal factors comprise the opinions of family members and authority figures about the patient's driving safety. Family members may encourage driving cessation by expressing concerns about driving safety or even by taking away the keys [9, 18], however, about half of the family members with doubts about the patient's driving safety were found not to attempt promoting driving cessation [42]. If family members do bring up the topic, older drivers may not be willing to follow up their advice [18]. Moreover, there is a minority of family members who encourage continuation of driving because they believe the patient still drives safely or they benefit from the patient's driving [11, 22, 23, 41]. In the majority of cases, patients with dementia and their family members need support from physicians regarding counselling and evaluation of the patient's fitness to drive [13, 18]. There are indications that recommendations to cease driving from authority figures, such as physicians, facilitate driving cessation [18, 22, 39, 42].

Environmental factors include traffic accidents and availability of alternative transportation. Traffic accidents and near misses have been reported as reasons for driving cessation [9, 22, 29]. Nevertheless, some patients with dementia continue driving for up to three years after experiencing a traffic accident [40, 43]. Additionally, *not* having caused any accident may also be a reason to continue driving [29]. Byszewski and colleagues [27] suggested that discussing alternative transportation may enhance acceptance of driving cessation, but mixed results have been obtained about the use of alternative transportation by patients with cognitive impairment. Talbot and colleagues [30] reported that patients living in a city, i.e. where alternative modes of transport are available, are more likely to cease driving. However, Taylor and Tripodes [44] found that the majority of patients with dementia may depend on rides of their partners, relatives, or friends and observed no increase in walking, using public transport, taxis, or van services after driving cessation.

This study has four aims. The first aim of this study is to evaluate how many patients with dementia adhere to the recommendation given after a fitness-to-drive assessment. The second aim is to identify which factors play a role in driving cessation of patients with dementia who underwent a fitness-to-drive assessment. Based on the literature, major factors hypothesized to be related to driving cessation are increasing severity of cognitive impairment and recommendations to cease driving. The third aim is to investigate whether patients with different aetiologies of dementia show a different likelihood of driving cessation. Based on the study of Seiler and colleagues [9], patients with DLB are expected to cease driving more frequently compared to patients with other aetiologies of dementia. The final aim is to evaluate transportation options for patients with dementia beyond driving. Eventually, implications will be provided of how driving cessation and alternative transportation could be addressed in clinical practice.

Methods
Participants
Participants with cognitive impairment were recruited via multiple health care centres and from the general

community. Inclusion criteria were an age above 30, a diagnosis of mild cognitive impairment, dementia, or Parkinson's disease (PD) with self-reported cognitive decline, a current valid driver's licence and a wish to continue driving. Exclusion criteria were the diagnosis of other neurological or psychiatric conditions that may influence driving performance and usage of medications with a severe influence on driving ability (International Council on Alcohol, Drugs and Traffic Safety Category III). Since not all participants had a diagnosis of dementia, they will be referred to as patients with cognitive impairment.

One hundred and seventy-two patients with cognitive impairment completed the study. Patients were aged 49 to 91 years (mean = 71.3 years; SD = 8.8 years) and 128 (74.4%) of the patients were men. Patients had held a driver's licence for 11 to 73 years (mean = 49.7 years; SD = 9.0 years) and the estimation of their total distance driven ranges from 87,000 to 12,183,000 km (mean = 1,720,000 km; SD = 2,692,000 km). Eighty-three (48.3%) patients were diagnosed with AD, 15 (8.7%) with VaD, 10 (5.8%) with AD and VaD, 13 (7.6%) with FTD, 8 (4.7%) with DLB, 17 (9.9%) with PD and 12 (7.0%) with other aetiologies of cognitive impairment. The aetiology of cognitive impairment was unclear in 14 (8.2%) cases.

Measures

The measures used for the present study represent a selection of measures as obtained from a comprehensive fitness-to-drive assessment following the protocol as described by Piersma and colleagues [1]. The pre-selection of measures was based on the literature and intended to cover relevant factors for driving cessation [10, 11, 13, 18, 22, 27, 29–35, 37, 39, 41, 42, 44].

Intrapersonal factors

Intrapersonal factors used for the prediction of driving cessation included age, gender, diagnosis (AD vs. other), level of cognitive impairment, decline in health, visual acuity (range 0–1), visual contrast sensitivity (range 0–16), importance of driving for the individual patient, and the opinion of patients about their own driving safety. The level of cognitive impairment was measured by the total score of the Clinical Dementia Rating (CDR) scale [45] and the total score of the Mini-Mental State Examination (MMSE) [46, 47]. Decline in health was determined by asking the patients during a follow-up interview whether they experienced changes in their health since their fitness-to-drive assessment. Answers were coded into three categories: (1) no, (2) to some extent, and (3) yes. During clinical interviews, patients were asked whether driving was important to them. Answer options were: (1) very important, (2) important, (3) practical but not important, and (4) unimportant. During the same interviews, patients were asked how they experienced their driving safety.

Answers were divided into three categories: (1) still driving as safely as when they were middle-aged, (2) driving less safely compared to when they were middle-aged or (3) driving unsafely.

Interpersonal factors

Interpersonal factors included the recommendation given by a researcher after the fitness-to-drive assessment, whether an authority figure (e.g. physician, driving instructor) recommended driving cessation, and the opinion of an informant about the patient's driving safety. The recommendation after completion of the fitness-to-drive assessment was given by one of the researchers involved and represented either (1) cease driving, (2) follow driving lessons and sign up for an official relicensing procedure or (3) continue driving. Besides the recommendation of a researcher after the fitness-to-drive assessment, also a recommendation to cease driving from an authority figure could be reported during the follow-up interview. Lastly, the opinion of an informant about the driving safety of the patient was asked during a clinical interview. Answers were divided into three categories: (1) still driving as safely as when the patient was middle-aged, (2) driving less safely compared to when the patient was middle-aged or (3) driving unsafely.

Environmental factors

Three environmental factors were considered, i.e. the opportunity to be passenger of another private car (*yes* or *no*), the number of other modes of transport used (e.g. walking, cycling, public transport, and taxis), and the number of car accidents. Accidents included accidents in the twelve months prior to study participation and (almost) accidents after the fitness-to-drive assessment prior to the follow-up interview.

Indications of driving reduction, restriction, and cessation

Driving reduction and restriction were considered as indications of a process of driving cessation. The variables were based on questions in a driving questionnaire. Driving reduction was derived from the patients' estimations of their driving experience in the previous twelve months minus the patient's estimations of their average driving experience per year since they obtained their driving licence. The questions for driving experience had the following answer options: (1) less than 1.000 km, (2) 1.000–5.000 km, (3) 5.000–10.000 km, (4) 10.000–20.000 km, (5) 20.000–30.000 km, (6) 30.000–50.000 km, (7) more than 50.000 km. Driving restriction was calculated by summing up the number of driving situations that were being avoided (range 0–9). The patients answered a multiple-choice question: 'Do you attempt to avoid the following traffic situations?'. Answer options were *peak hours/crowded roads, motorways, adverse weather conditions (like rain, fog or snow), slippery roads/ snow on the road, driving when it is dark, turning left, driving unfamiliar roads, driving abroad, another traffic situation,* and *none.* The final outcome measure was whether the patient was still driving or not (*StillDriving*), which was asked during a follow-up interview.

Procedure

Patients with cognitive impairment participated on a voluntary basis. Patients received no direct reward for participation, but patients who passed the on-road driving assessment could use this outcome in an official relicensing procedure. Failing the on-road driving assessment did *not* lead to revocation of the patients' driving licences.

The fitness-to-drive assessment consisted of two sessions. On the first occasion, clinical interviews with the participant and an informant were conducted, as well as a comprehensive neuropsychological assessment and driving simulator rides. Participants invited an informant of their choice, usually their partner. During the first session, participants were also screened to assure that they met the minimum legal requirements for an on-road driving assessment with regard to visual functions (visual acuity of 0.5, horizontal field of view of 120 degrees) and motor functions (no major impairments of both hands, or legs). The first session lasted approximately four hours in total, including around half an hour driving simulation. On the second occasion, the on-road driving assessment took place, which lasted around 45 min.

After the fitness-to-drive assessment, a driving recommendation was given by one of the researchers involved based on both the off-road and on-road assessments as well as clinical judgment. If patients were recommended to continue driving, this was communicated via postal mail. These patients received an overview of their personal fitness-to-drive assessment results corroborated with an explanation of the findings and the recommendation in writing. If patients were recommended to follow driving lessons or to cease driving, they were called and invited for an appointment with a neuropsychologist to discuss the results and the recommendation. After this appointment, these patients also received an overview of their personal fitness-to-drive assessment results, an explanation of the findings, the recommendation, and a summary of the conversation with the neuropsychologist in writing.

The follow-up interview took place by telephone three to twenty months (M = 7.3 months, SD = 3.6 months) after participation in the fitness-to-drive assessment. Questions were asked to the patient ($n = 78$), to the patient and the patient's partner together ($n = 29$) or to an informant only ($n = 65$). Informants were the partners of the patients ($n = 57$), or other relatives. Questions regarded whether the health of the patient declined, whether or not the patient ceased driving including reasons for this choice as well as use of alternative transportation. This interview lasted around 30 min per patient.

Statistical analyses

Values were missing in less than 3% of cases per variable, and were not replaced.

Adherence to the recommendation

Adherence to the recommendations given after the fitness-to-drive assessment was investigated using driving cessation rates and information from the follow-up interview on whether patients followed driving lessons and signed up for an official relicensing procedure. Reported reasons for non-adherence were recorded.

Factors related to driving cessation

Factors related to driving cessation were explored in two ways, i.e. first by describing reported reasons for driving cessation in the follow-up interviews using percentages and second by predicting driving cessation in a logistic regression analysis. Current and retired drivers were statistically compared on predictor variables. These variables included intrapersonal factors, interpersonal factors, environmental factors, and two factors related to the process of driving cessation (see Measures). Predictor variables correlating significantly ($p < 0.05$) (point biserial correlation coefficients) with *StillDriving* were selected for the binary logistic regression analysis with forced entry of predictor variables.

Driving cessation per aetiology

To evaluate differences in driving cessation rates between patients with different aetiologies of cognitive impairment, the numbers and percentages of patients who ceased driving at follow-up were calculated per aetiology.

Mobility of patients with cognitive impairment

It was examined which modes of transport were important for patients with cognitive impairment to continue to use and which modes of transport were used by current and retired drivers. In addition, changes in frequencies of walking, cycling, and public transport use after the fitness-to-drive assessment were compared between current and retired drivers based on the question "Do you walk/cycle/use public transport less or more since the fitness-to-drive assessment?". Finally, reasons for *not* walking, cycling, or using public transport were examined.

Results

Adherence to the recommendation

The vast majority of patients who were recommended to continue driving adhered to this recommendation (92.4%) (Table 1). Six (7.6%) patients decided to cease driving for one or two reasons: family members advocated driving cessation ($n = 3$), the patient felt driving was no longer safe ($n = 2$), an authority figure recommended driving cessation ($n = 1$), perceived health decline ($n = 1$), perceived

Table 1 Driving continuation and cessation by patients with cognitive impairment per recommendation given after the fitness-to-drive assessment

Recommendation	Driving at follow-up	
	Yes	No
Continue driving ($n = 79$)	73 (92.4%)	6 (7.6%)
Driving lessons ($n = 31$)	18 (58.1%)	13 (41.9%)
Cease driving ($n = 62$)	13 (21.0%)	49 (79.0%)
Total ($n = 172$)	104 (60.5%)	68 (39.5%)

stress related to the official relicensing procedure ($n = 1$), feeling uncomfortable driving or afraid to drive ($n = 1$), and a near miss occurred ($n = 1$).

Thirty-one patients with cognitive impairment were recommended to follow driving lessons and sign up for the official relicensing procedure. Of the thirteen patients who ceased driving, one (7.7%) patient followed driving lessons, but was recommended to cease driving by the driving instructor, and two (15.4%) patients signed up for the official relicensing procedure. The procedure was still pending for one patient while the other patient failed the on-road driving assessment for driving license renewal. Of the eighteen patients who were still driving, twelve (66.7%) patients followed driving lessons and eight (44.4%) patients signed up for the official relicensing procedure. This procedure was still pending in five cases, and three patients renewed their driving license. Five patients who continued to drive (27.8%) did not follow driving lessons and also did not sign up for the official relicensing procedure. Notably, several patients reported that they restricted or reduced their driving after the fitness-to-drive assessment. Moreover, two patients had planned to sign up for the official relicensing procedure in a few months depending on their health status.

The majority of patients with cognitive impairment who were recommended to cease driving, adhered to this recommendation (79.0%). Nevertheless, thirteen patients did not. Two of them were considering driving cessation and reduced driving very much already. One more patient was willing to cease driving in the future, when the partner would advocate driving cessation. However, ten patients were not considering to cease driving at all, with five patients giving reasons for driving continuation (driving is going well ($n = 2$), having a partner as co-pilot ($n = 2$), because of mobility needs ($n = 1$)).

Factors related to driving cessation
Reported reasons for driving cessation
Patients with cognitive impairment reported one up to five reasons for driving cessation (Fig. 1). Two patients who were not driving did not report a reason for driving cessation, since they did not make a definite choice about whether they would never drive anymore.

Prediction of driving cessation
Retired drivers were significantly older, had more often a diagnosis of AD, a higher CDR-score, a lower MMSE-score, more pronounced health decline, and a lower visual contrast sensitivity than current drivers (Table 2). Moreover, retired drivers were more often recommended to cease driving, both after the fitness-to-drive assessment and by authority figures, than current drivers. Furthermore, retired drivers used less alternative modes of transport than current drivers. Lastly, trends ($.05 < p < .10$) were found for retired drivers being more often female, finding driving less important, and being more often a passenger of other car drivers than current drivers.

Intrapersonal factors that correlated significantly with *StillDriving* were age ($r = -.156$, $p = .041$), gender ($r = -.153$, $p = .045$), CDR-score ($r = -.437$, $p < .001$), MMSE-score ($r = .309$, $p < .001$), health decline ($r = -.254$, $p = .001$), and contrast sensitivity ($r = .171$, $p = .025$). Interpersonal factors that correlated with *StillDriving* included the recommendation given after the fitness-to-drive assessment ($r = .657$, $p < .001$) and recommendations of driving cessation from authority figures ($r = -.309$, $p < .001$). One environmental factor correlated with *StillDriving*, i.e. the sum of modes of transport used other than the private car ($r = .188$, $p = .015$) with retired drivers using less modes of transport than current drivers. Subsequently, the factors correlating significantly with *StillDriving* were entered in a binary logistic regression analysis to determine the validity of the factors in predicting *StillDriving*. A significant model emerged to predict *StillDriving*, $\chi^2(9, N = 167) = 104.8$, $p < .001$. The model explained 46.6% of the total variance (Cox & Snell R^2) and classified 85.6% of the patients correctly as still driving or not. The factors that contributed significantly to the prediction were gender, CDR-score, health decline, and the recommendation given after the fitness-to-drive assessment, and there was a trend found for recommendations of driving cessation from authority figures (Table 3).

Driving cessation rates per aetiology of cognitive impairment
At the time of follow-up, 104 (60.5%) patients with cognitive impairment were still driving whereas 68 (39.5%) patients with cognitive impairment had ceased driving. The lowest rate of driving cessation was found in patients with DLB (1 of 8 patients; 12.5%). In patients with PD, the rate of driving cessation was similar (3 of 17 patients; 17.6%). Driving cessation rates were 30.8% (4 of 13 patients) in patients with FTD and 38.2% (32 of 83 patients) in patients with AD. The driving cessation rates were higher in patients with VaD (10 of 15 patients; 66.7%) and AD plus VaD (8 of 10 patients; 80.0%). Of the patients with other or unclear diagnoses, 38.5% ceased driving (10 of 26 patients).

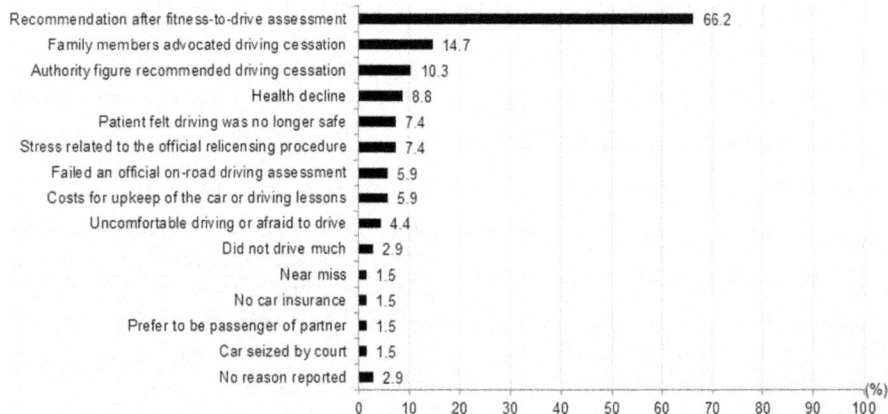

Fig. 1 Percentages of reported reasons for driving cessation by patients with cognitive impairment who ceased driving (multiple answers possible, *n* = 68)

Mobility of patients with cognitive impairment

Important modes of transportation

Patients with cognitive impairment (*n* = 170) reported none until up to six modes of transport they found important to continue to use. Driving (i.e. driving themselves or being passenger of other drivers) was by far the most important mode of transportation followed by cycling (Fig. 2).

Used modes of transportation

Of the current drivers with cognitive impairment, 86.5% reported also being passenger of other drivers: their partners (63.5%), other family members (28.8%), friends (22.1%), and other drivers such as neighbours or colleagues (3.8%). They also used other modes of transport, especially walking and cycling (Table 4). Of the retired drivers with cognitive impairment, 95.6% reported being passenger of other drivers: their partners (58.8%), other family members (47.1%), friends (17.6%), and other drivers such as a former colleague or a professional caretaker (4.4%). In comparison to current drivers, a smaller proportion of retired drivers was walking, cycling and using public transport and a larger proportion of retired drivers used taxis (Table 4).

Changes in frequencies of walking, cycling, and public transport use The percentages of retired drivers cycling (58.8%) and using public transport (35.3%) were low compared with current drivers (84.5% respectively 52.0%), however, the percentage of retired drivers who increased the frequency of cycling (42.5%) and public transport use (41.7%) after the fitness-to-drive assessment was higher compared with current drivers (10.6% respectively 17.0%) (Fig. 3). These retired drivers mentioned using these modes of transport instead of the car. Nevertheless, the majority did not increase or even decreased the frequency of walking, cycling, and public transport use.

Reasons for not walking, cycling, and using public transport Patients reported each none up to three reasons for not walking (*n* = 23), not cycling (*n* = 44), and/or not using public transport (*n* = 93) (Fig. 4). Not walking and not cycling was mostly associated with physical difficulties and falls. Dislike was another major reason for not walking for transport, whereas unfamiliarity and cognitive difficulties were other limiting factors for cycling. Not using public transport was largely explained by having no need to use public transport, because of using other modes of transportation. It is noteworthy that inconvenience of public transport was often reported, which could be related to physical difficulties, but also to cognitive difficulties (e.g. impairments in orientation) as well as unfamiliarity and distance from home.

Discussion

In this study, 172 patients with cognitive impairment were interviewed about their adherence to a driving recommendation received after participation in a comprehensive fitness-to-drive assessment. The vast majority of patients adhered to a recommendation to either continue driving, to follow driving lessons and undergo an official relicensing procedure, or to cease driving after the fitness-to-drive assessment. This indicates that fitness-to-drive assessments promote driving continuation in patients who are fit to drive while stimulating driving cessation in patients who are unfit to drive. Almost 40% of the patients with cognitive impairment ceased driving at follow-up. Nonetheless, some patients were reluctant to cease driving, which concurs with previous studies [46, 47]. In attempt to promote adherence, previously suggested practical strategies were applied in this study, i.e. providing details about the test results and a letter of explanation about how the fitness-to-drive assessment resulted in the driving recommendation, and discussing alternative transportation with those who were recommended to cease driving [27]. Despite the implementation

Table 2 Comparison of current and retired drivers with cognitive impairment on predictor variables

	Group		p Value (df)
	Current drivers (n = 104)	Retired drivers (n = 68)	
Intrapersonal factors			
Age in years, mean (SD), y	70.2 (8.7)	73.0 (8.7)	.032 (171)[a]*
Male sex, No. (%)	83 (79.8%)	45 (66.2%)	.051 (1)[b]
Diagnosis of AD, No. (%)	53 (51.0%)	40 (58.8%)	.035 (1)[b]*
CDR-score, No. (%)			
0	15 (14.4%)	1 (1.5%)	<.001 (2)[c]*
0.5	86 (82.7%)	44 (64.7%)	
1	3 (2.9%)	23 (33.8%)	
MMSE-score, mean (SD)	24.9 (3.5)	22.4 (4.2)	<.001 (171)[a]*
Health decline, No. (%)			
No	76 (73.1%)	33 (49.2%)	.004 (2)[c]*
To some extent	7 (6.7%)	5 (7.5%)	
Yes	21 (20.2%)	29 (43.3%)	
Visual acuity (0–1), mean (SD)	.88 (0.21)	.84 (0.21)	.181 (169)[a]
Contrast sensitivity (0–16), mean (SD)	12.84 (0.68)	12.55 (0.96)	.022 (170)[a]*
Importance of driving, mean (SD)	1.57 (0.73)	1.78 (0.83)	.091 (171)[a]
Patient's judgement of driving safety, No. (%)			
Safe	88 (85.4%)	52 (76.5%)	.136 (2)[c]
Less safe than when middle-aged	15 (14.6%)	16 (23.5%)	
Unsafe	0 (0.0%)	0 (0.0%)	
Interpersonal factors			
Recommendation given after fitness-to-drive assessment, No. (%)			
Continue driving	73 (92.4%)	6 (7.6%)	<.001 (2)[c]*
Driving lessons	18 (58.9%)	13 (41.9%)	
Cease driving	13 (21.0%)	49 (79.0%)	
Authority figure recommended driving cessation, No. (%)	1 (1.0%)	12 (17.6%)	<.001 (1)[b]*
Informant's judgement of driving safety, No (%)			
Safe	68 (66.6%)	42 (64.6%)	.190 (2)[c]
Less safe than when middle-aged	32 (31.4%)	18 (27.7%)	
Unsafe	2 (2.0%)	5 (7.7%)	
Environmental factors			
Passenger of other drivers, No. (%)	90 (86.5%)	65 (95.6%)	.067 (1)[b]
Sum of modes of transport used other than the private car, mean (SD)	2.48 (0.83)	2.12 (1.04)	.013 (168)[a]*
Car accidents, mean (SD)	0.10 (0.33)	0.16 (0.51)	.484 (171)[a]
Process of driving cessation			
Driving reduction, mean (SD)	−1.49 (1.49)	− 1.83 (1.72)	.151 (168)[a]
Driving restriction, mean (SD)	1.85 (1.77)	2.34 (2.30)	.343 (170)[a]

[a]Mann-Whitney U test
[b]Fisher's Exact test
[c]χ2 test
Statistical significance (p < .05) is indicated by*
Abbreviations: AD Alzheimer's disease, CDR-score Clinical Dementia Rating Total Score, MMSE-score Mini Mental State Examination Total Score

of these strategies, 21% of the patients who were recommended to cease driving did not cease driving, which is a matter of concern..

Driving cessation occurred in most cases in response to a recommendation to cease driving, which was given after the fitness-to-drive assessment, by family members

Table 3 Summary of binary logistic regression analysis for the prediction of driving continuation ($n = 101$) versus driving cessation ($n = 66$) in patients with cognitive impairment

Predictor variable	B	SE B	Wald	P	Odds ratio
Age	0.002	0.002	0.800	.371	1.002
Gender	−1.149	0.575	3.991	.046*	0.317
CDR-score	−4.512	1.498	9.075	.003*	0.011
MMSE-score	−0.026	0.070	.137	.712	0.975
Health decline	−0.658	0.288	5.211	.022*	0.518
Contrast sensitivity	0.201	0.340	.348	.555	1.222
Authority figure recommended driving cessation	−2.149	1.249	2.961	.085	0.117
Recommendation after fitness-to-drive assessment	1.748	0.321	29.724	<.001*	5.743
Sum of other used modes of transport	−0.234	.290	.649	.420	0.792
Constant	−1.101	5.568	.039	.843	0.333
Total $R^2 = 0.466$*					

Statistical significance ($p < .05$) is indicated by *

or by authority figures. These results indicate that interpersonal factors are very important for patients with cognitive impairment in the decision making process, which is in correspondence with previous studies in patients with dementia [22, 42]. Hence family members and physicians may have a crucial role in imposing the decision to cease driving on patients who ignore a negative outcome of a fitness-to-drive assessment [20, 48]. Future research should focus on how this can be established effectively without harming the relationship with the patient [24, 49].

Personal factors, i.e. gender, CDR-score, and health decline also play a role in driving cessation. The observed gender effect supports findings from previous studies in which women have been found to cease driving earlier than men [31, 32], but this gender difference was not always found [30]. Future studies should clarify if men are more likely to continue driving when it is no longer safe and if women are more likely to cease driving when it is still safe. Based on the current study, men and women should still be treated equally, because the group of patients who neglected a driving cessation recommendation included both men and women. Cognitive impairment and self-rated health have also been found to predict driving cessation in other studies in which no driving recommendation was given [10, 30, 31, 33]. This implicates that when a decline in health is observed, this should be discussed with the car driver with cognitive impairment. If patients can evaluate their own health decline as incompatible with driving, they might be willing to cease driving. In brief, patients with cognitive impairment who underwent a fitness-to-drive assessment were more likely to cease driving if they were recommended to cease driving, were female, and had relatively severe cognitive impairment and/or pronounced health decline.

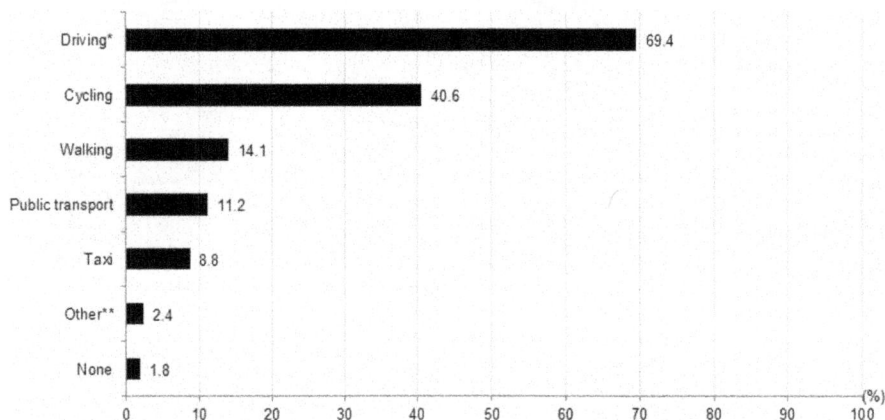

Fig. 2 Percentages of patients indicating the importance to continue to use certain modes of transportation (multiple answers possible, $n = 170$). *Driving included both being a driver and being a passenger of a private car. **Other included motorised quadricycles, a motorcycle, and a transportation service of day care

Table 4 Modes of transportation used by current and retired drivers with cognitive impairment (multiple answers possible)

Mode of transportation	Current drivers (n = 104)	Retired drivers (n = 68)
Passenger of other driver(s)	86.5%	95.6%
Walking	91.1%	79.4%
Cycling	84.5%	58.8%
Public transport	52.0%	35.3%
Taxis	10.7%	25.0%
Other modes[a]	11.7%	13.2%

[a]Other modes included an airplane, a boat, moped, motorcycle, motorised quadricycle, mobility scooter, buggy at a golf court, and transportation service of day care

Consistent with previous studies [8–10], a considerable proportion of patients with various aetiologies of cognitive impairment continued to drive. Driving cessation was most common among patients with VaD (66.7%) and patients with AD and VaD (80.0%). Contrary to the study of Seiler and colleagues [9] in which patients with DLB had the highest rate of driving cessation (90.9%), in this study patients with DLB had the lowest rate of driving cessation (12.5%). In both studies, the time since diagnosis varied between patients from very recent to several years ago, therefore the patients in this study might have been in a milder stage of DLB than the patients in Seiler and colleagues' study [9]. An explanation for the discrepancy in findings might be that the severity of cognitive impairment is more important for driving cessation than the aetiology of cognitive impairment. In line with this reasoning, CDR-scores were predictive of driving cessation, which corresponds with previous studies [30, 33]. Nonetheless, patients with different aetiologies of dementia may become unfit to drive due to different driving difficulties resulting from different symptoms [8, 14, 15, 50].

Patients with cognitive impairment preferred to use the private car for transportation, as a driver but also as passenger. This preference was expected because patients were selected on their wish to continue driving, as they are the target group for fitness-to-drive assessments. Especially family members (other than the partner) started to drive retired drivers with cognitive impairment, which is in line with Liddle and colleagues' argument that driving cessation is a family matter [11]. Remarkably, only a quarter of retired drivers with cognitive impairment used taxis. The group of retired drivers used less alternative modes of transportation than the group of current drivers, which may indicate that cognitive impairment may not only impact on driving but also on feasibility of using alternative transportation. An alternative explanation might be that retired drivers are less healthy in general leading to limitations in mobility. Even though the patient sample as used for the present study was characterized by cognitive impairment, physical difficulties were equally often reported as reason for not cycling or not using public transport, and as the major reason for not walking. On the one hand, retired drivers with cognitive impairment as a group may be frailer than current drivers with cognitive impairment, and the independent mobility of especially retired drivers may be limited and decreasing. On the other hand, around 40% of retired drivers using alternative transportation was able to sustain mobility by increasing their frequency of cycling and public transport use. These patients may represent a physically healthy group within the group of retired drivers with cognitive impairment. Research on traffic safety of patients with cognitive impairments using non-car modes of transportation is lacking, but would be helpful in order to indicate which alternative modes of

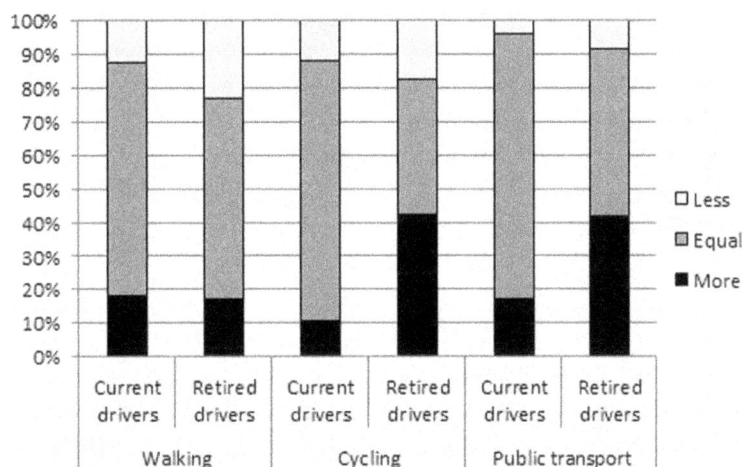

Fig. 3 Percentages of current and retired drivers with cognitive impairment who increased, did not change, or decreased their frequency of walking (n = 134), cycling (n = 125), and use of public transport (n = 77) after a fitness-to-drive assessment

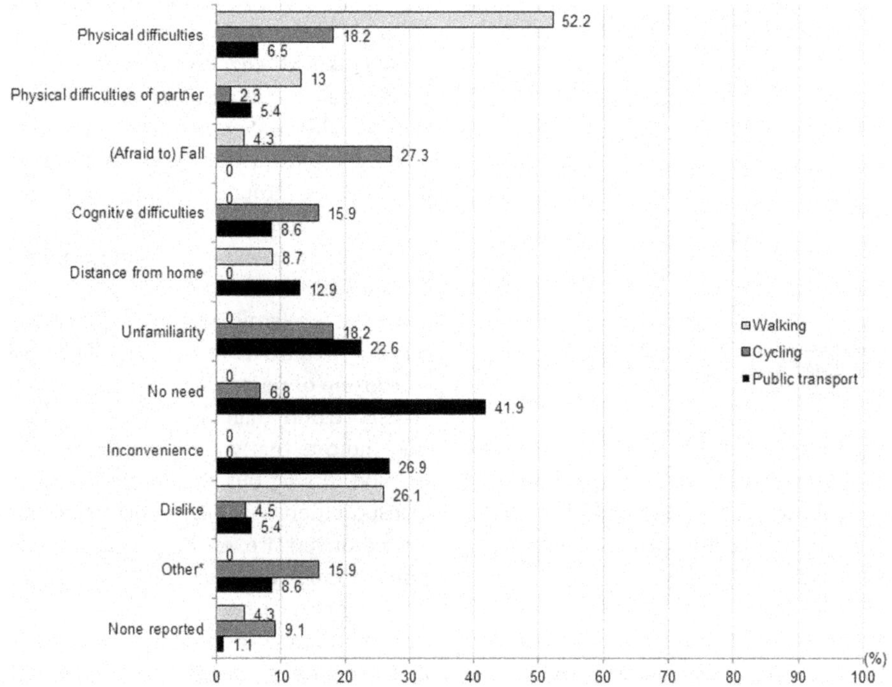

Fig. 4 Percentages of reported reasons for not walking ($n = 23$), not cycling ($n = 44$), and not using public transport ($n = 93$) (multiple answers possible). *Other included for cycling: feeling insecure on a bicycle, bicycle got stolen, a cycling accident, being hospitalized, and passiveness, and for public transport: costs, being hospitalized, partner dislikes public transport, experience with severe delay, feels nauseous in public transport, cannot take mobility scooter along, and maintaining driving skills

transport should be advised for patients with cognitive impairment. It is important to note that cyclists and pedestrians are vulnerable road users compared to car drivers, therefore traffic safety of retired drivers with cognitive impairments may be compromised. In conclusion, there is a lot of variation in mobility of patients with cognitive impairment, ranging from having no options for transportation anymore after driving cessation to sustaining mobility through driving or increasing use of alternative modes of transportation.

Limitations

Driving cessation is a process for many patients with cognitive impairment, but there was only one follow-up moment. Therefore, the eventual consequences of the fitness-to-drive assessment were not fully known yet for all patients, i.e. additional patients might have ceased driving soon after follow-up.

A second limitation is that impairments other than in cognition were not investigated thoroughly. The predictor variable 'health decline' is a broad term that includes declines in any aspect related to physical and mental health, however, these aspects were not analysed in more detail. Moreover, patients were screened for minimum visual and motor requirements for driving, but impairments in these domains that are not severe enough to lead to immediate revocation of a driving

license could still impact on driving. While two visual variables were included, this study failed to consider variables of motor behaviour. This is problematic as patients with PD, but also DLB and VaD, commonly suffer from motor impairments which could impair driving.

Another limitation concerns the use of the CDR for all patients with cognitive impairment. The CDR was originally developed to determine the severity of AD, and was also shown to be applicable to other aetiologies [51]. Nevertheless, for specific aetiologies of cognitive impairment other cut-offs or specific scales may be more appropriate, such as the Frontotemporal Dementia Rating Scale for FTD [52, 53].

Conclusions

Severity of cognitive impairment is very relevant for fitness to drive and predictive for driving cessation. Therefore, clinical tools such as the CDR should be used to stage the severity of cognitive impairment in the context of driving recommendations. There is consensus that patients with a CDR-score of 2 or 3 should be recommended to cease driving [12]. Patients with a CDR-score of 1 are less likely to be fit to drive than patients with a CDR-score of 0.5, but for both groups assessments are needed to investigate fitness to drive on an individual basis. Besides patients with more severe cognitive impairment, patients who perceive their health decline, and female patients, are more likely to cease driving, and also recommendations of driving cessation stimulate to do so.

Physicians have a very important role in informing patients about the impact of cognitive impairment on driving, because patients may be compromised in the evaluation of their own functioning and abilities. Physicians should explain that driving cessation will probably become inevitable with the progression of their disease and support patients and their family members in adapting to this change. A proportion of patients will have a wish to continue driving. It is difficult to judge fitness to drive of individual patients in clinical practice [24], therefore referral to fitness-to-drive assessments (e.g. to driving license authorities) is advised. This study showed that adherence to recommendations given after fitness-to-drive assessments is high, thus promoting driving cessation in patients who are unfit to drive while stimulating driving continuation in patients who are fit to drive. Still, physicians should discuss driving and mobility again after a fitness-to-drive assessment to assure that non-adherers are less likely to ignore the given driving recommendation, but also to acknowledge consequences of driving cessation. Depending on the personal situation, patients and their family members may need help in finding alternative modes of transportation to sustain their mobility, or might desire recognition of negative emotions related to driving cessation. Patients with cognitive impairment may benefit from social support groups to ease the process of driving cessation, and from alternative transportation tailored to their needs, e.g. dementia-friendly taxi services.

Abbreviations
AD: Alzheimer's disease; CDR: Clinical Dementia Rating; DLB: Dementia with Lewy Bodies; FTD: Frontotemporal dementia; MMSE: Mini-Mental State Examination; Non-AD: Non-Alzheimer's disease; PD: Parkinson's disease; VaD: Vascular dementia

Acknowledgements
We thank all referring physicians, all participants for their participation, and the students who were involved in the data collection. We also acknowledge the general support of the FitCI project group.

Funding
This work was funded by the Ministry of Infrastructure and the Environment (NL). The funders had no role in study design, data collection, analysis, interpretation of data, and writing of the manuscript.

Authors' contributions
DP was the primary investigator, leading the study, involved in conception and design, data collection, analysis and writing of the manuscript. ABMF contributed to the conceptualization, analysis and interpretation of data, and drafting of the manuscript. DDW, WHB, and OT were involved in conceptualization and study design, interpretation of data, and drafting the manuscript. RJD, JDG, MD, RP, and PPDD helped with conceptualization and study design, interpretation of data, and revising the manuscript. All authors read and approved the final manuscript.

Competing interests
The authors declare that they have no competing interests.

Author details
[1]Department of Clinical and Developmental Neuropsychology, University of Groningen, Groningen, The Netherlands. [2]SWOV Institute for Road Safety Research, The Hague, The Netherlands. [3]Department of Psychiatry and Neuropsychology, School of Mental Health and Neurosciences (MHeNS), Maastricht University, Maastricht, The Netherlands. [4]Department of Neurology and Alzheimer Research Center, University of Groningen and University Medical Center Groningen, Groningen, The Netherlands.

References
1. Piersma D, Fuermaier ABM, de Waard D, Davidse RJ, de Groot J, Doumen MJA, et al. Prediction of fitness to drive in patients with Alzheimer's dementia. PLoS One. 2016;11:e0149566.
2. Fox GK, Bowden SC, Bashford GM, Smith DS. Alzheimer's disease and driving: prediction and assessment of driving performance. J Am Geriatr Soc. 1997;45:949–53.
3. Friedland RP, Koss E, Kumar A, Gaine S, Metzler D, Haxby JV, et al. Motor vehicle crashes in dementia of the alzheimer type. Ann Neurol. 1988;24:782–6.
4. Drachman DA, Swearer JM. Driving and Alzheimer's disease: the risk of crashes. Neurology. 1993;43:2448–56.
5. Duchek JM, Carr DB, Hunt L, Roe CM, Xiong C, Shah K, et al. Longitudinal driving performance in early-stage dementia of the Alzheimer type. J Am Geriatr Soc. 2003;51:1342–7.
6. Hunt L, Morris JC, Edwards D, Wilson BS. Driving performance in persons with mild senile dementia of the Alzheimer type. J Am Geriatr Soc. 1993;41:747–52.
7. Marie Dit Asse L, Fabrigoule C, Helmer C, Laumon B, Berr C, Rouaud O, et al. Gender effect on driving cessation in pre-dementia and dementia phases: results of the 3C population-based study. Int J Geriatr Psychiatry. 2017;32: 1049–58.
8. Fujito R, Kamimura N, Ikeda M, Koyama A, Shimodera S, Morinobu S, et al. Comparing the driving behaviours of individuals with frontotemporal lobar degeneration and those with Alzheimer's disease. Psychogeriatrics. 2016;16:27–33.
9. Seiler S, Schmidt H, Lechner A, Benke T, Sanin G, Ransmayr G, et al. Driving cessation and dementia: results of the prospective registry on dementia in Austria (PRODEM). PLoS One. 2012;7:e52710.
10. Herrmann N, Rapoport MJ, Sambrook R, Hébert R, McCracken P, Robillard A, et al. Predictors of driving cessation in mild-to-moderate dementia. CMAJ. 2006;175:591–5.
11. Liddle J, Tan A, Liang P, Bennett S, Allen S, Lie DC, et al. "The biggest problem we've ever had to face": how families manage driving cessation with people with dementia. Int Psychogeriatrics. 2016;28:109–22.
12. Lundberg C, Johansson K, Ball K, Bjerre B, Blomqvist C, Braekhus A, et al. Dementia and driving: an attempt at consensus. Alzheimer Dis Assoc Disord. 1997;11:28–37.
13. Perkinson MA, Berg-Weger ML, Carr DB, Meuser TM, Palmer JL, Buckles VD, et al. Driving and dementia of the Alzheimer type: beliefs and cessation strategies among stakeholders. Gerontologist. 2005;45:676–85.
14. Piersma D, de Waard D, Davidse R, Tucha O, Brouwer W. Car drivers with dementia: different complications due to different aetiologies? Traffic Inj Prev. 2016;17:9–23.
15. Piersma D, Fuermaier ABM, De Waard D, Davidse RJ, De Groot J, Doumen MJABRA, et al. Assessing fitness to drive in patients with different types of dementia. Alzheimer Dis Assoc Disord. 2018;32:70–5.
16. Andrew C, Traynor V, Iverson D. An integrative review: understanding driving retirement decisions for individuals living with a dementia. J Adv Nurs. 2015;71:2728–40.
17. Davis RL, Ohman JM. Driving in early-stage Alzheimer's disease: an integrative review of the literature. Res Gerontol Nurs. 2016:1–15.
18. Persson D. The elderly driver: deciding when to stop. Gerontologist. 1993;33: 88–91.
19. Liddle J, Haynes M, Pachana NA, Mitchell G, McKenna K, Gustafsson L. Effect of a group intervention to promote older adults' adjustment to driving

cessation on community mobility: a randomized controlled trial. Gerontologist. 2014;54:409–22.

20. Adler G, Kuskowski M. Driving cessation in older men with dementia. Alzheimer Dis Assoc Disord. 2003;17:68–71.

21. Byszewski A, Aminzadeh F, Robinson K, Molnar F, Dalziel W, Man Son Hing M, et al. When it is time to hang up the keys: the driving and dementia toolkit - for persons with dementia (PWD) and caregivers - a practical resource. BMC Geriatr. 2013;13:117.

22. Croston J, Meuser TM, Berg-Weger M, Grant EA, Carr DB. Driving retirement in older adults with dementia. Top Geriatr Rehabil. 2009;25:154–62.

23. Friedland RP. Strategies for driving cessation in Alzheimer disease. Alzheimer Dis Assoc Disord. 1997;11(Suppl 1):73–5.

24. Gergerich EM. Reporting Policy Regarding Drivers with Dementia. Gerontologist. 2016;56:345–56.

25. Chacko EE, Wright WM, Worrall RC, Adamson C, Cheung G. Reactions to driving cessation: a qualitative study of people with dementia and their families. Australas Psychiatry. 2015;23:496–9.

26. Betz ME, Scott K, Jones J, Diguiseppi C. "Are you still driving?" Metasynthesis of patient preferences for communication with health care providers. Traffic Inj Prev. 2016;17:367–73.

27. Byszewski AM, Molnar FJ, Aminzadeh F. The impact of disclosure of unfitness to drive in persons with newly diagnosed dementia: patient and caregiver perspectives. Clin Gerontol. 2010;33:152–63.

28. Liddle J, Turpin M, Carlson G, McKenna K. The Needs and Experiences Related to Driving Cessation for Older People. Br J Occup Ther. 2008;71: 379–88.

29. Rudman DL, Friedland J, Chipman M, Sciortino P, Brayne C, Chipman ML, et al. Holding on and letting go: the perspectives of pre-seniors and seniors on driving self-regulation in later life. Can J Aging. 2006;25:65–76.

30. Talbot A, Bruce I, Cunningham CJ, Coen RF, Lawlor BA, Coakley D, et al. Driving cessation in patients attending a memory clinic. Age Ageing. 2005; 34:363–8.

31. Anstey KJ, Windsor TD, Luszcz MA, Andrews GR. Predicting driving cessation over 5 years in older adults: psychological well-being and cognitive competence are stronger predictors than physical health. J Am Geriatr Soc. 2006;54:121–6.

32. Rebok GW, Jones VC. Giving up driving: does social engagement buffer declines in mental health after driving cessation in older women? Int Psychogeriatrics. 2016;28:1235–6.

33. Foley DJ, Masaki KH, Ross GW, White LR. Driving cessation in older men with incident dementia. J Am Geriatr Soc. 2000;48:928–30.

34. Kowalski K, Love J, Tuokko H, MacDonald S, Hultsch D, Strauss E. The influence of cognitive impairment with no dementia on driving restriction and cessation in older adults. Accid Anal Prev. 2012;49:308–15.

35. Emerson JL, Johnson AM, Dawson JD, Uc EY, Anderson SW, Rizzo M. Predictors of driving outcomes in advancing age. Psychol Aging. 2012;27:550–9.

36. Huisingh C, McGwin G, Owsley C. Association of visual sensory function and higher-order visual processing skills with incident driving cessation. Clin Exp Optom. 2016;99:441–8.

37. MacLeod KE, Satariano WA, Ragland DR. The impact of health problems on driving status among older adults. J Transp Heal. 2014;1:86–94.

38. Freeman EE, Muñoz B, Turano KA, West SK. Measures of visual function and time to driving cessation in older adults. Optom Vis Sci. 2005;82:765–73.

39. Brayne C, Dufouil C, Ahmed A, Dening TR, Chi LY, McGee M, et al. Very old drivers: findings from a population cohort of people aged 84 and over. Int J Epidemiol. 2000;29:704–7.

40. Cooper PJ, Tallman K, Tuokko H, Beattie BL. Vehicle crash involvement and cognitive deficit in older drivers. J Saf Res. 1993;24:9–17.

41. Tuokko H, Sukhawathanakul P, Walzak L, Jouk A, Myers A, Marshall S, et al. Attitudes: mediators of the relation between health and driving in older adults. Can J Aging. 2016;35:44–58.

42. Mizuno Y, Arai A, Arai Y. Determination of driving cessation for older adults with dementia in Japan. Int J Geriatr Psychiatry. 2008;23:987–9.

43. Trobe JD, Waller PF, Cook-Flannagan CA, Teshima SM, Bieliauskas LA. Crashes and violations among drivers with Alzheimer disease. Arch Neurol. 1996;53:411–6.

44. Taylor BD, Tripodes S. The effects of driving cessation on the elderly with dementia and their caregivers. Accid Anal Prev. 2001;33:519–28.

45. Morris J. The clinical dementia rating (CDR): current version and scoring rules. Neurology. 1993;43:2412–4.

46. Kok R, Verhey F. [Dutch translation of the mini mental state examination (Folstein et al., 1975)]. 2002.

47. Folstein MF, Folstein SE, McHugh PR. "Mini-mental state". A practical method for grading the cognitive state of patients for the clinician. J Psychiatr Res. 1975;12:189–98.

48. Jett K, Tappen RM, Rosselli M. Imposed versus involved: different strategies to effect driving cessation in cognitively impaired older adults. Geriatr Nurs. 2005;26:111–6.

49. Jang RW, Man-Son-Hing M, Molnar FJ, Hogan DB, Marshall SC, Auger J, et al. Family physicians' attitudes and practices regarding assessments of medical fitness to drive in older persons. J Gen Intern Med. 2007;22:531–43.

50. De Simone V, Kaplan L, Patronas N, Wassermann EM, Grafman J. Driving abilities in frontotemporal dementia patients. Dement Geriatr Cogn Disord. 2007;23:1–7.

51. O'Bryant SE, Lacritz LH, Hall J, Waring SC, Chan W, Khodr ZG, et al. Validation of the new interpretive guidelines for the clinical dementia rating scale sum of boxes score in the National Alzheimer's coordinating center database. Arch Neurol. 2010;67:746–9.

52. Mioshi E, Hsieh S, Savage S, Hornberger M, Hodges JR. Clinical staging and disease progression in frontotemporal dementia. Neurology. 2010;74:1591–7.

53. Wyman-Chick KA, Scott BJ. Development of clinical dementia rating scale cutoff scores for patients with Parkinson's disease. Mov Disord Clin Pract. 2015;2:243–8.

3

Causes and correlates of 30 day and 180 day readmission following discharge from a Medicine for the Elderly Rehabilitation unit

Lloyd D. Hughes[1] and Miles D. Witham[2*]

Abstract

Background: Recently hospitalized patients experience a period of generalized risk of adverse health events. This study examined reasons for, and predictors of, readmission to acute care facilities within 30 and 180 days of discharge from an inpatient rehabilitation unit for older people.

Methods: Routinely collected, linked clinical data on admissions to a single inpatient rehabilitation facility over a 13-year period were analysed. Data were available regarding demographics, comorbid disease, admission and discharge Barthel scores, length of hospital stay, and number of medications on discharge. Discharge diagnoses for the index admission and readmissions were available from hospital episode statistics. Univariate and multivariate Cox regression analyses were performed to identify baseline factors that predicted 30 and 180-day readmission.

Results: A total of 3984 patients were included in the analysis. The cohort had a mean age of 84.1 years (SD 7.4), and 39.7% were male. Overall, 5.6% ($n = 222$) and 23.2% ($n = 926$) of the patients were readmitted within 30 days and 180 days of discharge respectively. For patients readmitted to hospital, 26.6% and 21.1% of patients were readmitted with the same condition as their initial admission at 30 days and 180 respectively. For patients readmitted within 30 days, 13.5% ($n = 30$) were readmitted with the same condition with the most common diagnoses associated with readmission being chest infection, falls/immobility and stroke. For patients readmitted within 180 days, 12.4% ($n = 115$) of patients were readmitted with the same condition as the index condition with the most common diagnoses associated with readmission being falls/immobility, cancer and chest infections. In multivariable Cox regression analyses, older age, male sex, length of stay and heart failure predicted 30 or 180-day readmission. In addition, discharge from hospital to patients own home predicted 30-day readmission, whereas diagnoses of cancer, previous myocardial infarction or chronic obstructive pulmonary disease predicted 180-day readmission.

Conclusion: Most readmissions of older people after discharge from inpatient rehabilitation occurred for different reasons to the original hospital admission. Patterns of predictors for early and late readmission differed, suggesting the need for different mitigation strategies.

Background

Readmission after discharge from hospital is common and has a considerable cost [1]. In the USA nearly one fifth of Medicare patients discharged from a hospital (approximately 2.6 million seniors), have an acute medical problem within 30 days that requires a further admission for treatment [2]. Furthermore, there is evidence that patients that are readmitted have a longer length of stay than for first admissions and a higher risk of complications [3].

The days and weeks after hospital discharge are a time of high risk not only for recurrence of the index medical condition, but for a wide range of other health and social care problems. Consequently, a majority of readmissions in older people are due to a diagnosis other than the index admission diagnosis [2]. This observation has led to the concept of a 'post-hospitalisation syndrome', described as an acquired transient period of vulnerability [4]. This syndrome may extend beyond the 30 days commonly

* Correspondence: m.witham@dundee.ac.uk
[2]Ageing and Health, University of Dundee, Ninewells Hospital, Dundee, UK
Full list of author information is available at the end of the article

used as the benchmark for readmission rates, perhaps as long as 6 months after the index admission [5].

Because of the risks and costs associated with readmission, there is considerable interest in identifying which patients are at risk of readmission, with a view to intervening to reduce readmission rates. The use of readmission rates as a quality standard in healthcare gives further impetus to these efforts. There has been some work developing predictive models to assist in the reduction in readmission rates, with varying degrees of success [6–9]. The majority of studies in this area to date have however excluded patients discharged to nursing homes and have focused on patient discharges from acute receiving hospitals. Indeed, predictive algorithms for readmission [1, 5, 6] have not specifically studied older patients, who may have differing reasons for readmission compared to younger patients.

There are also limited data on readmission rates for patients who have experienced a period of in-patient rehabilitation after a period of prolonged illness, with evidence to date from American studies. These patients typically remain in hospital for a number of weeks, and thus subsequent readmissions may be less likely to be related to hasty or incomplete discharge planning, allowing the impact of post-hospitalisation syndrome rather than incomplete discharge planning and community support to be dissected out.

Ottenbacher et al. reviewed centrally held data from 1365 post-acute inpatient rehabilitation facilities (*n* = 736,536), reported 30-day readmission rates of between 5.8 and 18.8% for different sub-groups of patients [10]. 50% of readmissions were within 11 days. The same research group have published further work focusing upon patients with 'debility', and reported higher rates of hospital readmission of 19% at 30 days and 34% at 90 days [11]. There are considerable differences between the manner in which rehabilitation is provided in the USA and in Europe (in relation to providers of care, differing financial incentives, type of rehabilitation facilities where care is provided) meaning that these findings may not be directly comparable.

This study therefore aimed to use routinely collected healthcare data to establish a) the reasons for readmission to acute care facilities in a cohort of older people discharged from inpatient rehabilitation after an acute illness, b) whether the reasons for readmission varied by the reason for the index admission, and c) what the predictors for 30 and 180 day readmission were in this cohort.

Methods
Service characteristics
The Dundee Medicine for the Elderly rehabilitation service offers inpatient rehabilitation to patients located

within Dundee (Scotland, United Kingdom) unitary authority (population 150,000). Patients over the age of 65 years, are accepted to the unit following an admission at acute receiving hospitals for acute medical or surgical illness from a variety of specialties including general medicine, general surgery, orthopedics, stroke medicine and neurosurgery. Patients are also accepted from sub-acute Medicine for the Elderly wards. Patients were selected following review by a consultant geriatrician; patients selected were those felt to have potential to achieve independence in domains of self-care who were medically stable after their acute admission. Patients who had limited to no expectation of functional improvement within a reasonable period of time or those felt unlikely to survive to discharge were not selected for transfer to the rehabilitation unit.

Inpatient rehabilitation is carried out on dedicated rehabilitation wards by a multidisciplinary team, including physiotherapists, occupational therapists, dieticians, social workers and speech and language therapists. This process is over-seen by a consultant geriatrician, with patient progress meetings at weekly intervals to discuss progress and any issues that may affect discharge success. The model of care on the rehabilitation unit remained unchanged throughout the analysis period.

Data sources
This analysis was conducted using linked, routinely collected clinical data in Tayside, Scotland. Anonymised data are held by the University of Dundee Health Informatics Centre (HIC) in an access-controlled Safe Haven environment. Analysis complied with HIC Standard Operating Procedures approved by the NHS East of Scotland Research Ethics Service and the NHS Tayside Caldicott Guardian. Separate ethics review for this project was therefore not required.

Data collected
Data used in this analysis were prospectively collected on all admissions to the Dundee Medicine for the Elderly rehabilitation unit between 1 January 1999 and 31 December 2011. Data were collected as part of routine clinical care and reviewed by the team caring for the patient during inpatient rehabilitation. The cohort was followed up until the end of May 2012. Mortality data were obtained using death certification information derived from Scottish Register Officer. This cohort has been described in detail previously [12–14].

Variables included age, sex, Scottish Index of Multiple Deprivation Quintile [15], discharge destination (home versus other options, which comprised long-stay hospital beds or care home), comorbid disease, admission and discharge 20-point Barthel scores, length of rehabilitation hospital stay, and number of medications on discharge.

Comorbid disease diagnoses were obtained in two different ways. A diagnosis of chronic kidney disease was coded based upon estimated glomerular filtration rate (eGFR) taken from linked clinical data using the MDRD equation [16]. Other diagnoses were obtained using International Classification of Diseases (ICD) 10 discharge diagnosis codes from hospital admissions prior to the index acute admission [17]. These included a diagnosis of previous myocardial infarction, stroke, congestive cardiac failure, and chronic obstructive pulmonary disease (COPD). The presence of diabetes mellitus was ascertained from the Scottish Care Information – Diabetes Collaborative (SCI-DC) database.

In addition, information on dynamic changes in C-reactive protein (CRP) was obtained as a measure of biological resilience [18], including maximum-recorded value during admission and time taken for elevated levels to halve in value.

Classification of admission and readmission diagnoses

The main diagnostic reason (recorded as ICD-10 codes) for admission to acute hospital prior to the rehabilitation referral for all patients was obtained from HIC datasets, alongside the main first readmission diagnosis to acute hospital for patients who were readmitted within 30 or 180 days. Only the first readmission was considered in this analysis.

These ICD codes were recorded, and collated into broader categories. For example, all cancer diagnoses were collated into 'Cancer Diagnoses' and different forms of dementia were collated into 'Dementia States'. In the 30-day and 180-day readmission groups, the 10 most common reasons for admission to hospital were established after reviewing collated diagnoses lists. The diagnoses for readmission were then charted by initial admission diagnosis for each of the two readmission groups in order to establish any relationships between initial admission and readmission diagnoses.

Data analysis

Statistical analyses were carried out in SPSS v22.0 (IBM, New York USA), and a two-sided p value of < 0.05 was taken as significant for all analyses. Individuals were excluded from the analysis if they died during their in-patient admission, or did not have a discharge Barthel score. The number of days between patients discharge from rehabilitation hospital discharge to next acute hospital admission was calculated, with readmission to acute hospital within 30 days and 180 days analysed separately. Cox regression analysis was used to examine the association between baseline factors and acute hospital readmission with dates censored at 30 days and 180 days after discharge (or at death if this was earlier). Analyses were adjusted for age, sex, and comorbid disease; variables

with a p-value < 0.3 on univariate analysis were also entered into the adjusted model.

Results

Of the 4449 patients in the complete medicine for the elderly rehabilitation dataset, 409 died during admission and were excluded from analysis, with a further 65 excluded due to the absence of a discharge Barthel score. A total of 3984 patients were included in the analysis.

Baseline characteristics

The characteristics of the overall patients group, patients readmitted to acute hospital care within 30 days and 180 days of discharge from the rehabilitation hospital are given in Table 1. Twenty-nine patients died within 30 days of discharge without being readmitted, and 325 died within 180 days of discharge without being readmitted. Patients readmitted to acute hospital facilities within 30 or 180 days were more likely to have a diagnosis of cancer, chronic obstructive pulmonary disease, congestive cardiac failure, previous myocardial infarction, a higher number of general hospitalizations over the period of data-collection (1999–2012) and a higher admission Barthel score.

Readmission to acute hospital diagnoses

For patients readmitted within 30 days, 27% ($n = 59/222$) of patients were readmitted with the same condition as their initial admission. For patients readmitted within 180 days, 21% ($n = 196/926$) of patients were readmitted with the same condition as their initial admission. The most common reasons for readmission for patients readmitted within 30 days were chest infection ($n = 20$), stroke ($n = 14$) and falls/immobility ($n = 13$). The most common reasons for readmission for patients readmitted within 180 days were admission secondary to falls/immobility ($n = 99$), chest infection ($n = 55$) or secondary to cancer ($n = 51$).

Figures 1 and 2 show how both deaths and readmissions for the 30 and 180 day time periods varied over the study period. Figures 3 and 4 show the main readmission diagnoses at 30 days and 180 days respectively, broken down by the original admission diagnosis.

Multivariate analyses for acute hospital readmissions

Table 2 shows the results of univariate analysis for readmissions within 30 days and 180 days. Tables 3 and 4 show the results of multivariate regression analyses, conducted firstly using time to readmission as the dependent variable and censoring at death or end of the follow up period, and secondly using time to either death or readmission (whichever came first) as the dependent variable. Multivariate analysis showed that for patients readmitted within 30 days, older age, male sex,

Table 1 Characteristics of overall cohort, patients readmitted within 30 days and patients readmitted within 180 days

	Whole cohort n = 3984	Readmitted by 30 days n = 222	Not readmitted and alive at 30 days (n = 3733)	Readmitted by 180 days N = 926	Not readmitted and alive at 180 days (n = 2733)	Died before readmission and before 180 days (n = 325)
Mean age (years) (SD)	84.1 (7.4)	82.7(7.3)*	84.2 (7.4)	83.6 (7.3)**	84.4 (7.4)	82.8 (7.5)
Male sex (%)	1582 (39.7)	112 (50.5)*	1459 (39.1)	419 (45.2)**	1017 (37.2)	146 (44.9)
Discharged to own home (%)	2982 (74.8)	161 (72.5)	2810 (75.3)	757 (81.7)**	2072 (75.8)	153 (47.1)
SIMD Quintiles (%)						
1 (most deprived)	1167 (29.3)	65 (29.3)	1090 (29.2)	277 (30.0)	784 (28.7)	106 (32.6)
2	572 (14.4)	31 (14.0)	536 (14.4)	127 (13.7)	388 (14.2)	57 (17.5)
3	490 (12.3)	27 (12.2)	459 (12.3)	109 (11.8)	333 (12.2)	48 (14.8)
4	1073 (26.9)	66 (29.7)	1002 (26.8)	241 (26.0)	758 (27.7)	74 (22.8)
5 (least deprived)	596 (15)	28 (12.6)	565 (15.1)	147 (15.9)	412 (15.1)	37 (11.4)
Missing Value	86 (2.2)	5 (2.3)	81 (2.2)	25 (2.7)	58 (2.1)	3 (0.9)
Mean Admission Barthel Score (SD)	10.4 (3.8)	11.1 (3.8)*	10.4 (3.8)	10.4 (3.6)	10.5 (3.8)	9.4 (4.3)
Mean Discharge Barthel Score (SD)	14.4 (4.6)	14.7 (4.4)	14.4 (4.6)	14.5 (4.3)	14.7 (4.5)	10.6 (6.0)
Median Length of Stay (days) (IQR)	33 (18–62)	28 (16–52)*	34 (18–62)	33 (20 – 56)	34 (18–64)	29 (18–55)
Median Number of Medications on Discharge (IQR)	2 (0–5)	2 (0–5)	2 (0–5)	3 (0–6)	3 (0–5)	0 (0–3)
Previous Myocardial Infarction (%)	683 (17.1)	52 (23.4)*	628 (16.8)	188 (20.3)**	435 (15.9)	60 (18.5)
Previous Stroke (%)	286 (7.2)	16 (7.2)*	266 (7.1)	67 (7.2)	189 (6.9)	30 (9.2)
Congestive Heart Failure (%)	342 (8.6)	33 (14.9)*	304 (8.1)	109 (11.8)**	183 (6.7)	50 (15.4)
eGFR < 60 ml/min/1.73m² (%)	2019 (50.7)	109 (49.1)	1891 (50.7)	482 (52.1)	1373 (50.2)	164 (50.5)
eGFR 30–59	1090 (27.4)	57 (25.7)	1023 (27.4)	251 (27.1)	762 (27.9)	77 (23.7)
eGFR 15–29	709 (17.8)	40 (18.0)	664 (17.8)	170 (18.4)	473 (17.3)	66 (20.3)
eGFR < 15	220 (5.5)	12 (5.4)	204 (5.5)	61 (6.6)	138 (5.0)	21 (6.5)
COPD (%)	553 (13.9)	46 (20.7)*	502 (13.4)	157 (17.0)**	338 (12.4)	58 (17.8)
Previous Diagnosis of Cancer (%)	467 (11.7)	34 (15.3)	428 (11.5)	125 (13.5)**	262 (9.6)	80 (24.6)
Diabetes Mellitus (%)	709 (17.8)	50 (22.5)	654 (17.5)	168 (18.1)	501 (18.3)	40 (12.3)

SIMD Scottish Index Multiple Deprivation Quintiles, *SD* standard deviation, *IQR* inter-quartile range, *eGFR* estimated glomerular filtration rate, *COPD* Chronic obstructive pulmonary disease
*p < 0.05 vs group not readmitted at 30 days
**p < 0.05 vs group not readmitted at 180 days

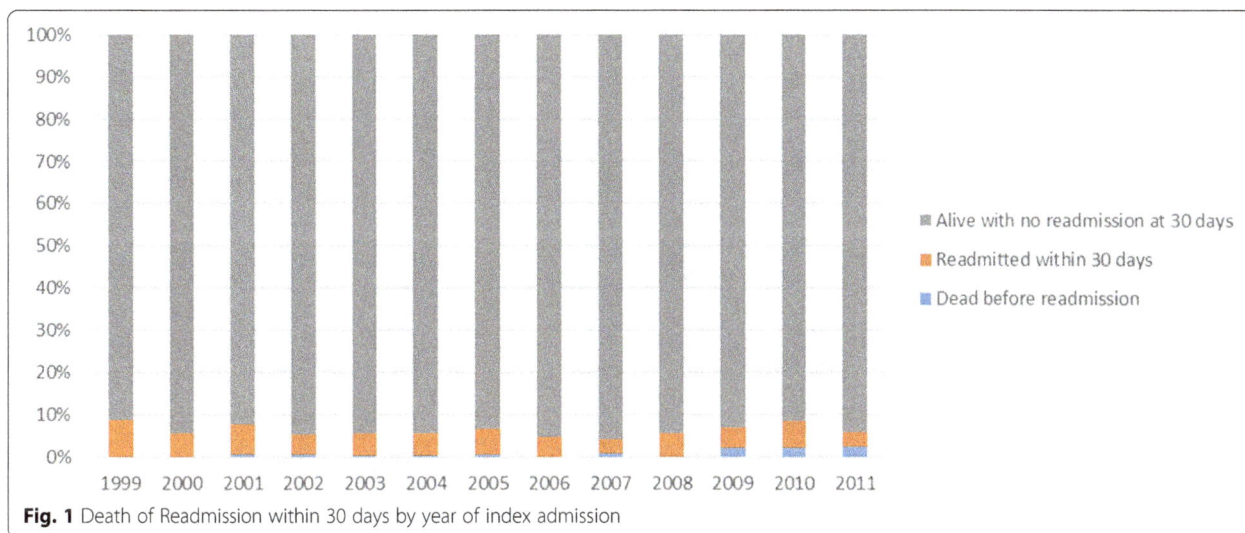

Fig. 1 Death of Readmission within 30 days by year of index admission

shorter length of hospital stay, discharge to own home and a previous diagnosis of chronic heart failure independent predictors of readmission within 30 days. For patients readmitted within 180 days, older age, male sex, shorter length of hospital stay and previous diagnosis of chronic heart failure were again independent predictors, but in addition previous myocardial infarction, previous diagnosis of cancer, and previous diagnosis of chronic obstructive pulmonary disease were additional independent predictors of readmission within 180 days. Results were very similar for readmission alone and for readmission or death as the outcome variable.

The ability of these sets of predictors to discriminate between those readmitted and those not readmitted was limited, with a c-statistic of 0.64 (95%CI 0.60 to 0.68) for readmission within 30 days, and 0.59 (95%CI 0.57 to 0.61) for readmission within 180 days.

Discussion

There are several key findings from this study. Readmissions to acute care in this cohort were due to a wide range of diagnoses, and were due to a different diagnosis to the index admission in over three-quarters of cases. Patterns differed between early and late readmission, and some index diagnoses (e.g. dementia, delirium, cardiovascular disease) were associated with a much higher chance of readmission with the same problem. The 30-day acute care readmission rate of 5.6% following a period of in-patient rehabilitation was lower than readmission rates reported in studies from the USA that ranged between 5.8–18.8% [10, 11, 19].

Risk factor patterns for early vs late readmission differed - for patients readmitted within 30 days a diagnosis of heart failure was the single factor increasing the likelihood of readmission, with discharge to the patients own home, and longer length of stay associated with reduced

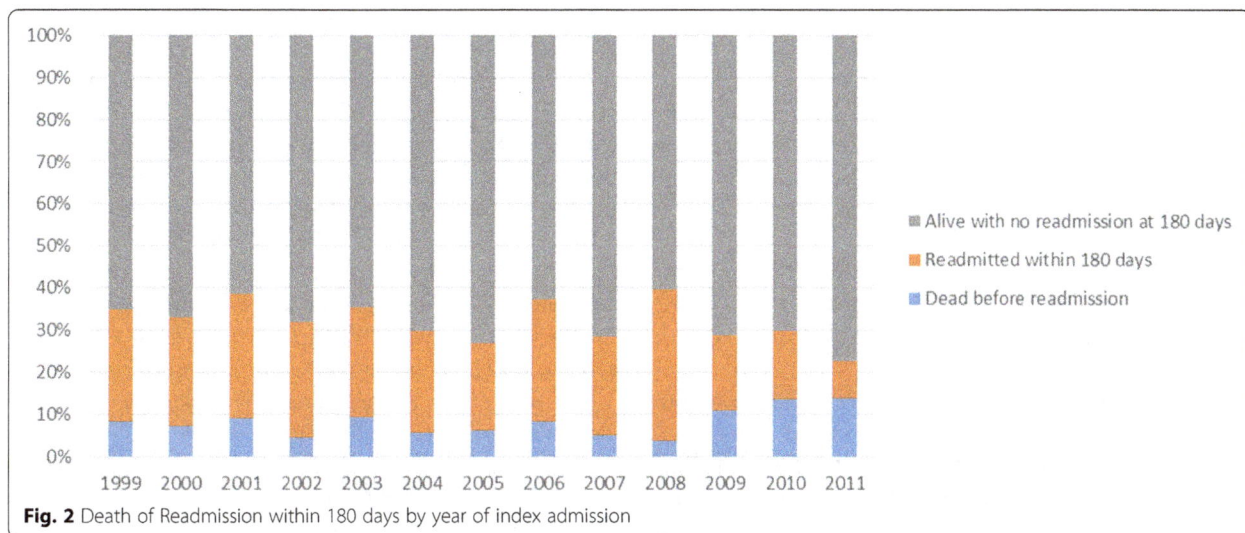

Fig. 2 Death of Readmission within 180 days by year of index admission

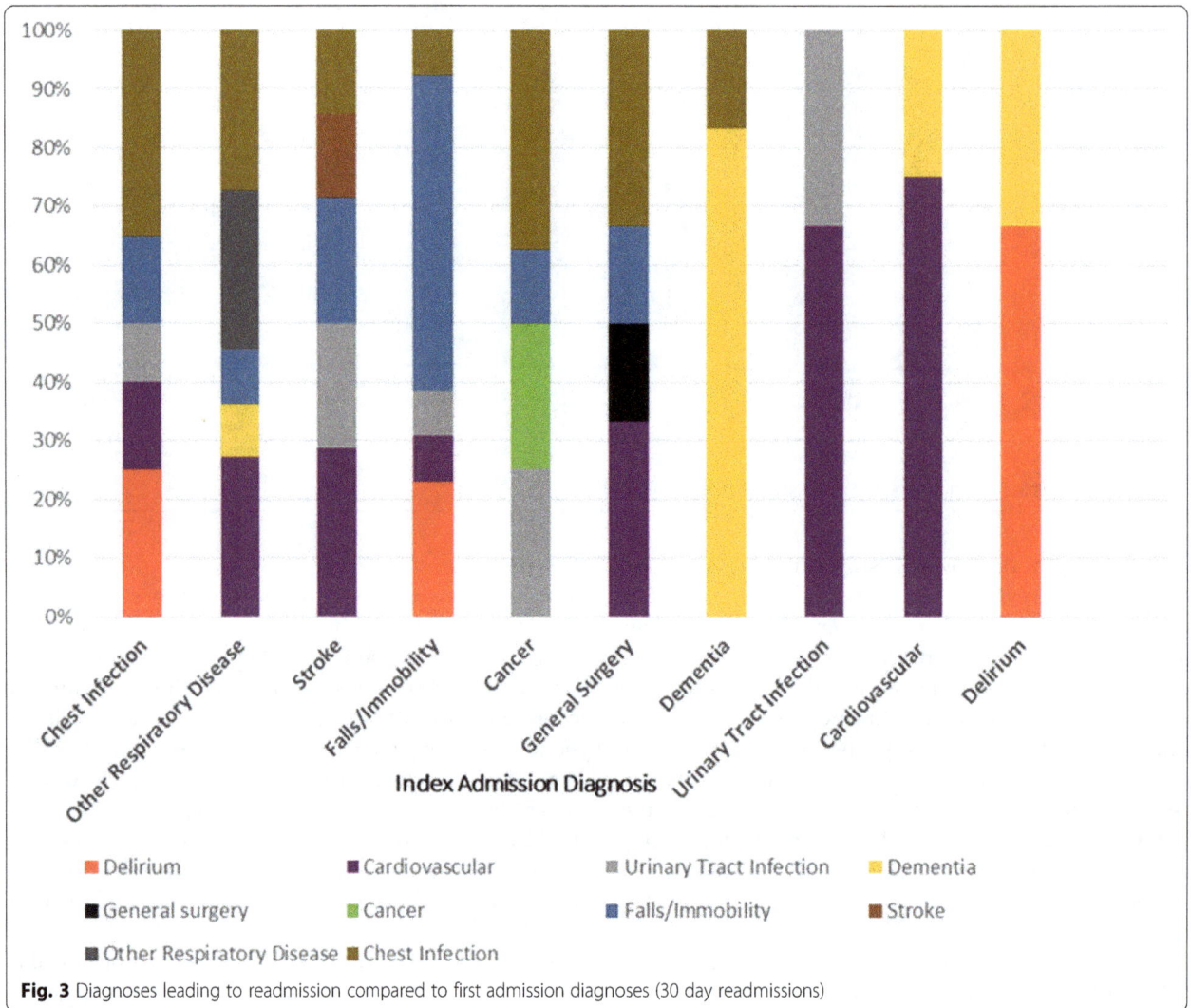

Fig. 3 Diagnoses leading to readmission compared to first admission diagnoses (30 day readmissions)

risk of readmission. In contrast, for patients readmitted within 180 days, the burden of comorbid disease as shown by a range of diagnoses and number of medications was associated with readmission. Although a longer length of stay was weakly associated with reduced risk of readmission to acute facilities, discharge to one's own home was not a protective factor. The discriminatory ability of a combination of the above factors for early or late readmission was only modest and is unlikely to be helpful in clinical practice, despite the inclusion of a measure of functional ability. Markers of inflammation and of biological resilience (maximum CRP and rate of CRP recovery) were not associated with the risk of readmission.

Our findings are consistent with previous work from the USA, where two-thirds of readmissions were for a different problem than the index admission [2]. The even higher rate of discrepant diagnoses seen in our analysis is likely to be due to the older age and increased comorbidity of our study population. A large number of comorbid diseases means more opportunity for a problem to arise in a different organ system. Furthermore, although we did not measure frailty in our study population, it is highly likely that frailty was prevalent as is the case in other groups of older inpatients. Analysis of trends in English hospitals reported that overall frailty burden, based on the coding of at least one frailty syndrome, has increased from 12 to 14% between 2005 and 2013 for older patients admitted electively or acutely [20]. Frailty denotes a loss of homeostatic reserve across multiple body systems. Thus a disturbance or illness in one system can easily precipitate failure of a different system, which would be consistent with our findings.

The risk factors for readmission that were significant in our cohort are similar to those seen in other studies. Cancer, COPD, ischaemic heart disease, heart failure and stroke have all been associated with high readmission rates [21–23], and our results are consistent with previous studies

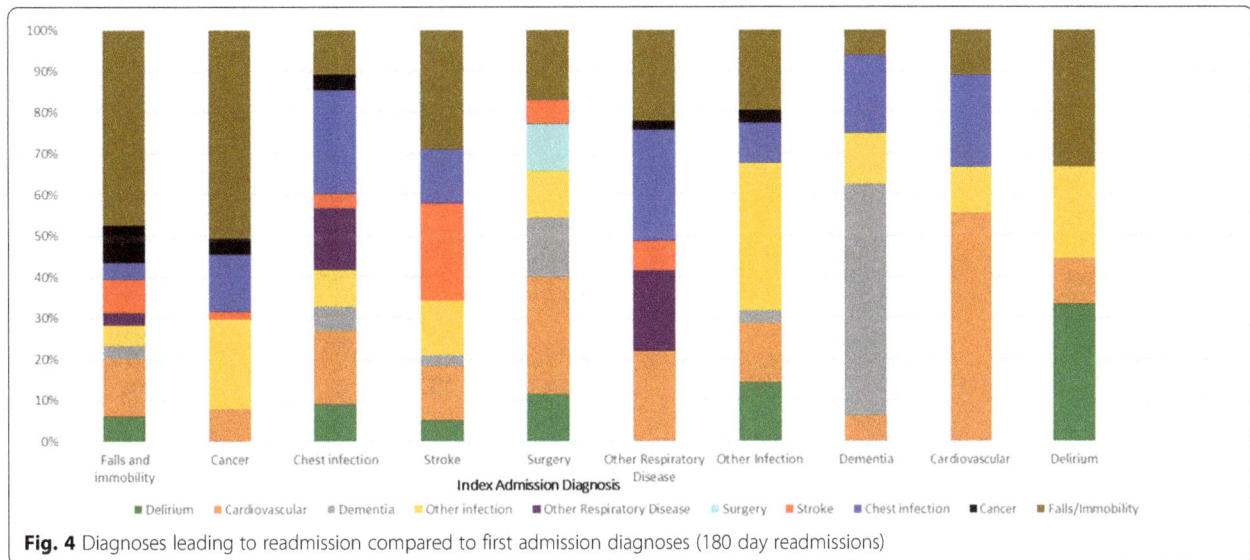

Fig. 4 Diagnoses leading to readmission compared to first admission diagnoses (180 day readmissions)

where multimorbidity and previous hospitalisations were risk factors for readmission [24–27]. A study from the USA looking at readmission following a period of in-patient rehabilitation reported that heart failure, infections, nutritional and metabolic disorders alongside digestive disorders were the most common reasons for readmission [10]. We did not find that these last two diagnoses were commonly associated with readmission to acute care in our cohort.

Previous work has also shown that men are more likely to be readmitted to hospital within 30 days of discharge, possibly due to reduced health-seeking behaviors [28]. Differences in health-seeking behaviors, the lower

role placed by men on preventative care and overly optimistic self-perceived health status may explain the apparent contradiction between higher morbidity in females in older age but higher risk of readmission for men after discharge [29, 30].

In contrast to previous studies from acute hospitals [9, 26, 27, 31], older age was associated with a reduced risk of readmission in our analysis. This may reflect patient selection – very old, very frail patients may not be selected for rehabilitation but may be transferred directly to nursing care facilities rather than the rehabilitation unit, whereas similarly frail younger patients may be

Table 2 Univariate Cox regression analyses – time to readmission

Variable in Analysis	Censored at 30 days		Censored at 180 days	
	Hazard Ratio (95% CI)	p	Hazard Ratio (95% CI)	p
Age (per year)	0.97 [0.96–0.99]	0.004	0.99 [0.98–0.99]	< 0.001
Female Sex	0.64 [0.49–0.83]	0.001	0.85 [0.80–0.90]	< 0.001
Admission Barthel score (per point)	1.05 [1.01–1.08]	0.01	1.01 [1.00–1.03]	0.13
Discharge Barthel score (per point)	1.01 [0.98–1.04]	0.34	1.01 [0.99–1.02]	0.39
Discharge Home	0.87 [0.65–1.16]	0.30	0.74 [0.64–0.85]	< 0.001
Length of Hospital stay (days)	0.997 [0.994–1.000]	0.04	0.998 [0.997–0.999]	< 0.001
Previous Myocardial Infarction	1.49 [1.09–2.03]	0.01	1.35 [1.17–1.56]	< 0.001
Previous Stroke	1.02 [0.61–1.69]	0.94	1.03 [0.82–1.29]	0.81
Congestive Cardiac Failure	1.90 [1.32–2.76]	0.001	1.68 [1.41–2.00]	< 0.001
Previous Diagnosis of Cancer	1.38 [0.96–1.99]	0.09	1.30 [1.10–1.53]	0.002
Diabetes Mellitus	1.11 [0.99–1.27]	0.09	1.04 [0.98–1.11]	0.19
Chronic Obstructive Pulmonary Disease	1.65 [1.19–2.28]	0.003	1.44 [1.24–1.68]	< 0.001
Medication Count on Discharge (per drug)	1.01 [0.98–1.05]	0.63	1.02 [1.00–1.03]	0.08
Maximum CRP Reading (per mg/L)	1.000 [0.998–1.001]	0.77	1.000 [0.999–1.001]	0.84
Time to half maximum CRP (per week)	0.997 [0.991–1.002]	0.23	1.000 [0.999–1.001]	0.87

Table 3 Multivariate Cox regression analysis – time to readmission censored at 30 days

Variable in Analysis	Risk of readmission (censored at 30 days or death)		Risk of readmission or death (censored at 30 days)	
	Hazard Ratio (95% CI)	p	Hazard Ratio (95% CI)	p
Age (per year)	0.98 [0.96–1.00]	0.04	0.98 [0.96–1.00]	0.06
Female Sex	0.76 [0.57–1.00]	0.05	0.76 [0.57–1.00]	0.05
Admission Barthel score (per point)	1.04 [1.00–1.08]	0.07	1.03 [1.00–1.07]	0.08
Discharge Home	0.54 [0.38–0.77]	0.001	0.51 [0.36–0.72]	< 0.001
Length of Hospital Stay (per day)	0.994 [0.991–0.998]	0.003	0.994 [0.990–0.998]	0.001
Previous Myocardial Infarction	1.25 [0.88–1.77]	0.21	1.19 [0.84–1.68]	0.32
Congestive Cardiac Failure	1.54 [1.02–2.34]	0.04	1.65 [1.10–2.47]	0.02
Previous Diagnosis of Cancer	1.33 [0.91–1.95]	0.14	1.30 [0.89–1.90]	0.18
Diabetes Mellitus	1.24 [0.89–1.72]	0.21	1.24 [0.89–1.72]	0.20
COPD	1.34 [0.94–1.90]	0.11	1.34 [0.95–1.90]	0.10

COPD Chronic obstructive pulmonary disease

selected for rehabilitation. Another possible explanation is that the rehabilitation team might view very old patients as at higher risk than younger patients, and accordingly plan discharges in such a way to mitigate this risk.

An association between shorter length of stay and increased risk of readmission has previously been reported for older patients discharged from acute hospitals [32–34]. However, we found only a small effect of length of stay on readmission risk; perhaps because patients admitted for rehabilitation have a relatively long length of stay, allowing comprehensive discharge planning and recovery from acute illness. The incremental benefit from an even longer stay may thus be minimal.

The discriminant ability of the risk factors we measured to predict future readmission was poor – too poor to be of use in planning clinical services. A systematic

review for risk prediction models for hospital readmission reported that most current readmission risk prediction models, whether designed for comparative or clinical purposes, perform poorly [8]. The review looked at 30 studies that assessed 26 unique models, and commented that few of these examined variables associated with overall health and function, illness severity, or social determinants of health. This lack may be particularly important for older patients where social determinants of health alongside broader markers of function are crucial in terms of planning both primary, secondary and social care services.

Reducing readmissions in this patient group will be challenging. A systematic review of both in-hospital (17 studies) and home-care (15 studies) interventions aimed at reducing readmissions for in older people (> 75 years old) found that most did not have any effect on readmission [34]. However, those interventions with home-care

Table 4 Multivariate Cox regression analysis – time to readmission, censored at 180 days

Variable in Analysis	Risk of readmission (censored at 180 days or death)		Risk of readmission or death (censored at 180 days)	
	Hazard Ratio (95% CI)	p	Hazard Ratio (95% CI)	p
Age (per year)	0.99 [0.98–1.00]	0.03	0.99 [0.98–1.00]	0.01
Female Sex	0.80 [0.71–0.91]	0.001	0.77 [0.69–0.87]	< 0.001
Admission Barthel score (per point)	0.99 [0.98–1.01]	0.44	0.98 [0.79–0.92]	0.03
Discharge Home	1.02 [0.86–1.21]	0.85	0.79 [0.68–0.92]	0.003
Length of Hospital Stay (per day)	0.997 [0.995–0.998]	< 0.001	0.995 [0.994–0.997]	< 0.001
Previous Myocardial Infarction	1.21 [1.03–1.42]	0.02	1.25 [1.07–1.45]	0.004
Congestive Cardiac Failure	1.48 [1.22–1.79]	< 0.001	1.57 [1.31–1.88]	< 0.001
Previous Diagnosis of Cancer	1.30 [1.10–1.55]	0.003	1.48 [1.27–1.73]	< 0.001
Diabetes Mellitus	1.00 [0.94–1.07]	1.00	0.99 [0.86–1.15]	0.93
COPD	1.24 [1.06–1.46]	0.009	1.23 [1.05–1.43]	0.009
Medication Count on Discharge	1.01 [0.99–1.03]	0.28	0.99 [0.98–1.01]	0.41

COPD Chronic obstructive pulmonary disease

components were more likely to be successful [34]. There is current work in the United Kingdom bringing together health and social care, in part to try and start addressing these concerns. However, the proportion of readmissions that are deemed avoidable after standardized and reliable review is not high; recent research reports less than 20% of readmissions are avoidable [27]. Furthermore, although readmission and hospitalization are important markers for disease severity, prognosis and quality of life there are clearly limits to any single metric as a surrogate for standard of care.

Our results reinforce the need to take a multisystem, holistic approach to reducing readmissions. Whilst some success has been noted with disease-specific interventions, e.g. for patients with heart failure [35], it is unlikely that interventions targeting a single disease (e.g. heart failure) will be successful in reducing readmissions due to other disease diagnoses after an index admission. Indeed, a focus on a single disease risks generating unintended knock-on consequences – rigorous control of heart failure may increase the risk of readmission with dehydration or acute kidney injury for example. Although a measure of biological resilience (CRP recovery rate) did not provide a useful way of predicting readmission in this analysis, similar measures of frailty or resilience may still provide both a way of predicting readmission and provide a target for intervention to reduce readmissions. Furthermore, other studies looking at readmission from rehabilitation units have suggested that information on functional status measures that are easily monitored by health care providers may improve plans for smooth transition of care delivery and aid the reduction of risk for hospital readmission [11].

Our analysis has a number of strengths. We used detailed health and functional outcomes data on a large set of patients undergoing rehabilitation in a medicine for the elderly unit. Studies to date have not assessed readmission following in-patient rehabilitation in a general older rehabilitation population, and there are differences between this group of patients compared to older adults discharged directly from acute hospitals [10, 11]. As this study analyzed routinely collected data, the data represents real-world clinical information that enables greater generalizability of the results.

There are several limitations that deserve comment. Our data were examined retrospectively and were not collected with this study in mind. Data quality is usually imperfect in datasets of routinely collected clinical data, and not all patients had Barthel scores available for analysis. Although the range of discharge diagnoses that we could classify from discharge coding data was wide, such data depends on both accurate diagnosis and accurate recording of the discharge diagnoses for coding, which is not always the case in routine clinical care. Use of this

source of diagnoses prevented us from including poorly-coded diagnoses such as dementia, and alternative sources (e.g. primary care records) were not available for linkage at the time of our analysis. The large number of reasons for the index hospital admissions precluded easy use of these reasons as a variable in the analyses of risk factors for readmission, but future work using larger datasets may be able to address this issue.

Patients who have been admitted to a rehabilitation unit have the ideal opportunity for discharge planning in a clinical environment geared towards optimizing hospital discharges. The results of our analysis may not necessarily be generalizable to other patients groups with shorter length of stay and less comprehensive discharge planning. Out of hospital care services have developed considerably since 2012 (the end of study period). Changes have included early community intervention services, Hospital @ Home teams and use of step-up intermediate care beds rather than admission to acute units. These changes have taken place in our locality after the end of the period studied in this analysis.

Conclusion

Our results confirm and extend previous work that readmissions of older people after hospital admission are due to a wide range of causes, and are often not due to a recurrence of the index problem. Work is needed to develop intervention packages that address readmission risks common to a range of diseases and syndromes of ageing, with a focus both on optimizing physiology, but also supporting patients and carers. In parallel, further work is required to identify those at highest risk of readmission so that such intervention packages can be targeted appropriately.

Abbreviations

CCF: Congestive cardiac failure; CKD: Chronic kidney disease; COPD: Chronic obstructive pulmonary disease; CRP: C – reactive protein; eGFR: estimated glomerular filtration rate; HIC: Health Informatics Centre; ICD: International Classification of Diseases; IQR: Inter-quartile range; MDRD: Modification of Diet in Renal Disease Study (MDRD) equation; NHS: National Health Service; NI: Not included; SCI-DC: Scottish Care Information Diabetes Collaborative; SD: Standard deviation; USA: United States of America

Funding

No specific funding was used to conduct these analyses. The original data linkage project that generated this dataset was funded by the Scottish Government, grant number SCPH/10.

Authors' contributions

LDH and MDW co-designed and performed the analysis, cowrote the manuscript and both critically revised the manuscript. Both authors agree to be accountable for all aspects of the work.

Competing interests

The authors declare that they have no competing interests.

Author details

[1]GP Registrar, Primary Care Directorate, NHS Education for Scotland, Edinburgh, UK. [2]Ageing and Health, University of Dundee, Ninewells Hospital, Dundee, UK.

References

1. Donze J, Aujesky A, Williams D, et al. Potentially avoidable 30-day readmissions in medical patients. Derivation and validation of a predictive model. JAMA Intern Med. 2013;173(8):632–8.

2. Jencks SF, Williams MV, Coleman EA. Rehospitalisations among patients in the Medicare fee-for service program. N Engl J Med. 2009;360:1418–28.

3. Reducing Readmissions. NHS Innovation & Improvement. Available from: http://webarchive.nationalarchives.gov.uk/20121108093302/http://www.institute.nhs.uk/quality_and_service_improvement_tools/quality_and_service_improvement_tools/discharge_planning.html Accessed: 13th Oct 2017.

4. Krumholz HM. Post-hospital syndrome- an acquired, Transient Condition of Generalised Risk. N Engl J Med. 2013;368(2):100–2.

5. van Walraven JA, Taljaard M, et al. Incidence of potentially avoidable urgent readmissions and their relation to all-cause urgent readmissions. CMAJ. 2011;183(14):E1067–72.

6. Billings J, Blunt I, Steventon A, Georghiou LG, Bardsley M. Development of a predictive model to identify inpatients at risk of re-admission within 30 days of discharge (PARR-30). BMJ Open. 2012;2:e001667.

7. Cotter PE, Bhalla VK, Wallis SJ, Biram RW. Predicting readmissions: poor performance of the LACE index in an older UK population. Age Ageing. 2012;41:784–9.

8. Kansagara D, Englander H, Salanitro A, et al. Risk prediction models for readmission rates: a systematic review. JAMA. 2011;306:1688–98.

9. van Walraven DIA, Bell C, et al. Derivation and validation of an index to predict early death or unplanned readmission after discharge after discharge from hospital to the community. CMAJ. 2010;182:551–7.

10. Ottenbacher KJ, Karmarkar A, Graham JE, et al. Thirty-day hospital readmission following discharge from post-acute rehabilitation in fee-for-service Medicare patients. JAMA. 2014;311(6):604–14.

11. Fisher SR, Graham JE, Krishnan S, Ottenbacher KJ. Predictors of 30-day readmission following inpatient rehabilitation for patients at high risk for hospital readmission. Phys Ther. 2016;96(1):62–70.

12. Witham MD, Ramage L, Burns SL, et al. Trends in function and Postdischarge mortality in a medicine for the rehabilitation Centre over a 10-year period. Arch Phys Med Rehabil. 2011;92:1288–92.

13. Lynch JE, Henderson NR, Ramage L, McMurdo MET, Witham MD. Association between statin medication and improved outcomes during inpatient rehabilitation in older people. Ageing and Ageing. 2012;41(2):260–2.

14. Beveridge LD, Ramage L, McMurdo MET, George J, Witham MD. Allopurinol use is associated with greater functional gains in older rehabilitation patients. Age Ageing. 2013;42(3):400–4.

15. Scottish Index of Multiple Deprivation. SIMD Results 2012. Available from: http://simd.scotland.gov.uk/publication-2012/. Accessed 10 Oct 2017.

16. Levey AS, Bosch JP, Lewis JB, Greene T, Rogers N, Roth D. A more accurate method to estimate glomerular filtration rate from serum creatinine: a new prediction equation. Modification of diet in renal disease study group. Ann Intern Med. 1999;130(6):461–70.

17. The ICD-10 Classification of Mental and Behavioural Disorders: Clinical descriptions and diagnostic guidelines. Geneva: World Health Organization, 1992.

18. Barma M, Goodbrand JA, Donnan PT, McGilchrist MM, Frost H, McMurdo ME, Witham MD. Slower decline in C-reactive protein after an inflammatory insult is associated with longer survival in older hospitalised patients. PLoS One. 2016;11(7):e0159412.

19. Dara LC, Ingber MJ, Carichner JBA, et al. Evaluating hospital readmission rates after discharge from inpatient rehabilitation. Arch Phys Med Rehabil. 2018;99(6):1049–59.

20. Soong J, Poots A, Scott S, et al. Quantifying the prevalence of frailty in English hospitals. BMJ Open. 2015;5:e008456.

21. Saunders ND, Nichols SD, Antiporda MA, Johnson K, et al. Examination of unplanned 30-day readmissions to a comprehensive cancer hospital. J Oncol Pract. 2015;11(2):e177–81.

22. Royal College of Physicians. National COPD audit Programme. COPD: who cares when it matters most? – outcomes report 2014. National Supplementary Report 2017. London.

23. Rao A, Barrow E, Vuik S, Darzi A, Aylin P. Systematic review of hospital readmissions in stroke patients. Stroke Res Treat. 2016;2016:9325368.

24. Donze J, Lipsitz S, Bates DW, Schnipper JL. Causes and patterns of readmissions in patients with common comorbidities: retrospective cohort study. BMJ. 2013;347:f7171.

25. Kahlon S, Pederson J, Majumdar SR, et al. Association between frailty and 30-day outcomes after discharge from hospital. CMAJ. 2015;187(11):799–804.

26. Marcantonio ER, McKean S, Goldfinger M, et al. Factors associated with unplanned hospital readmission among patients 65 years of age and older in a Medicare managed care plan. Am J Med. 1999;107(1):13–7.

27. Walraven v, Bennet C, Jennings A, et al. Proportion of hospital readmissions deemed avoidable: a systematic review. CMAJ. 2011;183:E391–402.

28. Woz S, Mitchell S, Hesko C, et al. Gender as risk factor for 30 days post-discharge hospital utilisation: a secondary data analysis. BMJ Open. 2012;2:e000428.

29. Courtenay WH. Constructions of masculinity and their influence on men's well-being: a theory of gender and health. Soc Sci Med. 2000;50:1385–401.

30. Kirchengast S, Haslinger B. Gender differences in health-related quality of life among healthy aged and old-aged Austrians: cross-sectional analysis. Gend Med. 2008;5(3):270–8.

31. Silverstein MD, Huanying Q, Mercer SQ, et al. Risk factors for 30-day hospital readmission in patients ≥65 years of age. Proc (Bayl Univ Med Cent). 2008; 21(4):363–72.

32. Dobrzanska L, Newell R. Readmissions: a primary care examination of reasons for readmission of older people and possible readmission risk factors. J Clin Nurs. 2006;15(5):599–606.

33. Preyde M, Brassard K. Evidence-based risk factors for adverse health outcomes in older patients after discharge home and assessment tools: a systematic review. J Evid Based Soc Work. 2011;8(5):445–68.

34. Linertova R, Garcia-Perez L, Vazquez-Diaz JR, et al. Interventions to reduce hospital readmissions in the elderly: in-hospital or home care. A systematic review. J Eval Clin Pract. 2011;17(6):1167–75.

35. Desai AS, Stevenson LW. Rehospitalization for heart failure – predict or prevent? Circulation. 2012;126:501–6.

4

Minimally invasive anterior muscle-sparing versus a transgluteal approach for hemiarthroplasty in femoral neck fractures-a prospective randomised controlled trial including 190 elderly patients

Franziska Saxer[1†] (iD), Patrick Studer[1,4†], Marcel Jakob[1*], Norbert Suhm[1], Rachel Rosenthal[3], Salome Dell-Kuster[2,5], Werner Vach[1] and Nicolas Bless[1]

Abstract

Background: The relevance of femoral neck fractures (FNFs) increases with the ageing of numerous societies, injury-related decline is observed in many patients. Treatment strategies have evolved towards primary joint replacement, but the impact of different approaches remains a matter of debate. The aim of this trial was to evaluate the benefit of an anterior minimally-invasive (AMIS) compared to a lateral Hardinge (LAT) approach for hemiarthroplasty in these oftentimes frail patients.

Methods: Four hundred thirty-nine patients were screened during the 44-months trial, aiming at the evaluation of 150 patients > 60 yrs. of age. Eligible patients were randomised using an online-tool with completely random assignment. As primary endpoint, early mobility, a predictor for long-term outcomes, was evaluated at 3 weeks via the "Timed up and go" test (TUG). Secondary endpoints included the Functional Independence Measure (FIM), pain, complications, one-year mobility and mortality.

Results: A total of 190 patients were randomised; both groups were comparable at baseline, with a predominance for frailty-associated factors in the AMIS-group. At 3 weeks, 146 patients were assessed for the primary outcome. There was a reduction in the median duration of TUG performance of 21.5% (CI [− 41.2,4.7], $p = 0.104$) in the AMIS-arm (i.e., improved mobility). This reduction was more pronounced in patients with signs of frailty or cognitive impairment. FIM scores increased on average by 6.7 points (CI [0.5–12.8], $p = 0.037$), pain measured on a 10-point visual analogue scale decreased on average by 0.7 points (CI: [− 1.4,0.0], $p = 0.064$). The requirement for blood transfusion was lower in the AMIS- group, the rate of complications comparable, with a higher rate of soft tissue complications in the LAT-group. The mortality was higher in the AMIS-group.

Conclusion: These results, similar to previous reports, support the concept that in elderly patients at risk of frailty, the AMIS approach for hemiarthroplasty can be beneficial, since early mobilisation and pain reduction potentially reduce deconditioning, morbidity and loss of independence. The results are, however, influenced by a plethora of factors. Only improvements in every aspect of the therapeutic chain can lead to optimisation of treatment and improve outcomes in this growing patient population.

(Continued on next page)

* Correspondence: Marcel.Jakob@usb.ch
†Franziska Saxer and Patrick Studer contributed equally to this work.
[1]Department of Orthopaedics and Traumatology, University Hospital Basel, Spitalstrasse 21, 4031 Basel, Switzerland
Full list of author information is available at the end of the article

(Continued from previous page)

Keywords: Femoral neck fracture, Orthogeriatrics, Gerontotraumatology, Fracture hemiarthroplasty, Minimal invasive hemiarthroplasty, Trauma surgery in geriatric patients, Randomized controlled trial in the elderly

Background

Femoral neck fractures (FNFs) are typically associated with old age and represent a major cause of morbidity, functional dependence and socio-economic burden. These fractures also represent a sign of frailty, associated with a one-year mortality of approximately 30% [1–3] The affected patient population is very heterogeneous [4–6], with pre-fracture characteristics like age, the number of independent activities of daily living (ADLs) or the presence of dementia [6] being prognostic factors for long-term outcome [4].

The treatment of FNFs is a matter of debate and varies with age, fracture pattern and general health [7, 8]. For elderly patients with FNFs, conservative treatment and osteosynthesis have mostly been abandoned [8–12]. At our institution, many elderly patients are treated with cemented [13] hemiarthroplasty (HA) due to better short-term results, avoidance of suffering, efficient restoration of functional capacities and preservation of independence [9–12, 14, 15] (see Fig. 1 for the institutional treatment algorithm).

Approaches for joint replacement though can differ considerably in their invasiveness [16]. The lateral trans-gluteal Hardinge (LAT) approach [17] has been one of the standard approaches for joint replacement of the hip for decades. In the twenty-first century, the anterior minimally invasive Hueter (AMIS) approach regained popularity [18–20]. This approach allows a muscle-sparing access to the hip joint using an inter-muscular and inter-nervous plane, while the transgluteal approach necessitates the transection of muscular tissue. The rationale for using the AMIS approach is a potential reduction of soft tissue damage, blood loss and postoperative pain, as well as an acceleration of postoperative mobilisation, with a consecutive reduction of length of stay (LOS) and duration of rehabilitation [21–25] compared to other approaches.

Despite several publications, there is no consensus on the optimal approach for total hip arthroplasty (THA) [26, 27]. Furthermore, the reported data after THA have typically been derived from a younger and healthier population of patients with osteoarthritis [21–24]. Evidence from geriatric patients suffering FNFs is scarce [28–32].

Therefore, the primary objective of the trial was the comparison of a minimally invasive to a more conventional approach for the implantation of cemented HA in elderly patients suffering from FNFs. The "Timed up and go" test (TUG) [33] at 3 weeks was chosen as the

primary endpoint due to its prognostic value for long-term mobility and independence [34, 35]. A reduction of 20% in the TUG duration was assumed to be clinically relevant [36]. The secondary objectives of the trial were an evaluation of the changes in functional independence and TUG performance during the first postoperative year; the description of differences in the surgical performance, complications and mortality between the two approaches; and a subgroup analysis on the influence of functional independence and cognitive impairment.

Methods

The trial was designed as a prospective single-centre randomised controlled trial (RCT) with a one-year follow-up period at a level-one orthopaedic and trauma centre. From 09/11 to 04/15, we screened all consecutive, previously ambulatory patients 60 years or older with an FNF eligible for HA according to our institutional algorithm (Fig. 1). For inclusion and exclusion criteria, see Table 1.

Eligible patients entered the informed consent process. Depending on their cognitive abilities (quantified using a mental status questionnaire [37], MSQ), they were individually or in the presence of a designated proxy informed about the diagnosis, the proposed treatment and the randomised trial. The surgeon on call included patients only if they consented in writing or – in case of relevant cognitive impairment – gave their verbal assent with written consent by a designated proxy according to Swiss civil code (Art. 378) or a legal guardian. The trial was approved by the ethics committee (Ethikkommission beider Basel) EKBB Reference No. 68/11) and followed good clinical practice, as well as the Declaration of Helsinki. The trial has been registered with clinicaltrials.gov, and the complete protocol is available as additional files.

After consent to surgery and trial participation, the surgeon on call randomised the patients using a web-based randomisation tool (randomizer.at) with the "Completely At Random" option. The randomised treatment was delivered as soon as possible (i.e., 31% of patients underwent operation on the day of randomisation, 48% the next day, and only 2% of the patients had to wait 2 or more days for surgery, including those waiting for medical reasons like oral anticoagulation, etc).

At baseline, the following patient characteristics were recorded: age, gender, body mass index (BMI), residential status, use of a walking aid, diagnosis of dementia,

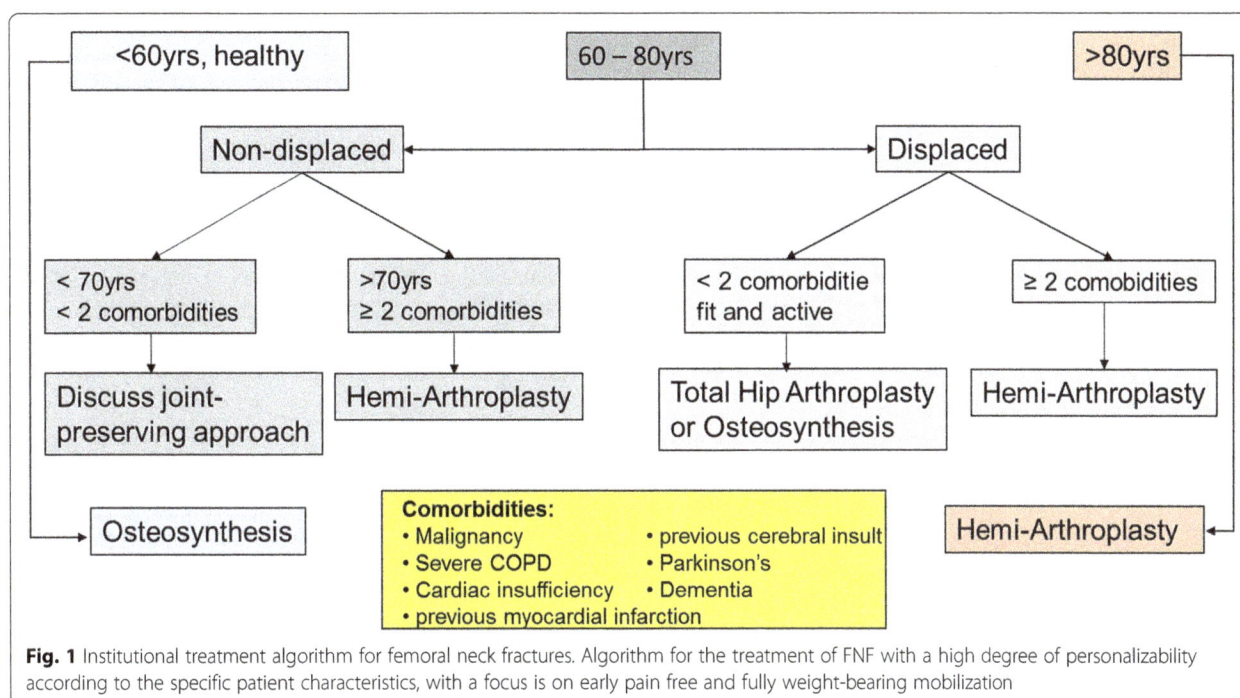

Fig. 1 Institutional treatment algorithm for femoral neck fractures. Algorithm for the treatment of FNF with a high degree of personalizability according to the specific patient characteristics, with a focus is on early pain free and fully weight-bearing mobilization

number of medications (substances), Charlson Comorbidity Index [38], and ASA (American Society of Anesthesiologists) grading [39]. Additionally, standard laboratory parameters were recorded. The pre-fracture Functional Independence Measure (pfFIM) [40] status was assessed retrospectively.

Surgery was performed after standard perioperative antimicrobial prophylaxis. Both groups were operated on using a cemented AMIS© stem (Medacta International, Castel San Pietro, Switzerland) and a monopolar head (Mathys AG, Bettlach, Switzerland) according to the manufacturer's instructions (including the use of monopolar heads by another manufacturer, since initially monopolar heads were not available in the shaft manufacturer's product range) and our standard operating procedures.

For the LAT approach, an incision of 8–14 cm is centred on the trochanter major to expose the fascia latae. After splitting this structure, the vasto-gluteal sling is exposed (the complex of the gluteus medius muscle proximally, the trochanter major and the vastus lateralis muscle distally). For the preparation of the capsule, the muscles are split in line with their fibres in the anterior third of the muscular body forming a musculo-tendineous flap.

For the AMIS approach, a 7- to 10-cm incision is made 2 cm latero-distally to the antero-superior iliac spine towards the fibular head. The interval between the sartorius muscle medially and the tensor fascia latae laterally is developed. The capsule is exposed between the rectus femoris muscle medially and the vastus intermedius muscle laterally.

All patients underwent the same postoperative aftercare with thrombo-embolic prophylaxis as well as mobilisation with full weight bearing under physiotherapeutic guidance from day one, using standard analgesia. As part of orthogeriatric care [41], patients were followed-up and treated for osteoporosis, fall prophylaxis, malnutrition and delirium. The latter was assessed by the nursing staff using a modified Delirium Observation Screening scale (DOS)

Table 1 In- and Exclusion Criteria

Inclusion Criteria	Exclusion Criteria
Age of 60 years or more, ambulatory with/without walking aid before trauma	Multiple fractures
Femoral neck fracture eligible for hemi-arthroplasty in accordance with the algorithm for femoral neck fractures	Suspicion of a pathological fracture in the context of known or unknown malignancy
	Previous surgery on the injured femur
Informed consent in surgery and trial- participation	Refusal of trial participation by the patient or legal representatives

In- and exclusion criteria chosen deliberately broad to increase the external validity of the results. The exclusion criteria based on the pattern of injury were defined to avoid an interference with early mobility by e.g. the inability to use walking aids due to fractures of the upper extremity, or lesions to the contralateral leg

[42] and – in case of pathology – the Confusion Assessment Method (CAM) [43].

Intraoperative data, such as the duration of surgery or intraoperative blood loss, were recorded. The latter was assessed via the number of erythrocyte concentrates ordered perioperatively up to 72 h post-surgery. Perioperative in-hospital complications were assessed as secondary outcome variables using the Clavien-Dindo classification [44] to differentiate general and surgery-related complications. After hospitalisation, only the occurrence of serious adverse events (SAE), surgery-related complications and implant-related infections were recorded. LOS was documented, as was the discharge destination (in-patient rehabilitation, nursing home, etc.). After discharge, follow-up was scheduled for 3 (only functional assessment), 6 and 12 weeks and one year postoperatively for clinical examination, functional assessment and X-rays as per the institutional standard.

The first assessment of functional recovery was performed in-hospital on day 5. At every follow-up TUG [33, 45], FIM [40] and pain scores were recorded by an independent study nurse blinded to the treatment allocation. TUG is an assessment of physical mobility validated in elderly patients with high discriminative potential at early time points [46] and a predictive value for the long-term functional outcome [34, 35]. The test measures the time needed by an individual to get up from a chair (seat height 45 cm, arm height 65 cm), walk a distance of 3 m with habitual shoes and a walking aid, and sit down again [33]. The FIM [40] is an assessment of ADL that evaluates 13 motor and 5 cognitive faculties. Pain was assessed using a 0- to 10-point visual analogue scale (VAS).

The literature describes unfavourable outcomes in patients affected by frailty. The definition of frailty remains controversial [47]. Frailty often is described as a multidimensional dynamic state of increased vulnerability and loss of resistance to external stressors, resulting in an increased risk of adverse outcomes [48]. The protocol envisaged a subgroup analysis based on the MSQ scores as a surrogate marker for frailty. This was complemented by visualising treatment effects in dependence on pfFIM status, given the inverse relationship between the baseline FIM and frailty [49].

At the time of submission, the authors became aware of a publication by Arjunan et al. [50], which described a frailty index based on the FIM, medication count and comorbidities, aspects that had all been assessed during the present trial. Therefore, an additional post hoc subgroup analysis based on the described frailty index was performed. The computation of this frailty index is outlined in the Additional file 1.

The sample size calculation used the original description of the test [33] to obtain information on the distribution to be expected for the primary outcome. This resulted in a sample size of 150 patients to be included in the analysis in order to demonstrate a percentage difference in medians of 20% (corresponding to 6 s) with 80% power. Assuming a drop-out rate of 20% after experience from trials in the same patient population, an inclusion of 190 patients was planned. A recent investigation on the minimum clinical important difference (MCID) of the TUG [36] identified an MCID of 6 s when using quality of life assessed by the EQ-5D as an anchor and the minimum detectable change approach, and even smaller differences when using other anchors and approaches.

Statistical analysis

The distribution of continuous variables is described by mean/SD or selected percentiles as appropriate. The distribution of ordinal and binary variables is described by absolute and relative frequencies. The significance of differences between the groups was assessed with the Wilcoxon rank sum test for continuous and ordinal variables and with Fisher's exact test for binary variables.

The outcome "duration of TUG performance" was compared between the two treatment arms using a regression model for the log-transformed values with adjustment for pfFIM status and age, allowing us to estimate a percentage difference in medians (details are given in the Additional file 2 and Additional file 3: Figure S1). Other continuous outcomes including VAS scores were analysed with a linear regression model, such that effects (delta) correspond to mean differences. Binary outcomes were analysed with a generalised linear model with log link and binomial outcome distribution reporting effects as relative risks. The one-year mortality is presented as percentages derived from a Kaplan-Meier-estimate, but effects are described as hazard ratios based on a Cox regression model. Treatment arms were defined according to randomisation, and adjustments were performed using the same covariates as in analysing the primary endpoint. The distribution of continuous outcomes was visualised in relation to treatment arm and pre-fracture FIM status by scatter plots mimicking the adjustment for this factor in the analyses. Boxplots were used in subgroup analyses, and the distribution of ordinal outcomes was visualised by pie charts.

Patients who declined to perform the TUG were excluded from the analysis; those who could not start or failed to complete the test were included in the analysis with a value of 300 s, which lies distinctly above the maximally observed value. To increase the rate of follow-up, patients who declined follow-up at our institution were offered an assessment at their location of residence.

TUG at 3 weeks postoperation was defined as the primary outcome in the protocol, with a list of secondary outcomes like LOS, intraoperative aspects, the performance of activities of daily living (FIM), mortality, etc. We added pain, implant-related infections and the return to pre-fracture ambulatory status (with or without a walking aid) after 3 and 12 months. The protocol furthermore suggested a subgroup analysis within the patient groups defined by MSQ scores ≤7 and MSQ scores ≥8 corresponding to abnormal vs normal values, respectively [37].

All computations were performed using Stata 14.2 (StataCorp. 2015. College Station, TX: StataCorp LP). A significance level of 5% was used.

Results

Patient flow and characteristics

Over 44 months (September 1st, 2011 to April 15th, 2015), 448 patients were screened for inclusion, 258 were not eligible (see Table 2), and 190 were randomised. The primary endpoint was assessed in 146 patients (for details, see Fig. 2). Participation in follow-up visits and the availability of TUG and FIM scores are depicted in Additional file 4: Table S1. The participation rate declined over time in both arms, and 75% attended the 3-month follow-up visit. Conversely, on day 5, 20% did not perform the TUG, and later the rate of TUG performance rose to 95%. Except for day 5, when TUG was more readily performed by LAT patients, the rates were similar between the two treatment arms. FIM scores were missing in 13 patients at baseline (equally

Table 2 Reasons for non-inclusion

Exclusion Criterion	n total 258
Total hip arthroplasty	53
Joint preserving strategy	5
Additional or other fracture	33
Non-ambulatory on admission	23
Underlying malignancy or neurologic disease	22
Death before inclusion	3
Refusal of surgery	7
Intercurrent contralateral femoral fracture	12
Patients' refusal of consent to trial	37
Guardians'/proxies' refusal of consent to trial	36
Unclear IC situation (demented but no guardian or family etc.)	10
Logistics (tourists, commuters not insured in Switzerland etc.)	17

The reasons for non-inclusion mirror the heterogeneity of the patient population. While some patients are active and un-burdened by comorbidity with the indication for total hip arthroplasty as personalized treatment strategy, others are non-ambulatory on admission. Also legitimate informed consent is a sensitive topic. In unclear situations, patients had to be excluded. All other patients either gave consent or proxy consent was obtained with patients' assent. Only 12 patients suffered an intercurrent femoral fracture which may be explained by the evaluation of all patients suffering FNF by a fracture liaison service that established basic prophylaxis, diagnostics and treatment for osteoporosis [35]

distributed between the treatment arms) and 6 patients at day 5 (only from the AMIS-arm). Investigations regarding predictors for drop-out are displayed in the Additional file 5 and Additional file 6: Table S2.

Table 3 shows the baseline patient characteristics in the two study arms. The patients were on average 84.2 years old and predominantly female. It should be noted that in spite of randomisation, there was a certain imbalance between the groups. The AMIS-arm had slightly more female patients (77% vs 66%), as well as a higher level of support in the living situation (65% vs 43%), more frequent use of walking aids (63% vs 46%) and a higher rate of dementia (32% vs 20%). However, both groups were comparable with respect to BMI, MSQ score [37], pfFIM status, number of medications, Charlson Comorbidity Index [51], ASA score [52], time until surgery and laboratory parameters.

Over time, 38 different surgeons performed 179 operations. Five surgeons performed 13 or more operations, and 19 surgeons operated 2–8 times. All surgeons were board-certified but had varying levels of experience. The surgeon on duty, who was always supervised by a senior surgeon experienced in both approaches, performed the intervention.

Primary endpoint

One-hundred and twenty-six patients (86%) performed the TUG at the 3-week follow-up with a duration of TUG performance between 11 and 266 s (median 30 s, mean 46 s). Twenty patients (12 LAT, 8 AMIS) could not start or finish the test and entered the analysis with a value set to 300 s:

2 patients had too poor of a performance status to start the test;
2 patients suffered from too much pain to start the test;
2 patients could not move without assistance;
5 patients could not move to a chair;
7 patients could not stand up from a chair; and
2 patients could not walk 3 m.

The analysis of the primary outcome, i.e., the duration of TUG, was adjusted for pfFIM status and age (cf. the Additional file 2). For two patients, pfFIM status was not available, so 144 patients remained in the adjusted analysis. Additional file 7: Table S3 shows the distribution of baseline characteristics among the patients entering this analysis. Compared to Table 3, the imbalance of some characteristics – in particular pfFIM – was more pronounced in this adjusted analysis.

The distribution of the primary endpoint is visualised in Fig. 3. The percentage difference in median was estimated as a 21.5% shorter duration of TUG performance (i.e., – 21.5%) favouring the AMIS-arm with a 95% CI of

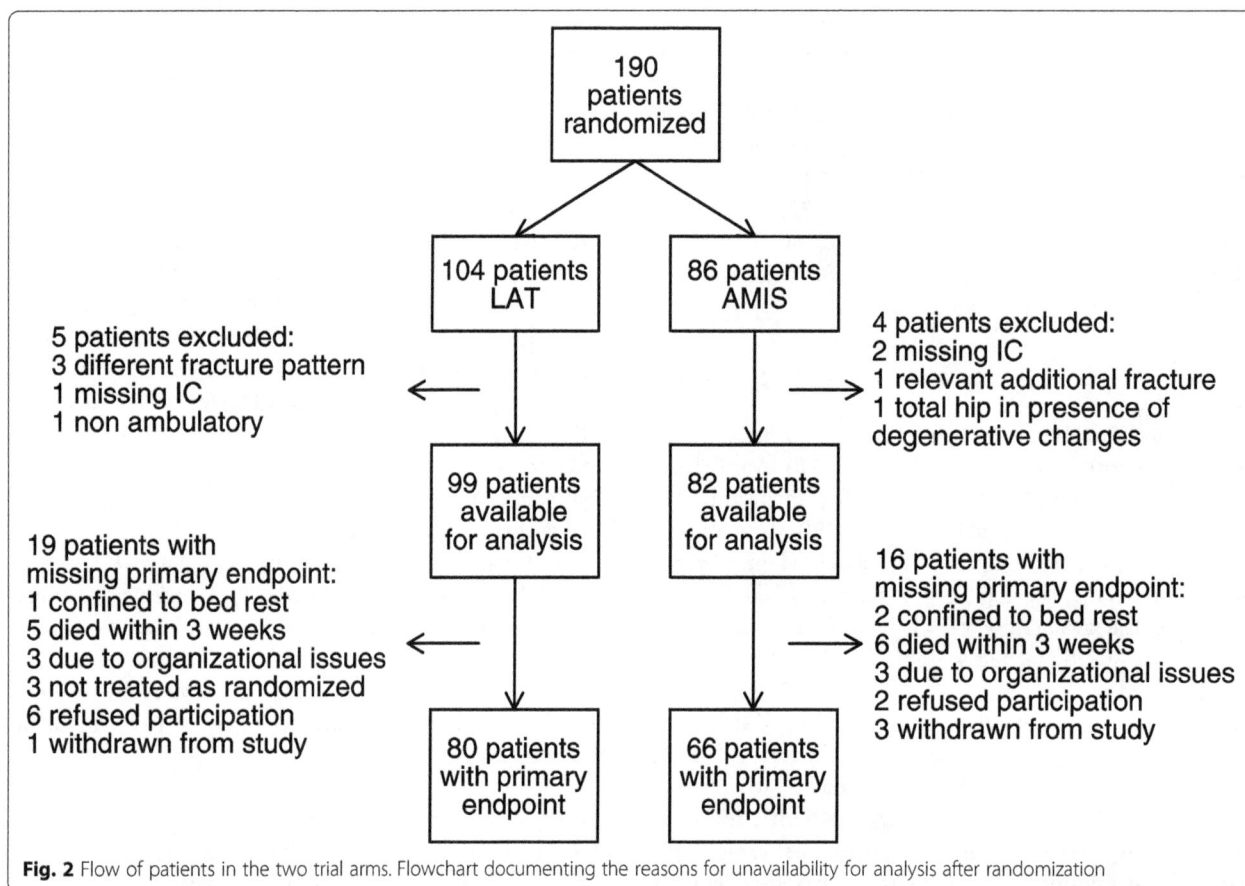

Fig. 2 Flow of patients in the two trial arms. Flowchart documenting the reasons for unavailability for analysis after randomization

[– 41.2, 4.7] and a *p*-value of 0.101. Analysing the same patients without adjustment for baseline variables resulted in a percentage difference of – 17.2% (CI [– 39.8, 14.0], *p* = 0.249). Investigations concerning the sensitivity of these results to the handling of missing values in the primary outcome and the pfFIM status are elaborated in the Additional file 8 and Additional file 9: Table S4. Figure 3 suggests a more pronounced treatment effect in patients with low pfFIM status.

Secondary outcomes

Figure 4 shows the distribution of the duration of TUG performance at all time points in relation to treatment arm and pfFIM status. The median duration was lower in the AMIS-arm at all time points, with a decreasing treatment difference over time (cf. Table 4). The advantage for patients with low pfFIM status is more pronounced at earlier time points.

Patients in the AMIS-arm had higher FIM values at almost all time points during the one-year follow-up after baseline, in particular for patients with low pfFIM status (see Additional file 10: Figure S2). The corresponding effect estimates in Table 4 suggest that the effect on the FIM was the largest at week 3 (difference in mean values 6.7 points, CI:[0.5,12.8], *p* = 0.037), but to

some degree, the effect was still present after 12 months (3.6, CI: [– 5.2,12.4], *p* = 0.427). During the first postoperative year, a substantial fraction of patients reached FIM levels comparable to their pfFIM status. This proportion at early time points was higher in the AMIS-arm, and the results were reversed at later time points (see Table 4). The complete individual trajectories for the duration of TUG performance and FIM scores are shown in Additional file 11: Figure S3.

AMIS patients suffered less pain at all time points, in particular those with low pfFIM values. The distribution of the VAS scores in relation to treatment and pfFIM status is detailed in Additional file 12: Figure S4. The corresponding effect estimates in Table 4 indicate a clinically relevant advantage, especially in the early postoperative period, when taking into account that the mean VAS score in the whole population was only 1.6 at day 5 and decreased thereafter.

The difference between AMIS and LAT with respect to other outcome variables is depicted in Table 5, indicating a lower degree of postoperative delirium, a shorter LOS, a lower need for blood transfusions, and a shorter operative time for the AMIS-arm. Infections and death were more frequent after AMIS, but SAEs during follow-up occurred less frequently. The chance of

Table 3 Baseline characteristics in the two treatment-arms

	LAT	AMIS	
Age			
N	99	82	p = 0.767
Mean (sd)	84.0 (6.6)	84.4 (6.7)	
Median (10%, 90%)	84.0 (75.0,92.0)	86.0 (74.0,92.0)	
Gender			
Male	33/99 33.3%	19/82 23.2%	p = 0.134
Female	66/99 66.7%	63/82 76.8%	
Body Mass Index			
N	94	72	p = 0.689
Mean (sd)	23.7 (4.9)	23.8 (4.8)	
Median (10%, 90%)	24.0 (18.0,29.0)	23.0 (18.0,29.0)	
Residential status			
Own home	56/98 57.1%	37/82 45.1%	p = 0.127
Own home supported	15/98 15.3%	12/82 14.6%	
Assisted living	4/98 4.1%	9/82 11.0%	
Nursing home	20/98 20.4%	23/82 28.0%	
Other	3/98 3.1%	1/82 1.2%	
Walking aid			
Yes	45/98 45.9%	51/81 63.0%	p = 0.023
Dementia			
Yes	20/98 20.4%	26/82 31.7%	p = 0.084
MSQ			
N	92	77	p = 0.312
Mean (sd)	7.9 (2.9)	7.5 (3.1)	
Median (10%, 90%)	9.0 (3.0,10.0)	9.0 (2.0,10.0)	
pfFIM			
N	93	75	p = 0.860
Mean (sd)	107.0 (26.6)	107.8 (24.5)	
Median (10%, 90%)	123.0 (63.0,126.0)	120.0 (67.0,126.0)	
Number of medications			
N	97	82	p = 0.524
Mean (sd)	6.9 (4.4)	6.5 (4.4)	
Median (10%, 90%)	6.0 (2.0,13.0)	6.0 (1.0,12.0)	
Charlson Comorbidity Score			
N	98	79	p = 0.952
Mean (sd)	2.3 (2.1)	2.3 (2.2)	
Median (10%, 90%)	2.0 (0.0,5.0)	2.0 (0.0,5.0)	
Frailty Index			
N	92	73	p = 0.739
Mean (sd)	0.18 (0.15)	0.17 (0.16)	
Median (10%, 90%)	0.12 (0.01,0.40)	0.13 (0.03,0.41)	
ASA score			
2	33/99 33.3%	23/82 28.0%	p = 0.436
3	62/99 62.6%	55/82 67.1%	
4	4/99 4.0%	4/82 4.9%	

Table 3 Baseline characteristics in the two treatment-arms *(Continued)*

	LAT	AMIS	
Time until surgery (hours)			
N	97	82	*p* = 0.943
Mean (sd)	27.4 (18.9)	25.6 (14.4)	
Median (10%, 90%)	23.0 (7.0,52.0)	24.0 (7.0,44.0)	
Haemoglobin			
N	98	82	*p* = 0.901
Mean (sd)	129.5 (16.1)	129.9 (15.7)	
Median (10%, 90%)	132.5 (109.0,149.0)	130.0 (107.0,149.0)	
Creatinine			
N	95	76	*p* = 0.596
Mean (sd)	19.8 (10.1)	19.5 (11.9)	
Median (10%, 90%)	17.0 (10.0,30.0)	17.0 (10.0,29.0)	
Albumin			
N	98	82	*p* = 0.674
Mean (sd)	33.7 (6.9)	34.0 (4.7)	
Median (10%, 90%)	35.0 (28.0,40.0)	34.0 (29.0,39.0)	
CRP			
N	98	82	*p* = 0.512
Mean (sd)	15.7 (29.7)	17.9 (27.1)	
Median (10%, 90%)	4.0 (1.0,58.0)	6.0 (0.0,49.0)	
Leukocytes			
N	98	82	*p* = 0.997
Mean (sd)	10.3 (3.7)	10.2 (3.6)	
Median (10%, 90%)	10.0 (6.0,15.0)	10.0 (6.0,15.0)	

Basic patient characteristics, although the groups are comparable there is a higher degree of frailty associated factors apparent in the AMIS- arm with a higher level of support (65% vs 43%), a more frequent use of walking aids (63% vs 46%) and a higher rate of diagnosed dementia (32% vs 20%)

returning to "No walking aid" was similar in both arms. The one-year mortality was 20% in the LAT-arm and 28% in the AMIS-arm (adj. HR 1.64, CI: [0.84,3.21], *p* = 0.149). Five patients died following implant-related infections, 3 of these from the LAT and 2 from the AMIS-arm, and all cases followed the patients' wishes for best supportive care.

In the LAT-arm, 5 patients showed wound healing problems, and 46 had documented significant postoperative haematoma. Five patients in the LAT-arm developed an implant-related infection. Seven patients from the AMIS-arm had implant-related infections. All of these cases were associated with soft tissue complications like haematoma or wound healing disturbance. In the AMIS-arm, no other patients with soft tissue complications were noted. All infections were diagnosed during the first 6 postoperative weeks. Treatment followed standard practice [53]. Severe complications during hospitalisation were more frequent in the AMIS-arm, but considering complications related to surgery, no difference was

observed, with 35% of LAT and 39% of AMIS patients suffering no surgery-related complications. Low-grade complications treatable with common medications, like antiemetics, analgesics, etc., were experienced by 52% and 47% of patients, respectively. Six percent of patients from each group needed transfusions or antibiotics, while 7% from the LAT-arm and 8% from the AMIS-arm needed surgical treatment for surgery-associated complications, mainly infection. Overall complications were similarly distributed between the groups (see Additional file 13: Figure S5 for details).

None of the differences in secondary outcomes reached significance, even after adjusting for baseline differences in age or pfFIM status.

Subgroup analyses

Figure 5 visualises the distribution of the variable "duration of TUG performance" by treatment arm after stratification by MSQ score. There were distinct differences favouring AMIS in patients with MSQ scores ≤7 (covering

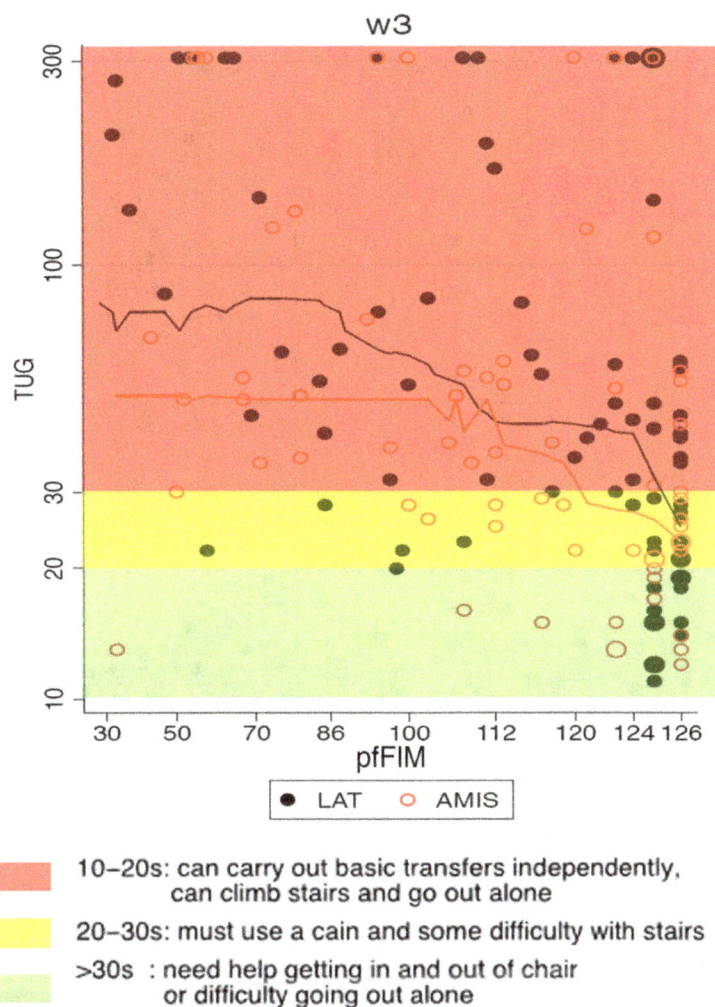

Fig. 3 The distribution of duration of TUG performance (DTP) at the 3 weeks follow up visit in relation to treatment arm and pfFIM. Visualisation of the duration of TUG performance in the context of its clinical relevance. The green background signifies independence, while the yellow and red imply an increasing degree of dependence for mobilisation (yellow) and basic activities of daily living (red)

26% of the population). However, there was nearly no difference in patients with MSQ scores ≥8, which was similar to the more pronounced effect in low-performing patients according to the pfFIM status observed above. Indeed, pfFIM status and MSQ score were highly correlated ($r = 0.72$). When using the frailty index of Arjunana et al. and a cut-off point of 0.25, the highly frail group included 26% of all patients, and we observed a similar pattern (Fig. 5). The frailty index was negatively correlated with pfFIM ($r = -0.90$) and MSQ ($r = -0.63$).

Discussion

The data presented here support the conclusion that the muscle-sparing AMIS approach to the hip joint for HA can be beneficial for an early return to function and performance in ADLs, especially in potentially frail elderly patients, even if statistical superiority cannot be demonstrated. This corresponds to the results after

THA, both considering the perceived benefit as well as the persistent lack of scientific evidence [22–27]. The dominance of differences at early time points between AMIS and traditional approaches might have a more significant impact in elderly patients with potentially reduced physical reserve because, unlike after THA, differences persisted over the first postoperative year in the population in our dataset. Renken et al. [31] reported similar results after HA for FNFs in 60 randomised elderly patients with better mobility and functioning in ADL at early time points after an AMIS approach compared to a Watson Jones approach, while other authors did not find differences [54–56] and concluded that there is an influence of surgeon proficiency, rather than the actual approach [55].

We observed a persistent influence of the treatment on function and ADL. This effect decreased over time, but this may be due to ceiling/floor effects, as many

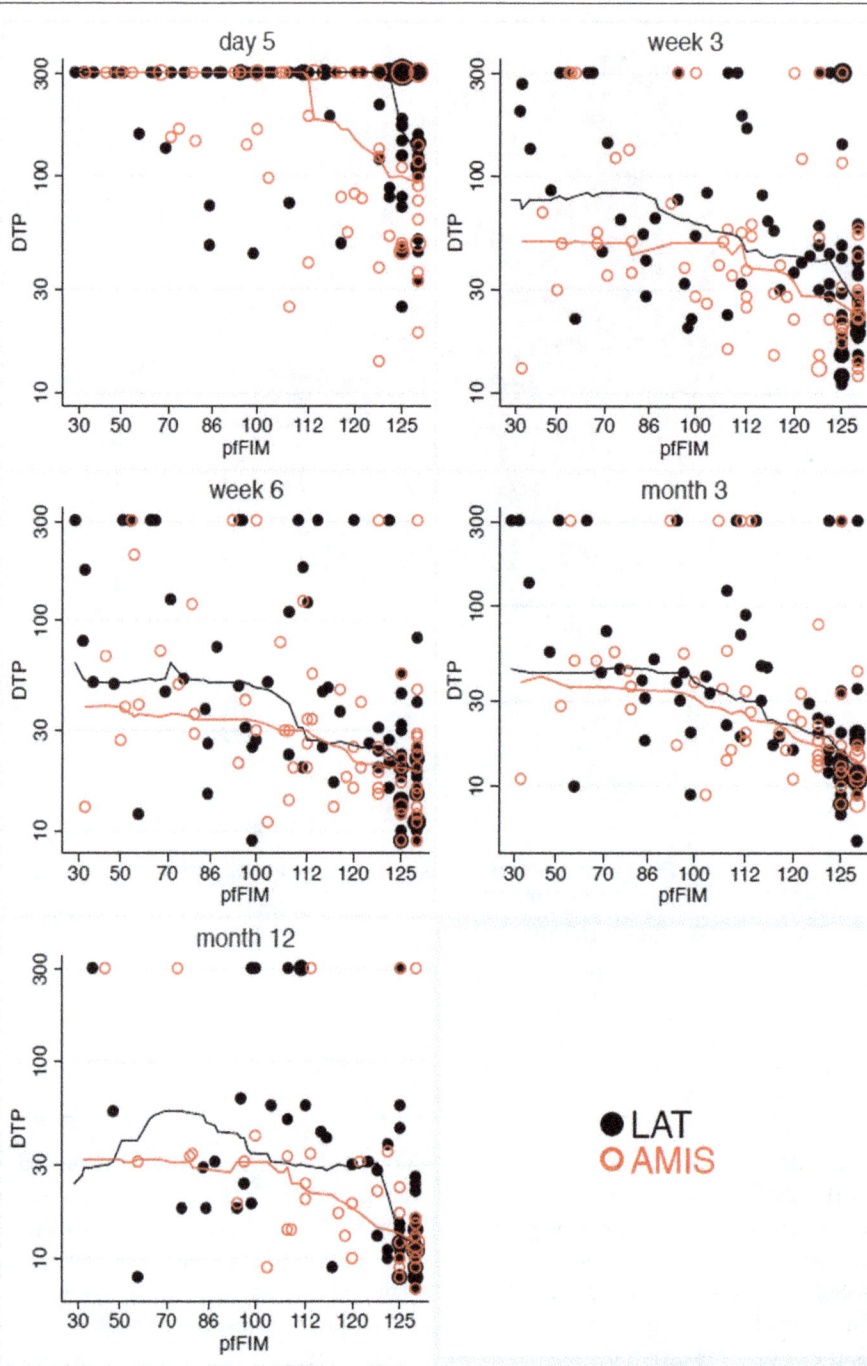

Fig. 4 Distribution of duration of TUG performance (DTP) at day 5 and at all follow up visits in relation to treatment and pfFIM. Individual values for patients' TUG performance in relation to their pfFIM and treatment. The running median curves are based on the next 25 neighbours on both sides of an observation and illustrate larger differences in patients with lower pfFIM. Note that the y-axis uses a logarithmic scale

patients reach normal values for TUG performance or FIM scores. It might be assumed that the rather early occurrence and – in our dataset – persistence of outcome differences was related to the impact of hardly reversible perioperative deconditioning due to persistent pain or immobilisation, which has been associated with the traditional approaches. This tendency could also be

an explanation for the more pronounced benefit of AMIS in patients with a higher risk of frailty, i.e. more frailty associated characteristics and potentially less reserve, to compensate for postoperative muscular hypotrophy.

This association points towards a methodological dilemma and might explain the current lack of high-level

Table 4 Treatment effects on duration of TUG performance (DTP), FIM and pain over time

	LAT	AMIS	effect	95% CI	p-value
	n	n			
DTP					
Day 5	83	62	−24.4	[−40.4, −4.2]	0.022
Week 3	79	65	−21.5	[−41.2, 4.7]	0.101
Week 6	80	63	−16.4	[−36.9, 10.8]	0.216
Month 3	75	58	−10.1	[−34.9, 24.2]	0.520
Month 12	55	42	−10.3	[−40.3, 34.9]	0.604
FIM					
Day 5	93	75	3.9	[−1.8, 9.7]	0.181
Week 3	89	72	6.7	[0.5, 12.8]	0.037
Week 6	84	66	5.5	[−1.1, 12.2]	0.106
Month 3	77	60	3.6	[−4.1, 11.4]	0.361
Month 12	59	47	3.6	[−5.2, 12.4]	0.427
VAS					
Day 5	68	51	−0.8	[−1.5,−0.1]	0.026
Week 3	86	70	−0.7	[−1.4,0.0]	0.064
Week 6	81	63	−0.2	[−0.8,0.3]	0.433
Month 3	76	59	−0.4	[−0.8,0.0]	0.075
Month 12	59	47	−0.0	[−0.5,0.4]	0.935
Back to pfFIM-level:					
Day 5	93	75	1.1	2.7	0.587
Week 3	89	72	4.5	6.9	0.515
Week 6	84	66	7.1	16.7	0.076
Month 3	77	60	33.8	26.7	0.456
Month 12	59	47	49.2	38.3	0.326

Treatment effects during the first postoperative year
Upper three panels: Effect-estimates with 95% confidence intervals and p-values for the outcomes DTP, FIM and pain at each time point. The effect for DTP is expressed as the percentage difference in median. The effect for FIM is the difference in the mean change from baseline. The effect for pain is the difference in mean VAS score. The effects refer to the difference AMIS minus LAT
Lower panel: Percentage of patients with FIM-values equal or above their pre-fracture values

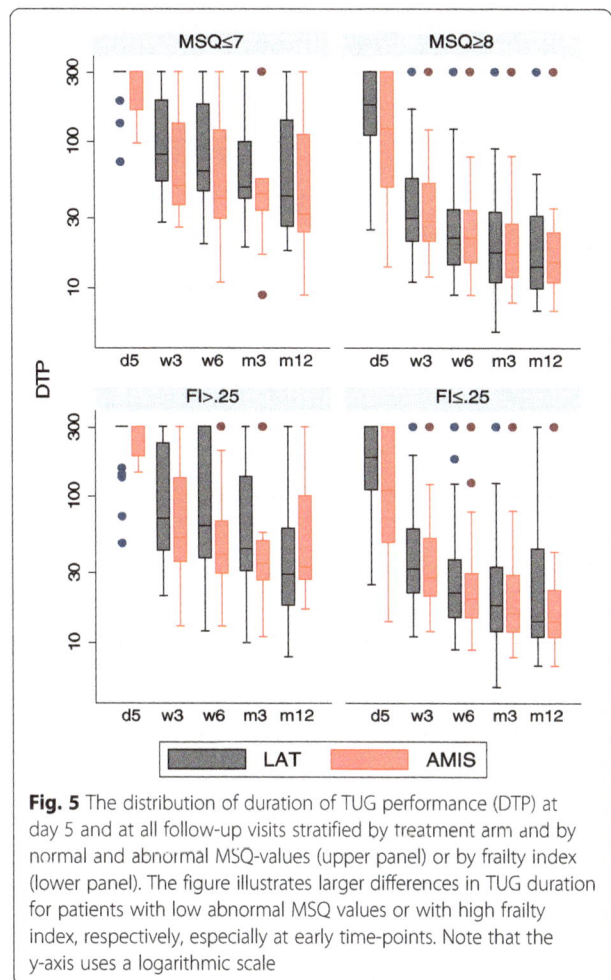

Fig. 5 The distribution of duration of TUG performance (DTP) at day 5 and at all follow-up visits stratified by treatment arm and by normal and abnormal MSQ-values (upper panel) or by frailty index (lower panel). The figure illustrates larger differences in TUG duration for patients with low abnormal MSQ values or with high frailty index, respectively, especially at early time-points. Note that the y-axis uses a logarithmic scale

evidence for the superiority of minimally invasive surgery in the treatment of FNFs. There are few recently published RCTs analysing the benefit of minimally invasive surgery in patients with FNFs [31, 54–57]. The analysed patient populations tend to be relatively small, and most trials exclude cognitively impaired patients, who make up a large proportion of the affected elderly population. The heterogeneity of the population in principle complicates the generation of valid generalisable data.

In addition, the aspects of old age and cognitive impairment present a conceptual difficulty in RCTs. Cognitively impaired patients or patients diagnosed with dementia are typically excluded from interventional trials given the complexity of legitimate inclusion as well as the potential difficulty of meaningful data acquisition [58–60]. In our institution, approximately one-third of patients presenting with an FNF suffer from dementia. The rate of more subtle cognitive impairment is significantly higher. In these patients, an early return to their previous residential status and function is especially important [61]. Our data show a strong correlation between surrogate markers for frailty like FIM and MSQ as measure of cognitive impairment. There is also a marked correlation with the calculated frailty index comprising FIM, medication and comorbidities that has been reported as predictor of mortality, 30-day residence and length of inpatient stay. All of these measures predicted a benefit of AMIS over LAT as an approach for HA, which was specifically pronounced in patients with MSQ scores ≤7, i.e., in the presence of cognitive impairment.

In a literature review on minimally invasive THA, Jung et al. [62] reported consistently lower levels of pain and use of analgesics. The same effect has been documented after HA for FNFs in retrospective and prospective analyses [30, 31, 63], and this effect was also present in our

Table 5 Differences in secondary outcomes between the two treatment groups

	LAT	AMIS	LAT	AMIS	Effect	p	Adjusted Effect	p
	n	n	Mean	Mean	Delta		Delta	
Postoperative delirium	89	77	0.94	0.87	−0.07	0.667	−0.12	0.468
LOS	96	78	11.39	10.97	−0.41	0.630	−0.70	0.393
Operative time	97	82	100.1	96.3	−3.8	0.419	−5.3	0.253
Erythrocyte concentrates within 72 h	97	82	0.73	0.50	−0.23	0.174	−0.31	0.078
			%	%	RR		RR	
Implant related infections	96	79	5.2	8.9	1.70	0.347	1.81	0.281
SAE during follow up	90	73	30.0	26.0	0.87	0.577	0.90	0.682
Return to no WA at 3 months	45	23	28.9	26.1	0.90	0.809	0.80	0.578
Return to no WA at 12 months	34	17	61.8	64.7	1.05	0.836	0.94	0.829
			%dead	%dead	HR		HR	
1 year mortality	99	82	20.2	28.0	1.46	0.205	1.64	0.149

The results are more favorable in the LAT arm for the avoidance of implant related infections and the one-year mortality. There is also an advantage for return to no walking aids at three months. The AMIS arm, on the other hand was more favorable for all the other aspects analyzed. However, none of the differences reached statistical significance. Adjustment was performed for pfFIM and age
WA Walking aid, *SAE* serious adverse event or surgery related complication

data set, with patients in the AMIS-arm on average suffering lower levels of pain. However, the effect did not reach significance, unlike in previous studies [31, 63], and must be interpreted with caution since the agreement between formal ratings and verbal expressions of pain or discomfort seems to decrease with advancing age [64], and the reliability with cognitive impairment might be additionally limited.

Another aspect reported as an advantage after minimally invasive surgery is lower blood loss. We documented intraoperative blood loss as well as haemoglobin levels at different postoperative time points. We found, however, that these parameters were not reliable (or consistent) in our data set due to lack of standardised documentation of the intraoperative blood loss and individualised fluid management, as reported by other authors [31]. As a surrogate marker, the need for transfusion was evaluated, which is handled uniformly at our institution. We observed a higher need for transfusion within the first 72 h for patients treated with LAT compared to patients after AMIS as reported after HA via the AMIS approach. This is an important aspect in a comorbid patient population, since patients are not only at high risk of fluid overload and cardiac complications as a consequence of blood transfusion but also at a high risk of complications from anaemia such as delirium, fatigue and prolonged immobilisation. The above-mentioned RCTs on the subject report conflicting results in this aspect.

We should finally note that we observed a non-significant increase in mortality under AMIS, corresponding to 8 more deaths in 100 patients, without being able to give a clear explanation for the result. Further investigations in larger populations are necessary to clarify the question of a true difference in mortality.

Strengths and limitations

The strength of the current trial is its RCT design with a relatively high number of patients, including patients with cognitive deficits, which reduces the potential for selection bias. The early assessment of TUG as a functional parameter for the primary outcome makes the current results predictive for performance in ADLs and for preservation of independence [34, 35], which are highly patient-relevant endpoints. However, we did not include instruments sensitive enough to catch such long-term differences. An additional strength is the large number of participating surgeons and their allocation by independent administrative procedures, resulting in a highly balanced allocation and avoiding a bias in treatment effect estimation due to experience-based selection of surgeons. A uniform level of surgical quality could be ascertained by the presence of a senior expert.

We included in the analysis of the primary outcome 144 patients, nearly reaching the intended sample size of 150 as planned by the power analysis. We also observed a difference in median duration of TUG performance of 6 s (LAT: 41 s, AMIS: 35 s), corresponding to the assumed effect in the sample size calculation and hitting the MCID reported for the TUG [36]. The failure to reach significance may be due to our decision to include in the analysis patients who failed to perform the TUG successfully with a duration of 300 s, which is in contrast to other studies ignoring these patients. In this way, we reduced the potential for bias, but we also increased the variability and hence reduced the power. Indeed, exclusion of these patients leads to a smaller treatment effect estimate of − 16.8%, with a smaller p-value of 0.089.

The current trial is limited by the high rate of screening failures, which is typical in prospective RCTs in elderly patients [59]. Furthermore, a certain loss to follow-up and failure to perform the TUG is problematic. However, sensitivity analyses suggest that the main findings are robust against different ways of handling missing values. The patient numbers in the two treatment arms show a distinct – but insignificant – difference, reflecting the lack of block randomisation. We also have to note that the FIM is constructed as an observational tool for nursing home staff with close contact to patients, but it was used in our trial by study nurses relying on patient or proxy narratives. We did not perform a specific assessment of the pre-fracture frailty in this trial, and hence we were forced to use surrogate measures to investigate a dependence of the treatment effect on frailty.

Conclusion

FNFs in elderly patients are frequent, and given demographic developments, their socio-economic impact will increase in coming decades. Every step contributing to a better outcome in these patients is beneficial for the individual patient and for society. In this regard, the present trial – despite failing to reach a significant difference in the primary outcome – adds to a growing body of evidence. These results support the implementation of a specifically designed treatment regimen for fragility fractures, taking into account the complexity of the heterogeneous patient population known as "the elderly".

Additional files

Additional file 1: Definition of Frailty Index. Description of the approach for the quantification of frailty.

Additional file 2: Statistical approach for analysing the primary outcome. Description of the analytical approach for the statistical analysis of the primary outcome with display of the primary outcome with and without a logarithmic transformation in Additional file 3: Figure S1.

Additional file 3: Figure S1. The distribution of the duration of TUG performance (DTP) at 3 weeks in the two treatment arms with and without a logarithmic transformation. Comparing the upper and lower part, we can observe that the logarithmic transformation implies a less skewed distribution of the primary outcome in both arms of the study.

Additional file 4: Table S1. Participation rates at follow-up visits and percentages of patients performing TUG or having assessed FIM, respectively. The percentages refer to the number of patients attending the visit.

Additional file 5: Predictors for drop out. Description of the analytic strategy for the evaluation of the potential influence of patient characteristics on the availability of outcome parameters with display of the results in Additional file 6: Table S2.

Additional file 6: Table S2. Association of patient characteristics and availability of the primary outcome. Association of patient characteristics and previous measurements with non-attendance at follow-up visits, non-availability of DTP or non-performance of TUG when attending. The observed ORs in each treatment arm, the p-value of an overall effect of the variable (p1), and the p-value of a test for equality across the two arms (p2) are given. For continuous variables, the OR refers to changing this variable by one standard deviation.

Additional file 7: Table S3. Distribution of baseline characteristics in the two treatment groups among patients entering the analysis of the primary endpoint. The table illustrates larger differences in baseline characteristics for patients with complete data for the analysis of the primary outcome compared to Table 3 showing the baseline characteristics of all patients.

Additional file 8: Sensitivity analyses. Description of the analytic strategy for the evaluation of the potential influence of different ways to handle missing values on the effect estimates with display of the results in Additional file 9: Table S4.

Additional file 9: Table S4. Variation of treatment effect estimates, confidence intervals and p-values for the outcomes DTP and FIM at 3 weeks and at day 5 across six different approaches to handle missing values.

Additional file 10: Figure S2. Distribution of FIM at all time-points in relation to treatment and prefecture FIM (prFIM). The lines refer to running medians based on the next 25 neighbours on both sides of an observation. The area of each point is proportional to the number of observations with the specific combination of FIM and prFIM value. With increasing time postoperative an increasing number of patients can reach their pre-fracture level of independence. The advantage of AMIS in comparison to FIM is more pronounced in patients with low prefracture FIM values.

Additional file 11: Figure S3. The individual trajectories of DTP and FIM for all patients. With respect to DTP the typical pattern is a continuous improvement over time. However, in both arms a few patients experience a sudden deterioration. With respect to FIM the typical pattern is a distinct deterioration due to the fracture/surgery and a continuous improvement afterwards. However, in both treatment arms some patients get stuck in the recovering process.

Additional file 12: Figure S4. Distribution of the VAS pain scores at all time-points in relation to treatment and pre-fracture FIM status (prFIM). The lines refer to running means based on the next 25 neighbours on both sides of an observation. The area of each point is proportional to the number of observations with the specific combination of VAS and prFIM value. We observe higher mean VAS values in the LAT arm compared to the AMIS arm in partucular for patients with low pre-fractureFIM values at week 3, week6 and month 3.

Additional file 13: Figure S5. Distribution of in-hospital complications according to the Clavien-Dindo classification. In this context, only in-hospital complications are presented as the rate of later complications was low and might reflect an underreporting especially of infections treated by the GP in this patient population.

Abbreviations

ADL: Activities of daily living; AMIS: Anterior minimally invasive surgery; BMI: Body mass index; CAM: Confusion Assessment Method; DOS: Delirium Observation Screening scale; FI: Frailty index; FIM: Functional independence measure; FNF: Femoral neck fracture; HA: Hemiarthroplasty; LAT: Lateral transgluteal Hardinge approach; LOS: Length of (hospital) stay; MSQ: Mental status questionnaire; pfFIM: Pre-fracture functional independence measure; RCT: Randomised controlled trial; SAE: Serious adverse events; THA: Total hip arthroplasty; TUG: "Timed up and go"-test; VAS: Visual analogue scale

Acknowledgements

We thank Anna Padiyath, Evelyn Kungler, Bojana Savic and Ilona Ahlborn for being a dedicated study team. We furthermore thank all consultants of the Department of Orthopaedics and Traumatology for bearing the burden of additional tasks during the conduct of the trial.

Funding

The study was financed by internal research means of the Department of Orthopaedics and Traumatology. No external funding has been received.

Authors' contributions

FS, PS, MJ, NS and NB conceptually designed the trial. RR and SDK were responsible for the statistical design of the trial as well as the methodologic aspects. The data acquisition was mainly performed by PS, supported by FS. WV had a main part in analysing the data set, while FS, PS, MJ, NS and NB interpreted the results. The manuscript was drafted by FS, WV, PS, and NB with critical revision by MJ, NS, RR and SDK. All authors have approved the submitted version of the manuscript and agree to be accountable for all aspects of the work in ensuring that questions related to the accuracy or integrity of any part of the work are appropriately investigated and resolved. We confirm that this work is original and has not been published elsewhere, nor is it currently under consideration for publication elsewhere.

Ethics approval and consent to participate

The trial was approved by the ethics committee (Ethikkommission beider Basel, EKBB Reference No. 68/11). Since 2014 the ethics committee incorporates several cantons under the name Ethikkommission Nordweistschweiz (EKNZ). The trial followed good clinical practice (GCP) as well as the tenets of the Declaration of Helsinki. Key personnel had appropriate training in GCP.

Eligible patients entered the informed consent process. Depending on their cognitive abilities (quantified using a mental status questionnaire), they were individually, or in the presence of a designated proxy, informed about the diagnosis, the proposed treatment and the randomised trial. Patients were only included by the surgeon on call if they consented in writing or – in the case of cognitive impairment – gave their verbal assent with written consent by a designated proxy according to the Swiss civil code (Art. 378) or a legal guardian.

Competing interests

Rachel Rosenthal has been an employee of F. Hoffmann-La Roche Ltd. since May 01, 2014. The present study was designed before Rachel Rosenthal joined F. Hoffmann-La Roche Ltd. and has no connection to her employment by the company. Rachel Rosenthal continues to be affiliated with the University of Basel. The other authors have no conflict of interest to declare.

Author details

[1]Department of Orthopaedics and Traumatology, University Hospital Basel, Spitalstrasse 21, 4031 Basel, Switzerland. [2]Basel Institute for Clinical Epidemiology and Biostatistics, University Hospital Basel, Spitalstrasse 12, 4031 Basel, Switzerland. [3]Faculty of Medicine, University of Basel, Klingelbergstr. 61, 4056 Basel, Switzerland. [4]Clinic for Orthopaedics and Trauma Surgery Stephanshorn, Brauerstrasse 95, 9016 St. Gallen, Switzerland. [5]Department of Department of Anaesthesiology, Surgical Intensive Care, Prehospital Emergency Medicine and Pain Therapy, University Hospital Basel, Spitalstrasse 21, 4031 Basel, Switzerland.

References

1. Hannan EL, Magaziner J, Wang JJ, et al. Mortality and locomotion 6 months after hospitalization for hip fracture: risk factors and risk-adjusted hospital outcomes. JAMA. 2001;285(21):2736–42. https://doi.org/10.1001/jama.285.21.2736.
2. Leibson CL, Tosteson ANA, Gabriel SE, Ransom JE, Melton LJ. Mortality, disability, and nursing home use for persons with and without hip fracture: a population-based study. J Am Geriatr Soc. 2002;50(10):1644–50. https://doi.org/10.1046/j.1532-5415.2002.50455.x.
3. Benetos IS, Babis GC, Zoubos AB, Benetou V, Soucacos PN. Factors affecting the risk of hip fractures. Injury. 2007;38(7):735–44. https://doi.org/10.1016/j.injury.2007.01.001.
4. Michel JP, Hoffmeyer P, Klopfenstein C, Bruchez M, Grab B, d'Epinay CL. Prognosis of functional recovery 1 year after hip fracture: typical patient profiles through cluster analysis. J Gerontol A Biol Sci Med Sci. 2000;55(9):M508–15. https://doi.org/10.1093/gerona/55.9.M508.
5. Eastwood EA, Magaziner J, Wang J, et al. Patients with hip fracture: subgroups and their outcomes. J Am Geriatr Soc. 2002;50(7):1240–9. https://doi.org/10.1046/j.1532-5415.2002.50311.x.
6. Penrod JD, Litke A, Hawkes WG, et al. Heterogeneity in hip fracture patients: age, functional status, and comorbidity. J Am Geriatr Soc. 2007;55(3):407–13. https://doi.org/10.1111/j.1532-5415.2007.01078.x.
7. Florschutz AV, Langford JR, Haidukewych GJ, Koval KJ. Femoral neck fractures: current management. J Orthop Trauma. 2015;29(3):121–9. https://doi.org/10.1097/BOT.0000000000000291.
8. Miyamoto RG, Kaplan KM, Levine BR, Egol KA, Zuckerman JD. Surgical Management of Hip Fractures I: An Evidence-based Review of Neck Fractures. J Am Acad Orthop Surg. 2008;16(10):596–607.
9. Rogmark C, Johnell O. Primary arthroplasty is better than internal fixation of displaced femoral neck fractures: a meta-analysis of 14 randomized studies with 2,289 patients. Acta Orthop. 2006;77(3):359–67. https://doi.org/10.1080/17453670610046262.
10. Rogmark C, Flensburg L, Fredin H. Undisplaced femoral neck fractures-no problems? A consecutive study of 224 patients treated with internal fixation. Injury. 2009;40(3):274–6. https://doi.org/10.1016/j.injury.2008.05.023.
11. Rogmark C, Leonardsson O. Hip arthroplasty for the treatment of displaced fractures of the femoral neck in elderly patients. Bone Joint J. 2016;98-B(3):291–7. https://doi.org/10.1302/0301-620X.98B3.36515.
12. Parker MJ, Pryor G, Gurusamy K. Hemiarthroplasty versus internal fixation for displaced intracapsular hip fractures: a long-term follow-up of a randomised trial. Injury. 2010;41(4):370–3. https://doi.org/10.1016/j.injury.2009.10.003.
13. Parker M, Selvan K, Azegami S. Arthroplasties with and without bone cement for proximal femoral fractures in adults. Cochrane Database Syst Rev. 2010;6:13–8. https://doi.org/10.1002/14651858.CD001706.pub4.www.cochranelibrary.com.
14. Ye CY, Liu A, Xu MY, Nonso NS, He RX. Arthroplasty versus Internal Fixation for Displaced Intracapsular Femoral Neck Fracture in the Elderly : Systematic Review and Meta - analysis of Short - and Long - term Effectiveness. 2016; 129(21) https://doi.org/10.4103/0366-6999.192788.
15. Gjertsen J-E, Vinje T, Lie SA, et al. Patient satisfaction, pain, and quality of life 4 months after displaced femoral neck fractures: a comparison of 663 fractures treated with internal fixation and 906 with bipolar hemiarthroplasty reported to the Norwegian hip fracture register. Acta Orthop. 2008;79(5):594–601. https://doi.org/10.1080/17453670810016597.
16. Howard JL, Lanting BL. Surgical approach in primary total hip arthroplasty: anatomy, technique and clinical outcomes 2015;58:128–139. doi:https://doi.org/10.1503/cjs.007214.
17. Hardinge K. The direct lateral approach for small incision total hip replacement. J Bone Jt Surg. 1982;64(1):17–9. https://doi.org/10.1053/j.sart.2004.08.005.
18. Matta JM, Shahrdar C, Ferguson T. Single-incision anterior approach for total hip arthroplasty on an orthopaedic table. Clin Orthop Relat Res. 2005;441:115–24. https://doi.org/10.1097/01.blo.0000194309.70518.cb.
19. Laude F, Moreau PVP. Arthroplastie totale de hanche par voie antérieure de Hueter mini-invasive. Maîtrise Orthop. 2008;178. https://www.docvadis.fr/files/all/2iJ5zwHEgLFBjQiPJvm2wg/la_voie_d_abord_mini_invasive_anterieure_pour_les_proth_ses_totales_de_hanche_voie_anterieure_pth.pdf.
20. Paillard P. Hip replacement by a minimal anterior approach. 2007;31:13–5. https://doi.org/10.1007/s00264-007-0433-7.
21. Moerenhout KG, Cherix S, Rüdiger HA. Prothèse totale de la hanche. Rev Med Suisse. 2012;8(367):2429–32.

22. Goebel S, Steinert AF, Schillinger J, et al. Reduced postoperative pain in total hip arthroplasty after minimal-invasive anterior approach. Int Orthop. 2012;36(3):491–8. https://doi.org/10.1007/s00264-011-1280-0.

23. Ilchmann T, Gersbach S, Zwicky L, Clauss M. Standard transgluteal versus minimal invasive anterior approach in hip arthroplasty: a prospective, consecutive cohort study. Orthop Rev (Pavia). 2013;5(4):31. https://doi.org/10.4081/or.2013.e31.

24. Mayr E, Nogler M, Benedetti MG, et al. A prospective randomized assessment of earlier functional recovery in THA patients treated by minimally invasive direct anterior approach: a gait analysis study. Clin Biomech. 2009;24(10):812–8. https://doi.org/10.1016/j.clinbiomech.2009.07.010.

25. Miller LE, Gondusky JS, Bhattacharyya S, Kamath AF, Boettner F, Wright J. Does surgical approach affect outcomes in Total hip Arthroplasty through 90 days of follow-up? A systematic review with Meta-analysis. J Arthroplast. 2017; https://doi.org/10.1016/j.arth.2017.11.011.

26. Konan S, Das R, Volpin A, Haddad FS. The direct anterior approach in total hip arthroplasty a systematic review of the literature:732–40. https://doi.org/10.1302/0301-620X.99B6.38053.

27. Jolles B, Bogoch E. Posterior versus lateral surgical approach for total hip arthroplasty in adults with osteoarthritis. Cochrane Database Syst Rev. 2003;(3) https://doi.org/10.1002/14651858.CD003828.pub2.

28. Butler M, Forte ML, Joglekar SB, Swiontkowski MF, Kane RL. Evidence summary: systematic review of surgical treatments for geriatric hip fractures. J Bone Joint Surg Am. 2011;93(12):1104–15. https://doi.org/10.2106/JBJSJ.00296.

29. Schneider K, Audigé L, Kuehnel SP, Helmy N. The direct anterior approach in hemiarthroplasty for displaced femoral neck fractures. Int Orthop. 2012;36(9):1773–81. https://doi.org/10.1007/s00264-012-1535-4.

30. Unger AC, Dirksen B, Renken FG, Wilde E, Willkomm M, Schulz AP. Treatment of femoral neck fracture with a minimal invasive surgical approach for hemiarthroplasty - clinical and radiological results in 180 geriatric patients. Open Orthop J. 2014;8:225–31. https://doi.org/10.2174/1874325001408010225.

31. Renken F, Renken S, Paech A, Wenzl M, Unger A, Schulz AP. Early functional results after hemiarthroplasty for femoral neck fracture: a randomized comparison between a minimal invasive and a conventional approach. BMC Musculoskelet Disord. 2012;13:141. https://doi.org/10.1186/1471-2474-13-141.

32. Parker MJ, Pervez H. Surgical approaches for inserting hemiarthroplasty of the hip. Cochrane Database Syst Rev. 2002;(3) https://doi.org/10.1002/14651858.CD001707.

33. Podsiadlo D, Richardson S. The timed "Up & Go": a test of basic functional mobility for frail elderly persons. J Am Geriatr Soc. 1991;39(2):142–8. http://www.ncbi.nlm.nih.gov/entrez/query.fcgi?cmd=Retrieve&db=PubMed&dopt=Citation&list_uids=1991946.

34. Rouleau DM. The timed up and go test is an early predictor of functional outcome after Hemiarthroplasty for femoral neck fracture. J Bone Jt Surg. 2012;94(13):1175. https://doi.org/10.2106/JBJSJ.01952.

35. Ingemarsson AH, Frändin K, Mellström D, Möller M. Walking ability and activity level after hip fracture in the elderly--a follow-up. J Rehabil Med. 2003;35(2):76–83. https://doi.org/10.1080/16501970306113.

36. Gautschi OP, Stienen MN, Corniola MV, et al. Assessment of the minimum clinically important difference in the timed up and go test after surgery for lumbar degenerative disc disease. Neurosurgery. 2016;80(3):380–5. https://doi.org/10.1227/NEU.0000000000001320.

37. Kahn RL, GOLDFARB AI, Pollack M, Peck A. Brief objective measures for the determination of mental status in the aged. Am J Psychiatry. 1960;117:326–8. https://doi.org/10.1176/ajp.117.4.326.

38. Charlson ME, Pompei P, Ales KL, MacKenzie CR. A new method of classifying prognostic comorbidity in longitudinal studies: development and validation. J Chronic Dis. 1987;40(5):373–83. https://doi.org/10.1016/0021-9681(87)90171-8.

39. Dripps RD. New classification of physical status. Anesthesiology. 1963;24(1):111. https://doi.org/10.1007/SpringerReference_222279.

40. Brautigam K, Flemming A, Schulz H, Dassen T. How reliable is the functional independence measure (FIM)? [German]. Pflege. 2002;15(3):131–6.

41. Suhm N, Kaelin R, Studer P, et al. Orthogeriatric care pathway: a prospective survey of impact on length of stay, mortality and institutionalisation. Arch Orthop Trauma Surg. 2014;134(9):1261–9. https://doi.org/10.1007/s00402-014-2057-x.

42. Schuurmans MJ, Shortridge-Baggett LM, Duursma SA. The delirium observation screening scale: a screening instrument for delirium. Res Theory Nurs Pract. 2003;17(1):31–50. https://doi.org/10.1891/rtnp.17.1.31.53169.

43. Inouye SK, Van Dyck CH, Alessi CA, Balkin S, Siegal AP, Horwitz RI. Clarifying confusion: the confusion assessment method: a new method for detection of delirium. Ann Intern Med. 1990;113(12):941–8. https://doi.org/10.7326/0003-4819-113-12-941.

44. Dindo D, Demartines N, Clavien P-A. Classification of surgical complications: a new proposal with evaluation in a cohort of 6336 patients and results of a survey. Ann Surg. 2004;240(2):205–13. https://doi.org/10.1097/01.sla.0000133083.54934.ae.

45. Yeung TSM, Wessel J, Stratford PW, MacDermid JC. The timed up and go test for use on an inpatient orthopaedic rehabilitation ward. J Orthop Sports Phys Ther. 2008;38(7):410–7. https://doi.org/10.2519/jospt.2008.2657.

46. Kennedy DM, Stratford PW, Hanna SE, Wessel J, Gollish JD. Modeling early recovery of physical function following hip and knee arthroplasty. BMC Musculoskelet Disord. 2006;7:100. https://doi.org/10.1186/1471-2474-7-100.

47. Junius-walker U, Onder G, Soleymani D, et al. European Journal of Internal Medicine The essence of frailty : A systematic review and qualitative synthesis on frailty concepts and de fi nitions. 2018:1–8. https://doi.org/10.1016/j.ejim.2018.04.023.

48. Conroy S, Elliott A. The frailty syndrome. Med (United Kingdom). 2017;45(1):15–8. https://doi.org/10.1016/j.mpmed.2016.10.010.

49. Kawryshanker S, Raymond W, Ingram K, Inderjeeth CA. Effect of frailty on functional gain, resource utilisation, and discharge destination: an observational prospective study in a GEM ward. Curr Gerontol Geriatr Res. 2014; https://doi.org/10.1155/2014/357857.

50. Arjunan A, Peel NM, Hubbard RE. Brief Report Feasibility and validity of frailty measurement in geriatric rehabilitation. 2018:144–6. https://doi.org/10.1111/ajag.12502.

51. Charlson M, Szatrowski TP, Peterson J, Gold J. Validation of a combined comorbidity index. J Clin Epidemiol. 1994;47(11):1245–51. https://doi.org/10.1016/0895-4356(94)90129-5.

52. Saklad M. Grading for Patients for Surgical Procedures. Anesthesiology. 1941;2(5):281–4.

53. Zimmerli W, Trampuz A, Ochsner PE. Prosthetic-joint infections. N Engl J Med. 2004;351(16):1645–54. https://doi.org/10.1056/NEJMra040181.

54. Roy L, Laflamme GY, Carrier M, Kim PR, Leduc S. A randomised clinical trial comparing minimally invasive surgery to conventional approach for endoprosthesis in elderly patients with hip fractures. Injury. 2010;41(4):365–9. https://doi.org/10.1016/j.injury.2009.10.002.

55. Auffarth A, Resch H, Lederer S, et al. Does the choice of approach for hip hemiarthroplasty in geriatric patients significantly influence early postoperative outcomes? A randomized-controlled trial comparing the modified smith-Petersen and Hardinge approaches. J Trauma. 2011;70(5):1257–62. https://doi.org/10.1097/TA.0b013e3181eded53.

56. Tsukada S, Wakui M. Minimally invasive intermuscular approach does not improve outcomes in bipolar hemiarthroplasty for femoral neck fracture. J Orthop Sci. 2010;15(6):753–7. https://doi.org/10.1007/s00776-010-1541-6.

57. Kaneko K, Mogami A, Ohbayashi O, Okahara H, Iwase H, Kurosawa H. Minimally invasive hemiarthroplasty in femoral neck fractures. Randomized comparison between a mini-incision and an ordinary incision: preliminary results. Eur J Orthop Surg Traumatol. 2005;15(1):19–22. https://doi.org/10.1007/s00590-004-0198-2.

58. Cherubini A, Del Signore S, Ouslander J, Semla T, Michel JP. Fighting against age discrimination in clinical trials, J Am Geriatr Soc. 2010; https://doi.org/10.1111/j.1532-5415.2010.03032.x.

59. Witham MD, McMurdo MET. How to get older people included in clinical studies. Drugs Aging. 2007; https://doi.org/10.2165/00002512-200724030-00002.

60. Van Deudekom FJ, Postmus I, Van Der Ham DJ, et al. External validity of randomized controlled trials in older adults, a systematic review. PLoS One. 2017;12(3):1–8. https://doi.org/10.1371/journal.pone.0174053.

61. Gill N, Hammond S, Cross J, Smith T, Lambert N, Fox C. Optimising care for patients with cognitive impairment and dementia following hip fracture. Z Gerontol Geriatr. 2017; https://doi.org/10.1007/s00391-017-1224-4.

62. Jung J, Anagnostakos K, Kohn D. Klinische ergebnisse nach minimal-invasiver Hüftendoprothetik. Orthopade. 2012;41(5):399–406. https://doi.org/10.1007/s00132-011-1895-2.

63. Auffarth A, Resch H, Lederer S, et al. Does the choice of approach for hip hemiarthroplasty in geriatric patients significantly influence early postoperative outcomes? A randomized-controlled trial comparing the modified smith-petersen and hardinge approaches. J Trauma Inj Infect Crit Care. 2011;70(5):1257–62. https://doi.org/10.1097/TA.0b013e3181eded53.

64. Bergh I, Sjostrom B, Oden A, Steen B. An application of pain rating scales in geriatric patients. Aging Clin Exp Res. 2000;12(5):380–7. https://doi.org/10.1007/BF03339864.

5

Low 25-hydroxyvitamin D levels and the risk of frailty syndrome

Sang Yhun Ju[1,2]* [iD], June Young Lee[3] and Do Hoon Kim[4]

Abstract

Background: Vitamin D deficiency and frailty are common with aging. Previous studies examining vitamin D status and frailty have produced mixed results, and in particular, the shape of the association has not been well established. We examined the association between 25-hydroxyvitamin D (25OHD) serum levels and frailty by performing a systematic review and dose-response meta-analysis.

Methods: We searched the PubMed, EMBASE and Cochrane Library databases of Elsevier through February 2017. Cross-sectional and cohort studies that reported adjusted risk ratios with 95% confidence intervals (CI) for frailty with ≥3 categories of 25OHD serum levels were selected. Data extraction was performed independently by two authors. The reported risk estimates for 25OHD categories were recalculated, employing a comprehensive trend estimation from summarized dose-response data.

Results: The pooled risk estimate of frailty syndrome per 25 nmol/L increment in serum 25OHD concentration was 0.88 (95% CI = 0.82–0.95, I^2 = 86.8%) in the 6 cross-sectional studies and 0.89 (95% CI = 0.85–0.94, I^2 = 0. 0%) in the 4 prospective cohort studies. Based on the Akaike information criteria (AIC), a linear model was selected (AIC for the nonlinear model: − 5.4, AIC for the linear model: − 6.8 in the prospective cohort studies; AIC for the linear model: − 13.6, AIC for the nonlinear model: − 1.77 in the cross-sectional studies).

Conclusions: This dose-response meta-analysis indicates that serum 25OHD levels are significantly and directly associated with the risk of frailty. Further studies should address the underlying mechanisms to explain this relationship and to determine whether vitamin D supplementation is effective for preventing frailty syndrome.

Keywords: Vitamin D, 25-hydroxyvitamin D, Frailty, Elderly, Cohort studies, Cross-sectional studies, Dose-response, Systematic review, Meta-analysis

Background

With increasing age, blood vitamin D concentrations decrease due to decreased kidney function, diminished sun exposure, intrinsic skin response to ultraviolet radiation and poor diet [1]. Vitamin D deficiency contributes to the development of osteoporosis and sarcopenia in older individuals, which increases the risk of fractures and falls and concomitant morbidity and mortality [2–4].

Frailty is a clinical state in which an individual's vulnerability to developing increased dependency and/or mortality when exposed to a stressor is increased [5–7]. Numerous frailty diagnostic tools have been proposed, with one recent systematic review [8] identifying 67 various frailty instruments. The Physical Frailty Phenotype [7], which includes indicators such as shrinking, weakness, poor endurance, slowness, and low physical activity, is a widely used instrument for assessing physical frailty in the research setting. However, the concept of frailty, i.e., general vulnerability to various external stressors, extends far beyond the physical dimension, resulting in a

* Correspondence: kolpos@daum.net
[1]Department of Family Medicine, Yeouido St. Mary's Hospital, College of Medicine, The Catholic University of Korea, 10, 63-Ro, Yeongdeungpo-Gu, Seoul 07345, Republic of Korea
[2]Hospice Palliative Medicine, Division of Spirituality, Yeouido St. Mary's Hospital, College of Medicine, The Catholic University of Korea, 10, 63-Ro, Yeongdeungpo-Gu, Seoul 07345, Republic of Korea
Full list of author information is available at the end of the article

multidimensional conceptualization of frailty based on interactions among various domains, including physical, psychological and social domains [5, 8–10]. Early detection of frailty may present an opportunity to introduce effective management strategies to improve outcomes [9].

An increasing number of studies investigating the association between 25-hydroxyvitamin D (25OHD) and frailty have yielded conflicting information. Although hypovitaminosis D can potentially increase the risk of frailty, not all observational studies have confirmed this relationship [11, 12]. Evidence from several cross-sectional studies supports a U-shaped [13] or linear inverse association between 25OHD levels and frailty [14, 15]. However, findings from longitudinal studies on the association between 25OHD levels and the development of frailty are inconsistent. Several studies have indicated that low vitamin D levels are significantly associated with frailty syndrome in the elderly, whereas others have found no association [16–19]. When the results were combined in a meta-analysis [12] published in 2016, the lowest 25OHD levels were associated with a 27% increase in the risk of frailty compared to the highest levels of 25OHD. However, the findings of the previous meta-analysis may be over- or underestimated due to variation in the 25OHD cutoff values used to define low and high 25OHD level categories as well as variation in the units used to measure serum levels of 25OHD.

Furthermore, the exact relationships, including whether a dose-response pattern exists, are currently unclear. Defining which levels of 25OHD are strongly associated with frailty syndrome is important for shaping elderly health recommendations about vitamin D supplementation considering the optimal serum 25OHD concentration. Furthermore, a recent prospective cohort study [20] in community-dwelling older women with a mean follow-up of 8.5 years did not identify a significant association between deficient (10–19 ng/mL) or insufficient (20–29.9 ng/mL) vitamin levels and incident frailty when compared to sufficient levels (≥30 ng/mL). Therefore, we conducted a systematic review and a dose-response meta-analysis of published cross-sectional and prospective cohort studies to further clarify the association between vitamin D and the risk of frailty.

Methods

Literature search

We searched the PubMed, Cochrane Library, and EMBASE databases via Elsevier through February 2017. A medical librarian together with the reviewers developed database-specific search strategies according to the particular subject headings and searching structure of the databases (Additional file 1). Furthermore, manual searches of the bibliographies of relevant articles were conducted to identify additional studies.

Eligibility criteria

Studies were included in the meta-analysis if they met the following inclusion criteria: 1) an observational design including cross-sectional studies and cohort studies in humans, 2) the inclusion of frailty as a specified outcome, 3) a baseline assessment of serum 25OHD levels, 4) the inclusion of data on relative risk (RR) and its corresponding 95% confidence interval (CI) or data to calculate these values for frailty syndrome for each category of serum 25OHD level, and 5) the inclusion of the most recent and complete study (i.e., the most detailed category classification) if cohorts were duplicated in more than one study.

Exclusion criteria, data extraction and quality assessment

Review articles, editorials, commentaries, and letters with no new data analysis, meta-analyses, and abstracts were excluded. The exclusion criteria for this study were as follows: 1) an experimental design was used, 2) the outcome was not frailty, and 3) only two serum 25OHD levels were specified. Two investigators (Sang Yhun Ju and Do Hoon Kim), coauthors of the present study, independently extracted the data from the original reports. The following information was extracted: the first author's family name, year of publication, country of origin, the mean or median age of the participants, gender, sample size, the number of participants for each serum 25OHD level, the number of cases for each serum 25OHD concentration category, adjusted covariates, definitions of frailty used, the method of 25OHD assessment, follow-up duration, and categories of serum 25OHD and their corresponding RRs with their 95% CIs for frailty. The adjusted risk estimates that reflected the most comprehensive control were extracted to avoid potential confounding variables. Disagreements between the two reviewers were resolved by consensus. We planned, conducted, and reported this systematic review according to the widely accepted quality standards (Additional file 2) for reporting meta-analyses of observational studies in epidemiology [21].

Statistical analysis

The methodology of the statistical analysis has been described in detail elsewhere [22]. In brief, the RR with 95% CI for each 25-nmol/L increase in the serum 25OHD in each study was calculated and was used for the meta-analysis. We performed a 2-stage random-effects dose-response meta-analysis to examine a potential nonlinear relationship between serum 25OHD levels and frailty [23]. We determined the best-fitting model, defined as the one with the smallest Akaike information criteria (AIC) [24]. The statistical heterogeneity of the studies was assessed using I^2 statistics [25]. We regarded I^2 values greater than 50% as indicators of high heterogeneity. The possibility of publication bias was assessed using Egger's tests [26] and visual inspection of the funnel plot. We also applied the trim-and-fill algorithm [27] to identify and correct for funnel plot asymmetry. In the presence of publication bias, the p values for Egger's tests were less than 0.1. All statistical analyses were performed using Stata software, version 14.0 (Stata Corp., College Station, TX, USA).

Results

Literature search and study selection

The process of identifying and selecting the studies is summarized in Fig. 1. A total of 895 articles were identified via Cochrane Central, PubMed, and EMBASE. Of these, 147 duplicate articles were excluded, and a further 677 articles were excluded based on their title and abstract, leaving 71 articles for further evaluation. After obtaining the full articles, we excluded a further 67 articles. Finally, we identified 8 articles including 10 studies that investigated the association between vitamin D status and frailty risk; 2 articles [16, 17] reported separate results for stratification by study design (i.e., cross-sectional and prospective cohort studies).

Study characteristics and quality

Table 1 presents the information extracted from all included studies. Four studies had a cross-sectional design [13–15, 28], two were prospective studies [18, 20], and two studies reported both cross-sectional and prospective evaluations [16, 17]. All four studies were prospective cohort studies in a total of 8209 participants who were free of frailty at baseline. Among the participants, 737 incident cases of frailty occurred during a follow-up duration from 2.9 to 8.5 years. A total of six cross-sectional studies provided data on 20,949 participants, including 1802 cases of frailty. Five studies were conducted in Europe [15–18, 28], and the other three studies were conducted in the United States [13, 14, 28]. The mean age of the participants ranged from 62.2 to 79.2 years. Two studies [13, 28] included males only, two studies [14, 20]

included females only, and four studies [16–18, 28] included both males and females. Most of the studies [13–15, 18, 20, 28] defined cases of frailty using frailty phenotypes, and the two studies by Puts et al. [16] and Schöttker et al. [17] used nine frailty indicators and the frailty index, respectively. Two studies [13, 14] used liquid chromatography tandem-mass spectrometry (LC-MS/MS), two studies [16, 18] used competitive binding protein assays, three studies [15, 17, 28] used immunoassays and one study [20] used radioreceptor assays. The selected studies reported their data on 25OHD levels in either nmol/L (three studies) [15–17] or ng/mL (five studies) [13, 14, 18, 20, 28]. We extracted the highest adjusted risk estimates from each study. Four studies adjusted for key covariates, including age, sex, timing of blood collection, BMI, smoking, and physical activity [13, 16, 18, 28]. The results of quality assessment are shown in Additional file 3. The average quality scores were 6.8 for the six cross-sectional studies and 8 for the four prospective cohort studies.

The reported risk estimates for the association between 25OHD level intervals and frailty are illustrated in Fig. 2. A roughly inverse linear relationship was found between 25OHD levels and frailty risk in most studies, with the exception of the cross-sectional study by Ensrud et al. [14], which identified a U-shaped association, and the cohort study by Vogt et al. [18], which found no association between 25OHD levels and frailty risk. In all the other studies, the group with the highest 25OHD levels had the lowest frailty risk.

Quantitative data synthesis

The reported effect estimates of the 25OHD groups were converted in the risk estimates for a 25-nmol/L increase in 25OHD levels and pooled for the meta-analysis. The meta-analysis summarized the results of six cross-sectional studies with 21,207 participants including 1802 cases of frailty and four prospective cohort studies accounting for a total of 8746 individuals and 864 frailty events during follow-up. 25OHD was significantly inversely associated with frailty in four of six cross-sectional studies and one of four cohort studies. The pooled risk estimates of frailty syndrome per 25-nmol/L increment in serum 25OHD concentration were 0.88 (95% CI = 0.82–0.95, I^2 = 86.8%) in the six cross-sectional studies and 0.89 (95% CI = 0.85–0.94, I^2 = 0.0%) in the four prospective cohort studies (Fig. 3).

For comparisons with results from other studies and reviews, the RRs for the 50 and 75 nmol/L increases in 25OHD levels were also estimated: 0.65 (95% CI = 0.50–0.85) and 0.52 (95% CI = 0.35–0.78), respectively, for cross-sectional studies and 0.76 (95% CI = 0.66–0.87) and 0.66 (0.53–0.82), respectively, for prospective cohort studies. The funnel plot of the linear dose-response slopes was somewhat asymmetric for the cross-sectional

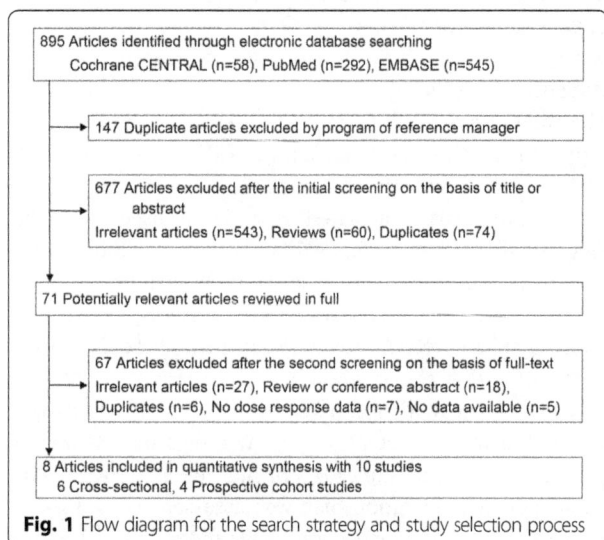

895 Articles identified through electronic database searching
Cochrane CENTRAL (n=58), PubMed (n=292), EMBASE (n=545)

147 Duplicate articles excluded by program of reference manager

677 Articles excluded after the initial screening on the basis of title or abstract
Irrelevant articles (n=543), Reviews (n=60), Duplicates (n=74)

71 Potentially relevant articles reviewed in full

67 Articles excluded after the second screening on the basis of full-text
Irrelevant articles (n=27), Review or conference abstract (n=18), Duplicates (n=6), No dose response data (n=7), No data available (n=5)

8 Articles included in quantitative synthesis with 10 studies
6 Cross-sectional, 4 Prospective cohort studies

Fig. 1 Flow diagram for the search strategy and study selection process

Table 1 Characteristics of studies and participants included in the meta-analysis of the association between serum 25-hydroxyvitamin D concentration and frailty

Author / Year / Study name	Country / Follow-up (years)	Gender / Age range (Mean age)	Participant (no.)	Case (no.)	Levels of 25OHD (Unit)	RR/OR (95% CI)	Definition (frailty) Assessment (25OHD)	Covariates / Key-set covariates (yes/no)
Prospective cohort studies of serum 25-hydroxyvitamin D levels in relation to frailty								
Puts et al [16] 2005 LASA	Netherlands 3,	M and F >65 (74.5, not frail; 79.2,frail)	66 305 514	20 51 54	<25 25-50 >50 (nmol/L)	1.90(0.92–3.95) 1.24 (0.77–2.00) 1.00 (Reference)	Nine Frailty indicators, competitive binding protein assay	aKey-sets of covariates, education, IL-6, CRP, alcohol, PTH, self-reported chronic disease, use of anti-inflammatory drugs, use of estrogen
Schöttker et al [17] 2014 ESTHER	Germany 8	M and F 50-74 (62.6)	866 2790 2515	92 230 188	<30 30-50 >50 (nmol/L)	1.18 (0.85–1.63) 1.12 (0.88–1.43) 1.00 (Reference)	Frailty Index, immunoassay	Age, sex, education, BMI, smoking, light physical activity and self-rated health
Vogt et al [18] 2015 KORA	Germany 2.9	M and F >65 (75.5)	107 100 160 137	21 4 7 3	<15 15-20 20-30 >30 (ng/mL)	2.84 (0.38–21.22) 0.46 (0.04–5.84) 1.01 (0.1–10.07) 1.00 (Reference)	Frailty Phenotype, competitive binding protein assay	aKey-sets of covariates, baseline frailty status, education, alcohol, CVD, diabetes, multimorbidity and PTH (yes)
Buta et al [20] 2017 WHAS II	United States 8.5	F 70-79 (73.8	28 135 141 65	9 29 21 8	<10 10-19.9 20-29.9 >30 (ng/mL)	2.29 (0.92–5.69) 1.44 (0.71–2.94) 1.08 (0.52–2.22) 1.00 (Reference)	Frailty Phenotype, radioreceptor assay	Age, race, education, smoking, season of blood draw, BMI, cardiovascular disease, diabetes mellitus, hyperlipidemia and hypertension
Cross-sectional studies of serum 25-hydroxyvitamin D levels in relation to frailty								
Puts et al [16] 2005 LASA	Netherlands	M and F >65 (74.5,not frail; 79.2,frail)	141 471 659	56 166 70	<25 25-50 >50 (nmol/L)	2.55 (1.56–4.17) 1.66 (1.15–2.40) 1.00 (Reference)	Nine Frailty Indicators, competitive binding protein assay	aKey-sets of covariates, education, IL-6, CRP, alcohol, PTH, self-reported chronic disease, use of anti-inflammatory drugs, use of estrogen
Ensrud et al [14] 2010 SOF	United States	F >65 (76.7)	1280 1233 2428 1366	301 217 329 218	<15 15-19.9 20.0-29.9 >30 (ng/mL)	1.47 (1.19–1.82) 1.24 (0.99–1.54) 1.00 (Reference) 1.32 (1.06–1.63)	Frailty Phenotype, LC-MS/MS	aKey-sets of covariates, site, self-reported health status, education, alcohol, comorbidity, and short MMSE
Ensrud et al [13] 2011	United States	M >65	408 803	54 55	<20 20-29.9	1.47 (1.07–2.02) 1.02 (0.78–1.32)	Frailty Phenotype, LC-MS/MS	Age, race, site, season of blood draw, BMI, self-reported health status,

Table 1 Characteristics of studies and participants included in the meta-analysis of the association between serum 25-hydroxyvitamin D concentration and frailty (*Continued*)

Author Year Study name	Country Follow-up (years)	Gender Age range (Mean age)	Participant (no.)	Case (no.)	Levels of 25OHD (Unit)	RR/OR (95% CI)	Definition (frailty) Assessment (25OHD)	Covariates Key-set covariates (yes/no)
MrOS		(73.8)	395	21	>30 (ng/mL)	1.00 (Reference)		education, living alone, smoking status, alcohol intake, comorbidity score, Teng 3MS score, and baseline frailty status
Tajar et al [15] 2013 EMAS	Italy, belgium, Poland, Sweden, UK, Spain, Hungary and Estonia	M ≥60 (69.5)	524 453 399	43 19 7	<50 50-75 >75 (nmol/L)	5.74 (2.12–15.6) 3.55 (1.27–9.90) 1.00 (Reference)	Frailty Phenotype, radioimmunoassay	Age, centre, smoking, co-morbid conditions and PTH
Schöttker et al [17] 2014 ESTHER	Germany	M and F 50–74 (62.2)	1444 4199 3936	52 120 87	<30 30-50 >50 (nmol/L)	1.90 (1.30–2.78) 1.48 (1.09–2.01) 1.00 (Reference)	Frailty Index, immunoassay	Age, sex, education, BMI, smoking, light physical activity and self-rated health
Pabst et al [28] 2015 KORA-Age	Germany	M and F 65–90 (75.6)	292 192 257	17 8 12	<15 15-20 20-30 (ng/mL)	1.00 (Reference) 0.71 (0.22–2.32) 0.60 (0.19–1.91)	Frailty Phenotype, enhanced chemiluminescence immunoassay	[a]Key-sets of covariates, years of education, self-perceived economic situation, co-morbidity score, MMSE

Abbreviations: *BMI* body mass index, *CRP* C-reactive protein, *ESTHER* Epidemiological investigations of the chances of preventing, recognizing early and optimally treating chronic diseases in an elderly population, *KORA* Cooperative Health Research in the Region of Augsburg, *IL-6* interleukin-6, *LASA* Longitudinal Aging Study Amsterdam, *LC-MS/MS* liquid chromatography tandem-mass spectrometry, *MrOS* Osteoporotic Fractures in Men Study, *PTH* parathyroid hormone, *SOF* Study of Osteoporotic Fractures, *WHAS II* Women's Health and Aging Study II, *25(OH)D* 25-hydroxyvitamin D. [a]Key-sets of covariates: age, sex, season of blood draw, body mass index (or obesity), smoking, and physical activity

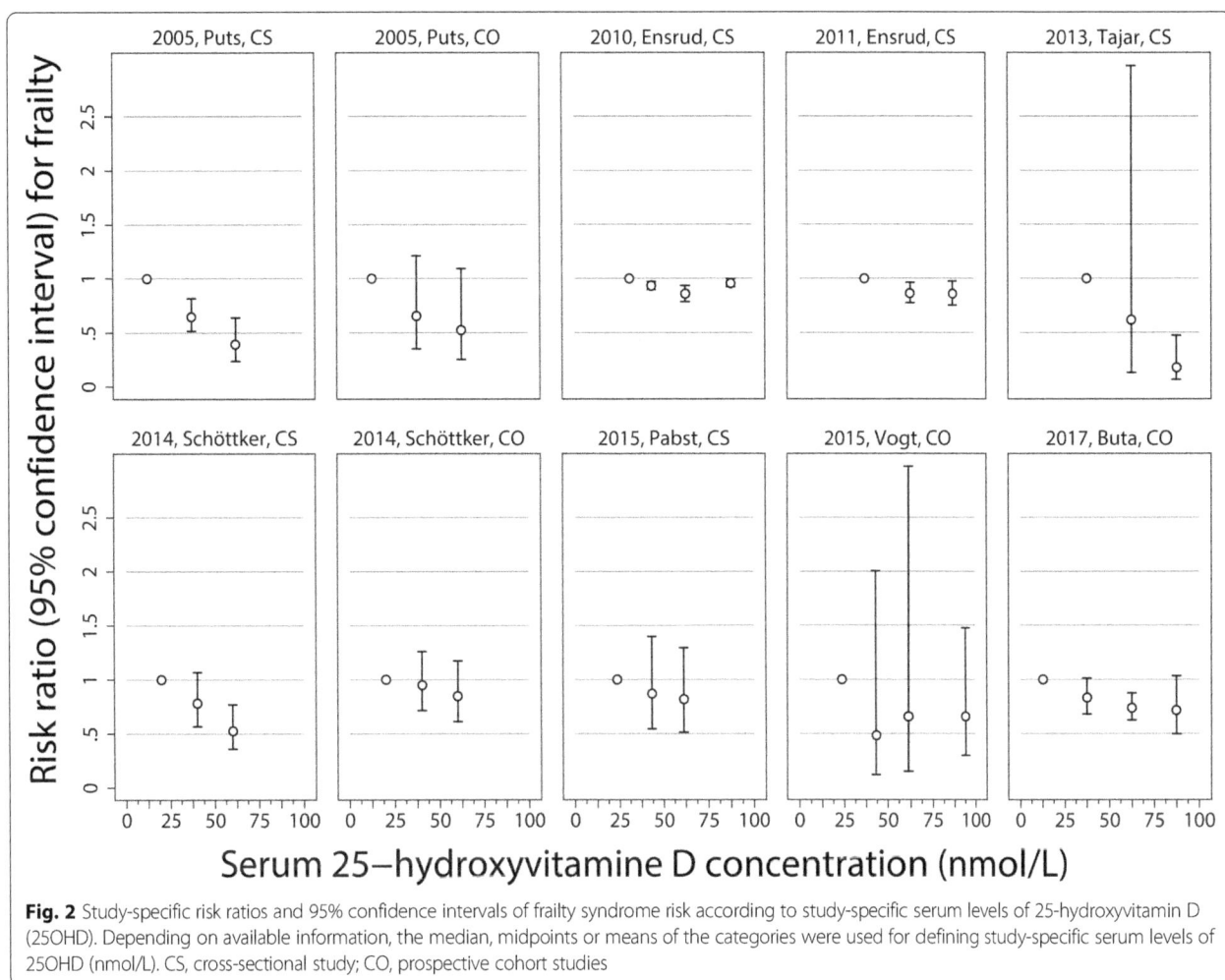

Fig. 2 Study-specific risk ratios and 95% confidence intervals of frailty syndrome risk according to study-specific serum levels of 25-hydroxyvitamin D (25OHD). Depending on available information, the median, midpoints or means of the categories were used for defining study-specific serum levels of 25OHD (nmol/L). CS, cross-sectional study; CO, prospective cohort studies

studies, with smaller studies tending to have larger risk estimates, suggesting publication bias. A publication bias was detected with Egger's test for the cross-sectional studies (Additional file 4: Figure S1; $p = 0.007$), but not for the prospective cohort studies (Additional file 4: Figure S2; $P = 0.693$). The trim-and-fill sensitivity method imputed estimates from three hypothesized negative un-published estimates. The corrected effect estimate for a 25-nmol/L increase in the 25OHD level was reduced to 0.98 (95% CI = 0.90–1.05, $I^2 = 88.9\%$), demonstrating no relationship between the risk of frailty and serum 25OHD levels after accounting for a potential publication bias.

Four prospective cohort studies were included in the restricted cubic spline models (Fig. 4a). Based on the AIC, a linear model was selected (AIC for the nonlinear model: – 5.4, AIC for the linear model: – 6.8). Compared with a serum 25OHD level of 12.5 nmol/L, the RR (95% CI) for frailty was 0.96 (0.94–0.98) for 20 nmol/L, 0.86 (0.80–0.94) for 40 nmol/L, 0.77 (0.67–0.88) for 60 nmol/L, and 0.64 (0.50–0.80) for 94 nmol/L. Six cross-sectional studies were included in the restricted cubic spline models (Fig. 4b). Based on the AIC, a linear model was selected

(AIC for the linear model: – 13.6, AIC for the nonlinear model: – 1.77). Compared with the serum 25OHD level of 12.5 nmol/L, the OR (95% CI) of frailty for the cross-sectional studies was 0.94 (0.90–0.98) for 20 nmol/L, 0.85 (0.77–0.94) for 31 nmol/L, 0.78 (0.68–0.91) for 40 nmol/L, 0.66 (0.52–0.86) for 60 nmol/L, and 0.52 (0.35–0.78) for 94 nmol/L.

Subgroup analyses

Subgroup analyses were performed based on geographic lo-cation (Europe vs. United States, definition frailty, key sets of covariates (yes vs. no), Newcastle-Ottawa Scale (≥7 vs < 7), and follow-up years (≥median vs. <median). The sub-groups are presented in Table 2. Overall, an inverse associ-ation between a 25 nmol/L increase in 25OHD levels and risk of frailty was consistently observed in each subgroup. In the subgroup analyses of cross-sectional studies, the in-verse association was statistically significant for the geo-graphic region of Europe (OR = 0.78, 95% CI = 0.68–0.88, $I^2 = 50.6\%$), the subgroup (nine frailty indicators and the frailty index) of frailty definition (OR = 0.76, 95% CI = 0.68–0.85, $I^2 = 0\%$), the subgroup of other 25OHD measurement

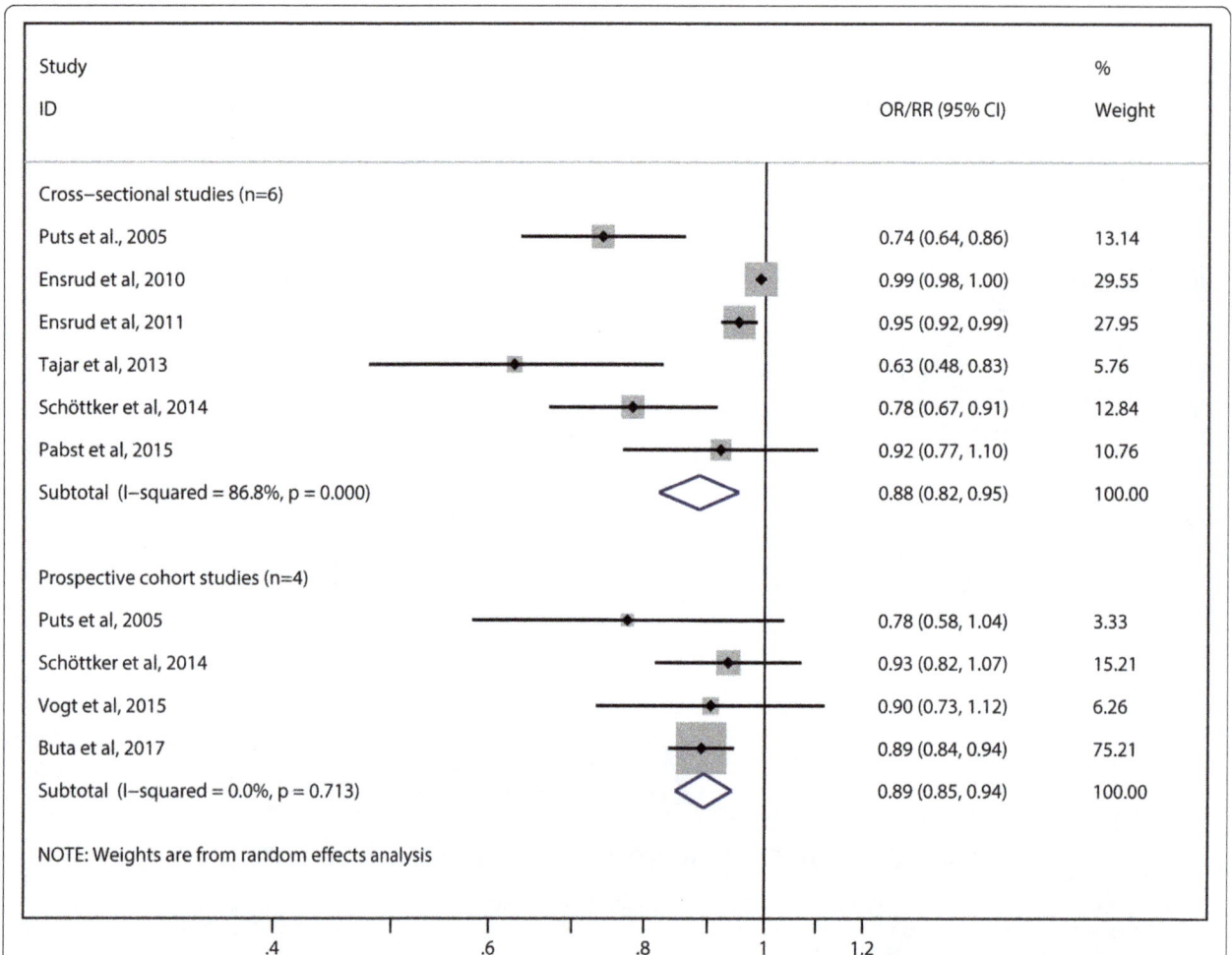

Fig. 3 Forest plots of the risk ratios (RRs) of frailty syndrome per 25 nmol/L increment in serum 25-hydroxyvitamin D concentration using a random-effects analysis. The squares represent study-specific RR (the square sizes are proportional to the weight of each study in the overall estimate); the horizontal lines represent 95% confidence intervals (CIs), and the diamond represents the overall RR estimate with 95% CI

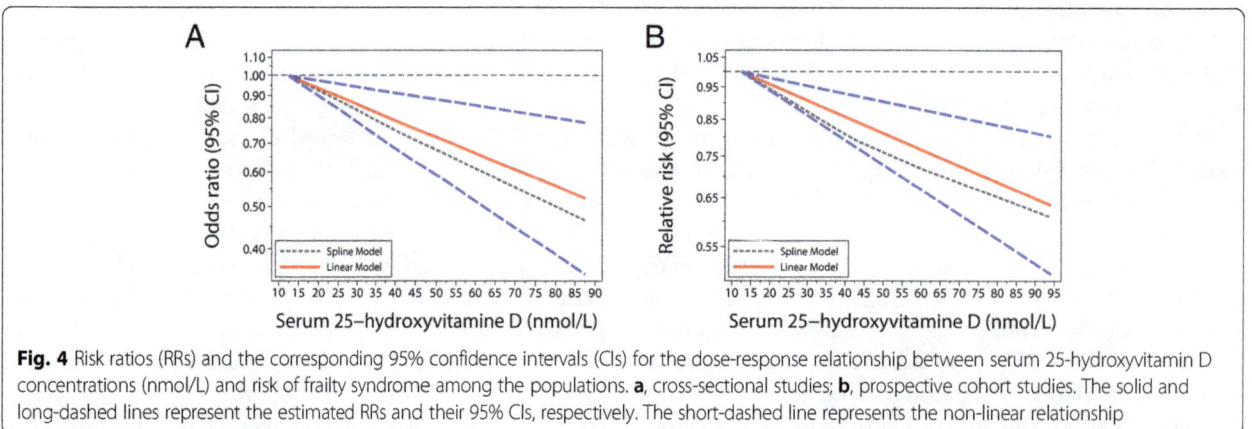

Fig. 4 Risk ratios (RRs) and the corresponding 95% confidence intervals (CIs) for the dose-response relationship between serum 25-hydroxyvitamin D concentrations (nmol/L) and risk of frailty syndrome among the populations. **a**, cross-sectional studies; **b**, prospective cohort studies. The solid and long-dashed lines represent the estimated RRs and their 95% CIs, respectively. The short-dashed line represents the non-linear relationship

methods (OR = 0.78, 95% CI = 0.68–0.88, I^2 = 50.6%) and the Newcastle-Ottawa scale ≥7 subgroup (OR = 0.71–0.91, I^2 = 41.4). In addition, within the prospective cohort studies, we found that the association was significant for phenotype definition of frailty (RR = 0.89, 95% CI = 0.84–0.94, I^2 = 0%), duration of follow-up ≥5.6 year (RR = 0.90, 95% CI = 0.85–0.95, I^2 = 0%) and the subgroup (yes) of key-set covariates (RR = 0.90, 95% CI = 0.85–0.95, I^2 = 0%).

Discussion

To our knowledge, this is the first dose-response quantitative systematic review of observational studies investing the effect of serum 25OHD levels on the risk of frailty using data from both cross-sectional and prospective cohort studies. This meta-analysis of data from more than 20,000 study participants demonstrates a statistically significant inverse association between serum 25OHD levels and the risk of frailty, and this finding was consistent across subgroups. A 25-nmol/L increase in 25OHD levels was associated with an 11% decrease in the incidence of frailty in prospective cohort studies and a 12% decrease in the risk of frailty in the cross-sectional studies. A statistically linear relationship between serum 25OHD levels and the risk of frailty was also found, even after adjustments for other known risk factors.

We estimated a protective effect of a 25-nmol/L increase in 25OHD levels against frailty because this number is the

difference between the upper limit of vitamin D deficiency, defined by most experts as a 25OHD level less than 50 nmol/L, and the lower limit of sufficient vitamin D levels above 75 nmol/L. Additionally, a daily intake of at least 1000 IU (25 μg/d; 1 μg = 40 IU) of vitamin D3 appears to be required to elevate vitamin D concentrations by 25 nmol/L, which would ensure that no less than 50% of the population has the recommended 25OHD level of at least 75 nmol/L [3, 18]. Several studies indicated increases in serum 25OHD levels of only ~ 7–10 nmol/L per 400 IU of daily vitamin D supplementation [29, 30]. Recently, a study reported that the extent of the 25OHD increase upon vitamin D supplementation depended on 25OHD baseline levels, age, and body weight [31]. Hence, a new guideline for the dosing requirement for vitamin supplementation in frail elderly persons, based on initial vitamin D levels, should be established after further investigation.

A previous meta-analysis [12] of seven prospective cohorts reported an inverse association between vitamin D deficiency and frailty. However, only data in the highest compared with the lowest categories of 25OHD were used rather than the use of all categories. This dose response meta-analysis allowed us to evaluate risk across the entire spectrum of observed 25OHD levels. We observed an inverse linear association between 25OHD levels and the risk of frailty among the elderly population, suggesting that any incremental increase in serum

Table 2 Frailty risk per 25 nmol/L increase in serum 25-hydroxyvitamin D in subgroup meta-analyses of the cross-sectional studies and the prospective cohort studies

Group	Subgroup	No.	OR/RR (95% CI)	I^2 (%)	P
Cross-sectional studies					
Geographic location	Europe	4	0.78 (0.68–0.88)	50.6	0.108
	United States	2	0.98 (0.94–1.01)	79.8	0.026
Definition of frailty	Phenotype	4	0.95 (0.89–1.01)	81.1	0.001
	Others	2	0.76 (0.68–0.85)	0.0	0.612
Method of [a]25OHD assessment	[b]LC-MS/MS	2	0.98 (0.94–1.01)	79.8	0.026
	Others	4	0.78 (0.68–0.88)	50.6	0.108
[c]Key-sets of covariates	Yes	3	0.87 (0.75–1.02)	80.1	0.007
	No	3	0.81 (0.63–1.04)	89.6	< 0.001
[d]Newcastle-Ottawa Scale	≥ 7	3	0.81 (0.71–0.91)	41.4	0.182
	< 7	3	0.95 (0.95–1.02)	86.9	< 0.001
Prospective cohort studies					
Definition of frailty	Phenotype	2	0.89 (0.84–0.94)	0.0	0.877
	Others	2	0.89 (0.76–1.04)	22.8	0.255
Follow-up (years)	≥ 5.6	2	0.90 (0.85–0.95)	0.0	0.510
	< 5.6	2	0.86 (0.72–1.02)	0.0	0.403
[c]Key-sets of covariates	Yes	2	0.90 (0.85–0.95)	0.0	0.510
	No	2	0.86 (0.72–1.02)	0.0	0.403

[a]25OHD 25-hydroxyvitmain D, [b]LC-MS/MS liquid chromatography tandem-mass spectrometry [c]Key-sets of covariates: age, sex, season of blood draw, body mass index (or obesity), smoking, and physical activity; [d]Newcastle-Ottawa Scale: Total score could range from 0 to 9

25OHD level was associated with a decreased risk of frailty. However, because serum 25OHD concentrations in the current data for the frailty study range from 12.5 to 95 nmol/L, we have not been able to investigate the dose-response relationship between higher levels of 25OHD, i.e., > 95 nmol/L and risk of frailty. It is too early to determine whether there is a specific cutoff level of serum 25OHD that increases or reduces the risk of developing frailty syndrome because a limited number of studies used serum 25OHD levels as a categorical variable and provided RR data for each category and because of the variation in the definition of frailty. Thus, the results of this analysis should be interpreted cautiously. We cannot rule out the possibility that the serum 25OHD level has a threshold rather than dose-response effect on the risk of frailty.

Our results suggest that high 25OHD levels are associated with a lower risk of frailty in elderly people. Conversely, frailty itself may contribute to lower 25OHD by reducing the levels of outdoor activity and sunlight exposure. Elderly individuals with frailty are at a high risk of developing vitamin D deficiency due to decreased dietary intake, less sun exposure, and a decreased capacity to produce sufficient amounts of calcitriol due to an age-related decline in hydroxylation by the kidney [1]. The causality of the association between low vitamin D levels and the frailty syndrome has not been completely elucidated. Nevertheless, there are several potential biological mechanisms that could explain the inverse association between vitamin D and frailty.

Considerable overlap exists between sarcopenia and frailty, especially in terms of the physical aspects of the frailty phenotype: low grip strength, gait speed and muscle mass [32]. While the underlying mechanisms and pathophysiology of sarcopenia remain to be clarified, inadequate nutritional intake in older individuals may contribute to the multifactorial pathogenesis of sarcopenia [33]. In particular, vitamin D, one of the most popular micronutrients, was reported to play important roles in muscle differentiation, stimulation of calcium and phosphorus transport and muscle contraction [34]. A muscle biopsy study revealed atrophy of type II muscle fibers in subjects with profound vitamin D deficiency [35]. During sudden movement, the fast and strong type II muscle fibers are the first to be recruited to avoid falling [36]. A meta-analysis observed that daily vitamin D doses in the range of 700 to 1000 IU or achieving serum concentrations between 60 and 95 nmol/L reduced the risk of falling by 19% in older individuals [3]. 1,25-Dihydroxyvitamin D (1,25OHD) can act on muscle fibers by binding to its nuclear vitamin D receptor (VDR) and thereby increasing the de novo synthesis of protein, which regulates muscle strength [36]. VDR number decreases with aging in several organs involved in calcium metabolism, and

1alpha-hydroxylase activity decreases mainly due to a decrease in renal function, reducing vitamin D activation [1]. An age-related decline in VDR expression is supported by studies in rats in which VDR expression declined with advancing age in both the intestine and bone [37, 38]. When 25OHD levels are low, active metabolite 1,25OHD levels and calcium absorption decrease [39]. This reduced serum calcium led to an increase in parathyroid hormone levels to stimulate 1,25OHD production, resulting in an increased risk of bone turnover and bone loss [39, 40]. Consequently, a decline in muscle function and strength caused by vitamin D could explain slowness, low physical activity and weakness.

The last pathway through which low vitamin D may affect frailty is related to its hypothesized anti-inflammatory properties [41]. Several studies [16, 17, 29] have demonstrated a heightened inflammatory state among frail older adults marked by high serum levels of inflammatory mediators, such as cytokines and acute phase proteins, supporting the existence of a dysregulated immune system in frailty. An increased susceptibility to infection and risk of autoimmune disease has been shown in 25OHD deficiency. Illness may be the beginning of a vicious cycle between 25OHD deficiency and frailty [5]. Individuals with illness tend to exhibit poor nutritional status, go outside less frequently and experience less sun exposure, which are underlying causes of low serum 25OHD concentrations [5, 6, 10, 33]. A recent study suggested that 1,25OHD may be an important regulator of the inflammatory response during bacterial infection [42]. Active vitamin D metabolites can downregulate inflammatory markers via the nuclear VDR expressed in antigen-presenting cells, and vitamin D deficiency may result in increased pro-inflammatory cytokines that impact muscle strength and performance [43, 44].

The findings of our study should be interpreted within its limitations. The included studies have no data regarding vitamin D supplementations evaluated through food frequency questionnaires or self-administered questionnaires, which could affect serum 25OHD concentrations; therefore, the present study may under- or overestimate our results. The definitions for frailty used in the included studies were different (i.e., Fried phenotype, modified phenotype, nine frailty indications, and frailty index), thus affecting our pooled analysis, although subgroup analysis was performed according to definitions of frailty. Because several eligible studies did not provide sufficient information for a dose-response analysis of 25OHD levels, the number of participants, cases, and logarithms of RRs and corresponding standard errors, we excluded the potential related studies [19, 45–49], which may introduce a potential selection bias in our analysis. Unlike those observed for prospective cohort studies, the results from cross-sectional studies were somewhat heterogeneous but consistently pointed to an inverse relationship despite the observation that the strength of the association differed substantially across studies. Additionally, publication bias seems to have occurred for cross-sectional but not for prospective cohort studies in the literature, which may contribute to the stronger inverse association observed among the former. Our meta-analysis only included studies published in English and did not search for unpublished studies that might contribute to the asymmetrical funnel plot. When we explored the influence of a potential publication bias trim-and-fill method, our findings revealed no significant association of 25OHD with frailty among the cross-sectional studies. However, detection and adjustment of publication bias is difficult and somewhat controversial when only a small number of trials is available [50]. The funnel plot suggests the presence of three negative, outlying studies that were not balanced by positive studies. Additional investigations including a reference review did not reveal any further peer-reviewed studies for inclusion. Although this may represent publication bias, it may also reflect a truly significant inverse relationship between vitamin D status and frailty.

Conclusion

Our findings suggest that 25OHD serum levels are independently associated with the risk of frailty, which is consistent with the results of a nonlinear analysis and a linear regression analysis. Further interventional research should investigate whether vitamin D supplementation can be useful for preventing frailty in the elderly population.

Additional files

Additional file 1: Search strategy.

Additional file 2: MOOSE Checklist for Meta-analyses of Observational Studies.

Additional file 3: Quality of the observational studies in the meta-analysis based on the Newcastle-Ottawa Scale.

Additional file 4: Publication bias for association between serum 25-hydroxyvitamin D concentration per 25-nmol/L increment and frailty syndrome. **Figure S1**. Begg's Funnel plot with 95% confidence intervals in the meta-analysis of the cross-sectional studies. **Figure S2**. Begg's Funnel plot with 95% confidence intervals in the meta-analysis of the prospective cohort studies.

Abbreviations

1,25OHD: 1,25-dihydroxyvitamin D; 25OHD: 25-hydroxyvitamin D; AIC: Akaike information criteria; CI: Confidence interval; OR: Odds ratio; RR: Relative risk

Acknowledgements

We thank Na Jin Kim from the Medical Library, College of Medicine, The Catholic University of Korea, for performing the database searches.

Funding

This research received no specific grant from any funding research agency in the public, commercial or not-for-profit sectors.

Authors' contributions

SYJ had full access to the entire study; took responsibility for the study's integrity and the accuracy of the data analysis; designed the study; reviewed and revised the final manuscript; and contributed to the conception, design, statistical analysis, data interpretation, and manuscript drafting of this study. SYJ and DHK contributed to the data extraction by evaluating the quality of each study's methodology using previously established criteria. JYL contributed to statistical analysis and the data interpretation. All the authors approved the final manuscript for submission.

Competing interests

The authors declare that they have no competing interests.

Author details

[1]Department of Family Medicine, Yeouido St. Mary's Hospital, College of Medicine, The Catholic University of Korea, 10, 63-Ro, Yeongdeungpo-Gu, Seoul 07345, Republic of Korea. [2]Hospice Palliative Medicine, Division of Spirituality, Yeouido St. Mary's Hospital, College of Medicine, The Catholic University of Korea, 10, 63-Ro, Yeongdeungpo-Gu, Seoul 07345, Republic of Korea. [3]Department of Biostatistics, Korea University College of Medicine, 145, Anam-Ro, Seongbuk-Gu, Seoul 02841, Republic of Korea. [4]Department of Family Medicine, Korea University Ansan Hospital, 70-9, Darigan 2-gil, Danwon-Gu, Ansan-Si, Gyeonggi-Do 15459, Republic of Korea.

References

1. de Jongh RT, van Schoor NM, Lips P. Changes in vitamin D endocrinology during aging in adults. Mol Cell Endocrinol. 2017;453:144–50.
2. Bischoff-Ferrari HA, Dawson-Hughes B, Staehelin HB, Orav JE, Stuck AE, Theiler R, Wong JB, Egli A, Kiel DP, Henschkowski J. Fall prevention with supplemental and active forms of vitamin D: a meta-analysis of randomised controlled trials. BMJ. 2009;339:b3692.
3. Bischoff-Ferrari HA, Giovannucci E, Willett WC, Dietrich T, Dawson-Hughes B. Estimation of optimal serum concentrations of 25-hydroxyvitamin D for multiple health outcomes. Am J Clin Nutr. 2006;84(1):18–28.
4. Smit E, Crespo CJ, Michael Y, Ramirez-Marrero FA, Brodowicz GR, Bartlett S, Andersen RE. The effect of vitamin D and frailty on mortality among non-institutionalized US older adults. Eur J Clin Nutr. 2012;66(9):1024–8.
5. Morley JE, Vellas B, van Kan GA, Anker SD, Bauer JM, Bernabei R, Cesari M, Chumlea WC, Doehner W, Evans J, et al. Frailty consensus: a call to action. J Am Med Dir Assoc. 2013;14(6):392–7.
6. Clegg A, Young J, Iliffe S, Rikkert MO, Rockwood K. Frailty in elderly people. Lancet. 2013;381(9868):752–62.
7. Fried LP, Tangen CM, Walston J, Newman AB, Hirsch C, Gottdiener J, Seeman T, Tracy R, Kop WJ, Burke G, McBurnie MA, et al. Frailty in older adults: evidence for a phenotype. J Gerontol A Biol Sci Med Sci. 2001;56(3): M146–156.
8. Buta BJ, Walston JD, Godino JG, Park M, Kalyani RR, Xue QL, Bandeen-Roche K, Varadhan R. Frailty assessment instruments: systematic characterization of the uses and contexts of highly-cited instruments. Ageing Res Rev. 2016;26:53–61.
9. Sacha J, Sacha M, Sobon J, Borysiuk Z, Feusette P. Is it time to begin a public campaign concerning frailty and pre-frailty? A Review Article. Front Physiol. 2017;8:484.
10. Dent E, Lien C, Lim WS, Wong WC, Wong CH, Ng TP, Woo J, Dong B, de la Vega S, Hua Poi PJ, et al. The Asia-Pacific clinical practice guidelines for the Management of Frailty. J Am Med Dir Assoc. 2017;18(7):564–75.
11. Wong YY, Flicker L. Hypovitaminosis D and frailty: epiphenomenon or causal? Maturitas. 2015;82(4):328–35.
12. Zhou J, Huang P, Liu P, Hao Q, Chen S, Dong B, Wang J. Association of vitamin D deficiency and frailty: a systematic review and meta-analysis. Maturitas. 2016;94:70–6.

13. Ensrud KE, Blackwell TL, Cauley JA, Cummings SR, Barrett-Connor E, Dam TT, Hoffman AR, Shikany JM, Lane NE, Stefanick ML, et al. Circulating 25-hydroxyvitamin D levels and frailty in older men: the osteoporotic fractures in men study. J Am Geriatr Soc. 2011;59(1):101–6.

14. Ensrud KE, Ewing SK, Fredman L, Hochberg MC, Cauley JA, Hillier TA, Cummings SR, Yaffe K, Cawthon PM. Circulating 25-hydroxyvitamin D levels and frailty status in older women. J Clin Endocrinol Metab. 2010;95(12):5266–73.

15. Tajar A, Lee DM, Pye SR, O'Connell MD, Ravindrarajah R, Gielen E, Boonen S, Vanderschueren D, Pendleton N, Finn JD, et al. The association of frailty with serum 25-hydroxyvitamin D and parathyroid hormone levels in older European men. Age Ageing. 2013;42(3):352–9.

16. Puts MT, Visser M, Twisk JW, Deeg DJ, Lips P. Endocrine and inflammatory markers as predictors of frailty. Clin Endocrinol. 2005;63(4):403–11.

17. Schottker B, Saum KU, Perna L, Ordonez-Mena JM, Holleczek B, Brenner H. Is vitamin D deficiency a cause of increased morbidity and mortality at older age or simply an indicator of poor health? Eur J Epidemiol. 2014;29(3):199–210.

18. Vogt S, Decke S, de Las Heras Gala T, Linkohr B, Koenig W, Ladwig KH, Peters A, Thorand B. Prospective association of vitamin D with frailty status and all-cause mortality in older adults: results from the KORA-age study. Prev Med. 2015;73:40–6.

19. Wong YY, McCaul KA, Yeap BB, Hankey GJ, Flicker L. Low vitamin D status is an independent predictor of increased frailty and all-cause mortality in older men: the health in men study. J Clin Endocrinol Metab. 2013;98(9):3821–8.

20. Buta B, Choudhury PP, Xue QL, Chaves P, Bandeen-Roche K, Shardell M, Semba RD, Walston J, Michos ED, Appel LJ, et al. The Association of Vitamin D Deficiency and Incident Frailty in older women: the role of Cardiometabolic diseases. J Am Geriatr Soc. 2017;65(3):619–24.

21. Stroup DF, Berlin JA, Morton SC, Olkin I, Williamson GD, Rennie D, Moher D, Becker BJ, Sipe TA, Thacker SB. Meta-analysis of observational studies in epidemiology: a proposal for reporting. Meta-analysis of observational studies in epidemiology (MOOSE) group. JAMA. 2000;283(15):2008–12.

22. Ju SY, Jeong HS, Kim DH. Blood vitamin D status and metabolic syndrome in the general adult population: a dose-response meta-analysis. J Clin Endocrinol Metab. 2014;99(3):1053–63.

23. Orsini N, Bellocco R, Greenland S. Generalized least squares for trend estimation of summarized dose-response data. Stata J. 2006;6(1):40–57.

24. Akaike H. A new look at the statistical model identification. IEEE Trans Autom Control. 1974;19(6):716–23.

25. Higgins JP, Thompson SG. Quantifying heterogeneity in a meta-analysis. Stat Med. 2002;21(11):1539–58.

26. Egger M, Davey Smith G, Schneider M, Minder C. Bias in meta-analysis detected by a simple, graphical test. BMJ. 1997;315(7109):629–34.

27. Duval S, Tweedie R. Trim and fill: a simple funnel-plot-based method of testing and adjusting for publication bias in meta-analysis. Biometrics. 2000;56(2):455–63.

28. Pabst G, Zimmermann AK, Huth C, Koenig W, Ludwig T, Zierer A, Peters A, Thorand B. Association of low 25-hydroxyvitamin D levels with the frailty syndrome in an aged population: results from the KORA-age Augsburg study. J Nutr Health Aging. 2015;19(3):258–64.

29. Barger-Lux MJ, Heaney RP, Dowell S, Chen TC, Holick MF. Vitamin D and its major metabolites: serum levels after graded oral dosing in healthy men. Osteoporosis Int. 1998;8(3):222–30.

30. Heaney RP, Davies KM, Chen TC, Holick MF, Barger-Lux MJ. Human serum 25-hydroxycholecalciferol response to extended oral dosing with cholecalciferol. Am J Clin Nutr. 2003;77(1):204–10.

31. Lehmann U, Riedel A, Hirche F, Brandsch C, Girndt M, Ulrich C, Seibert E, Henning C, Glomb MA, Dierkes J, et al. Vitamin D3 supplementation: Response and predictors of vitamin D3 metabolites - A randomized controlled trial. Clini Nutr. 2016;35(2):351–8.

32. Cederholm T. Overlaps between frailty and sarcopenia definitions. Nestle Nutr Inst Workshop Ser. 2015;83:65–9.

33. Artaza-Artabe I, Saez-Lopez P, Sanchez-Hernandez N, Fernandez-Gutierrez N, Malafarina V. The relationship between nutrition and frailty: effects of protein intake, nutritional supplementation, vitamin D and exercise on muscle metabolism in the elderly. A systematic review. Maturitas. 2016;93:89–99.

34. Garcia LA, King KK, Ferrini MG, Norris KC, Artaza JN. 1,25(OH)2vitamin D3 stimulates myogenic differentiation by inhibiting cell proliferation and modulating the expression of promyogenic growth factors and myostatin in C2C12 skeletal muscle cells. Endocrinology. 2011;152(8):2976–86.

35. Yoshikawa S, Nakamura T, Tanabe H, Imamura T. Osteomalacic myopathy. Endocrinol Jpn. 1979;26(Suppl):65–72.

36. Pfeifer M, Begerow B, Minne HW. Vitamin D and muscle function. Osteoporosis Int. 2002;13(3):187–94.

37. Gonzalez Pardo V, Boland R, de Boland AR. Vitamin D receptor levels and binding are reduced in aged rat intestinal subcellular fractions. Biogerontology. 2008;9(2):109–18.

38. Horst RL, Goff JP, Reinhardt TA. Advancing age results in reduction of intestinal and bone 1,25-dihydroxyvitamin D receptor. Endocrinology. 1990;126(2):1053–7.

39. Seamans KM, Hill TR, Scully L, Meunier N, Andrillo-Sanchez M, Polito A, Hininger-Favier I, Ciarapica D, Simpson EE, Stewart-Knox BJ, et al. Vitamin d status and indices of bone turnover in older European adults. Int J Vitam Nutr Res. 2011;81(5):277–85.

40. Ebeling PR. Vitamin D and bone health: epidemiologic studies. Bonekey Rep. 2014;3:511.

41. Bruyere O, Cavalier E, Buckinx F, Reginster JY. Relevance of vitamin D in the pathogenesis and therapy of frailty. Curr Opin Clin Nutr Metab Care. 2017;20(1):26–9.

42. Hoe E, Nathanielsz J, Toh ZQ, Spry L, Marimla R, Balloch A, Mulholland K, Licciardi PV. Anti-Inflammatory Effects of Vitamin D on Human Immune Cells in the Context of Bacterial Infection. Nutrients. 2016;8(12):806.

43. Cesari M, Penninx BW, Pahor M, Lauretani F, Corsi AM, Rhys Williams G, Guralnik JM, Ferrucci L. Inflammatory markers and physical performance in older persons: the InCHIANTI study. J Gerontol A Biol Sci Med Sci. 2004;59(3):242–8.

44. van Etten E, Mathieu C. Immunoregulation by 1,25-dihydroxyvitamin D3: basic concepts. J Steroid Biochem Mol Biol. 2005;97(1–2):93–101.

45. Chang CI, Chan DC, Kuo KN, Hsiung CA, Chen CY. Vitamin D insufficiency and frailty syndrome in older adults living in a northern Taiwan community. Arch Gerontol Geriatr. 2010;50(Suppl 1):S17–21.

46. Krams T, Cesari M, Guyonnet S, Abellan van Kan G, Cantet C, Vellas B, Rolland Y. Is the 25-Hydroxy-vitamin D serum concentration a good marker of frailty? J Nutr Health Aging. 2016;20(10):1034–9.

47. Lapid MI, Cha SS, Takahashi PY. Vitamin D and depression in geriatric primary care patients. Clin Interv Aging. 2013;8:509–14.

48. Shardell M, D'Adamo C, Alley DE, Miller RR, Hicks GE, Milaneschi Y, Semba RD, Cherubini A, Bandinelli S, Ferrucci L. Serum 25-hydroxyvitamin D, transitions between frailty states, and mortality in older adults: the Invecchiare in chianti study. J Am Geriatr Soc. 2012;60(2):256–64.

49. Shardell M, Hicks GE, Miller RR, Kritchevsky S, Andersen D, Bandinelli S, Cherubini A, Ferrucci L. Association of low vitamin D levels with the frailty syndrome in men and women. J Gerontol A Biol Sci Med Sci. 2009;64(1):69–75.

50. Lau J, Ioannidis JP, Terrin N, Schmid CH, Olkin I. The case of the misleading funnel plot. BMJ. 2006;333(7568):597–600.

6

The importance of trust-based relations and a holistic approach in advance care planning with people with dementia in primary care: a qualitative study

Bram Tilburgs[1]* [iD], Myrra Vernooij-Dassen[1], Raymond Koopmans[2,3,4], Marije Weidema[5], Marieke Perry[2,3,6] and Yvonne Engels[7]

Abstract

Background: ACP enables individuals to define and discuss goals and preferences for future medical treatment and care with family and healthcare providers, and to record these goals and preferences if appropriate. Because general practitioners (GPs) often have long-lasting relationships with people with dementia, GPs seem most suited to initiate ACP. However, ACP with people with dementia in primary care is uncommon. Although several barriers and facilitators to ACP with people with dementia have already been identified in earlier research, evidence gaps still exist. We therefore aimed to further explore barriers and facilitators for ACP with community-dwelling people with dementia.

Methods: A qualitative design, involving all stakeholders in the care for community-dwelling people with dementia, was used. We conducted semi-structured interviews with community dwelling people with dementia and their family caregivers, semi structured interviews by telephone with GPs and a focus group meeting with practice nurses and case managers. Content analysis was used to define codes, categories and themes.

Results: Ten face to face interviews, 10 interviews by telephone and one focus group interview were conducted. From this data, three themes were derived: development of a trust-based relationship, characteristics of an ACP conversation and the primary care setting.
ACP is facilitated by a therapeutic relationship between the person with dementia/family caregiver and the GP built on trust, preferably in the context of home visits. Addressing not only medical but also non-medical issues soon after the dementia diagnosis is given is an important facilitator during conversation. Key barriers were: the wish of some participants to postpone ACP until problems arise, GPs' time restraints, concerns about the documentation of ACP outcomes and concerns about the availability of these outcomes to other healthcare providers.

Conclusions: ACP is facilitated by an open relationship based on trust between the GP, the person with dementia and his/her family caregiver, in which both medical and non-medical issues are addressed. GPs' availability and time restraints are barriers to ACP. Transferring ACP tasks to case managers or practice nurses may contribute to overcoming these barriers.

Keywords: Advance care planning, General practitioner, Dementia, Primary care

* Correspondence: Bram.Tilburgs@radboudumc.nl
[1]Department of IQ healthcare, Radboudumc, Nijmegen, The Netherlands
Full list of author information is available at the end of the article

Background

People with dementia face a progressive decline in functional and mental capacity, with a median survival of 7 to 10 years from the first symptoms of the disease [1–3]. Because of its chronic and life limiting nature and the expected cognitive decline, timely advance care planning (ACP) is advised [4].

A recently published international consensus statement from the European Association of Palliative Care defined ACP as the process which enables people to define goals and preferences for future medical treatment and care, to discuss these goals with family and healthcare providers, and to record and review these preferences if appropriate [5]. Although ACP is recommended by dementia experts, for people with dementia it is uncommon in daily practice and futile medical treatments, avoidable hospitalisations and poor quality of life often occur [2, 4, 6–8].

Research on the effectiveness of ACP for people with dementia is scarce. However, in adult populations, ACP improved the concordance of preferred and delivered care and the communication between patients, their family and healthcare professionals [9, 10]. In frail elderly, ACP reduced anxiety, depression and stress. When ACP was initiated, frail elderly also received less aggressive treatments, were less often admitted to the hospital and more often died in their trusted environment [11]. Dementia-specific research in long-term care settings showed that ACP reduced healthcare costs and hospital admissions [12].

Compared to people with dementia who are institutionalized, community-dwelling people with dementia more often have the mental capacity to express their preferences for future care and to actively participate in ACP. In the Netherlands, over two third of the people with dementia live in the community with general practitioners (GP), often assisted by a practice nurse, as primary healthcare providers [13]. In many cases, case managers are also involved to coordinate different aspects of care and provide emotional support [14]. Because most people with dementia and their family caregivers have long-lasting relationships with their GPs, GPs seem suited and willing to initiate ACP [15, 16]. In primary care however, ACP with people with dementia hardly takes place or takes place very late [12, 17, 18].

Previous research identified uncertainties about the timing, future, evaluation and decisional capacities of people with dementia to contribute to the limited initiation of ACP [19]. A timely start, facilitates ACP, because in the beginning of the disease process when cognitive decline is still mild, participating in decision making is still possible. Involving people with dementia and family caregivers and regularly reviewing and documenting ACP outcomes facilitates ACP as well [19].

Because of the difficult subjects being discussed, it can be assumed that the communication and relationship with the GP are also important facilitators for ACP [20]. Dementia-specific knowledge about this topic is however limited [21, 22]. Previous research also showed that people with dementia favour discussing non-medical issues within ACP [23]. This holistic approach were the psychological, social and spiritual domains, next to the physical domain are included, fits the definition palliative care and the broad definition of ACP as proposed by Rietjens et al. [5, 24]. Evidence on this potential facilitator is however also limited.

As ACP with people with dementia by GPs is still rarely practiced, we aimed to further explore barriers and facilitators concerning this subject. We thereby especially focused on the evidence gaps concerning the communication between the GP and people with dementia, the relationship of GPs with people with dementia and the inclusion of non-medical preferences within ACP.

Methods
Research design

A qualitative design was used in order to reach our research aim [25]. We included people with dementia, living independently in the community or a in a residential home and receiving care from a GP, together with their family caregivers. GPs, practice nurses and case managers were included because they are important stakeholders in the care for people with dementia [26].

Case managers and practice nurses were interviewed during a focus group, which method is particularly useful to explore the participants' knowledge and experiences [27]. Because of their busy time schedule, GPs were interviewed by telephone, as this facilitated flexibility in scheduling the interview. People with dementia, together with their family caregivers, were interviewed face to face in their own homes, as their cognitive decline might impede group discussions.

Recruitment of participants

We recruited GPs by contacting the GP peer review group of the department of primary and community care of the Radboudumc and through the professional contacts of the researchers involved in our study (MP, BT and YE). We strived for a sample of GPs which contained males and females and a variety of experience with dementia care, as both characteristics influence general practitioners' attitudes towards dementia [28].

People with dementia, their family caregivers, case managers and practice nurses were recruited during several community meetings for people with dementia and family caregivers (Alzheimer café's) in the region of Nijmegen and through the professional contacts of one of the researchers (MP). We decided to interview people with dementia accompanied by their family caregivers because earlier research showed that they prefer making decisions about future care together [23, 29]. Furthermore, we considered it very important for participating people with dementia to feel safe discussing such a delicate topic. GPs and case managers and practice nurses could participate if they were involved in the care for people with dementia. Potential participants were informed by letter about the study and were requested to sign an informed consent before the interview.

Data collection

The main researcher (BT), a male PhD candidate, psychologist and nurse, trained in conducting and analysing qualitative interviews, was present during all interviews. Two additional interviewers were: a female researcher in palliative care, trained in conducting and analysing qualitative interviews (YE) and a female medical student, with no prior experience in qualitative research (MW). No relationship existed with the respondents prior to the interviews.

The interviews with the GPs were conducted by one researcher (BT). The face to face interviews with people with dementia and family caregivers were conducted by two researchers (BT, MW) as was the focus group (BT, YE). Field notes were made during each interview and participants gave their consent to audio-tape the interviews.

A similar topic guide was used for all three forms of interviewing. This guide was developed during several sessions with the members of the research team (BT, MP, YE, MVD, RK) and pilot tested with a family caregiver and a person with dementia (Additional file 1). All people with dementia and family caregivers received a written summary of their interview and were invited to give comments.

Data analysis

All interviews were transcribed verbatim. Data analysis started directly after the first interview using content analysis [30]. After each interview had been coded, the topic list was adapted where required. Researchers independently open coded all interviews within each group of stakeholders (people with dementia/family care givers: BT and MW; GPs/case managers and practice nurses: BT and EB or RT or PL). Results were compared until consensus was reached. In case of disagreement, this was discussed with a senior researcher (YE, MP). After the last interview within each group of stakeholders, the researchers made an affinity diagram to cluster codes and define categories and themes [30, 31]. All data were then combined to create definitive categories and themes. Because we wanted to focus on new findings, codes already thoroughly described in earlier research were marked. The codes concerning new findings will

be described in the results section. The codes already known from earlier research will only be presented in a table.

Ethical consent

The study was approved by the research ethics committee (CMO) of the region Arnhem-Nijmegen in accordance with the Medical Research Involving Human Subjects Acts and the declaration of Helsinki (NL52613.091.15). Anonymity was assured by removing all participant information that could lead to identification from the transcripts.

Results

GPs aged 31 to 64 years and their work experience varied between one to 33 years. Sixty percent of the GPs was female. The number of patients within each practice ranged between 1700 and 7370 and the percentage of persons with dementia in their practice varied between 0.1 and 10%. One GP was trained as an expert GP elderly care. Case managers/practice nurses aged 46 to 63 years. Their work experience ranged between 5 and 25 years with a case load between 55 and 75 people with dementia. All were female and trained in dementia care. People with dementia aged 79 to 90 years and 70% was male. The time since diagnosis ranged from 6 months to 6 years. Family caregivers aged 24 to 85 years and 77% was female. Nine people with dementia lived in their own home with their family caregiver. One lived in a residential home, separately from her family caregiver.

One focus group of 90 min with case mangers and practice nurses was conducted. The interviews by telephone with GPs lasted 30 min. The interviews with people with dementia and family caregivers lasted 90 min. With the GPs, people with dementia and family caregivers, no new codes emerged after eight interviews. To confirm saturation two additional interviews were conducted. In three interviews with people with dementia and their family caregivers, an extra family caregiver was present. One person with dementia passed away after we already made the appointment for the interview. Because the widow of this person explicitly asked to participate and seemed capable to express her husband's view as well as her own, we decided to keep her included in this study. Field notes were made during each interview and participants gave their consent to audio-tape the interviews.

Content analysis revealed barriers and facilitators for initiating ACP by GPs with people with dementia in three themes: development of a trust based therapeutic relationship, characteristics of an ACP conversation, the primary care setting and eight categories: the relationship with the general practitioner, home visits, starting ACP, stakeholder involvement, discussing goals, evaluation and documentation, time availability, organisation of the general practice. These themes, categories and codes are displayed in Table 1.

Several codes within the categories of the relationship with the GP, starting ACP, stakeholder involvement and evaluation and documentation were identical to barriers and facilitators described in earlier research (Table 1) and were therefore not described in the result section.

Theme 1: Development of a trust based therapeutic relationship
The relationship with the general practitioner
Facilitators GPs, people with dementia and family caregivers stated that it is important that the GP knows the person with dementia personally, is empathic, supportive and provides information respectfully. People with dementia and their family caregivers added that, when discussing preferences for the future, they want their GP to listen to them, is easy to talk to and knows what they find important in life.

"A connection, an invisible connection, but that is a feeling, a feeling you have that you are at ease because she (GP) is there. He (person with dementia) did not have to be afraid anymore. He did not have to worry. He did not have to be nervous If he couldn't remember something, well... he could get his thoughts of his mind so to speak..... There was a trusting relationship which was beautiful to see" (family caregiver, interview 2).

Barriers Several family caregivers and people with dementia stated that their GP trivialized their situation, was too distant and did not listen to them. This made them hesitant to discuss sensitive topics. GPs, people with dementia, family caregivers and case managers and practice nurses also found that GPs had too little contact with people with dementia and their family caregivers. According to some GPs, having infrequent contacts was due to either a capable family caregiver or the person with dementia living in a residential home.

Home visits
Facilitators People with dementia, family caregivers, case managers and practice nurses preferred to have ACP at the home of the person with dementia. In this trusted environment, people with dementia are more at ease to talk about sensitive topics and feel less hurried by the GP's time schedule. People with dementia, family caregivers, case managers and practice nurses found that during such home visits, GPs get more insight in the person with dementia's living situation.

"I would prefer to have the conversation here (at home) and not at an impersonal office. The home environment is different; than you can sit in your own chair and communicate about personal topics" (family caregivers, interview 9).

According to the GPs, ACP conversations ideally should take place at the location preferred by the person with dementia and family caregiver.

Barriers Case managers and practice nurses and GPs doubted if home visits for ACP would be feasible because of the GP's busy schedule. This corresponded with the fact that, according to most people with dementia and family caregivers their GPs rarely conduct home visits.

Theme 2: Characteristics of an ACP conversation
Starting ACP
Facilitators Some GPs, people with dementia, family caregivers and all case managers and practice nurses wanted to start ACP immediately after the diagnosis was given. Starting early has the advantage of being able to choose the moment of initiation and ACP under stressful circumstances can be avoided.

"Yes, uh.... it also depends on the co-morbidities but for me pretty soon... That is difficult because what is pretty soon... But I would say that from diagnosis, you want to start to discuss what peoples wishes are....." (general practitioner, interview 2).

Other GPs also stated that dyads should first be given time after the disclosure of the diagnosis, because this is often a difficult experience. Case managers and practice nurses, people with dementia and family caregivers added that people with dementia and family caregivers should be given time before an ACP conversation to think about what they want to discuss.

According to several GPs, some types of information received from other healthcare professionals or family caregivers could trigger them to start ACP. According to some people with dementia, ACP is initiated sooner when a wish for euthanasia was expressed. One GP added that using the Surprise Question (a question the general practitioner asks himself in silence to identify those patients with an increased chance to die or deteriorate within a year) stimulated his proactive behaviour.

Barriers Part of the GPs, people with dementia and family carers only wanted to discuss preferences for the future when problems actually arise. Some GPs said to postpone ACP until the cognitive deterioration becomes problematic, and for that reason monitored the person

Table 1 Themes, categories and codes

Themes	Categories	Codes	
		Facilitators	Barriers
Development of a trust based therapeutic relationship	The relationship with the GP	The GP knows what PWD find important in life (PWD)	The GP is to distant (FC,PWD)
		The GP is easy to talk to (PWD)	The GP does not listen to PWD (FC)
		An open relationship with the GP is important (PWD)	The GP has little contact with PWD (PWD, FC,GP, CM)
		A trusting relationship with the GP is important (CM, FC, PWD, GP)	The GP trivialises the situation (PWD, FC)
		The GP listens to the PWD (PWD, FC)	
		The GP knows the PWD/FC personally (PWD, FC, GP)	
		The GP provides empathic support (FC, PWD, GP)	
		The GP understands the PWD (PWD)	
		Providing information respectful is important (PWD, GP)	
		The GP provides the right information (PWD)[a] [52]	
		Good communication makes ACP easier (GP)[a] [21, 22]	
		A good relationship with the GP is important (PWD, FC)[a] [21]	
	Home visits	ACP should take place at home (CM, FC, PWD)	The GP does not conduct home visits (FC, PWD)
		ACP should take place at a quiet moment (FC, PWD)	The GP does not know the living situation (CM, FC)
		More time available during home visits (FC)	
		By conducting home visits, the GP knows the living situation (CM, FC)	
		ACP should be held at the PWD's preferred location (GP)	
Characteristics of an ACP conversation	Starting ACP	ACP starts after providing the diagnosis (GP)	Not all PWD/FC want ACP (PWD, GP)
		ACP should not start under stress (CM, GP)	GP's lack knowledge/experience of ACP (GP)
		PWD/FC should first cope with the diagnosis before the start of ACP (GP)	The diagnosis is not always clear (GP)
		ACP should start when the PWD/FC states the need to do so (GP)	GP doesn't take the initiative to start ACP (CM, FC, PWD)
		FC takes the initiative to start ACP (FC)	Healthcare professionals find discussing end of life issues difficult (CM)
		Because of a wish for euthanasia, ACP is started (PWD)	Dementia does not give complaints (PWD)
		PWD must be followed from diagnosis on (GP)	Start ACP when problems arise (CM, GP, PWD, FC)
		Information from family and healthcare providers stimulates the start of ACP (GP)	*The assessment of decisional competency is difficult*[a] [46]
		Surprise Question helps to start ACP (GP)	
		ACP should start early because of the cognitive decline (GP, FC, PWD, CM)[a] [21, 22, 45–47]	
		GPs should take the initiative for ACP (GP, CM, PWD, FC)[a] [16, 21, 22]	
		The GP's positive attitude stimulates the	

Table 1 Themes, categories and codes (Continued)

Themes	Categories	Codes	
		Facilitators	Barriers
		start of ACP (GP)[a] [22]	
	Stakeholder involvement	Provide choices instead of open questions (GP)	ACP is confronting for PWD (GP)
		ACP should not be confronting (GP)	Religion limits discussions about future care (GP)
		ACP content must be adjusted to PWD level of understanding (FC, GP)	Social status influences ACP (GP)
		All healthcare providers should be present during ACP (GP)	PWD's/FC's IQ and self-knowledge influences ACP (GP)
		ACP with the FC and GP without PWD sometimes takes place (FC)	Multiple healthcare providers present during ACP limits ACP (GP)
		End of life decisions are made together (FC, PWD)[a] [45, 53, 54]	Preferences of FC and PWD can differ (CM, GP)
		FC must present within ACP (CM, FC, PWD, GP)[a] [45, 53, 54]	ACP is difficult to explain (GP)
		FC makes ACP decisions (PWD, FC)[a] [45, 53]	*The assessment of decisional competency is difficult (GP)*[a] [46]
		PWD must be present when ACP is discussed (GP, FC, CM, PWD)[a] [45, 53–55]	
Characteristics of an ACP conversation	Discussing goals	PWD's preferences are the starting point of ACP (GP CM)	Not all problems can be discussed upfront (GP)
		FC respects PWD choices (FC)	
		PWD/FC want to be able to prepare ACP (CM, PWD, FC)	
		ACP decisions provide clarity and peace (FC, PWD, GP)	
		The GP sometimes must be authoritarian (GP)	
		ACP should deal with current issues (GP)	
		Supporting FCs should be discussed during ACP (FC)	
		Medical subjects should be discussed during ACP (CM, PWD,FC)	
		social subjects should be discussed during ACP (PWD,FC)	
		PWD know what they want for their future (FC, PWD)	
		ACP prevents moments of crisis and over treatment (GP)	
		ACP stimulates autonomy (GP)	
		Through ACP the GP can explain care possibilities (GP)	
	Evaluation and documentation	ACP should not be evaluated to often (CM)	ACP documentation not always available for all stakeholders (GP, FC, PWD, CM)
		ACP must be evaluated regularly (GP)[a] [45, 54]	ACP decisions are considered final (FC)
		ACP outcomes must be documented and available for all stakeholders (GP, CM)[a] [21, 45–47]	The PWD's current will counts (CM, GP, FC)
		ACP must be a cyclical process (PWD,FC,CM, GP)[a] [45, 54]	*When to evaluate ACP is unclear (GP)*[a] [54]
The primary care setting	Time availability	The GP should take enough time for ACP (FC)	ACP consultations are often to short (GP, MC, PWD, FC)

Table 1 Themes, categories and codes *(Continued)*

Themes	Categories	Codes	
		Facilitators	Barriers
		The GP is easily available (FC)	GP has limited time for ACP (FC)
		ACP saves time in the long term (GP)	Because of limited time only medical subjects are discussed (PWD, FC, CM)
			The GP is rushed during ACP (FC)
			ACP doesn't save time in the long term (GP)
			ACP takes time in the short term (GP)
			Planning an ACP conversation is sometimes difficult (GP)
	Organisation of the general practice	regular appointments with GP/CM/PN facilitates ACP (FC, PWD, GP)	Casemanager is often involved to late (GP, CM, PWD, FC)
		CM/PN discusses medical and social subjects (FC)	PWD have limited contact with their CM/PN (FC)
		CM/PN has more knowledge of living situation compared to GP (FC,GP, PWD)	PN/CM cannot discuss medical issues (GP)
		CM/PN has more knowledge of dementia compared to GP (CM, PWD)	Inadequate reimbursement limits ACP (GP)
		The therapeutic relationship with the CM/PN facilitates ACP (PWD, FC)	
		ACP can also be provided by a CM/PN (FC)	
		GPs and CMs/PNs should have regular contact (FC, GP)	
		Specialized training in dementia/elderly care stimulates ACP (GP)	
		PN/CM can support GP in ACP process (GP)	
		GP should coordinate ACP (GP)	
		Special care programs for dementia facilitate ACP (GP)	
		ACP should be structurally implemented (GP)	

GP stated by general practitioner, *CM* stated by casemanager/practice nurse, *PWD* stated by person with dementia, *FC* stated by family caregiver
[a]codes which already have been described in earlier research

with dementia after the diagnosis had been provided. A lack of knowledge and experience with ACP, an unclear diagnosis and the fact that ACP is a difficult concept to explain were other reasons to postpone ACP, as mentioned by GPs. Finally, according to case managers and practice nurses, GPs do not initiate ACP as they fear talking about difficult subjects.

Stakeholder involvement
Facilitators Some GPs wanted all healthcare professionals involved in the care for a person with dementia to participate in ACP so that all knew what had been discussed and decided. Some GPs also stated that, if the person with dementia approved, ACP consultations sometimes took place without the person with dementia. For example, when the person with dementia denied or

did not accept the dementia diagnosis. Family caregivers and GPs found that, in order to stimulate involvement of people with dementia, the GP should tailor ACP to the cognitive level of the person with dementia and make sure that the conversation is not confronting. When GPs asked closed instead of open questions, participation of people with dementia within ACP also becomes easier.

Barriers Some GPs mentioned that people with dementia's and family caregivers' low social status, low IQ, limited self-knowledge or strong religious beliefs sometimes made involving dyads in ACP difficult. According to some GPs, the presence of multiple family caregivers during ACP was a disturbance and therefore only wanted ACP with the person with dementia and their family caregiver.

Discussing goals

Facilitators According to GPs, case managers and practice nurses, people with dementia's life values, wishes and goals must be the starting point of ACP and such a conversation should therefore begin with what they find important in life. People with dementia, family caregivers, case managers and practice nurses explicitly mentioned that during ACP not only medical (e.g. do not resuscitate statements, hospital admissions) but also non-medical subjects (e.g. daytime activities, social contacts, what bothers him or her at this moment) should be discussed. Case managers and practice nurses, people with dementia and family caregivers agreed that if people with dementia express a wish for euthanasia, this topic should be addressed as well.

> "We discussed the human aspect..........but also if we can still keep on living in this house and if more care has to be provided. He (person with dementia) doesn't want to move........ He himself is the driving force behind this (ACP). He wants to anticipate..." (family caregiver, interview 8).

The discussion of goals had additional advantages. According to GPs, it gave them the opportunity to explain possible care options and in addition provide clarity, peace, stimulate mourning and prevent overtreatment, which often happened when decisions had to be made all of a sudden in moments of crisis. Some GPs added that discussing goals fostered autonomy. However, sometimes a paternalistic approach was found necessary.

Barriers If the preferences of people with dementia and family carers differed, GPs, case managers and practice nurses found the discussion of goals more difficult. GPs also expressed that it is not always possible to openly discuss all potential future problems.

Evaluation and documentation

Facilitators In the opinion of case managers and practice nurses, reviewing ACP too often made it seem artificial. In their opinion, reviewing ACP every 6 to 12 months was sufficient.

Barriers Most family caregivers and GPs agreed that the current wishes of people with dementia should be leading, even if this would contradict earlier decisions. One family caregiver considered ACP decisions to be binding and therefore found ACP evaluation unnecessary.

People with dementia, family caregivers, GPs and case managers and practice nurses doubted if important ACP outcomes are documented in a structured way by GPs and raised concerns about the availability of such outcomes for other healthcare professionals.

Theme 3: The primary care setting
Time availability

Facilitators According to family caregivers, the GP should be easily available and should take enough time for ACP consultations. According to part of the GPs, although ACP requires short term time investments, it saves time in the long run.

Barriers All interviewees found the usual duration of a consultation too short for ACP. Consequently, according to people with dementia, family caregivers and case managers and practice nurses, GPs mainly address medical subjects and are rushed during ACP.

> "When we came in, the first thing she (the GP) said was; I don't have much time and then she said: good afternoon. She sat down and started to fire all sorts of questions at my mother. My mother didn't know what was going on... At a certain moment I said; stop!.... This doesn't make her happy at all." (family caregiver, interview 9).

According to part of the GPs, ACP demands short term time investments while time is scarce and they were not convinced that ACP would save time in the long term. Moreover, some GPs stated that they do not have time to plan and regularly review ACP decisions.

Organisation of the general practice

Facilitators GPs found guidelines and the use of specialised care programs for dementia useful. These helped them to initiate ACP in a structured manner. The involvement of a case manager and practice nurse could further accommodate ACP. According to case managers and practice nurses and family caregivers, case managers and practice nurses have more knowledge of dementia. They also have more time to plan, prepare and carry out ACP than GPs do. Case managers and practice nurses, compared to GPs, also have more opportunities to monitor people with dementia and family caregivers and thereby identify problems early.

> Quote: "We use a certain score and when somebody is frail,......our practice nurse visits them at home.... more in a general sense.... to see...... how are you doing? What are the problems now, but also what do you expect in the future?" (general practitioner, interview 6).

People with dementia and family caregivers confirmed this and added that regular contact and the therapeutic relationship they develop with a case manager and practice nurse helped them to discuss preferences for future care.

Barriers Some GPs stated that case managers and practice nurses cannot make medical decisions and therefore can only partly conduct ACP. Some GPs stated that they occasionally forgot to make use of a case manager and practice nurse. This was confirmed by case managers and practice nurses who as a result were often involved late.

Difficulties with reimbursing ACP within the Dutch healthcare system were also mentioned as a problem by GPs. Solving this would stimulate them to initiate ACP, also because some believe that ACP will reduce healthcare costs.

Discussion

In this study we aimed to further explore barriers and facilitators for ACP with people with dementia by GPs, with a focus on the evidence gaps concerning the communication between the GP and people with dementia, the relationship of GPs with people with dementia and the inclusion of non-medical preferences within ACP. Newly found facilitators are: having a relationship with the GP that is built on trust and mutual understanding, and the discussion of ACP in the comfort of people with dementia's homes. Explicitly addressing non-medical issues in ACP discussions, with a focus on discussing people with dementia's current and short-term goals was considered a facilitator by all stakeholders. The involvement of a case managers and practice nurse also facilitates ACP. GPs' lack of time is an important barrier for ACP. To two other barriers known from earlier research nuances could be added: Some participants wanted ACP to start early, while others wanted to wait until problems actuality arise. Stakeholders raised concerns about the availability of ACP documentation to all professionals involved. They were willing to review ACP but not often.

The importance of the relationship with the GP, as stressed by the participants in this study, is in line with earlier research in primary care [32]. Patients who suffer from more severe diseases or who have problems with psychosocial or existential impact, such as people with dementia, appraise their relationship with the GP as more important [33]. Unfortunately, the focus during consultations still seems to be on treatment compliance with little attention to social, psychological or spiritual issues, even when advance directives are discussed [34, 35]. Particularly in dementia, with its high psychosocial and existential burden and specific relational and communicational needs, this can be considered an omission [3, 36, 37].

As shown in our results and in a systematic review on GP communication, home visits and taking time are important when difficult subjects are discussed [38]. When GPs take more time, more psychosocial problems are attended and patient satisfaction rises [39]. However, it is also known that GPs are busy, and time per consultation is limited. This time restraints seems an important reason for the limited number of home visits, for the GPs' main focus on medical problems and for the inadequate assessment of care needs [40–42]. The lack of ACP by GPs therefore seems, at least partly, caused by how GPs are organized.

Recommendations for future practice

Participants in our study mentioned the use of case managers or practice nurses as a possible solution for overcoming problems concerning the development of a therapeutic relationship and the available time. Case managers and practice nurses have more opportunities to visit people with dementia and thereby develop a therapeutic relation which seems so important [43]. When using collaborative care models, in which case managers or practice nurses take on certain tasks of the GP, regular consultations between GPs and case managers and practice nurses are advised and division of tasks regarding ACP should be explicitly addressed [44]. This facilitates a combined medical, psychosocial and spiritual and thus holistic approach. Also, when multiple disciplines are involved, it is essential that preferences for future care are clearly documented and made available to all [21, 45–47]. Because case managers and practice nurses also have time constraints their caseload must be monitored [43].

In recent years ACP has shifted from a document driven conversation where mainly options for medical treatments and end-of-life preferences were discussed, to a broader scope where the physical, psychosocial and spiritual domains are all included [5, 48]. Previous research and this paper showed that a broad approach to ACP including non-medical issues is a facilitator for people with dementia. When their valued abilities or activities are used to justify their choices, their participation in ACP can be established despite of their cognitive decline [29]. This holistic approach which starts with the person's with dementia current wishes and concerns, therefore contributes to their autonomy and can also be used to guide further decision making about future care [49, 50]. ACP then is extended to something more than just a 'checkbox' for medical decisions. It becomes an open encounter between people with dementia, family caregivers and healthcare professionals during which a wide array of preferences concerning future care can be discussed that may contribute to living well with dementia [51].

Strengths and limitations

The inclusion of all important stakeholders involved in ACP with people with dementia in primary care is the main strength of this study. By integrating the findings from different perspectives, robust and all-embracing insights were built [25]. As we chose to interview people with dementia and family caregiver dyads in their own homes, we were able to discuss delicate topics in their trusted environment without any rush or disturbance. This gave the participants the opportunity to provide in depth information which enriched our data and conclusions.

The study also has some limitations. Because of recruitment difficulties, the number of case managers and practice nurses participating in this is study was limited and we were not able to conduct ideal purposive sampling. As a result, some beliefs or experiences may not be represented in our data [25]. However, as we reached saturation in the interviews with people with dementia, family caregiver dyads and GPs, and no new themes emerged within the focus group with case managers and practice nurses, we assume that all themes concerning our research aim were exposed.

The fact that we choose to conduct the interviews with people with dementia accompanied by their family caregiver may have influenced our study outcomes. As our results show, their preferences for future care sometimes differ. For that reason both parties may possibly have expressed some different views when interviewed alone. This therefore might be addressed during future research. However, our interview strategy is similar to the situation in daily practice, in which GPs usually discuss future care with patients and informal caregivers together.

Our study outcomes may also be influenced by the specific region in which we conducted our research. This may therefore also be addressed during future research.

Conclusion

When people with dementia and family caregivers discuss preferences for future care with their GP, home visits, an open relation built on trust and addressing non-medical issues, particularly those in the near future, are key facilitators to ACP.

GPs' busy time schedule is an important barrier. Case managers and practice nurses have more opportunities to regularly conduct home visits, gain insight in the living situation and to start an open trust-build relationship with people with dementia and their family caregivers. This provides them with the opportunity to use a goal-oriented approach and discuss a broad range of topics. Collaborative care models might therefore help to overcome the time barrier and contribute to exploiting the newly found facilitators to ACP and contribute to living well with dementia.

Abbreviations
ACP: Advance care planning; GP: General practitioner

Acknowledgements
The authors would like to thank: Renee Tuinte, Petra Lohof and Eline Bijl, form the Radboud University, Nijmegen, the Netherlands, for their contributions to this study.

Funding
The author(s) disclose receipt of the following financial support for the research, authorship, and/or publication of this article: This study was supported by the ZonMw Memorabel program, project number 79-73305-98-420.

Authors' contributions
BT contributed to the conception and design, data analysis and data interpretation, writing of the manuscript. MW contributed to the data analyses and data interpretation and writing of the manuscript. YE contributed to the design, data analyses and data interpretation and writing of the manuscript. MP: contributed to the design, data analyses and data interpretation and writing of the manuscript. MvD contributed to the design and writing of the manuscript. RK contributed to the design and writing of the manuscript. All authors read and approved the final manuscript.

Competing interests
The authors declare that they have no competing interests.

Author details
[1]Department of IQ healthcare, Radboudumc, Nijmegen, The Netherlands. [2]Department of Primary and Community Care, Radboudumc, Nijmegen, The Netherlands. [3]Radboudumc Alzheimer Centre, Nijmegen, The Netherlands. [4]Joachim en Anna, Centre for Specialized Geriatric Care, Nijmegen, The Netherlands. [5]Department of Medical Oncology, Radboudumc, Nijmegen, The Netherlands. [6]Department of Geriatric Medicine, Radboudumc, Nijmegen, The Netherlands. [7]Department of Anesthesiology, Pain and Palliative Medicine, Radboudumc, Nijmegen, The Netherlands.

References
1. Todd S, et al. Survival in dementia and predictors of mortality: a review. Int J Geriatr Psychiatry. 2013;28(11):1109–24.
2. Mitchell SL, et al. The clinical course of advanced dementia. N Engl J Med. 2009;361(16):1529–38.
3. World Health Organization. Dementia fact sheet. 2017. [cited 2017 28-12-2017]; Available from: http://www.who.int/mediacentre/factsheets/fs362/en/.
4. van der Steen JT, et al. White paper defining optimal palliative care in older people with dementia: a Delphi study and recommendations from the European Association for Palliative Care. Palliat Med. 2014;28(3):197–209.
5. Rietjens JAC, et al. Definition and recommendations for advance care planning: an international consensus supported by the European Association for Palliative Care. Lancet Oncol. 2017;18(9):e543–51.
6. Blasi ZV, Hurley AC, Volicer L. End-of-life Care in Dementia: a review of problems, prospects, and solutions in practice. J Am Med Dir Assoc. 2002;3(2):57–65.
7. van der Steen JT. Dying with dementia: what we know after more than a decade of research. J Alzheimers Dis. 2010;22(1):37–55.
8. Hendriks SA, et al. Dying with dementia: symptoms, treatment, and quality of life in the last week of life. J Pain Symptom Manag. 2014;47(4):710–20.
9. Houben CH, et al. Efficacy of advance care planning: a systematic review and meta-analysis. J Am Med Dir Assoc. 2014;15(7):477–89.
10. Tamayo-Velazquez MI, et al. Interventions to promote the use of advance directives: an overview of systematic reviews. Patient Educ Couns. 2010;80(1):10–20.
11. Detering KM, et al. The impact of advance care planning on end of life care in elderly patients: randomised controlled trial. BMJ. 2010;340:c1345.

12. Robinson L, et al. A systematic review of the effectiveness of advance care planning interventions for people with cognitive impairment and dementia. Age Ageing. 2012;41(December 2011):263–9.

13. Alzheimer Nederland. Cijfers en feiten over dementie. 2015. Retrieved from hhttps://www.alzheimer-nederland.nl/sites/default/files/directupload/factsheet-dementie-algemeen.pdf. Last visited on 10-11-2015.

14. Reilly S, et al. Case management approaches to home support for people with dementia. Cochrane Database Syst Rev. 2015;1:CD008345.

15. Schers H, et al. Familiarity with a GP and patients' evaluations of care. A cross-sectional study. Fam Pract. 2005;22(1):15–9.

16. Brazil K, et al. General practitioners perceptions on advance care planning for patients living with dementia. BMC Palliat Care. 2015;14(1):14.

17. Abarshi E, et al. Discussing end-of-life issues in the last months of life: a nationwide study among general practitioners. J Palliat Med. 2011;14(3):323–30.

18. Evans N, et al. End-of-life care in general practice: a cross-sectional, retrospective survey of 'cancer', 'organ failure' and 'old-age/dementia' patients. Palliat Med. 2014;28(7):965–75.

19. Tilburgs B, et al. Barriers and facilitators for GPs in dementia advance care planning: a systematic integrative review. PLoS One. 2018;13(6):e0198535.

20. De Vleminck A, et al. Barriers and facilitators for general practitioners to engage in advance care planning: a systematic review. Scand J Prim Health Care. 2013;31(4):215–26.

21. Poppe M, Burleigh S, Banerjee S. Qualitative evaluation of advanced care planning in early dementia (ACP-ED). PLoS ONE. 2013;8(4):e60412.

22. De Vleminck A, et al. Barriers to advance care planning in cancer, heart failure and dementia patients: a focus group study on general practitioners' views and experiences. PLoS ONE. 2014;9(1):e84905.

23. Hamann J, et al. Patient participation in medical and social decisions in Alzheimer's disease. J Am Geriatr Soc. 2011;59(11):2045–52.

24. European Association for Palliative Care. 2010. [cited 2018 19.06.2018]; Available from: http://www.eapcnet.eu/Themes/AbouttheEAPC/DefinitionandAims.aspx.

25. Kuper A. An introduction to reading and appraising qualitative research. BMJ. 2008;337(7666):404.

26. Robinson L, et al. Primary care and dementia: 2. Long-term care at home: psychosocial interventions, information provision, carer support and case management. Int J Geriatr Psychiatry. 2010;25(7):657–64.

27. Kitzinger J. Qualitative research. Introducing focus groups. BMJ. 1995;311(7000):299–302.

28. Turner S, et al. General practitioners' knowledge, confidence and attitudes in the diagnosis and management of dementia. Age Ageing. 2004;33(5):461–7.

29. Karel MJ, et al. Reasoning in the capacity to make medical decisions: the consideration of values. J Clin Ethics. 2010;21(1):58–71.

30. Graneheim UH, Lundman B. Qualitative content analysis in nursing research: concepts, procedures and measures to achieve trustworthiness. Nurse Educ Today. 2004;24(2):105–12.

31. Johnson JK, et al. Conducting a multicentre and multinational qualitative study on patient transitions. BMJ Qual Saf. 2012;21(Suppl 1):i22–8.

32. Wensing M, et al. A systematic review of the literature on patient priorities for general practice care. Part 1: description of the research domain. Soc Sci Med. 1998;47(10):1573–88.

33. Delgado A, et al. Patient expectations are not always the same. J Epidemiol Community Health. 2008;62(5):427–34.

34. Dooley J, Bailey C, McCabe R. Communication in healthcare interactions in dementia: a systematic review of observational studies. Int Psychogeriatr. 2015;27(8):1277–300.

35. Tulsky JA, et al. Opening the black box: How do physicians communicate about advance directives? Ann Intern Med. 1998;129:441–9.

36. Chiao CY, Wu HS, Hsiao CY. Caregiver burden for informal caregivers of patients with dementia: a systematic review. Int Nurs Rev. 2015;62(3):340–50.

37. Lloyd A, et al. Physical, social, psychological and existential trajectories of loss and adaptation towards the end of life for older people living with frailty: a serial interview study. BMC Geriatr. 2016;16(1):176.

38. Slort W, et al. Perceived barriers and facilitators for general practitioner–patient communication in palliative care: a systematic review. Palliat Med. 2011;25(6):613–29.

39. Howie JG, et al. Long to short consultation ratio: a proxy measure of quality of care for general practice. Br J Gen Pract. 1991;41(343):48–54.

40. Bruce DG, et al. Communication problems between dementia carers and general practitioners: effect on access to community support services. Med J Aust. 2002;177(4):186–8.

41. Schoenmakers B, Buntinx F, Delepeleire J. What is the role of the general practitioner towards the family caregiver of a community-dwelling demented relative? Scand J Prim Health Care. 2009;27(1):31–40.

42. van Hout H, et al. General practitioners on dementia: tasks, practices and obstacles. Patient Educ Couns. 1999;39(2):219–25.

43. Backhouse A, et al. Stakeholders perspectives on the key components of community-based interventions coordinating care in dementia: a qualitative systematic review. BMC Health Serv Res. 2017;17(1):767.

44. McInnes S, et al. An integrative review of facilitators and barriers influencing collaboration and teamwork between general practitioners and nurses working in general practice. J Adv Nurs. 2015;71(9):1973–85.

45. Dickinson C, et al. Planning for tomorrow whilst living for today: the views of people with dementia and their families on advance care planning. Int Psychogeriatr. 2013;25(12):2011–21.

46. Robinson L, et al. A qualitative study: Professionals' experiences of advance care planning in dementia and palliative care, 'a good idea in theory but'. Palliat Med. 2013;27(5):401–8.

47. Hirschman KB, Kapo JM, Karlawish JH. Identifying the factors that facilitate or hinder advance planning by persons with dementia. Alzheimer Dis Assoc Disord. 2008;22(3):293.

48. Romer AL, Hammes BJ. Communication, trust, and making choices: advance care planning four years on. J Palliat Med. 2004;7(2):335–40.

49. Oresanya LB, Lyons WL, Finlayson E. Preoperative assessment of the older patient: a narrative review. JAMA. 2014;311(20):2110–20.

50. van de Pol MH, et al. Expert and patient consensus on a dynamic model for shared decision-making in frail older patients. Patient Educ Couns. 2016;99(6):1069–77.

51. Delden JJM. The goal of advance care planning (het doel van advance care planning). Ned Tijdschr Geneeskd. 2017;45

52. Stirling C, et al. A qualitative study of professional and client perspectives on information flows and decision aid use. BMC Med Inform Decis Mak. 2012;12:26.

53. Livingston G, et al. Making decisions for people with dementia who lack capacity: qualitative study of family carers in UK. BMJ. 2010;341:c4184.

54. Horton-Deutsch S, Twigg P, Evans R. Health care decision-making of persons with dementia. Int J Soc Res Pract. 2007;6(1):105–20.

55. Dening KH, Jones L, Sampson EL. Preferences for end-of-life care: a nominal group study of people with dementia and their family carers. Palliat Med. 2013;27(5):409–17.

7

Evaluating the social fitness Programme for older people with cognitive problems and their caregivers: lessons learned from a failed trial

H W Donkers[1,2]* ⓘ, D J Van der Veen[1,2], S Teerenstra[3], M J Vernooij-Dassen[1,2], M W G Nijhuis-vander Sanden[1,4] and M J L Graff[1,2,4]

Abstract

Background: This process evaluation article describes the lessons learned from a failed trial which aimed to assess effectiveness of the tailor-made, multidisciplinary Social Fitness Programme to improve social participation of community-dwelling older people with cognitive problems (clients) and their caregivers (couples).

Methods: A process evaluation was performed to get insight in 1) the implementation of the intervention, 2) the context of intervention delivery from professionals' point of view, and 3) the potential impact of intervention delivery from participants' perspectives. Data was gathered using mixed-methods: questionnaires, focus group discussions, interviews, medical records.

Results: *1) Implementation.* High study decline (65,3%) was mainly caused by a lack of internal motivation to increase social participation expressed by clients. 17 couples participated, however, intervention delivery was insufficient. *2) Context.* Barriers during intervention delivery were most often related to client (changing needs), caregiver (increased burden) and health professional factors (delivery of integrated care lacked routine). *3) Impact* Qualitative analyses revealed participants to be satisfied with intervention delivery, we were unable to capture these results through our primary outcome measure.

Conclusions: This process evaluation revealed the Social Fitness study did not fit in three ways. First, framing the intervention on social participation promotion was as threatening to clients. The feeling of being unable to adequately contribute to social interactions seemed to be causing embarrassment. Second, the intervention seemed to be too complex to implement in the way it was designed. Third, there is a tension between the offering of a personalised tailor-made intervention and evaluation through a fixed study design.

Keywords: Cognitive functioning, Process evaluation, Psychosocial care, Social health, Social participation

* Correspondence: Hanneke.Donkers@radboudumc.nl
[1]Radboud university medical center, Radboud Institute for Health Sciences, IQ healthcare, P.O. Box 9101, 6500, HB, Nijmegen, The Netherlands
[2]Radboud university medical center, Donders Institute for Brain, Cognition and Behaviour, Radboudumc Alzheimer Center, Nijmegen, The Netherlands
Full list of author information is available at the end of the article

Background

Social participation is a central theme in psychosocial dementia care [1], and as part of social health it is considered important for successful and healthy ageing [2, 3]. The definition for social participation used in this study is: involvement in social activities in which there is interaction with others in the society which makes one feels valued, attached to the community and gives meaning to someone's life [4–6]. Six levels of involvement are: 1) doing an activity in preparation for connecting with others, 2) being with others, 3) interacting with others without doing a specific activity with them, 4) doing an activity with others, 5) helping others, and 6) contributing to society [4]. Social participation is a potentially modifiable factor, however, effective person-centred interventions focused on social participation promotion for people with cognitive problems and their caregivers are scarce [7, 8]. We therefore developed the Social Fitness Programme (SF Programme); an intervention aimed at enabling social participation [9].

The SF Programme is a tailor-made multidisciplinary intervention combining guidance by an occupational therapist (OT; applying the evidence-based COTiD-intervention [10, 11]) physiotherapist (PT; through the evidence-based person-centred Coach2Move-protocol [12–14]) and welfare professional [9]. The SF Programme combines active treatment methods, including exercises and training of bodily functions and the effective use of skills and strategies to improve participation in social activities of the client and caregiver. Our starting point was to incorporate effective elements of psychosocial interventions in dementia as the preconditions in the Social Fitness Programme. The *multi-component* [15, 16] intervention therefore is aimed at empowering and enabling clients and caregivers to participate socially through a *patient-centred* [17, 18] approach. This *community-based* [19] intervention consists of a *tailor-made* intervention plan which includes *feasible goals* [20, 21] that represent the social activities which are relevant and important to the individual person. To achieve this, *shared-decision making* principles are incorporated during goal setting and intervention delivery [22–24]. Intervention delivery takes place in the *own environment* to enable the removal of barriers and to facilitate the execution of activities in the social and physical environment (*the context*). The professionals use a personalised approach to *empower* participants to *optimise compensatory and environmental strategies* and make *use of adaptations* to enable clients and caregivers to participate socially in their own context. The intervention addresses *needs, preferences and abilities* of the person with cognitive problems, the caregiver and their social environment. The professionals involved in intervention delivery used coaching methods focused on improving their self-confidence and self-management.

The welfare professionals provided practical support in achieving participants' goals, such as active guidance towards clients' activities and caregiver support.

Enhancing social participation of people with cognitive problems and their caregivers is challenging, as our previous studies [9, 25] revealed. We found barriers, on acceptability, demand, implementation and practicability. Also, interdisciplinary collaboration between healthcare and welfare professionals was suboptimal. However, the Social Fitness Programme seemed feasible according to stakeholders and limited efficacy showed promising results: 78,6% percent of the participants with cognitive problems attended new (social) activities during the SF Programme, with or without their caregivers. However, we found barriers influencing feasibility [26].

While results on feasibility were promising, we aimed to perform a Randomised Controlled Trial (RCT) as suggested in the Medical Research Council (MRC) guidance [27, 28]. We aimed to include 92 couples for a full RCT; however after an inclusion period of 15 months it appeared that 32 couples declined participation and only 17 were included. Recruitment difficulties are often seen in research. As a result, recruitment is often slower than expected and required sample sizes are not obtained within funding deadlines. This makes under-recruitment a problem or trials with negative consequences for patients, science and economy [29–33].

As a result of the high amount of study decline in relation to the participants who gave informed consent, study inclusion was terminated. Additional file 1 contains the study protocol of the trial and descriptive results of our primary and secondary outcomes. To get insight in the implementation of the intervention, the context of intervention delivery from professionals' point of view, and the potential impact of intervention delivery from participants' perspectives, we performed a mixed-method process evaluation according to the guide by Saunders and colleagues [34]. This article describes this process evaluation and the lessons learned from a failed trial.

Methods
Study design

We used a mixed-methods design for our process evaluation. Data for this process evaluation was gathered in parallel to the effectiveness study through questionnaires, focus group discussions, face-to-face and telephone interviews, and medical records. Data was gathered at different moments: before the start of the intervention, during intervention delivery, and after study termination.

We applied a comprehensive and systematic approach in which we focussed on three areas: implementation, context of intervention delivery and impact of intervention delivery [34]. *Implementation* captures the process of intervention delivery and consists of different elements, including: reach (participation rate), recruitment of participants (reasons to participate and reasons to decline participation), intervention adherence (dose delivered and dose received), fidelity (the quality of intervention delivery) and adaptations (changes that undermine intervention fidelity). The *context* of intervention delivery refers to external elements influencing implementation or effects, both positively and negatively. The potential *impact of intervention delivery* on participants was investigated from both clients and caregivers point of view.

Participants

People with cognitive problems (clients) were eligible for study participation if they lived at home, wished to improve their social participation and suffered from cognitive problems defined as: dementia diagnosis (Mini-Mental State Examination; MMSE ≥10; [35] or memory problems signalled by the referring professional (MMSE 10–24) or with a primary caregivers' score of ≥3.6 on the Informant Questionnaire on COgnitive Decline in the Elderly (IQCODE-N [36] (only for clients with high intelligence or high levels of education resulting in an MMSE-score between 25 and 30). Moreover, also *clients' primary caregivers* who wished to maintain or improve their own social participation or the social participation of the people they cared for were eligible. Participants' wish to improve their social participation was established during intake by their ability to formulate at least one social participation goal on level two (being with others) of our operational definition for social participation.

Intervention and implementation

The SF Programme is a multidisciplinary intervention which consists of an integration of community occupational therapy (OT) following the Community Occupational Therapy in Dementia (COTiD) programme [10, 11, 37], physiotherapy (PT) following the Coach2-Move programme [12–14], and guidance by welfare professionals. For a more detailed description see our feasibility study [9]. After a thorough problem analysis by OT and PT, the OT discussed with the client and caregiver personal goals, including goals on social activities. The OT consecutively discussed with the PT and welfare professional what was needed in the intervention and support to reach these goals, and converted this information into an intervention plan. The intervention plan included a combination of information and instruction combined with exercises to improve the use of strategies, skills, bodily functions and movement capacity using coaching methods focused on improving the self-confidence, self-efficacy, and self-management skills. Clients were supported and trained to use compensational strategies effectively, and caregivers were supported and trained in problem solving and communication skills.

Welfare professionals aimed to elicit positive experiences in social activities, by guiding participants towards activities that were tailored to personal motivation, routines and abilities, and to enhance their personal and environmental resources. The SF Programme was goal-oriented and contained up to two interdisciplinary professional home visits a week during three months, and less frequent continued guidance after three months of intervention. During the multidisciplinary intervention, the General Practitioner (GP) and other professionals continued to provide primary care as usual.

Study procedures and data collection

Table 1 provides an overview of the data collection. 1. Implementation: *Reach and recruitment* of participants were evaluated by research assistant through analysing records from telephone interviews with referring professionals and with people who seemed willing to participate. *Intervention adherence* was determined before the start of the intervention by using case vignettes, and after intervention delivery by assessing the medical records using a predefined checklist. The case vignettes included a case description based on a real case. OTs and PTs were asked to answer open ended questions regarding problem analysis, goal setting, and interdisciplinary cooperation. To evaluate *fidelity and adaptations* OT and PT medical records of participants allocated to the intervention group were studied. Involvement of welfare professionals was addressed as part of OT records.

2. To gain understanding in the *context of intervention delivery*, all healthcare and welfare professionals involved in intervention delivery were interviewed: they participated in a focus group and those unable to join were interviewed face-to-face. The focus groups were structured using a topic guide and conducted by the researcher (HD; trained as moderator) and observed by the research assistant (DV).

3. To get insight in the *impact of intervention delivery* from clients and caregivers who were assigned to the RCTs' intervention group and who completed all measurements were interviewed. These structured interviews were conducted by the research assistant (DV; trained as interviewer) at the clients' or caregivers' home.

Data analysis

We performed quantitative and qualitative drop-out analysis for our intervention (Table 1). Regarding *implementation*, a content analysis was performed on telephone interview records to get information on recruitment. The focused analysis of adherence, fidelity and adaptations was performed on the case vignettes and medical records by the two researchers (HD,DV) independently.

Table 1 Mixed method process evaluation of the Social Fitness Programme

Focus and operationalisation	Method	Analysis
1.Implementation *Reach & Recruitment: Reasons for participation and reasons to decline participation.*	Records from telephone interviews	Content analysis of records from telephone interviews by research assistant with referring professionals and with people who seemed willing to participate.
Adherence: Intervention dose delivered and intervention dose received by participants.	Case vignettes and medical records	Focussed analysis through predefined checklists to assess case vignettes and medical records. The checklist focussed on: elements of the problem analysis, use of shared-decision making during goal setting, intervention delivery (consistency between treatment plan and intervention goals, consistency between goals and intervention delivery, and interdisciplinary cooperation)
Fidelity: Quality of intervention delivery. Adaptations: Changes that undermine fidelity.	Medical records from OT and PT professionals involved in intervention delivery using checklists	Analysis of medical records, focused on: - Description of intervention delivery and adaptations - Consistence of the intervention goals with the problem analysis - Professionals' evaluation of intervention delivery
2.Context of intervention delivery: *External elements influencing implementation or effects.*	Focus groups and interviews with professionals involved in intervention delivery, using a structured topic list	Content analysis on elements influencing implementation or effects Focus group evaluation of the Social Fitness Programme, topics: - The guideline - Individual knowledge, skills and behaviour - Client and caregiver factors - Interactions with other professionals - Incentives and recourses - Required organisational changes
3.Impact of intervention delivery: Potential *impact of intervention delivery* on participants	Interviews with client-caregiver couples assigned to the intervention group, using a structured topic list	Content analysis on participants' evaluations on participating in the study. Interview topic list: - How did you evaluate participation in the Social Fitness Programme? - Did you gain anything? - Were your expectations met? - What should be changed to improve the programme?

OT Occupational Therapy, PT Physiotherapy

The answers on the open-ended questions of the case vignettes were scored on a predefined list of possible answers, creating a total percentage of intervention delivery. The OT and PT medical records were scored using a predefined list with quality criteria for the SF Programme. Scores were discussed until consensus was reached.

Focus groups and interviews on the *context of intervention delivery* and on *the impact of intervention delivery* were recorded, transcribed and analysed by two researchers (HD;DV) using Atlas.ti 7.1.4. The transcripts were thematically analysed through a content analysis [38]. The main researcher (HD) coded the focus groups and interview transcripts, and coding was checked by the research assistant (DV). The initial coding results were reviewed, discussed, and refined until consensus was reached on all codes. This resulted in identification of main themes and categories, which were discussed in project team meetings with all authors. Consecutively, we applied a checklist [39] to map professionals' experiences and opinions regarding the *context of intervention delivery*. Qualitative data on participants' *impact of intervention delivery* was compared to their intervention goals and medical records to get insight in the reasons for not finding effects on our primary outcome measure.

Results
1) implementation
Reach and recruitment
Within a time frame of fifteen months 60 client/caregiver couples were informed on the study; 11 of them did not meet inclusion criteria and study participation was declined by 32 couples, which is a decline rate of 65,3% (qualitative drop-out analysis). In all, seventeen couples were included in the intervention and they were randomly assigned to the intervention group (n = 8) or the control group (n = 9).

Analysis revealed the recruitment difficulties originate from two main causes (quantitative drop-out analysis). First, a lack of internal motivation to increase social participation expressed by people with cognitive problems. Second, caregivers were often overburdened and referring professionals feared that this burden would increase if they would participate in this study. Other reasons for study decline mentioned were acute physical problems which required frequent hospital visits and denial of cognitive problems by the client.

Adherence

Adherence to intervention guidelines was on average sufficient for Occupational Therapists (OTs) both before and after intervention delivery (Table 2). Physiotherapists (PTs) scored insufficient before intervention delivery, however average scores after intervention delivery were sufficient.

Fidelity and adaptations

All couples from the intervention group ($n = 8$) completed OT training within six months of intervention delivery (Table 3). Only three clients (38%) received PT training within the SF Programme, while based on frailty and mobility scores PT was indicated for all eight clients. One client was referred to PT but declined participation, and four clients continued their own regular PT treatment independent from the SF programme. Four couples already received guidance from a Dementia Casemanager before the start of the intervention, and one couple was assigned to a one during the intervention. Therefore, the coordinating OT discussed these cases with Welfare Professionals and decided together to involve the Dementia Casemanager instead of the welfare professional.

2) context of intervention delivery

All professionals involved in intervention delivery participated in one of two organised focus groups, in Nijmegen ($n = 8$ participants) or Deventer ($n = 5$ participants), or they were interviewed face-to-face ($n = 3$). In total, five OTs, three PTs, four Dementia Casemanagers, three Welfare Professionals and one Practice Nurse participated. Analysis of the data revealed barriers and facilitators influencing implementation and effects of the Social Fitness programme (Table 4). Emerging themes and categories were in agreement with the checklist designed by Flottorp and colleagues [39], which is a comprehensive integrated checklist of determinants of practise (TICD-checklist).

Most barriers were related to client and caregiver factors: lack of clients' motivation to increase social participation and to transfer to an intervention PT, increased caregiver burden, changing needs and decrease of capacity causing a focus shift and adding intervention goals during intervention delivery. Also, because of limited inclusion, professionals had little experience in intervention delivery

Table 2 Adherence to intervention guidelines

	Before intervention delivery: Range% (average%)	After intervention delivery: Range% (average%)
Occupational Therapy (OT)	4 OTs: 61–75 (70)	8 OT records: 48–86 (69)
Physiotherapy (PT)	3 PTs: 35–58 (46)	3 PT records: 58–82 (68)

Table 3 Fidelity of intervention delivery

	Participants receiving intervention elements/ total number of participants in the intervention group
Received Occupational Therapy intervention (COTiD)	8/8
Received Physiotherapy intervention (Coach2Move)	3/8
Received welfare intervention	3/8

and they were unable to get a routine. Moreover, working together in a multidisciplinary team with several different professionals was challenging. In most cases, the involved PTs where other people than the PTs who were trained in the SF protocol and involved in our study, because clients were unwilling to switch to a different PT. Additionally, the Dementia Casemanagers and the Practise Nurse were not trained in the SF protocol, although they were involved in guiding SF programme participants instead of the Welfare professionals. Most important facilitators for intervention delivery were related to client and caregivers' motivation to accept support for enabling to function in their own home environment, and their motivation to contribute to research by participating in the study. Also, involved professionals who were highly motivated to participate in the study, were facilitators for intervention delivery.

3) impact of intervention delivery

To get insight in the impact of intervention delivery, we interviewed the participants who were allocated to the intervention group and who completed t2 measurements: one caregiver (i7) and four couples (i2- i3- i4-i6). All participants but one (the caregiver form couple i6) were satisfied with the results from the intervention after t2. These fairly positive evaluations with regard to intervention delivery did not result in improvements on group level in terms of results on the primary outcome which was used in this study (results are shown in Additional file 1). To get insight in the reasons for this incongruence, we performed additional qualitative analysis on the interview data as part of this process evaluation.

For all participants except one caregiver (i4), quantitative analyses revealed a (partially) mismatch between formulated goals and activities initiated during the SF Programme. This mismatch was for four clients (i2, i3, i4, i7) related to the deterioration of their cognitive and/or physical problems, which led to a shift in intervention goals and adaptation of the intervention plan. For two participants (caregiver i3, client i6) it was associated with difficulties to formulate and evaluate own personal goals. For two caregivers (i2 and i7), not all personal goals formulated at baseline were given attention during the SF Programme. Table 5 illustrates the mismatch between goal

Table 4 Professionals' experiences with intervention delivery

	Barriers for intervention delivery[a]	Facilitators for intervention delivery[a]
Theme 1	Social Fitness Programme guideline factors	
Categories theme 1	- Intervention length too short for structural behaviour change	- Professionals were motivated to participate in the SF study - *Goal setting focused the intervention* - *Additional attention for caregiver*
Theme 2	Individual health professional factors	
Categories theme 2	- Lack of clarity regarding own role during intervention delivery - Reservations in referring clients to welfare professionals - Little experience in SF programme performance - *Illness of volunteer*	- Professionals put more effort into treatment as a result of their clients participating in research - *GP supported participation in the SF programme and coordinated all care initiatives*
Theme 3	Client and caregiver factors	
Categories theme 3	- Lack of internal motivation to increase social participation expressed by people with cognitive problems - Increased caregiver burden during intervention delivery - Changing needs (i.e. as a result of physical problems) - Client was unwilling to transfer from own PT to intervention PT - *Caregiver had limited time available* - *Caregiver/client had difficulties in handling cognitive decline* - *Client had difficulties in prioritising*	- Expressed need for support to maintain or increase functioning in the home environment - Clients' motivation to contribute in research and therefore participate in the SF programme (i.e. contribute to society) - *Client was motivated to participate (i.e. to prevent necessity of client for going to day-care; happy to share her story)*
Theme 4	Professional interactions	
Categories theme 4	- Suboptimal sharing of information among SF professionals - *Lack of coordination, too many people involved alongside SF Programme* - *Difficulties in reaching WP*	- Collaboration improved during the study - *Professionals were already used to working together* - *Dementia Casemanager motivated clients for OT*
Theme 5	Incentives and resources	
Categories theme 5	- Limited availability of organised social activities in the community which suit the participants with cognitive problems - *Lack of PT reimbursement by health insurance*	- Not applicable
Theme 6	Organisational resources	
Categories theme 6	- Rearrangement resulted in discontinuity of welfare professionals	- Not applicable

[a]*Italic barriers and facilitators originate from OT and PT medical records*
SF Social fitness, GP General Practitioner, OT Occupational Therapy, PT Physiotherapy

setting and intervention delivery for two clients who participated in the Social Fitness study, which contributed to the fact we did not find effects on group level.

Discussion

Although the Social Fitness Programme was developed using scientific evidence, expert opinions and stakeholder needs (involving healthcare and welfare professionals, and caregivers of people with cognitive problems), and although results on feasibility seemed promising [9], we were unable to overcome implementation barriers: over 65% of the people who were referred to the effectiveness study declined participation As a result, our intervention reach was minimal and we felt the necessity to stop the inclusion and to analyse the process and barriers thoroughly. Our analysis during the process evaluation revealed the high decline rate during recruitment was mainly caused by a lack of internal motivation to increase social participation expressed by people with cognitive

problems. From our previous studies [9, 25], we knew this mechanism played a role. However, we were unaware of the scale of this problem and we expected that caregivers, as they were often dissatisfied with the decreased social participation of the people they cared for, would be willing to participate and would persuade the person they cared for to participate in the study.

While recruitment difficulties are often seen in research [29–33], and interventions on social participation more often only reach only a small minority of the targeted population [40], the decline rate of our study was very high. While the single OT [10, 11, 37] and PT interventions [12–14], which were incorporated in the Social Fitness programme dealt with implementation difficulties as well, sufficient participants could be included and effectiveness of these interventions was established. Besides the single interventions being less complex, another possible reason for their success was the focus on activities of daily living, taking into account the relevance for social

Table 5 Examples of the mismatch between goal setting and intervention delivery

- Client i2 described positive experiences with participating in a fall-prevention training as part of the SF Programme, however this was not reflected in the primary outcome score as they did not change. Analysing the personal goals revealed that these did not target decreasing fall accidents but they focused instead on the clients' wish of being in charge and making own decisions, riding a bike and travelling. This revealed a mismatch between goal setting and intervention delivery.
- Client i3 described participation in new social activities, but this was not reflected in primary outcome scores. The increase in participation concerned an activity (day care) different from the activities on which goals were formulated (walking, riding a bike, playing a pool game, travelling). The formulated goals were too difficult to attain due to deterioration of the clients' situation. This revealed a mismatch between goal setting and intervention delivery; the formulated goals were not realistic and therefore goals were changed during intervention delivery.

interaction, which is experienced as less threatening by participants with cognitive problems. We therefore hypothesize the way we framed the intervention during recruitment (social participation improvement) was suboptimal and too direct, threatening peoples' autonomy because they are 'accused' of being unable to self-manage and seem to be in need for help [41]. The feeling of being unable to adequately contribute to social interactions seemed to be causing embarrassment. Framing the intervention on managing abilities in daily life in the context of decline would probably have appealed to people more. Activities of daily living such as getting dressed and preparing breakfast act as a precondition to the performance of social participation [4, 25], and therefore the focus of intervention delivery can remain unchanged. However, based on recent evidence we do suggest to incorporate behavioural coping strategies, as this is recently shown to be effective in social participation promotion [42].

Our process evaluation also revealed that besides minimal reach and recruitment difficulties, we faced more problems with regard to implementation which made it inadequate: although adherence Other implementation difficulties were related to barriers on all known healthcare levels, which was confirmed by participating professionals. A major problem in measuring effects was the shift from initial intervention goals during intervention delivery, as our primary measurement focussed on the recurrent measurement of the initial set goals.. Also, in many cases, other professionals (PTs and Dementia Casemanagers) who were not involved in the study and therefore not trained in the SF protocol, were involved in intervention delivery, which acted as a barrier for good intervention delivery. Implementation was insufficiently incorporated in existing networks.

The lack of participants to meet power calculations inhibited the effectiveness evaluation of this complex intervention. This process evaluation revealed the lack of effect was the result of a major implementation failure,

rather than genuine ineffectiveness [28]. To our knowledge, no other studies aiming at social participation improvement of people with cognitive problems and their caregivers through a person-centred, individualised and community-based intervention exist.Only few effective social participation interventions really reach vulnerable populations and are implemented in practice [43]. These effective interventions were not directed at people with dementia, and resulted more in facilitating of daily activities than older adults'empowerment or community integration. Also, effects on social participation were often not considered. For example, a person-centred activity-focused case management intervention study directed at frail older adults, did not establish effectiveness recently [44]. This study showed that an intervention directed at promoting physical activity does not automatically increase social participation. More research on person-centred and community-based interventions to improve social participation in elderly people with dementia and their caregivers is therefore recommended Our intervention, the Social Fitness study, incorporates only elements known to be effective in psychosocial interventions in dementia care. We therefore believe in the potential effectiveness of our programme, but we do have to find solutions to overcome the implementation barriers we were faced with. This study adds new knowledge to this field of research, which should be used in further research to prevent and overcome these implementation barriers.

In all, the tailor-made Social Fitness Programme did not fit in three ways. *First*, offering an intervention explicitly focused at improving social participation did not fit with clients and caregivers. Managing and coping with the inevitable decline on daily basis could be a better starting point for intervention, instead of directly focussing on active social participation. *Second*, the intervention seems to be too complex to implement in the way it was designed, and as a result implementation was inadequate. This is a result of involvement and interactions between three different professionals at one hand, and changing needs, increased decline and interactions between clients and their caregivers at the other hand. Difficulties arose especially when goals on social participation which were set at the start of the intervention appeared to be too difficult to attain. We therefore suggest to incorporate one leading professional who analyses the situation on all domains, including social participation, and sets priorities, and who then involves other professionals no sooner than possible: a step-by-step approach, for goal setting and intervention delivery. *Third*, there is a tension between the offering of a tailor-made intervention and evaluating it through a fixed study design. As a result, the follow-up measurements evaluated merely unfinished treatments and overall outcomes at fixed times. A participatory design would have fitted the effectiveness evaluation of this intervention better [45]. Participatory Action Research focuses on social processes and collaboration with participants to get insight in actual changes in practise [46].

Conclusions

The Social Fitness study did not fit in three ways. First, framing the intervention on social participation promotion was as threatening to clients. The feeling of being unable to adequately contribute to social interactions seemed to be causing embarrassment. Second, the intervention seemed to be too complex to implement in the way it was designed. Third, there is a tension between the offering of a personalised tailor-made intervention and evaluation through a fixed study design.

Abbreviations

COPM: Canadian Occupational Performance Measure; COTiD: Community Occupational Therapy in Dementia; GP: General Practitioner; IQCODE-N: Informant Questionnaire on COgnitive Decline in the Elderly; MMSE: Mini-Mental State Examination; MRC: Medical Research Council; OT: Occupational Therapist; PT: Physiotherapist; RCT: Randomised Controlled Trial; SF Programme: Social Fitness Programme

Acknowledgements

We want to thank the persons with cognitive problems and their caregivers for participating in this study. The professionals from the development group are thanked for their valuable input during intervention development. We also would like to thank the Social Fitness Professionals from both communities for participating in our research. Nijmegen: Ergotherapie Hoogland, Fysiotherapie Theunissen, Fysiotherapie Dukenburg, SWON. Deventer: ErgoCentraal, Fysiotherapie Borgele, Groepspraktijk fysiotherapie Deventer, Raster groep.

Funding

This work was supported by the Dutch Alzheimer Association, under grant number WE03.2011–21. The funders had no role in study design, data collection and analysis, decision to publish, or preparation of the manuscript.

Authors' contributions

HD, MVD, MN, and MG designed the study; DV was instrumental in the data collection; and HD and DV performed the analyses. HD and MG compiled the draft manuscript; and ST, DV, MN and MVD commented. All authors read and approved the final manuscript.

Competing interests

All author declare to have no conflicts of interest in the manuscript including financial, consultant, institutional or other relationships that might lead to bias or a conflict of interest.

Author details

[1]Radboud university medical center, Radboud Institute for Health Sciences, IQ healthcare, P.O. Box 9101, 6500, HB, Nijmegen, The Netherlands. [2]Radboud university medical center, Donders Institute for Brain, Cognition and Behaviour, Radboudumc Alzheimer Center, Nijmegen, The Netherlands. [3]Department for Health Evidence, section Biostatistics, Radboud university medical center, Radboud Institute for Health Sciences, Nijmegen, The Netherlands. [4]Department of Rehabilitation, Radboud university medical center, Donders Institute for Brain, Cognition and Behaviour, Nijmegen, The Netherlands.

References

1. Vasse E, Moniz-Cook E, Rikkert MO, Cantegreil I, Charras K, Dorenlot P, Fumero G, Franco M, Woods B, Vernooij-Dassen M. The development of quality indicators to improve psychosocial care in dementia. Int Psychogeriatr. 2012;24(6):921–30.
2. Huber M, Knottnerus JA, Green L, van der Horst H, Jadad AR, Kromhout D, Leonard B, Lorig K, Loureiro MI, van der Meer JW, et al. How should we define health? Bmj. 2011;343:d4163.
3. Vernooij-Dassen M, Jeon YH. Social health and dementia: the power of human capabilities. Int Psychogeriatr. 2016;28(5):701–3.
4. Levasseur M, Richard L, Gauvin L, Raymond E. Inventory and analysis of definitions of social participation found in the aging literature: proposed taxonomy of social activities. Soc Sci Med. 2010;71(12):2141–9.
5. Berkman LF. Social support, social networks, social cohesion and health. Soc Work Health Care. 2000;31(2):3–14.
6. Law M. Participation in the occupations of everyday life. Am J Occup Ther. 2002;56(6):640–9.
7. Cohen-Mansfield J, Perach R. Interventions for alleviating loneliness among older persons: a critical review. Am J Health promot. 2015;29(3):e109–25.
8. Pitkala KH, Raivio MM, Laakkonen ML, Tilvis RS, Kautiainen H, Strandberg TE. Exercise rehabilitation on home-dwelling patients with Alzheimer's disease--a randomized, controlled trial. Study protocol. Trials. 2010;11:92.
9. Donkers HW, van der Veen DJ, Vernooij-Dassen MJ, der Sanden MWG N-v, MJL G. Social participation of people with cognitive problems and their caregivers: a feasibility evaluation of the social fitness Programme. Int J Geriatr Psychiatry. 2017;32(12):e50–63.
10. Graff MJ, Vernooij-Dassen MJ, Thijssen M, Dekker J, Hoefnagels WH, Rikkert MG. Community based occupational therapy for patients with dementia and their care givers: randomised controlled trial. Bmj. 2006;333(7580):1196.
11. Graff MJL, Melick, M, van Thijssen M, Verstraten P, & Zajec J.: Ergotherapiebijouderen met dementieenhunmantelzorgers: Het EDOMAH-programma. Houten, NL: Bohn Stafleu van Loghum; 2010.
12. de Vries NM, Staal JB, Teerenstra S, Adang EM, Rikkert MG, Nijhuis-van der Sanden MW. Physiotherapy to improve physical activity in community-dwelling older adults with mobility problems (Coach2Move): study protocol for a randomized controlled trial. Trials. 2013;14:434.
13. de Vries NM, van Ravensberg CD, Hobbelen JS, van der Wees PJ, Olde Rikkert MG, Staal JB, Nijhuis-van der Sanden MW. The Coach2Move approach: development and acceptability of an individually tailored physical therapy strategy to increase activity levels in older adults with mobility problems. J Geriatr Phys Ther. 2015;38(4):169–82.
14. de Vries NS, Staal JB, van der Wees PJ, Adang, EMM; Akkermans R, Olde Rikkert MGM, Nijhuis-van der Sanden MWG.: Patient-centred physical therapy is (cost-) effective in increasing physical activity and reducing frailty in older adults with mobility problems: a randomized controlled trial with 6 months follow-up. J Cachexia, Sarcopenia Muscle 2015.
15. Brodaty H, Green A, Koschera A. Meta-analysis of psychosocial interventions for caregivers of people with dementia. J Am Geriatr Soc. 2003;51(5):657–64.
16. Brodaty H, Arasaratnam C. Meta-analysis of nonpharmacological interventions for neuropsychiatric symptoms of dementia. Am J Psychiatry. 2012;169(9):946–53.
17. Gitlin LN, Hodgson N, Jutkowitz E, Pizzi L. The cost-effectiveness of a nonpharmacologic intervention for individuals with dementia and family caregivers: the tailored activity program. Am J Geriatr Psychiatry. 2010;18(6):510–9.
18. Van Mierlo LD, Van der Roest HG, Meiland FJ, Droes RM. Personalized dementia care: proven effectiveness of psychosocial interventions in subgroups. Ageing Res Rev. 2010;9(2):163–83.
19. Gitlin LN, Winter L, Burke J, Chernett N, Dennis MP, Hauck WW. Tailored activities to manage neuropsychiatric behaviors in persons with dementia and reduce caregiver burden: a randomized pilot study. Am J of Geriatr Psychiatry. 2008;16(3):229–39.
20. Chee YK, Gitlin LN, Dennis MP, Hauck WW. Predictors of adherence to a skill-building intervention in dementia caregivers. J Gerontol A Biol Sci Med Sci. 2007;62(6):673–8.
21. Cooper C, Mukadam N, Katona C, Lyketsos CG, Ames D, Rabins P, Engedal K, de Mendonca LC, Blazer D, Teri L, et al. Systematic review of the effectiveness of non-pharmacological interventions to improve quality of life of people with dementia. Int psychogeriatr. 2012;24(6):856–70.
22. Olazaran J, Reisberg B, Clare L, Cruz I, Pena-Casanova J, Del Ser T, Woods B, Beck C, Auer S, Lai C, et al. Nonpharmacological therapies in Alzheimer's disease: a systematic review of efficacy. Dement Geriatr Cogn Disord. 2010;30(2):161–78.

23. Spijker A, Vernooij-Dassen M, Vasse E, Adang E, Wollersheim H, Grol R, Verhey F. Effectiveness of nonpharmacological interventions in delaying the institutionalization of patients with dementia: a meta-analysis. J Am Geriatr Soc. 2008;56(6):1116–28.

24. Droes RM, Breebaart E, Ettema TP, van Tilburg W, Mellenbergh GJ. Effect of integrated family support versus day care only on behavior and mood of patients with dementia. Int Psychogeriatr. 2000;12(1):99–115.

25. Donkers H, Vernooij-Dassen M, van der Veen D, Nijhuis-van der Sanden M, Graff M. Social participation perspectives from persons with cognitive problems and their caregivers: a descriptive qualitative study. Submitted.

26. Donkers HW, van der Veen DJ, Vernooij-Dassen MJ, Nijhuis-van der Sanden MW, Graff MJ. Social participation of people with cognitive problems and their caregivers: a feasibility evaluation of the social fitness Programme. Int J Geriatr Psychiatry. 2017.

27. Craig P, Dieppe P, Macintyre S, Michie S, Nazareth I, Petticrew M. Medical Research Council G: developing and evaluating complex interventions: the new Medical Research Council guidance. Bmj. 2008;337:a1655.

28. Craig P, Dieppe P, Macintyre S, Michie S, Nazareth I, Petticrew M. Developing and evaluating complex interventions: the new Medical Research Council guidance. Int J Nurs Stud. 2013;50(5):587–92.

29. McMurdo ME, Roberts H, Parker S, Wyatt N, May H, Goodman C, Jackson S, Gladman J, O'Mahony S, Ali K, et al. Improving recruitment of older people to research through good practice. Age Ageing. 2011;40(6):659–65.

30. Crombie IK, McMurdo ME, Irvine L, Williams B. Overcoming barriers to recruitment in health research: concerns of potential participants need to be dealt with. Bmj. 2006;333(7564):398.

31. Campbell MK, Snowdon C, Francis D, Elbourne D, McDonald AM, Knight R, Entwistle V, Garcia J, Roberts I, Grant A et al: Recruitment to randomised trials: strategies for trial enrollment and participation study. The STEPS study. Health techno assess 2007, 11(48):iii, ix-105.

32. Paramasivan S, Strong S, Wilson C, Campbell B, Blazeby JM, Donovan JL. A simple technique to identify key recruitment issues in randomised controlled trials: Q-QAT - Quanti-qualitative appointment timing. Trials. 2015;16:88.

33. Sawhney V, Graham A, Campbell N, Schilling R. Does modification to the approach to contacting potential participants improve recruitment to clinical trials? J Clin Med Res. 2014;6(5):384–7.

34. Saunders RP, Evans MH, Joshi P. Developing a process-evaluation plan for assessing health promotion program implementation: a how-to guide. Health Promot Pract. 2005;6(2):134–47.

35. Vertesi A, Lever JA, Molloy DW, Sanderson B, Tuttle I, Pokoradi L, Principi E: Standardized Mini-Mental State Examination. Use and interpretation. Can fam physician 2001, 47:2018–2023.

36. Ayalon L. The IQCODE versus a single-item informant measure to discriminate between cognitively intact individuals and individuals with dementia or cognitive impairment. J Geriatr Psychiatry Neurol. 2011;24(3):168–73.

37. Graff M, Vernooij-Dassen M, Zajec J, Olde-Rikkert M, Hoefnagels W, Dekker J. How can occupational therapy improve the daily performance and communication of an older patient with dementia and his primary caregiver? A case study. Dementia. 2006;5(4):503–32.

38. Graneheim UH, Lundman B. Qualitative content analysis in nursing research: concepts, procedures and measures to achieve trustworthiness. Nurse Educ Today. 2004;24(2):105–12.

39. Flottorp SA, Oxman AD, Krause J, Musila NR, Wensing M, Godycki-Cwirko M, Baker R, Eccles MP. A checklist for identifying determinants of practice: a systematic review and synthesis of frameworks and taxonomies of factors that prevent or enable improvements in healthcare professional practice. Implement Sci. 2013;8:35.

40. Levasseur M, Lefebvre H, Levert MJ, Lacasse-Bedard J, Desrosiers J, Therriault PY, Tourigny A, Couturier Y, Carbonneau H. Personalized citizen assistance for social participation (APIC): a promising intervention for increasing mobility, accomplishment of social activities and frequency of leisure activities in older adults having disabilities. Arch Gerontol Geriatr. 2016;64:96–102.

41. Lloyd LIZ, Calnan M, Cameron A, Seymour J, Smith R. Identity in the fourth age: perseverance, adaptation and maintaining dignity. Ageing Soc. 2012;34(1):1–19.

42. Provencher V, Desrosiers J, Demers L, Carmichael PH. Optimizing social participation in community-dwelling older adults through the use of behavioral coping strategies. Disabil Rehabil. 2016;38(10):972–8.

43. Levasseur M, Dubois MF, Filliatrault J, Vasiliadis HM, Lacasse-Bedard J, Tourigny A, Levert MJ, Gabaude C, Lefebvre H, Berger V, et al. Effect of personalised citizen assistance for social participation (APIC) on older adults' health and social participation: study protocol for a pragmatic multicentre randomised controlled trial (RCT). BMJ Open. 2018;8(3):e018676.

44. Granbom M, Kristensson J, Sandberg M. Effects on leisure activities and social participation of a case management intervention for frail older people living at home: a randomised controlled trial. Health Soc Care Community. 2017;25(4):1416–29.

45. Neuhauser Linda L. Integrating participatory design and health literacy to improve research and interventions. Stud health technol and inform. 2017;240:303–29.

46. Stringer ET. Action research, fourth edition. Edn. SAGE: Thousand Oaks, California; 2014.

8

Does social participation reduce the risk of functional disability among older adults in China? A survival analysis using the 2005–2011 waves of the CLHLS data

Min Gao[1], Zhihong Sa[2*], Yanyu Li[3], Weijun Zhang[1], Donghua Tian[1], Shengfa Zhang[1] and Linni Gu[1]

Abstract

Background: Existing studies in developed countries show that social participation has beneficial effects on the functional ability of older adults, but research on Chinese older people is limited. This study examined the effects of participating in different types of social activities on the onset of functional disability and the underlying behavioral and psychosocial mechanisms among older adults aged 65 and older in China.

Methods: The 2005, 2008, and 2011 waves of the Chinese Longitudinal Health Longevity Study were used. Life table analysis and discrete time hazard models were adopted to examine the relationship between social participation and functional disability. Social participation was defined as the frequencies of engaging in group leisure-time activities (i.e., playing cards/mahjong) and organized social activities, involving in informal social interactions (i.e., number of siblings frequently visited), and participating in paid jobs. Extensive social participation was measured by a composite index by adding up the four types of social activities that an older person was engaged in.

Results: After controlling for the effect of socio-demographic characteristics, health status, and health behavioral factors, extensive social participation is associated with a significant reduced risk for the onset of functional disability (hazard ratio [HR] = 0.92, $p < 0.001$). Different types of social participation affect the risk of functional decline through different mechanisms. Frequent playing of cards/mahjong is a protective factor for functional decline (HR = 0.78, $p < 0.001$), and the relationship is partially mediated by cognitive ability and positive emotions (accounting for 18.9% and 7.0% of the association, respectively). Frequent participation in organized social activities is significantly related to a reduced risk of functional decline (HR = 0.78, $p < 0.001$), and the association is mediated by physical exercises and cognitive ability (accounting for 25.7% and 17.7% of the association, respectively). Frequent visits from siblings has a strong inverse relationship with functional decline (HR = 0.75, $p < 0.001$). However, no significant association between paid job and functional decline is observed.

Conclusion: Extensive social participation, regular engagement in group leisure-time activities, organized social activities, and informal social interactions in particular may have beneficial effects on the functional health of older adults through behavioral and psychosocial pathways. The findings shed light for the importance of promoting social participation among older adults.

Keywords: Chinese older adults, Onset of functional disability, Social participation

* Correspondence: zsa@bnu.edu.cn
[2]School of Sociology, Beijing Normal University, No.19, Xinjiekou wai Street, Beijing 100875, China
Full list of author information is available at the end of the article

Background

China has entered a period of accelerated population aging that is accompanied by an increasing prevalence of chronic diseases and functional disability among older adults. In 2017, people aged 60 and over accounted for 17.3% of China's total population of 1.39 billion [1]. In 2013, more than 100 million older adults had at least one chronic noncommunicable disease, of whom more than 37 million had significant declines in physical function [2, 3]. The number of older adults with functional disability is expected to increase to 66 million by 2050 [4]. The large size of older population with chronic diseases and functional disability has created a tremendous challenge for China's health and social care systems. Encouraging social participation among older adults is an essential part of the active aging strategy [5]. In 2002, the United Nations considered "active aging" a policy framework for addressing population aging in the 21st century. The Chinese government has also adopted the policy of active aging as one of the important means of achieving successful aging for older people.

Numerous studies in developed countries show that social participation has beneficial effects on various health outcomes, including mortality, morbidities, psychological well-being, functional and cognitive abilities, and quality of life [6–8]. Recent studies have also indicated that the relationship between social participation and functional disability varies by participating in different types of social activities or organizations [8]. However, the underlying mechanisms through which different types of social participation affect the risk of functional disability among older adults are not well understood [9].

Despite the potential importance of social participation for the various health outcomes of older adults, existing studies among Chinese older adults tend to focus on the relationship between social participation and mental health or mortality [10, 11]. Only a few studies focus on the relationship between social participation and functional disability. The studies that used cross-sectional data reveal that participation in social activities is inversely associated with functional disability among Chinese older adults [12, 13]. However, the findings based on cross-sectional data may suffer from reverse causality. Moreover, the social and structural contexts of social participation among older adults in China are different from those in developed countries. The Chinese cultural tradition of familism encourages bonds within family and kinship, and civil society in China is still in its early stage of development. Thus, chances for social participation for Chinese older

people are rather limited. The present study aimed to investigate the effects of participation in various types of social activities on functional decline and the underlying behavioral and psychosocial mechanisms among Chinese adults aged 65 years and older. This study improved upon previous studies in China by using large representative longitudinal data collected between 2005 and 2011, examining social activities and social relationships, and employing a survival analysis method that treats social participation and the mediating factors as time-varying variables.

Social participation and functional disability

The influence of social participation on functional ability has been widely discussed in developed countries. According to social integration theory, social engagement gives meaning to an individual's life by enabling him or her to participate in it fully, to be obligated, to feel attached to one's community, and to feel fulfilled, which are all beneficial to health. Social relationship can also shape health-related resources that are available and increase motivation and social pressure to take good care of one's health [14, 15].

In support of social integration theory, existing studies in developed countries consistently show that extensive engagement in social activities is associated with a low likelihood of functional disability among older adults [16–19]. For instance, a study on older Japanese reveals that membership in multiple social organizations is associated with a reduced risk of having incident functional disability possibly because participation in various social activities enables older people to take on multiple social roles [17]. Moreover, these studies indicate that social participation benefits the functional ability of older adults through psychosocial, behavioral, and physiological pathways. First, engagements in social activities may benefit the health of older adults by helping them find social and spiritual supports, thereby reducing mental health problems. Studies provide sufficient evidence that high levels of social participation reduce the likelihood of having mental health problems [20] and self-destructive habits [21], and that mental distress has negative effects on physical health. Moreover, involvement in social activities can help older adults lower the risk of functional disability by maintaining cognitive ability [15]. Second, the underlying linkage between social participation and one's functional health can be explained by engaging in protective health behaviors [22]. For instance, participation in community voluntary works can benefit the functional health of older adults by staying physically active [23]. Third, social participation may exert direct physiological benefits, such as buffering stress, boosting host resistance, and lowering the biomarkers of disease risks [24].

While most studies use an aggregated indicator of social participation (i.e., number of social activities) [25] or focus on one of its particular types, recent studies have also shown that the relationship between social participation and functional decline differs by types of social activities probably because different social activities play different roles in health prevention [17]. Engagement in leisure-time activities may encourage people to stay physically active and reduce the risk of developing functional disabilities [26]. In addition, participating in organized social activities, such as church attendance and group voluntary activities, could confer health-enhancing benefits through psychosocial pathways, such as having considerable chances to socialize with others aside from family members and obtaining a sense of motivation, inner direction, and purposefulness [27]. A longitudinal study indicates that older adults who engage in volunteering activities have good self-rated health, few depressive symptoms, and good functional abilities possibly because volunteering provides them a chance to take on new roles that are psychologically rewarding [28]. Furthermore, participating in productive activities, such as paid work, is negatively related to the onset of functional decline probably by preserving one's physical and cognitive abilities [29]. Engagement in paid work also means having considerable individual/social resources, which may help in maintaining good health [30]. Although the empirical investigations into the mechanisms through which different types of social participation affect the risk of functional disability among older adults can provide evidence for health promotion, this important issue is understudied in the existing literature.

Social participation and functional disability in China

Research on the relationship between social participation and functional disability among Chinese older adults is limited. A cross-sectional study based on the nationally representative data reveals that the frequency of participation in various social activities, such as interacting with friends, playing mahjong, volunteering, and other activities, is positively related to the functional ability of older adults. Positive social interactions gained from involving in these activities may provide one of the explanations for the beneficial effects of social participation on functional ability [13]. Another cross-sectional study contends that

re-entering into the labor force after retirement is positively related to the functional health of Chinese older adults [31]. These studies provide important evidence for the relationship between social participation and functional health among Chinese older adults, but research based on cross-sectional data may have the problem of reverse causality. Losses in physical function and self-care capacities may lead to reduced social participation; hence, social participation may be more of a consequence of functional disability than it is a cause.

The social and structural contexts of social participation among older adults in China are different from those in developed countries, and the observed relationship between various types of social participation and functional disability in developed countries may not be applicable to Chinese older adults. The Chinese cultural tradition of familism encourages bonds within family and kinship. Thus, informal social interactions among immediate family members and relatives are the most important aspects of social relationships for Chinese older adults. Civil society is still at its early stage of development such that voluntary activities organized by social organizations or self-help groups are rather limited. Cultural and leisure-time activities, such as group dancing, singing, and playing cards/mahjong that are organized by older adults themselves, and formal social or voluntary activities, such as health lectures, trainings on using smartphones, and security patrols organized by residential committees, are the major forms of social activities that Chinese older adults are involved in [32]. Although participation in paid work is an indispensable part of social participation among Chinese older adults, their level of participation in the paid employment is low. China has an early mandatory retirement age such that men retire at 60 years old and women retire between 50 and 55 years old. The opportunities for relocating paid jobs are rather limited among retirees. Although some studies show that participation in paid job is beneficial to health among older adults in China, other studies indicate that Chinese older adults who remain in the paid job after retirement tend to have insufficient financial support and poor health conditions [33, 34]. Older adults who participate in paid jobs available to them after retirement are likely to experience burnout that offsets the beneficial effects of employment on health. On the basis of the existing literature and Chinese social and cultural backgrounds, the present study hypothesized that informal social interactions, group leisure-time activities, and organized social activities are negatively related to functional decline and that paid work is not related to functional ability among Chinese older adults. We also anticipated that extensive social participation has a strong negative relationship with functional decline because taking on multiple social roles may have overlapping health benefits.

Methods
Data

Data for this study were obtained from the 2005, 2008, and 2011 waves of the Chinese Longitudinal Healthy Longevity Survey (CLHLS). The CLHLS is a randomly selected sample of rural and urban older adults in 631 countries/cities of 22 provinces, which represents 85% of the total population in China. A detailed description of the sampling design and data quality of the CLHLS has been reported elsewhere [35]. The 1998 baseline and 2000 follow-up surveys of the CLHLS included approximately 10,000 respondents aged 80 years and over. The CLHLS started to interview younger-old persons in 2002. At each wave, survivors were re-interviewed, and the deceased interviewees were replaced by additional participants. The CLHLS collected information on socio-demographic characteristics, physical and mental health status, chronic diseases, family and social supports, and health behaviors.

This study used the fourth, fifth, and sixth waves because the wording of the questions on social participation and functional ability was consistent in the three waves. The CLHLS conducted face-to-face interviews with 15,638, 16,540, and 9765 individuals in 2005 (baseline), 2008 (Time 2), and 2011 (Time 3), respectively. To select an initially nondisabled group, we excluded 25 respondents whose age was below 65 and 3929 respondents who reported having problems with at least one activity of daily living in 2005. We also dropped 840 cases with missing information for independent and dependent variables, leaving a baseline sample of 10,844. After merging the baseline data with 2008 and 2011 waves, the number of respondents who survived and were surveyed in all three waves was 3731 (38.6% of the baseline sample). Compared with those who dropped out of the sample, the remaining participants were significantly more likely to be younger and married, reside in rural areas, have more children, have better education and cognitive and emotional conditions, and engage in all types of social activities and informal social interactions more actively (results shown in Appendix). Therefore, the observed association between social participation and functional disability in the present study may be underestimated.

Variables
Functional disability

Functional disability was measured by six activities (i.e., eating, dressing, indoor mobility, bathing, using the toilet, and continence) from the activities of daily living (ADL) scale. Individuals were asked if she/he had any difficulties with each of the activities. This study focused on the onset of functional disability. Respondents who reported having had no ADL problem at the baseline but experienced some difficulties with or were unable to perform at least one of the ADL activities at Time 2 or Time 3 were defined to have functional disability (coded as 1), and those who reported having had no ADL problem between 2005 and 2011 were defined to have no functional disability (coded as 0). This definition of ADL disability was consistent with that in previous studies [36, 37].

The survey further asked functional disabled respondents about the duration of being unable to perform the activities of daily living at each wave. On the basis of the information, we calculated age at which a respondent became functionally disabled. An individual was considered to have an onset of ADL disability if she/he changed from the status of having no ADL problems to having at least one ADL problem at a certain age.

Social participation

Given the social context for the social participation of Chinese older adults and the data limitation, we measured social participation with four indicators, including frequencies of engagement in group leisure-time activities (i.e., playing cards/mahjong) and organized social activities, informal social interactions (i.e., number of siblings frequently visited), and participation in paid jobs. The participants were asked about how often they played cards/mahjong and engaged in organized social activities. Each of the question has five responses: almost every day (coded as 4), not every day but at least once in a week (coded as 3), not every week but once in a month (coded as 2), not every month but sometimes (coded as 1), and never (coded as 0). Informal social interactions were measured by a continuous variable reflecting the number of living siblings frequently visited. Participation in paid work was measured by a dichotomous variable reflecting one's involvement in a paid job (coded as 1) or not (coded as 0). To further assess the influence of extensive participation in social activities on functional health, we used a composite measure of social participation by adding up the four types of social activities that an older person was engaged in. Each activity was coded as a dichotomous variable reflecting whether an individual participated or not.

Mediating variables

To assess the behavioral and psychosocial pathways through which social participation affected the risk of functional decline, health behaviors and cognitive and emotional health conditions were considered potential mediating factors. Physical exercise was used as an indicator of health behavior and was dichotomized into "not doing exercise" (coded as 0) and "doing exercise" (coded as 1). Cognitive ability and positive emotions were included as indicators of psychosocial factors. We measured cognitive ability following the Chinese version of the Mini-Mental Status Examination Index. The range for the cognitive ability index (Cronbach's α = 0.86) was between 0 and 23, with high scores reflecting good cognitive ability. Positive emotions were assessed by three questions: "Do you usually feel nervous or afraid?," "Do you usually feel lonely?," and "Do you usually feel more and more useless?" The response for each of the questions ranged between "never" (coded as 5) and "always" (coded as 1). We created a composite measure by summing up the three variables (ranging between 3 and 15), with high scores indicating good emotional condition.

Covariates

Three sets of covariates related to functional ability were included in the analysis. The first set of covariates comprised the indicators of demographic characteristics such as age, gender (male coded as 1), marital status (being married coded as 1), and rural/urban residence (urban coded as 1). Age was classified into six categories: 65–69, 70–74, 75–79, 80–84, 85–89, and 90 and above.

The second set of covariates included socioeconomic status, measured by education and self-perceived economic conditions. Given the relatively low level of education among Chinese older adults, education was classified into two categories: illiterate (coded as 0) and literate (coded as 1). The self-perceived economic condition was assessed by the question "How do you rate your economic status compared with other local people?" The variable included three categories: poor, fair, and good.

The third set of covariates consisted of self-rated health status and informal social support. The respondents were asked if they were ever diagnosed with any of the 15 chronic conditions, namely, hypertension, diabetes, heart diseases, stroke (or cardiovascular disease), bronchitis, tuberculosis, cataract, glaucoma, cancer, prostate tumor, gastric or duodenal ulcer, Parkinson's disease, bedsore, arthritis, and dementia. The number of chronic diseases was calculated by summing up the diseases they had been diagnosed with. Informal social support was indicated by a continuous variable reflecting the number of living children.

Statistical analysis

The survival analysis method was used given its advantage in predicting the influence of social participation on the onset of functional disability. The 7-year follow-up period was divided into 3-month intervals, and the respondents who did not have incident functional disability during the period were censored. First, a description of sample characteristics was presented. Second, we estimated the bivariate association between the different types of social participation and the onset of functional disability using life table analyses. Third, given that the dependent variable (i.e., time for the onset of functional disability) was a dichotomous measure, we used discrete hazard models to estimate the effect of social participation on the onset of functional disability after adjusting for the mediating factors and other covariates. A nested modeling approach was used to assess the mediating effect of the behavioral and psychosocial factors in the relationship between social participation and functional decline. We sequentially added behavioral and psychosocial factors in models 3 and 4 to identify the changes in HR estimates associated with various types of social participation. Finally, we calculated the mediating effects by using Sobel's test. The proportion of risk reduction for the onset of functional disability that was explained by each potential mediating factor was computed as follows: [(HR$_{basic model}$ − HR$_{adjusted model}$) / (HR$_{basic model}$ − 1)] * 100% [38]. Given the possible reciprocal relationship between social participation and functional disability, social participation, behavioral and psychosocial mediating factors, and some covariates were treated as time-varying variables, which can provide accurate prediction for the relationship between social participation and functional decline.

Results
Sample characteristics
Table 1 presents the distribution of sample characteristics. Respondents aged 80 years or older accounted for 44.6% of the entire sample. More than half of the respondents were women (51.7%), unmarried (51.2%), and residents of rural areas (53.2%). A total of 44.2% of the older adults were illiterate. Most of the respondents perceived their economic conditions as "fair" (68%), whereas 16% considered their economic status as "poor." The average number of living children was 3.9. The respondents reported having 1.2 diagnosed chronic diseases on average.

The overall level of social participation was low with an average number of social activities participated of 0.9 out of a total score of 4 (Table 1). The mean scores

Table 1 Description of sample characteristics among older adults aged 65 and over, CLHLS 2005, 2008, and 2011

Variables	% or mean (s.d.)
Social participation	
Extensive social participation (0–4)	0.9 (0.9)
Playing cards/mahjong (0–4)	0.6 (1.3)
Organized social activities (0–4)	0.4 (0.9)
Number of siblings frequently visited (0–8)	0.7 (1.3)
Paid job	
Not involved	94.2
Involved	5.8
Mediating variables	
Health behavior	
Physical exercise	
No	57.2
Yes	42.8
Psychosocial factors	
Cognitive ability (0–23)	20.0 (3.9)
Positive emotions (3–15)	11.5 (2.4)
Control variables	
Rural/urban residence	
Rural	53.2
Urban	46.8
Gender	
Female	51.7
Male	48.3
Age	
65–69	9.0
70–74	24.0
75–79	22.3
80–84	16.3
85–89	12.0
90 and above	16.3
Marital status	
Widowed/divorced/never married	51.2
Married	48.8
Education	
Illiterate	44.2
Literate	55.8
Self-perceived economic conditions	
Poor	16.0
Fair	68.0
Good	16.0
Number of living children	3.9 (1.8)
Number of chronic diseases	1.2 (1.3)
N	104,468

for group leisure-time activities (i.e., playing cards/mahjong) and organized social activities were 0.6 and 0.4 (out of a range between 0 and 4), respectively. The level of informal social interactions was also low with an average number of siblings frequently visited of 0.7 (out of a range of 0 and 8). Only 5.8% of the respondents were involved in paid jobs. Table 1 also shows that 42.8% of the respondents engaged in physical exercise. The average scores of the cognitive ability and positive emotion indices were 20 (for a range between 0 and 23) and 11.5 (for a range between 3 and 15), respectively, reflecting good overall cognitive and emotional conditions among older adults.

Life table analyses

Figures 1, 2, 3 and 4 provide graphical displays of cumulative survival probability for the onset of functional disability by different types of social participation among older adults over the 7-year period. The figures illustrate that the cumulative survival steeply declined among those who lack of or had low levels of social participation, and that the pattern was consistent for four types of social activities. Particularly, Figs. 1 and 2 depict that the cumulative survival for older persons who never played cards/mahjong or who did not participate in organized social activities declined more rapidly than that for those who participated in these activities frequently. Figure 3 shows that people who were not frequently visited by siblings had a higher probability of having functional disability compared with those whose siblings frequently visited. Figure 4 indicates that the cumulative survival probability for older persons who were not involved in paid jobs was smaller than that for people who were involved in paid jobs.

Regression results

The results from the univariate discrete time hazard regression models were consistent with the results from life table analyses (Table 2). The first column of Table 2 shows that extensive social participation had a strong negative association with the onset of functional disability. Moreover, playing cards/mahjong, engaging in organized social activities, and being frequently visited by siblings were all significantly related to the reduced risk of having incident functional disability, whereas participation in paid jobs was not significantly associated with the risk of functional decline.

In multivariate discrete time hazard regression analyses (Table 2), extensive social participation was significantly associated with a decreased risk of functional decline after adjusting for socio-demographic characteristics, health status, and behavioral and psychosocial factors (HR = 0.92, p < 0.001) (**Model 1**). In **Model 2**, regular participation in cards/mahjong playing (HR = 0.78, p < 0.001) and organized social activities (HR = 0.78, p < 0.001) and frequent visits by several siblings (HR = 0.75, p < 0.001) were all

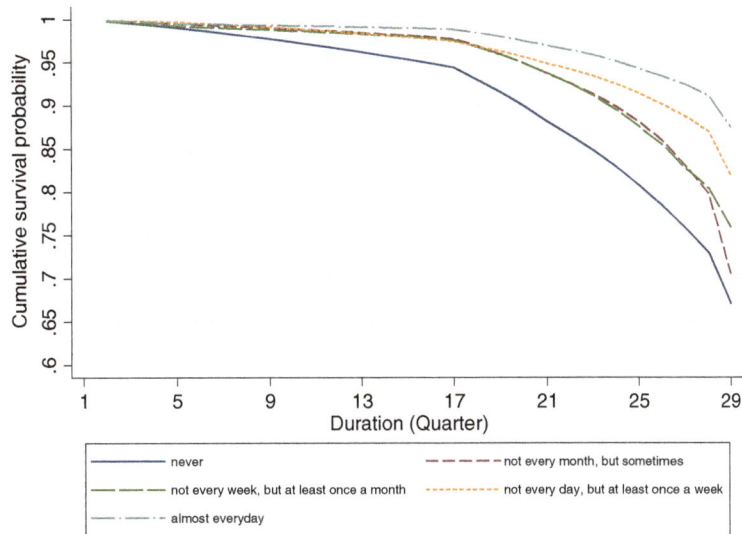

Fig. 1 Cumulative survival for the onset of functional disability by participation in group leisure-time activities

significantly associated with decreased risks of functional decline after controlling for socio-demographic characteristics and health status. However, involving in paid jobs was not significantly related to functional decline. **Model 3** indicates that, after adding physical exercise in the model, the significant association between participation in group leisure-time activities (HR = 0.79, $p < 0.001$) and organized social activities (HR = 0.83, $p < 0.01$) with functional disability still remained, but the magnitude of the associations was slightly reduced. **Model 4** shows that, when cognitive ability and positive emotions were added in the model, the magnitude of the association between participation in group leisure-time activities (HR = 0.84, $p < 0.001$) and

organized social activities (HR = 0.86, $p < 0.05$) with functional decline was further reduced but still remained significant. A significant inverse relationship between frequent visits by siblings (HR = 0.76, $p < 0.001$) and the onset of functional disability was observed even after controlling for the effects of behavioral and psychosocial factors and other covariates, and the magnitude of the association remained similar across **Models 2** and **4**.

Moreover, engagement in physical exercise (HR = 0.61, $p < 0.001$) was associated with a low risk of functional decline. Having good cognitive ability (HR = 0.92, $p < 0.001$) and a high degree of positive emotions (HR = 0.89, $p < 0.001$) were both significantly related to a reduced risk of

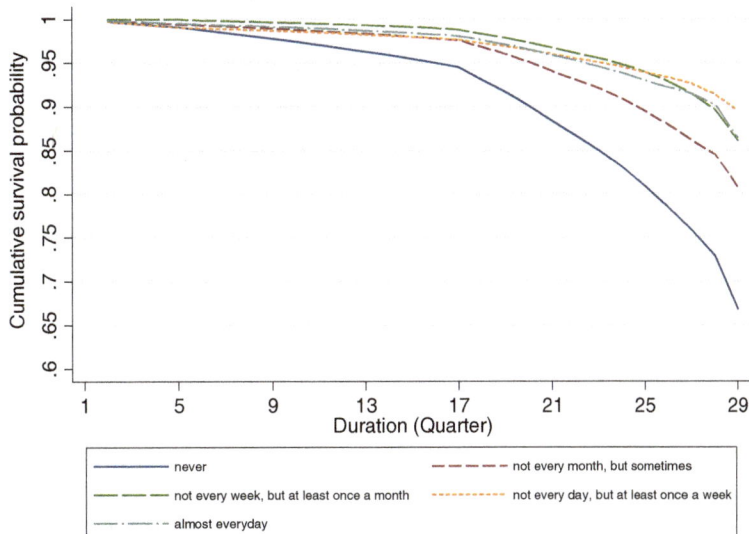

Fig. 2 Cumulative survival for the onset of functional disability by participation in organized social activities

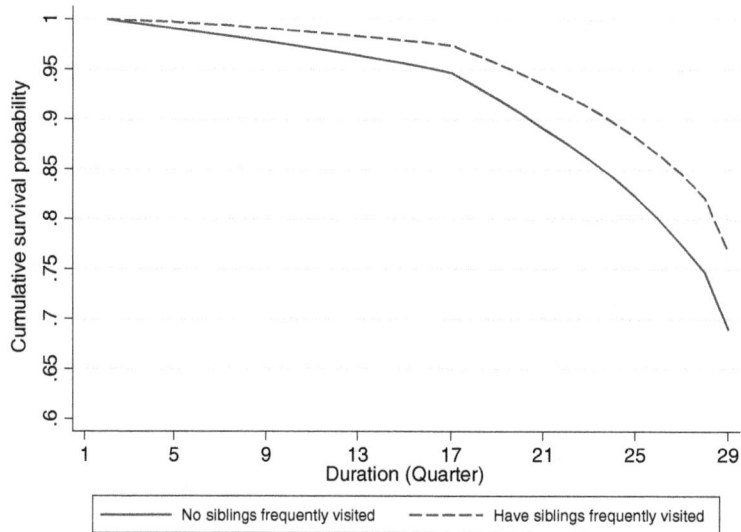

Fig. 3 Cumulative survival for the onset of functional disability by informal social interactions

functional disability (**Model 4**). **Model 4** also indicates that older adults who were 70 years or older or literate (HR = 1.37, $p < 0.01$), who lived in urban areas (HR = 1.78, $p < 0.001$), or who had more chronic diseases (HR = 1.25, $p < 0.001$) tended to have higher risks for the onset of functional disability than those in reference groups.

Mediating effect analyses

We further explored the potential mediating effects of behavioral and psychosocial factors on the relationship between various types of social activities and functional decline. Table 3 reveals that cognitive ability had the strongest mediating effect for the association between playing cards/mahjong and the onset of

functional disability, accounting for 18.9% of the association, followed by positive emotions (7.0%) and physical exercise (5.4%). The inverse relationship between engaging in organized social activities and the risk of functional decline was largely explained by physical exercise (25.7%) and cognitive ability (17.7%). Behavioral and psychosocial factors also had significant mediating effects for the association between the number of siblings frequently visited and the onset of functional disability, but the magnitude of the mediating effect was modest. Thus, further studies are needed to explore possible intervening factors between informal social interactions and functional disability among older adults.

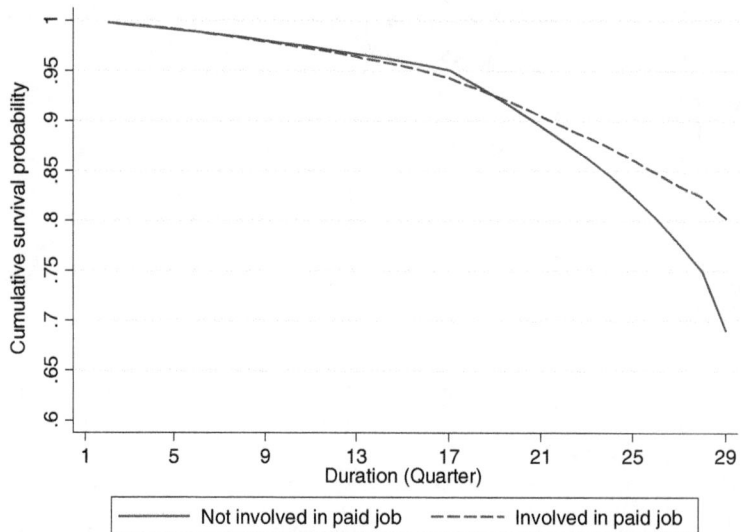

Fig. 4 Cumulative survival for the onset of functional disability by participation in paid job

Table 2 Discrete time hazard models predicting the onset of functional disability

	Crude HRs	Model 1 HRs	Model 2 HRs	Model 3 HRs	Model 4 HRs
Extensive social participation	0.62***	0.92***	–	–	–
Playing cards/mahjong	0.71***	–	0.78***	0.79***	0.84***
Organized social activities	0.72***	–	0.78***	0.83**	0.86*
Paid job (vs. Not involved)	0.86	–	0.92	0.97	1.13
Number of siblings frequently visited	0.59***	–	0.75***	0.75***	0.76***
Residence (vs. Rural)	1.65***	1.78***	1.61***	1.74***	1.78***
Gender (vs. Female)	0.84	1.06	0.93	0.95	1.07
Age (vs. 65–69)					
70–74	4.39**	4.11**	3.88**	3.95**	3.70*
75–79	6.13***	5.27**	4.95**	5.04**	4.44**
80–84	11.58***	9.41***	9.19***	9.22***	7.80***
85–89	12.58***	8.89***	10.09***	9.72***	7.16***
90 and above	27.23***	17.12***	21.26***	20.09***	13.63***
Educated (vs. Illiteracy)	0.80*	1.33**	1.15	1.23*	1.37**
Married (vs. Unmarried)	0.58***	1.20	1.12	1.12	1.22
Self-perceived economic conditions (vs. Poor)					
Fair	0.77*	1.04	0.82	0.83	1.07
Good	0.82	1.13	0.76	0.78	1.16
Number of living children	1.01	1.02	1.03	1.02	1.03
Number of chronic diseases	1.24***	1.26***	1.24***	1.24***	1.25***
Physical exercise (vs. No)	0.47***	0.59***		0.51***	0.61***
Cognitive ability index	0.88***	0.92***			0.92***
Positive emotion index	0.85***	0.89***			0.89***
Constant		0.01***	0.00***	0.00***	0.00***
N	104,468	104,468	104,468	104,468	104,468

*p < 0.05; **p < 0.01; ***p < 0.001

Discussion

Although social participation is related to low risks of having functional disability among older adults, the mechanisms underlying this inverse association are unclear. To the best of our knowledge, this study is one of the few studies that explores the relationship between various types of social activities and the onset of functional disability and the underlying behavioral and psychosocial mechanisms among older adults in China. In support of our hypothesis, the present study demonstrates that extensive social participation had a strong negative relationship with the risk of functional decline. The beneficial effects of participating in various social activities on functional ability are consistent with those in existing studies in developed countries [17, 18]. High levels of social participation are associated with low risks of functional decline by enabling older people to

Table 3 Mediating effects between social participation and the onset of functional disability

	Crude HRs	Physical exercise		Cognitive ability		Positive emotions	
		Adjusted HRs	Mediating effect (%)	Adjusted HRs	Mediating effect (%)	Adjusted HRs	Mediating effect (%)
Playing cards/mahjong	0.78***	0.79***	5.4	0.82***	18.9	0.79***	7.0
Organized social activity	0.78***	0.83***	25.7	0.82***	17.7	0.78***	0.3
Number of siblings frequently visited	0.75***	0.75***	1.9	0.76***	2.8	0.76***	1.4
Paid job[a]	0.91	0.96	–	1.03	–	0.97	–

***p < 0.001

[a]The variable paid job was not significantly associated with functional disability, so the mediating effect was not calculated

take on multiple social roles that are psychologically rewarding [12]. Moreover, social participation may exert direct health benefits by keeping them physically [23] or cognitively active [39].

The present study also reveals that frequent participation in group leisure-time activities, such as playing cards/mahjong, is protective against functional decline among older adults. The finding is consistent with a previous longitudinal study of Chinese older adults, which also indicates that involving in entertaining activities is associated with a low likelihood of having incidence of disability and death [40]. In this study, the association between playing cards/mahjong and the onset of functional disability is partially mediated by cognitive ability (accounting for 18.9% of the association). Playing cards/mahjong is an important part of leisure-time activities among Chinese older adults. The cognitively demanding nature of these activities might help them exercise reaction ability and memory, thereby delaying deterioration. Existing research provides evidence that the higher the level of participating in intellectual activities, the greater the benefit for cognitive ability among older people [41]. Studies also show that playing mahjong or cards can produce consistent gains across many cognitive performance measures among older adults [42]. Improvements in cognitive ability may result in changes in behaviors that promote broad-based engagement in functional activities [43]. Our further analysis reveals that older adults who play cards/mahjong more frequently are also significantly more likely to be involved in physical exercise compared with those who do not play cards/mahjong or play less frequently.

In addition, engagement in group leisure-time activities may be helpful for older adults in resolving negative emotions through positive social interactions. This study indicates that positive emotions explain 7% of the association between playing cards/mahjong and the onset of functional disability. A previous study reveals that engagement in group leisure-time activities is an effective way to alleviate negative emotions and obtain psychological well-being [44]. A Chinese study also shows that playing chess or cards is protective against the negative effects of stressful life events [45]. People may be willing to talk about problems they encounter with and try to seek emotional supports while playing with friends or relatives. Engagement in leisure-time activities is also associated with a low level of depression [46], which is a known risk factor for functional disability among older adults.

The present study also demonstrates that engagement in organized social activities is protective against the risk for the onset of functional disability among older people in China mainly by remaining physically active and maintaining cognitive ability. Some studies show that participation in organized social activities can encourage older people to do sufficient physical exercises together with others or on their own [13, 29]. Moreover, social networks built by engaging in organized social activities increase the motivation of older adults to take good care of one's health, provide considerable opportunities for companionship, and give meaning to life, which are all beneficial to physical and emotional health. Participating in group dancing and singing, listening to health promotion lectures, or playing cards/mahjong and attending workshops on how to use computers and cell phones are the most popular social activities that Chinese older people engage in. The former activities may help older adults gain significant health-related information and self-efficacy for keeping physically or cognitively active, whereas the latter activities may stimulate the brain functioning of older adults in the process of playing, learning, and memorizing new information and practicing new skills [41].

Despite of the beneficial effects of engaging in organized social activities on functional ability, participation in organized social activities is uncommon among older people in China. In our study, only 17.6% of the respondents report having engaged in organized social activities. Civil society is still in its early stage of development in China, and cultural, recreational, and voluntary activities organized by residential committees are the major forms of organized social activities engaging older people. Studies have indicated that most Chinese older adults are willing to participate in community life, but barriers, such as social exclusion, age discrimination, limited social connectedness, lack of access to information, and low socioeconomic status, hinder their participation. In addition, some of the formally organized social activities aim to accomplish various governmental goals, which may not be able to increase motivation and encourage active participation [47]. Thus far, the elite group of older adults tends to be the most socially active ones, and those with low socioeconomic status generally have limited participation in organized social activities.

Being frequently visited by siblings is significantly associated with reduced risks for the onset of functional disability. As an indispensable part of the social life among Chinese older adults, frequent visits from siblings appear to provide them with emotional support [48]. Accordingly, the risk of functional disability among older adults may be further reduced. The mediating effect of behavioral and psychosocial factors for the association between informal social interactions and functional disability is significant but weak. Thus, informal social interactions may affect the risk of functional disability among older adults through other mechanisms, such as by reducing stress.

Unlike some existing studies in China and other countries, which contend that engagement in paid work in old age benefits functional health [30, 49], our study shows that paid job is not significantly related to the functional disability of older adults. In this study, only 5.3% of the respondents have engaged in paid jobs during the 7-year period. One possible reason for this lack of association is that, in a social context with early mandatory retirement age and limited access to well-positioned paid jobs, the participation of older adults in paid jobs after retirement is likely to be out of financial necessity [47]. Moreover, although the engagement of older adults in paid jobs could bring them beneficial psychological effects [31], it may also exert adverse health consequences that offset the gains from social participation.

The present study has some strengths, such as the use of large panel data, which allows for the investigation of the relationship between change in various types of social participation and the onset of functional disability and its underlying mechanisms. Nonetheless, our study has certain limitations. First, the findings cannot be generalized to the entire old population in China because the sample only represents 85% of the total population. Second, although we consider the reciprocal relationship between social participation and functional ability by treating social participation and medicating factors as time-varying variables, possible reverse causality cannot be fully avoided. Third, measures of social activities are somewhat limited such that they cannot capture the variety of social activities that Chinese older people engage in. Fourth, future research should include additional intervening variables, such as mastery over life and stress, which may mediate the relationship between social participation and the onset of functional disability. Finally, the relatively high attrition rate of the panel data may bias the observed relationship between social participation and functional disability. Older adults who remain in the sample are significantly more likely to participate in social activities than those who are excluded in the follow-up surveys. Thus, the observed relationship between social participation and functional disability may be underestimated.

Conclusion

In conclusion, extensive social participation, regular engagement in group leisure-time activities and organized social activities, and active involvement in informal social interactions may provide functional health benefits to Chinese older adults through behavioral and psychosocial pathways to a certain extent. Clarifying the effect of different types of social participation on the onset of functional disability may shed important light on the development of policies and intervention programs to promote active social participation among older adults. Given the limited access of Chinese older adults in participating in social life, considerable efforts are needed by the government to develop supportive and effective policies to eliminate ageism and structural barriers for the broad social participation of older adults. Community and social organizations should play highly active roles in building a lively community life for older people.

Appendix

Table 4 Baseline characteristics of survivors and respondents who dropped out between 2005 and 2011

	Survivors in 2011 (N = 3731)	Drop-outs between 2005 and 2011 (N = 7113)	p-value[1]
	% or mean (s.d.)	% or mean (s.d.)	
Playing cards/ mahjong	0.7 (1.3)	0.6 (1.2)	< 0.001
Organized social activities	0.43 (1.0)	0.4 (0.9)	0.003
Paid job			0.02
Yes	6.6	5.6	
No	93.4	94.4	
Number of siblings frequently visited	0.9 (1.3)	0.5 (1.1)	< 0.001
Gender			0.97
Female	52.3	52.3	
Male	47.7	47.7	
Age			< 0.001
65–69	25.6	9.0	
70–74	21.9	10.0	
75–79	18.0	11.2	
80–84	11.3	9.6	
85–89	12.2	19.6	
90 +	11.1	40.6	
Residence			< 0.001
Rural	61.3	55.6	
Urban	38.7	44.4	
Education			< 0.001
Illiterate	52.1	58.2	
Literate	47.9	41.8	
Marital status			< 0.001
Unmarried	46.2	67.5	
Married	53.8	32.5	
Self-perceived economic conditions			0.13
Poor	14.9	16.0	
Fair	68.8	67.0	
Good	16.3	17.0	
Number of living children	3.9 (1.8)	3.5 (1.9)	< 0.001
Number of chronic diseases	1.2 (1.3)	1.2 (1.3)	0.68
Physical exercise			0.14
No	62.5	63.9	
Yes	37.5	36.1	
Cognitive ability index	20.6 (3.4)	18.8 (5.0)	< 0.001
Positive emotion index	11.6 (2.3)	11.3 (2.4)	< 0.001

[1]Significant difference in baseline characteristics between survivors in 2011 and those who dropped out between 2005 and 2011 was estimated using the Pearson χ^2 test for categorical variables and the T test for continuous variables

Abbreviations
ADL: Activities of daily living; CLHLS: Chinese Longitudinal Healthy Longevity Survey; MMSE: Mini-mental status examination

Acknowledgments
The authors are grateful to Bianca Suanet whose suggestions significantly improved the paper and to Lijun Yang from Beijing Normal University for his useful comments.

Funding
We gratefully acknowledge the funding support of the "Fundamental Research Funds for the Central Universities" (grant number SKZZB2014010) to this study.

Authors' contributions
ZS and MG conceived and designed the study. MG and YL analyzed the data. MG, ZS, YL, WZ, DT, SZ and LG were involved in the manuscript writing. ZS revised the manuscript. All the authors read and approved the final manuscript.

Competing interests
The authors declare that they have no competing interests.

Author details
[1]School of Social Development and Public Policy, China Institute of Health, Beijing Normal University, Beijing 100875, China. [2]School of Sociology, Beijing Normal University, No.19, Xinjiekou wai Street, Beijing 100875, China. [3]School of Humanities and Social Sciences, North China Electric Power University, Baoding 071000, China.

References
1. The number of elderly people aged 60 and over in China amounts to 241 million, accounting for 17.3% of the total population [http://www.gov.cn/xinwen/2018-02/26/content_5268992.htm] Accessed 2 Sept 2018 (In Chinese).
2. Wu Y, Dang J. China report of the development on aging cause: social sciences academic press; 2013. (In Chinese).
3. Wang X-Q, Chen P-J. Population ageing challenges health care in China. Lancet. 2014;383(9920):870.
4. WHO. China country assessment report on ageing and health. 2015.
5. WHO. Social determinants of health. WHO regional Office for South-East Asia. 2008.
6. Levasseur M, Desrosiers J, DS-C T. Subjective quality-of-life predictors for older adults with physical disabilities. Am J Phys Med Rehabil. 2008;87(10): 830–41.
7. Bourassa KJ, Memel M, Woolverton C, Sbarra DA. Social participation predicts cognitive functioning in aging adults over time: comparisons with physical health, depression, and physical activity. Aging Ment Health. 2017;21(2):133–46.
8. Takagi D, Kondo K, Kawachi I. Social participation and mental health: moderating effects of gender, social role and rurality. BMC Public Health. 2013;13(1):701.
9. WHO. Active ageing: A policy framework. Geneva: World Health Organization; 2002.
10. Chen N. The influence of social participation on the successful aging of middle-aged and elderly people. Chin J Gerontol. 2017;23:5962–4. (In Chinese)
11. Wei X, Wu R. The influence of the Elderly's social participation on their death hazard rate in China. South China Population. 2015;2:57–69. (In Chinese)
12. Li Y, Xu L, Chi I, Guo P. Participation in productive activities and health outcomes among older adults in urban China. Gerontologist. 2014;54(5):784–96.
13. Zhang C, Zhang D. The Influences of Social Activities on Urban Elderly People's Health: Based on CHARLS 2011. Populat Econ. 2016;5:55–63. (In Chinese)
14. Bauld L. The impact of smokefree legislation in England: Evidence review. 2011. https://assets.publishing.service.gov.uk/government/uploads/system/uploads/attachment_data/file/216319/dh_124959.pdf. Accessed 28 Jan 2018.
15. House JS, Landis KR, Umberson D. Social relationships and health. Science. 1988;241(4865):540–5.
16. Holt-Lunstad J, Smith TB, Layton JB. Social relationships and mortality risk: a meta-analytic review. PLoS Med. 2010;7(7):e1000316.
17. Kanamori S, Kai Y, Aida J, Kondo K, Kawachi I, Hirai H, Shirai K, Ishikawa Y, Suzuki K, Group J. Social participation and the prevention of functional disability in older Japanese: the JAGES cohort study. PLoS One. 2014;9(6): e99638.
18. James BD, Boyle PA, Buchman AS, Bennett DA. Relation of late-life social activity with incident disability among community-dwelling older adults. J Gerontol A Biol Sci Med Sci. 2011;66((4):467–73.
19. Hirai H, Kondo K, Ojima T, Murata C. Examination of risk factors for onset of certification of long-term care insurance in community-dwelling older people: AGES project 3-year follow-up study. Jap J Public Health. 2009;56(8):501–12.
20. Griffin J. The lonely society?: Mental Health Foundation; 2010.
21. Norstrand JA, Xu Q. Social capital and health outcomes among older adults in China: the urban–rural dimension. Gerontologist. 2011;52(3):325–34.
22. Cohen S, Underwood LG, Gottlieb BH. Social support measurement and intervention: a guide for health and social scientists: Oxford University Press; 2000.
23. Choi LH. Factors affecting volunteerism among older adults. J Appl Gerontol. 2003;22(2):179–96.
24. Glei DA, Goldman N, Ryff CD, Lin Y-H, Weinstein M. Social relationships and inflammatory markers: an analysis of Taiwan and the US. Soc Sci Med. 2012; 74(12):1891–9.
25. Avlund K, Lund R, Holstein BE, Due P. Social relations as determinant of onset of disability in aging. Arch Gerontol Geriatr. 2004;38(1):85–99.
26. Arem H, Moore SC, Patel A, Hartge P, De Gonzalez AB, Visvanathan K, Campbell PT, Freedman M, Weiderpass E, Adami HO. Leisure time physical activity and mortality: a detailed pooled analysis of the dose-response relationship. JAMA Intern Med. 2015;175(6):959–67.
27. Baltes MM, Wahl HW, Schmidfurstoss U. The daily life of elderly Germans: activity patterns, personal control, and functional health. J Gerontol. 1990; 45(4):173–9.
28. Morrow-Howell N, Hinterlong J, Rozario PA, Tang F. Effects of volunteering on the well-being of older adults. J Gerontol Ser B Psychol Sci Soc Sci. 2003; 58(3):S137–45.
29. Rubio E, Lázaro A, Sánchez-Sánchez A. Social participation and independence in activities of daily living: a cross sectional study. BMC Geriatr. 2009;9(1):26.
30. Hsu H. Does social participation by the elderly reduce mortality and cognitive impairment? Aging Ment Health. 2007;11(6):699–707.
31. Song B, Yu T. The influence on happiness of urban elderly reemployment. Populat J. 2011;1:42–6. (In Chinese)
32. Pei X. From alienation to participation: an discussion to the relationship between the elderly and social development. J Xuehai. 2004;1:113–20. (In Chinese)
33. Zhang Y. The effects of education level on reemployment of retired elders. Chin J Popul Sci. 1999;4:27–34. (In Chinese)
34. Shi L, Xie X. A study on the influence factors of reemployment of urban retired elderly people -a case of shanghai. China Labor. 2017;9: 56–60. (in Chinese)
35. Zeng Y. Reliability of age reporting among the Chinese oldest-old in the CLHLS datasets. Demog Methods Popul An. 2008;20:61–78.
36. Paterson DH, Warburton DE. Physical activity and functional limitations in older adults: a systematic review related to Canada's physical activity guidelines. Int J Behav Nutr Phys Act. 2010;7(1):38.
37. Takeda T, Kondo K, Hirai H. Psychosocial risk factors involved in progressive dementia-associated senility among the elderly residing at home. AGES project--three year cohort longitudinal study. Jap J Public Health. 2010; 57(12):1054–65.
38. Sobel ME. Asymptotic confidence intervals for indirect effects in structural equation models. Sociol Methodol. 1982;13:290–312.
39. Sakamoto A, Ukawa S, Okada E, Sasaki S, Zhao W, Kishi T, Kondo K, Tamakoshi A. The association between social participation and cognitive function in community-dwelling older populations: Japan Gerontological

Does social participation reduce the risk of functional disability among older adults in China? A survival...

89

evaluation study at Taisetsu community Hokkaido. Int J Geriatric Psychiatr. 2017;32(10):1131–40.

40. Zeng Y, Gu D, Purser J, Hoenig H, Christakis N. Associations of environmental factors with health and mortality among Chinese elderly: a sample survey in 22 provinces in China. Chin J Health Policy. 2014;7(6):53–62. (In Chinese)

41. Glei DA, Landau DA, Goldman N, Chuang Y-L, Rodríguez G, Weinstein M. Participating in social activities helps preserve cognitive function: an analysis of a longitudinal, population-based study of the elderly. Int J Epidemiol. 2005;34(4):864–71.

42. Stern C, Munn Z. Cognitive leisure activities and their role in preventing dementia: a systematic review. Int J Evid Based Healthcare. 2010;8(1):2–17.

43. Rebok GW, Ball K, Guey LT, Jones RN, Kim HY, King JW, Marsiske M, Morris JN, Tennstedt SL, Unverzagt FW. Ten-year effects of the ACTIVE cognitive training trial on cognition and everyday functioning in older adults. J Am Geriatr Soc. 2014;62(1):16–24.

44. Umberson D, Karas Montez J. Social relationships and health: a flashpoint for health policy. J Health Soc Behav. 2010;51(1_suppl):S54–66.

45. Fu W, Jiang Z, Zou L, Liu B. The impact of interest and social support on negative life events among community-dwelling older adults. Chin J Nurs Educ. 2016;13(11):867–70. (In Chinese)

46. Li Z. Literature review on social participation of the elderly in the past 30 years. Dongyue Tribune. 2009;30(8):60–4. (In Chinese)

47. Xu Q, Perkins DD, Chow JC. Sense of community, neighboring, and social capital as predictors of local political participation in China. Am J Community Psychol. 2010;45(3–4):259–71.

48. Chen F, Short SE. Household context and subjective well-being among the oldest old in China. J Fam Issues. 2008;29(10):1379–403.

49. Haider SJ, Loughran D. Elderly labor supply: work or play? Working Papers 2001.

9

Interventions for frail community-dwelling older adults have no significant effect on adverse outcomes

Michael Van der Elst[1*], Birgitte Schoenmakers[1], Daan Duppen[2], Deborah Lambotte[2], Bram Fret[2], Bert Vaes[1,3], Jan De Lepeleire[1] and D-SCOPE Consortium

Abstract

Background: According to some studies, interventions can prevent or delay frailty, but their effect in preventing adverse outcomes in frail community-dwelling older people is unclear. The aim is to investigate the effect of an intervention on adverse outcomes in frail older adults.

Methods: A systematic review and meta-analysis of Medline, Embase, the Cochrane Library, and Social Sciences Citation Index. Randomized controlled studies that aimed to treat frail community-dwelling older adults, were included. The outcomes were mortality, hospitalization, formal health costs, accidental falls, and institutionalization. Several sub-analyses were performed (duration of intervention, average age, dimension, recruitment).

Results: Twenty-five articles (16 original studies) were included. Six types of interventions were found. The pooled odds ratios (OR) for mortality when allocated in the experimental group were 0.99 [95% CI: 0.79, 1.25] for case management and 0.78 [95% CI: 0.41, 1.45] for provision information intervention. For institutionalization, the pooled OR with case management was 0.92 [95% CI: 0.63, 1.32], and the pooled OR for information provision intervention was 1.53 [95% CI: 0.64, 3.65]. The pooled OR for hospitalization when allocated in the experimental group was 1.13 [95% CI: 0.95, 1.35] for case management. Further sub-analyses did not yield any significant findings.

Conclusion: This systematic review and meta-analysis does not provide sufficient scientific evidence that interventions by frail older adults can be protective against the included adverse outcomes. A sub-analysis for some variables yielded no significant effects, although some findings suggested a decrease in adverse outcomes.

Keywords: Frailty - Intervention - Community-dwelling - RCT - Review - Older adults

Background

The population in the European Union is aging rapidly [1], and studies show that 30% of this population will be over age 65 by 2060 [1]. Therefore, the number of frail older adults with a high need for care and support will increase, and resource optimization is necessary [2, 3]. The literature describes two approaches to frailty [4–6]. The first, often designated as physical frailty, emphasizes frailty as a biological/medical concept, defined as *"a medical syndrome with multiple causes and contributors that is characterized by diminished strength, endurance, and reduced physiologic function that increases an individual's vulnerability for developing increased dependency and/or death"* [7]. The second approach investigates frailty in a multidimensional way. In addition to strength or endurance, this perspective emphasizes cognitive, social, and psychological factors as defined by Gobbens et al.: *"Frailty is a dynamic state affecting an individual who experiences losses in one or more domains of*

* Correspondence: michael.vanderelst@kuleuven.be
[1]Department of Public Health and Primary Care, University of Leuven, Kapucijnenvoer 33 bus 7001, B-3000 Leuven, Belgium
Full list of author information is available at the end of the article

human functioning (physical, psychological, social), which is caused by the influence of a range of variables and which increases the risk of adverse outcomes" [8].

Many studies suggest that frailty is associated with adverse outcomes including mortality, institutionalization, hospitalization, and accidental falls [7, 9–12]. Some authors assume that early detection and intervention are important to prevent or delay frailty, improve quality of life, and reduce costs of care [7, 13]. Nevertheless, it is unclear if interventions in frail community-dwelling older adults can be protective against adverse frailty outcomes [14–18].

This systematic literature review and meta-analysis examines the following three questions: Which interventions are applied to protect frail community-dwelling older adults against adverse outcomes? What effect do interventions have on frail community-dwelling older adults in terms of mortality, hospitalization, formal health costs, accidental falls, and institutionalization? Finally, how do age, study duration, and the multi- versus unidimensional approaches of frailty and recruitment influence the effect of an intervention?

Methods

A systematic review and meta-analysis was performed. Four electronic databases were consulted: Medline, Embase, The Cochrane Library (CL), and Social Sciences Citation Index (SSCI). The SSCI was consulted to assure that articles with a multidimensional approach to frailty would be found. The recommendations of the Cochrane Handbook for Systematic Reviews for Interventions 5.1.0 were used [19], and the protocol was registered (Prospero registration CRD42016035429).

Search strategy

The search strategy used four key terms: aged, frail elderly, independent living, and randomized controlled trial (RCT). The final search strategy was developed with the help of a librarian (Additional file 1: Data S1). The search for articles was carried out for the first time in September 2015 and the second time on June 17, 2016. The references for the selected articles were screened for other potentially relevant publications.

Inclusion and exclusion criteria

Within the scope of this study, the population in the included articles had to be 60 years or older, diagnosed as frail, and community-dwelling. Concerning the intervention and methodology, all studies had to be RCTs, frailty had to have been operationalized (regardless of the frailty operationalization), all types of intervention were allowed, there was no recruitment after hospital discharge (inpatient and outpatient), and the intervention must have been compared with care as usual. The

studies needed to have one or more of the following outcomes: mortality, institutionalization, hospitalization, formal health costs, and accidental falls. Pilot studies and studies not written in English, French, German, or Dutch were excluded.

Selection of studies

Retrieval and selection of studies were performed in a stepwise way. After duplicate records were removed, titles and abstracts were screened. Two reviewers assessed a sample of 12% (MVDE and DD). If their agreement reached 95%, the first author continued the inclusion process alone. In the next step, two researchers (MVDE and DD) independently read the full text of the selected articles for the inclusion and exclusion criteria. In cases of doubt or disagreement, a third researcher (BV) was asked to judge.

Critical appraisal

Two independent researchers (DL and BF) assessed the quality of each article with the Cochrane risk of bias tool [19]. An evaluation was made in seven areas (sequence generation, allocation concealment, blinding participants and personnel, blinding of outcome assessment, incomplete outcome data, selective outcome reporting, and other bias). If an article met two or fewer criteria, it was defined as low quality; meeting three or four criteria was defined as medium quality; and if it met more than four criteria, it was considered a high-quality paper.

Data extraction

The first author preformed the data-extraction by preparing an excel sheet including all the necessary data to answer the research questions like average age of a study, number of participants. Subsequently two researchers (DL and BF) controlled the accuracy of the data-extraction. Information concerning average age, percentage of male participants, type of intervention, operationalization of frailty, and method of recruitment of participants (e.g. participants could be recruited through census records, a service center or a care center, etc.) were subsequently collected and categorized (Additional file 2: Text S1). Frailty was defined unidimensionally if it included solely biological aspects (i.e., nutritional status, physical activity, mobility, strength, and energy). Frailty was defined multidimensionally if it also included variables such as cognition, mood, and social relations/social support [20].

Statistics

The statistical analysis was performed with SPSS 23.0 (IBM Corp., Armonk, NY, USA) and Review Manager 5.3 [21]. For the outcomes of mortality, institutionalization (residential home/nursing home/long-term care facility), and hospitalization (inpatients), the odds ratio (OR) was calculated for every intervention; for the outcome of accidental falls, the incidence rate ratio (IRR) was presented; for formal health costs a percentage was calculated, the sum of all the presented formal health costs in the intervention group (IG) was divided by the sum of all the presented formal health costs in the control group (CG). Raw data were used for the variables mortality, institutionalization and hospitalization, for accidental falls the IRR scores were used reported in the articles. If data were unclear the first author was contacted If possible, a pooled meta-analysis was executed to measure the odds ratio. A random effect model was applied because one can assume no common effect size exist, the study population may differ from each other in ways that could affect the treatment effect (e.g., differences in the average age of the study population). Differences among included studies were assessed and described in terms of heterogeneity. A sub-analysis was performed for duration of intervention, a multi- versus unidimensional approach to frailty, average age, recruitment method of the participants, and studies with a moderate or high quality. A sub-analysis also was performed for studies that used the Fried criteria or the Frailty Index. Funnel plots were inspected, and studies with multiple research arms were analyzed separately.

Results

The details of the search process are presented (Additional file 3: Figure S1). After the databases were searched, 25 articles were included for review representing 16 original studies. Duplicate data were excluded. All included papers are listed in Table 1 with study characteristics. The 16 original studies involved the following: nine with a case management intervention [2, 22–37], three with information provision interventions [38–41], one with physical intervention [42], one with psychosocial intervention [43], one with a pharmaceutical intervention [44], and one with a technological intervention [45]. Six articles approached frailty in an unidimensional way [2, 22–26, 37, 42, 44, 45], nine articles approached frailty in a multidimensional way [27, 29–36, 38–41, 43], and in one article the approach of frailty was unclear [28]. Two papers were of low quality (≤2) [39, 45]. For the interventions of case management and information provision, pooled meta-analyses were performed. For case management, sub-analyses also were performed.

The effects of an intervention

The effects of an intervention in the original studies are listed in Table 2. Two results were significantly better in the IG in comparison with the CG. In Hall et al. [29], the intervention of case management resulted in a lower institutionalization, with an OR of 0.32 [95% confidence interval (CI): 0.12, 0.87]. Perttila et al. performed a study with a physical intervention, this resulted in a lower number of accidental falls with an IRR of 0.43 [42]. Four

articles also offered an economic evaluation of the intervention, with one involving an information provision intervention showing a decrease in formal health costs in the IG of 11.84% in comparison with the CG [39].

For case management and information provision intervention, a pooled meta-analysis was performed (Table 3). The pooled ORs for mortality when allocated in the experimental group were 0.99 [95% CI: 0.79, 1.25] for case management and 0.78 [95% CI: 0.41, 1.45] for provision information intervention. The mortality ORs for the other interventions (pharmaceutical, 3.19 [95% CI: 0.13, 81.25]; psychosocial, 1.20 [95% CI: 0.41, 3.49]; technological, 7.48 [95% CI: 0.35, 157.76]) were greater than one.

For institutionalization, the pooled OR with case management was 0.92 [95% CI: 0.63, 1.32], and the pooled OR for information provision was 1.53 [95% CI: 0.64, 3.65]; they were not significant. The pooled OR for hospitalization when allocated in the experimental group was 1.13 [95% CI: 0.95, 1.35] for case management. The funnel plots, statistical heterogeneity and forest plots can be found in the appendix (Additional file 4: Figure S2: Funnel plot and Forest plot).

Sub-analysis

The influence of duration of intervention, average age, multi- versus unidimensional approach to frailty, and recruitment on the effect of an intervention was explored. Various sub-analyses were performed but with no significant results (Table 4). For the variable of age in the category ≤80, the risk for an adverse outcome was lower. Several methods to operationalize frailty were allowed, and a sub-analysis was performed. When frailty was operationalized with the Fried criteria [5] or the Frailty Index [6], the OR for mortality was 1.12 [95% CI: 0.52, 2.41].

Two papers had a low quality (≤2) (Additional file 5: Figure S3: critical appraisal) [39, 45]. For information provision, a sub-analysis was performed, and the pooled OR for mortality increased from 0.76 to 0.94 [95% CI: 0.42, 2.11]. For institutionalization, the pooled OR decreased from 1.53 to 1.35 [95% CI: 0.34, 5.29] (Additional file 4: Figure S2: Funnel plot and Forest Plot).

Discussion

The aim of this study was to investigate the effect of interventions to prevent adverse outcomes in frail community-dwelling older people. This systematic review and meta-analysis does not provide sufficient scientific evidence that interventions can be protective against the included adverse outcomes. A sub-analysis for some variables (duration of intervention, average age, dimension, recruitment) yielded no significant effects, although some findings suggested a decrease in adverse outcomes.

The results of this systematic review are in line with previous studies: the effect is unclear and inconsistent.

Interventions for frail community-dwelling older adults have no significant effect on adverse...

93

Table 1 Descriptive information included articles (N = 16 original studies, 25 articles) continued

OS. Author	arms	N	Frailty	Dim	Intervention	Duration	Age	QA
1. Aggar (2012), Cameron (2013), Fairhall (2012, 2014 & 2015)		237	Fried	1	Case management	12	83.3	4
2. De Vriendt (2016)		168	BEL-profile scale	1	Case management	2,5	80.4	4
3. Dorrestein (2016)		359	Poor self-perceived general health, concerns about falls and related activity avoidance	2	Psychosocial intervention	4	78.3	6
4. Favela (2013)	4.1	89	Rockwood	2	Case management	9	76	3
	4.2	88	Rockwood	2	Case management	9	76	3
5. Hall (1992)		167	≥ 65 and admitted by the Long Term Care program to personal care at home	–	Case management	36	77.9	4
6. Kehusmaa (2010), Ollonqvist (2008)		708	Meet the criteria for entitlement to the SII Pensioners' Care Allowance	2	Case management	8	78.4	4
7. Kim (2015)		66	Fried	1	Pharmaceutical intervention	3	80.7	5
8. Kono (2012 & 2013)		323	Being classified into the two lowest care need levels in the LTCI system: Support Levels 1 and 2 (out of 7)	2	Information provision intervention	24	79.9	2
9. Kono (2016)		360	Being classified into the two lowest care need levels in the LTCI system: Support Levels 1 and 2 (out of 7)	2	Information provision intervention	24	79.2	5
10. Metzelthin (2013, 2014 & 2015)		346	GFI	2	Case management	24	77.2	3
11. Monteserin (2010)		285	Meet 2 of following criteria:≥85y, > = 9 the Gijon Social Scale, ≥2 the Pfeiffer test, ≥2 the Charlson comorbidity index, ≥1 the Yesavage Depression Scale, ≥91 the Barthel index, ≥12 the Mini-Nutritional Assessment Short Form, polymedication, > 1 fall in the last 6 months and daily urinary incontinence in the last 6 months.	2	Information provision intervention	0	81.2	3
12. Perttila (2016)		83	Fried	1	Physical intervention	12	78.8	3
13. Upatising (2013)		32	Fried	1	Technological intervention	12	–	2
14. Van Hout (2010)		651	Self-reported score in the worst quartile of at least two of six COOP–WONCA charts	2	Case management	18	81.4	4
15. Van Leeuwen (2015), Hoogendijk (2016)	15.1	683	Identified by primary care physician as frail	2	Case management	6	80.6	3
	15.2	694	Identified by primary care physician as frail	2	Case management	12	80.4	3
	15.3	682	Identified by primary care physician as frail	2	Case management	18	80.8	3
16. Williams (1987)		117	No medical evaluation during the preceding year, significant decline in functional ability, unstable medical problem, unmet needs in the performance of ADL, taking three or more medications who had not had a medical evaluation within the past year, dissatisfied with current medical care, seeking a second opinion	1	Case management	8	76.5	6

Dim dimension of frailty: 1 = unidimensional physical/medical; 2 = multidimensional (social, cognitive, psychological) - = missing. Duration in months, age in years. Van Leeuwen et al. and Favela et al. are studies with several arms. *Ref.* = reference. *QA* Quality assessment, *OS* original study

In a systematic review, You et al. examined the effect of case management on mortality/survival days, and two out of seven articles reported a significant result [16]. Also, Hallberg and Kristerisson found in their systematic review that the effect of an intervention differed among studies: some found no effect on hospital admission, length of stay, or number of hospital days whereas others reported fewer hospital admissions and/or shorter lengths of stay [46]. Mayo-Wilson et al. concluded in their systematic review that home visiting is not consistently associated with a higher risk of mortality [47].

A pooled meta-analysis should lead to more significant and consistent results, yet this analysis did not. However, the literature provides evidence that a pooled meta-analysis

Table 2 Results intervention on adverse outcomes

OS. Author	Mortality [CI]	Institutionalization [CI]	Health costs [CI]	Accidental falls[CI]	Hospitalization [CI]
01.Cameron et al.	1.28 [0.53, 3.09]	–	–	–	–
01.Fairhall et al.	–	–	–	1.12 [0.78, 1.63]	–
01.Fairhall et al.	–	0.83 [0.46, 1.53]	4.8%	–	1.47 [0.87, 2.47]
02.De Vriendt et al.	2.89 [0.12, 72.08]	–	–	–	–
03.Dorrestein et al.	1.20 [0.41, 3.49]	–	–	0.86 [0.65, 1.13]	–
04.Favela et al.	0.98 [0.13, 7.26]	–	–	–	–
04.Favela et al.	0.49 [0.04, 5.59]	–	–	–	–
05.Hall et al.	0.79 [0.36, 1.71]	0.32 [0.12, 0.87]	–	–	–
06.Kehusmaa et al.	0.85 [0.39, 1.83]	1.28 [0.79, 2.06]	30%	–	1.03 [0.77, 1.39]
07.Kim et al.	3.19 [0.13, 81.25]	–	–	–	–
08.Kono et al.	0.52 [0.24, 1.13]	1.70 [0.40, 7.23]	-11.8%	–	–
09.Kono et al.	1.35 [0.69, 2.64]	2.41 [0.61, 9.49]	–	–	–
10.Metzelthin et al.	1.21 [0.53, 2.76]	–	–	–	–
10.Metzelthin et al.	–	0.65 [0.20, 2.18]	29%	–	0.92 [0.55, 1.55]
11.Monteserin et al.	0.59 [0.24, 1.43]	0.59 [0.10, 3.56]	–	–	–
12.Perttila et al.	–	–	–	0.43 [0.33, 0.57]	–
13.Upatising et al.	7.48 [0.35, 157.7]	–	–	–	–
14.Van Hout et al.	0.86 [0.54, 1.37]	1.12 [0.60, 2.08]	–	–	1.23 [0.90, 1.68]
15.Van Leeuwen et al.	1.11 [0.50, 2.48]	–	–	–	–
15.Van Leeuwen et al.	0.88 [0.49, 1.56]	–	–	–	–
15.Van Leeuwen et al.	1.37 [0.75, 2.48]	–	–	–	–
16.Williams et al.	–	1.30 [0.33, 5.09]	–	–	1.11 [0.51, 2.42]

mortality, institutionalization, and hospitalization as odds ratio [Confidence Interval]; formal health costs as ratio intervention group relative to control group; accidental falls as IRR; double data are not reported. OS = original study. - = missing. Van Leeuwen et al. and Favela et al. are studies with several arms

could produce significant findings. For example, Elkan et al. reported that mortality and institutionalization are significantly lower after a home-based support intervention for frail older adults in comparison with a control group [48]. Thomas et al. concluded that a physical intervention reduces mortality in older community-dwelling adults, but the inclusion criteria did vary among the included studies in these two analyses, which may explain the differences in outcome. Elkan et al. included non-randomized studies and studies with older adults recently discharged from the hospital [48] whereas the older adults in Thomas et al. are not defined as frail [49].

Remarkably, the data in the current work show that the odds of being hospitalized are higher in the intervention group than in the control group (Table 2). Berglund et al. reported in their RCT that after the intervention, participants in the experimental group were much more aware of whom to contact with questions about care and services [50]. This effect could explain why the odds of being hospitalized were higher in the intervention group than in the control group and is a likely reason why the results for the outcome of formal health cost in the experimental group were not significantly lower than in the control group.

The studies in the current analysis showed heterogeneity for average age, duration, etc., which could explain the inconsistency in the results [51]. A sub-analysis should lead to significant and consistent results. For example, Stuck et al. concluded that a preventive program reduces mortality in a younger study population (mean age < 80 years) but not in older populations [52]. However, in this study, a sub-analysis for the variable average age ≤ 80 years (Table 3) was not significant, and neither were the results of other sub-analyses. Our findings confirm Elkan et al.: population type, duration, and age have no significant effect on mortality and institutionalization [48].

Considerations for future research

A plausible reason for the lack of evidence is the heterogeneity within studies. Within studies, the contextual factors of the population in the experimental group was heterogeneous, with differences in age, educational level, morbidities, and context, etc. If frailty is operationalized with a multidimensional approach, however, the question that arises is: 'which dimensions were problematic?' Also the local setting within studies was heterogeneous, Van Leeuwen et al. used two regions, and Kono et al.

Table 3 Odds ratio and meta-analysis of case management and information intervention provision

	Mortality [CI]	Institutionalization [CI]	Hospitalization [CI]
Case management			
Cameron et al. (2013)	1.28 [0.53, 3.09]	–	–
De Vriendt et al. (2016)	2.89 [0.12, 72.08]	–	–
Fairhall et al. (2015)	–	0.83 [0.46, 1.53]	1.47 [0.87, 2.47]
Favela et al. (2013)	0.98 [0.13, 7.26]	–	–
Favela et al. (2013)	0.49 [0.04, 5.59]	–	–
Hall et al. (1992)	0.79 [0.36, 1.71]	0.32 [0.12, 0.87]	–
Kehusmaa et al. (2014)	0.85 [0.39, 1.83]	1.28 [0.79, 2.06]	1.03 [0.77, 1.39]
Metzelthin et al. (2015)	1.21 [0.53, 2.76]	0.65 [0.20, 2.18]	0.92 [0.55, 1.55]
Van Hout et al. (2010)	0.86 [0.54, 1.37]	1.12 [0.60, 2.08]	1.23 [0.90, 1.68]
Van Leeuwen et al. (2015)	1.11 [0.50, 2.48]	–	–
Van Leeuwen et al. (2015a)	0.88 [0.49, 1.56]	–	–
Van Leeuwen et al. (2015b)	1.37 [0.75, 2.48]	–	–
Williams et al. (1987)	–	1.30 [0.33, 5.09]	1.11 [0.51, 2.42]
Total (95% CI)	0.99 [0.79, 1.25]	0.92 [0.63, 1.32]	1.13 [0.95, 1.35]
Information provision intervention			
Kono et al. (2013)	0.52 [0.24, 1.13]	1.70 [0.40, 7.23]	–
Kono et al. (2016)	1.35 [0.69, 2.64]	2.41 [0.61, 9.49]	–
Monteserin et al. (2010)	0.59 [0.24, 1.43]	0.59 [0.10, 3.56]	–
Total (95% CI)	0.78 [0.41, 1.45]	1.53 [0.64, 3.65]	–

Total = meta-analysis. - = missing. [CI] = confidence interval

Table 4 Odds ratio or pooled odds ratio of the sub-analyses for a case management intervention for the outcomes of mortality, institutionalization, and hospitalization

	Mortality [CI]	Institutionalization [CI]	Hospitalization [CI]
Duration (months)			
≤6	1.18 [0.54, 2.56]	–	–
> 6 & ≤12	0.93 [0.62, 1.38]	1.10 [0.77, 1.58]	1.12 [0.88, 1.43]
> 12	1.00 [0.74, 1.37]	0.75 [0.47, 1.19]	1.14 [0.88, 1.49]
Dimension			
Unidimensional	1.37 [0.59, 3.18]	0.90 [0.52, 1.56]	1.35 [0.87, 2.08]
Multidimensional	0.99 [0.77, 1.27]	1.15 [0.80, 1.65]	1.09 [0.90, 1.33]
Age (years)			
≤80	0.90 [0.58, 1.40]	0.94 [0.65, 1.38]	1.01 [0.79, 1.29]
> 80	1.03 [0.78, 1.35]	0.96 [0.63, 1.48]	1.29 [0.99, 1.68]
Recruitment			
Primary health care center	1.03 [0.79, 1.36]	1.00 [0.58, 1.73]	1.14 [0.88, 1.49]
Health services	0.85 [0.50, 1.46]	0.96 [0.63, 1.45]	1.03 [0.77, 1.39]
Register	0.73 [0.16, 3.37]	–	–
Rehabilitation	1.28 [0.53, 3.09]	0.83 [0.46, 1.53]	1.47 [0.87, 2.47]
Combination	–	1.30 [0.33, 5.09]	1.11 [0.51, 2.42]

A sub-analysis was made for duration intervention, dimensional approach frailty, average population, and recruitment of the older adults. - = missing.
[CI] = confidence interval

and Perttila et al. used three regions [36, 39, 40, 42]. It is plausible that an intervention within a subgroup is effective. Analyzing the results of an experiment on an aggregated level might lead to an ecological fallacy [53].

Future research should not solely focus on the effect of an intervention but also address the question: why did interventions work when they did or why not, for who did they work and what contextual factors triggered the mechanisms required to make them work. This is described by Pawson and Tilley in 'realistic evaluation' (1997). They suggest that a realistic evaluation approach might provide a better understanding of the effect of an intervention [54]. This approach is a theory-driven method that not only addresses the outcome of an intervention, but also why interventions worked, when they worked or for who they worked [54].

A consensus about the concept of frailty is necessary for future research and would enable comparison, evaluation, and replication of interventional studies. Some authors have made valuable efforts toward reaching a consensus [7]; for example, 'The White Book on Frailty' has delivered an important contribution to this understanding [13].

Several other explanations are possible for the current results. The selected population may have been detected too late and already have been too frail [13, 15]. In addition, societal trends, such as changes in structure and function of families, might have aggravated the incidence or severity of frailty and complicated its effective management [13]. A lack of mindfulness for these societal trends also may be an explanation for the non-significant results. Several authors have discussed the difficulties of implementing the intervention [32, 34]. As a last consideration, future research making an economic evaluation must consider the extra awareness of services that older adults gain through an intervention [50].

Strengths and limitations
Previous systematic reviews have focused on the effect of one intervention in comparison with care as usual [55–58]. A strength of the current analysis is the overview of interventions for frail community-dwelling older adults in the context of several adverse outcomes. A second strength is that only RCTs were included whereas several other systematic reviews have also included non-RCTs [46, 51]. In this analysis, differences among studies were assessed (heterogeneity) in terms of duration of the intervention, average participant age, dimensional approach to frailty, recruitment of participants, and frailty operationalization, constituting a third strength. A fourth strength is that three of the five outcome measures – mortality, institutionalization, and hospitalization – are collected primarily through registers and can be seen as objective data, which decreases the risk for bias [2].

The analysis also has some weaknesses, so that the results should be interpreted with caution. A first weakness is the small number of original studies, which led to meta-analyses only for case management and information provision and reduced the reliability of the results. One reason for the small numbers of included publications is the lack of operationalization of 'frailty' in studies. An absence of an operationalization of frailty is also a feature in other studies [15, 17]. Other reasons for exclusion were a lack of usual care, no relevant outcomes, and the recruitment of non-community-dwelling participants. A second weakness is the concept of frailty. Several methods are used to operationalize frailty, and some may not be accurate enough to recruit frail older adults, making study comparison and evaluation difficult [56]. A third weakness is that several concepts, such as case management, information provision, institutionalization, and formal health costs, have different operationalizations, leading to heterogeneity among studies. In the current analysis, mortality, institutionalization, accidental falls, formal health costs, and hospitalization were used because they are often cited as adverse outcomes. Other outcomes not included in this systematic review include functional status, physical performances, quality of life, mastery, disability, etc. [14], which can be seen as a weakness. These outcomes are not included because of the different methods to operationalize these concepts.

Conclusion
The number of frail older adults with a high need of care and support is increasing. According to some studies, interventions can prevent or delay frailty, but their effect in preventing adverse outcomes in frail community-dwelling older people is unclear. The aim of this article was to investigate if interventions for frail community-dwelling older adults can be protective against adverse outcomes. This systematic review and meta-analysis does not provide sufficient scientific evidence that supports this assumption, even though some results suggest a decrease in adverse outcomes.

Future research must consider that the research population of older adults is very heterogeneous, also within studies. A good breakdown of all of these characteristics is necessary, and sub-analyses might avoid ecological fallacies. Each patient's specific needs and how to deliver these services are probably essential for the effectiveness of an intervention. New methods/approaches, for example the realist approach might provide a better understanding of the effect of an intervention. Future research must also consider new societal trends, implementation problems, and heightened awareness about services that may influence the results.

Abbreviations
CG: Control group; CI: Confidence interval; CL: The Cochrane Library; IG: Intervention group; IRR: Incidence rate ratio; OR: Odds ratio; OS: Original studies; RCT: Randomized controlled trial; SSCI: Social Sciences Citation Index

Acknowledgements
I would like to thank Michels Marleen (KU Leuven), who helped with the development of the search strategy. The D-SCOPE consortium is an inter-national research consortium and is composed of researchers from Vrije Universiteit Brussel, Belgium (dr. A.-S. Smetcoren, dr. S. Dury, prof. dr. L. De Donder, prof. dr. N. De Witte, prof. dr. E Dierickx, D. Lambotte, B. Fret, D. Duppen, prof. dr. M. Kardol, prof.dr. D. Verté); College University Ghent, Belgium (L. Hoeyberghs, prof. dr. N. De Witte); University Antwerpen, Belgium (dr. E De Roeck, prof. dr. S Engelborghs, prof. dr. P. P. Dedeyn); KU Leuven, Belgium (M. Van der Elst, prof. dr. B. Schoenmakers, prof. dr. J. De Lepeleire) and Maastricht University, The Netherlands (A. Van der Vorst, dr. G.A.R. Zijlstra, prof. dr. G.I.J.M Kempen, prof. dr. J.M.G.A Schols) .

Funding
Funding was provided by the instituut voor Innovatie door Wetenschap en Technologie (IWT). IWT-project number: IWT-140027 with the title "D-SCOPE: Detection - Support and Care of Older People in their Environment". The instituut voor Innovatie door Wetenschap en Technologie (IWT) had no role in study design, data collection, data-analysis, data interpretation, or writing of the report.

Authors' contributions
MVDE: study concept, data collection and data-analysis, drafting the manuscript. BS: study concept data-analysis, drafting manuscript, DD: data collection, critical revision of manuscript for intellectual content. DL: data extraction, critical revision of manuscript for intellectual content. BF: data extraction, critical revision of manuscript for intellectual content. BV: data collection, critical revision of manuscript for intellectual content. JDL: study concept, data-analysis, drafting the manuscript. All authors approved the final manuscript submitted for publication.

Competing interests
The authors declare that they have no competing interests.

Author details
[1]Department of Public Health and Primary Care, University of Leuven, Kapucijnenvoer 33 bus 7001, B-3000 Leuven, Belgium. [2]Department of Educational Sciences, Vrije Universiteit Brussel, Pleinlaan 2, B-1050 Brussels, Belgium. [3]Institute of Health and Society, Université Catholique de Louvain, Clos Chapelle-aux-champs 30, B-1200 Brussels, Belgium.

References
1. Eurostat. Active Ageing and Solidarity between Generations A statistical portrait of the European Union 2012. Luxembourg: Publications Office of the European Union; 2012.
2. Fairhall N, Sherrington C, Kurrle SE, et al. Economic evaluation of a multifactorial, interdisciplinary intervention versus usual care to reduce frailty in frail older people. J Am Med Dir Assoc [Internet]. 2015;16(1):41–8.
3. European Social Network Services for older people in Europe: Facts and figures about long term care services in Europe. 2008.
4. Lally F, Crome P. Understanding frailty. Postgrad Med J. 2007;83(975):16–20.
5. Fried LP, Tangen CM, Walston J, et al. Frailty in older adults: evidence for a phenotype. J Gerontol A Biol Sci Med Sci. 2001;56(3):146–56.
6. Mitnitski AB, Mogilner AJ, Rockwood K. Accumulation of deficits as a proxy measure of aging. ScientificWorldJournal. 2001;1:323–36.
7. Morley JE, Vellas B, van Kan GA, et al. Frailty consensus: a call to action. J Am Med Dir Assoc. 2013;14(6):392–7.
8. Gobbens RJJ, Luijkx KG, Wijnen-Sponselee MT, Schols JMGA. In search of an integral conceptual definition of frailty: opinions of experts. J Am Med Dir Assoc. 2010;11(5):338–43.
9. Kojima G. Frailty as a predictor of future falls among community-dwelling older people: a systematic review and meta-analysis. J Am Med Dir Assoc. 2015;16(12):1027–33.
10. Kelaiditi E, Andrieu S, Cantet C, et al. Frailty index and incident mortality, hospitalization, and institutionalization in Alzheimer's disease: data from the ICTUS study. J Gerontol A Biol Sci Med Sci. 2016;71(4):543–8.
11. Rockwood K, Fox RA, Stolee P, et al. Frailty in elderly people: an evolving concept. CMAJ. 1994;150(4):489.
12. Mosquera C, Spaniolas K, Fitzgerald TL. Impact of frailty on surgical outcomes: the right patient for the right procedure. Surgery. 2016;160(2):272–80.
13. Vellas B. White book on frailty. 2016. Available at: https://www.jpn-geriat-soc.or.jp/gakujutsu/pdf/whitebook.pdf. Accessed 26 Oct 2016.
14. Daniels R, van Rossum E, de Witte L, et al. Interventions to prevent disability in frail community-dwelling elderly: a systematic review. BMC Health Serv Res. 2008;8:1–8.
15. Theou O, Stathokostas L, Roland KP, et al. The effectiveness of exercise interventions for the management of frailty: a systematic review. J Aging Res. 2011;2011:1–19.
16. You EC, Dunt D, Doyle C, Hsueh A. Effects of case management in community aged care on client and carer outcomes: a systematic review of randomized trials and comparative observational studies. BMC Health Serv Res [Internet]. 2012;12:1–14.
17. Clegg AP, Barber S, Young JB, et al. Do home-based exercise interventions improve outcomes for frail older people? findings from a systematic review Rev Clin Gerontol. 2011;22(1):66–78.
18. Chin APMJ, van Uffelen JG, Riphagen I, van Mechelen W. The functional effects of physical exercise training in frail older people : a systematic review. Sports Med. 2008;38(9):781–93.
19. Collaboration TC. Cochrane handbook for systematic reviews of. Interventions. 2011.
20. de Vries NM, Staal JB, van Ravensberg CD, et al. Outcome instruments to measure frailty: a systematic review. Ageing Res Rev. 2011;10(1):104–14.
21. Review Manager (RevMan) [Computer program]. Version 5.3. Copenhagen: The Nordic Cochrane Centre TCC; 2014.
22. Aggar C, Ronaldson S, Cameron ID. Reactions to caregiving during an intervention targeting frailty in community living older people. BMC Geriatr. 2012;12:1–11.
23. Cameron ID, Fairhall N, Langron C, et al. A multifactorial interdisciplinary intervention reduces frailty in older people: randomized trial. BMC Med. 2013;11:1–10.
24. De Vriendt P, Peersman W, Florus A, et al. Improving health related quality of life and independence in community dwelling frail older adults through a client-centred and activity-oriented program. A pragmatic randomized controlled trial. J Nutr Health & Aging [Internet]. 2016;20(1):35–40.
25. Fairhall N, Sherrington C, Lord SR, et al. Effect of a multifactorial, interdisciplinary intervention on risk factors for falls and fall rate in frail older people: a randomised controlled trial. Age Ageing [Internet]. 2014; 43(5):616–22.
26. Fairhall N, Sherrington C, Kurrle SE, et al. Effect of a multifactorial interdisciplinary intervention on mobility-related disability in frail older people: randomised controlled trial. BMC Med [Internet]. 2012;10:1–13.
27. Favela J, Castro LA, Franco-Marina F, Sánchez-García S, Juárez-Cedillo T, Bermudez CE, et al. Nurse home visits with or without alert buttons versus usual care in the frail elderly: a randomized controlled trial. Clin Interv Aging. 2013;8:85–95.
28. Hall N, De Beck P, Johnson D, et al. Randomized trial of a health promotion program for frail elders. Can J Aging. 1992;11(1):72–91.
29. Hoogendijk EO, van der Horst HE, van de Ven PM, et al. Effectiveness of a geriatric care model for frail older adults in primary care: results from a stepped wedge cluster randomized trial. Eur J Intern Med. 2016;28:43–51.
30. Kehusmaa S, Autti-Rämö I, Valaste M, et al. Economic evaluation of a geriatric rehabilitation programme: a randomized controlled trial. J Rehab Med [Internet]. 2010;42(10):949–55.
31. Metzelthin SF, van Rossum E, de Witte LP, et al. Effectiveness of interdisciplinary primary care approach to reduce disability in community dwelling frail older people: cluster randomised controlled trial. BMJ. 2013; 347:1–12.

32. Metzelthin SF, Van Rossum E, De Witte LP, et al. Frail elderly people living at home; effects of an interdisciplinary primary care programme. Ned Tijdschr Geneeskd. 2014;158(17).

33. Metzelthin SF, van Rossum E, Hendriks MR, et al. Reducing disability in community-dwelling frail older people: cost-effectiveness study alongside a cluster randomised controlled trial. Age Ageing. 2015;44(3):390–6.

34. van Hout HP, Jansen AP, van Marwijk HW, et al. Prevention of adverse health trajectories in a vulnerable elderly population through nurse home visits: a randomized controlled trial. J Gerontol A Biol Sci Med Sci. 2010; 65(7):734–42.

35. Ollonqvist K, Aaltonen T, Karppi SL, et al. Network-based rehabilitation increases formal support of frail elderly home-dwelling persons in Finland: randomised controlled trial. Health Soc Care Community [Internet]. 2008; 16(2):115–25.

36. Van Leeuwen KM, Bosmans JE, Jansen AP, et al. Cost-effectiveness of a chronic care model for frail older adults in primary care: economic evaluation alongside a stepped-wedge cluster-randomized trial. J Am Geriatr Soc. 2015;63(12):2494–504.

37. Williams ME, Williams TF, Zimmer JG, et al. How does the team approach to outpatient geriatric evaluation compare with traditional care: a report of a randomized controlled trial. J Am Geriatr Soc [Internet]. 1987;35(12):1071–8.

38. Kono A, Kanaya Y, Fujita T, et al. Effects of a preventive home visit program in ambulatory frail older people: a randomized controlled trial. J Gerontol A Biol Sci Med Sci [Internet]. 2012;67(3):302–9.

39. Kono A, Kanaya Y, Tsumura C, Rubenstein LZ. Effects of preventive home visits on health care costs for ambulatory frail elders: a randomized controlled trial. Aging clin exp res [Internet]. 2013;25(5):575–81.

40. Kono A, Izumi K, Yoshiyuki N, et al. Effects of an updated preventive home visit program based on a systematic structured assessment of care needs for ambulatory frail older adults in Japan: a randomized controlled trial. J Gerontol A Biol Sci Med Sci. 2016:1–7.

41. Monteserin R, Brotons C, Moral I, et al. Effectiveness of a geriatric intervention in primary care: a randomized clinical trial. Fam Pract. 2010; 27(3):239–45.

42. Perttila NM, Ohman H, Strandberg TE, et al. Severity of frailty and the outcome of exercise intervention among participants with Alzheimer disease: a sub-group analysis of a randomized controlled trial. Eur Geriatr Med. 2016;7(2):117–21.

43. Dorresteijn TA, Zijlstra GA, Ambergen AW, et al. Effectiveness of a home-based cognitive behavioral program to manage concerns about falls in community-dwelling, frail older people: results of a randomized controlled trial. BMC Geriatr. 2016;16:1–11.

44. Kim H, Suzuki T, Kim M, et al. Effects of exercise and milk fat globule membrane (MFGM) supplementation on body composition, physical function, and hematological parameters in community-dwelling frail Japanese women: a randomized double blind, placebo-controlled, follow-up trial. PloS one [Internet]. 2015;10(2):1–20.

45. Upatising B, Hanson GJ, Kim YL, et al. Effects of home telemonitoring on transitions between frailty states and death for older adults: a randomized controlled trial. Int j Gen Med [Internet]. 2013;6:145–51.

46. Hallberg IR, Kristerisson J. Preventive home care of frail older people: a review of recent case management studies. J Clin Nurs. 2004;13(6B):112–20.

47. Mayo-Wilson E, Grant S, Burton J, et al. Preventive home visits for mortality, morbidity, and institutionalization in older adults: a systematic review and meta-analysis. PLoS One. 2014;9(3):e89257.

48. Elkan R, Kendrick D, Dewey M, et al. Effectiveness of home based support for older people: systematic review and meta-analysis. BMJ. 2001;323(7315): 719–24.

49. Thomas S, Mackintosh S, Halbert J. Does the 'Otago exercise programme' reduce mortality and falls in older adults?: a systematic review and meta-analysis. Age Ageing. 2010;39(6):681–7.

50. Berglund H, Wilhelmson K, Blomberg S, et al. Older people's views of quality of care: a randomised controlled study of continuum of care. J Clin Nurs. 2013;22(19–20):2934–44.

51. Low LF, Yap M, Brodaty H. A systematic review of different models of home and community care services for older persons. BMC Health Serv Res. 2011;11:1–15.

52. Stuck AE, Egger M, Hammer A, et al. Home visits to prevent nursing home admission and functional decline in elderly people: systematic review and meta-regression analysis. JAMA. 2002;287(8):1022–8.

53. Billiet J, Waege H. Een samenleving onderzocht: methoden van sociaal-wetenschappelijk onderzoek. 2005.

54. Pawson R, Tilley N. Realist evaluation. Monograph prepared for British Cabinet Office 2004.

55. De Labra C, Guimaraes-Pinheiro C, Maseda A, et al. Effects of physical exercise interventions in frail older adults: a systematic review of randomized controlled trials. BMC Geriatr. 2015;15:1–16.

56. Gustafsson S, Edberg A-K, Johansson B, Dahlin-Ivanoff S. Multi-component health promotion and disease prevention for community-dwelling frail elderly persons: a systematic review. Eur J Ageing. 2009;6(4):315–29.

57. Barlow J, Singh D, Bayer S, Curry R. A systematic review of the benefits of home telecare for frail elderly people and those with long-term conditions. J Telemed Telecare. 2007;13(4):172–9.

58. Eklund K, Wilhelmson K. Outcomes of coordinated and integrated interventions targeting frail elderly people: a systematic review of randomised controlled trials. Health Soc Care Community. 2009;17(5):447–58.

10

Characteristics and predictors for hospitalizations of home-dwelling older persons receiving community care: a cohort study from Norway

Martha Therese Gjestsen[1,2*], Kolbjørn Brønnick[3,4] and Ingelin Testad[1,5]

Abstract

Background: Older persons are substantial consumers of both hospital- and community care, and there are discussions regarding the potential for preventing hospitalizations through high quality community care. The present study report prevalence and factors associated with admissions to hospital for community-dwelling older persons (> 67 years of age), receiving community care in a Norwegian municipality.

Methods: This was a cohort study of 1531 home-dwelling persons aged ≥67 years, receiving community care. We retrospectively scrutinized admissions to hospital for the study cohort over a one-year period in 2013. The frequency of admissions was evaluated with regard to association with age (age groups 67–79 years, 80–89 years and ≥ 90 year) and gender. The hospital admission incidence was calculated by dividing the number of admissions by the number of individuals included in the study cohort, stratified by age and gender. The association between age and gender as potential predictors and hospitalization (outcome) was first examined in univariate analyses followed by multinomial regression analyses in order to investigate the associations between age and gender with different causes of hospitalization.

Results: We identified a total of 1457 admissions, represented by 739 unique individuals, of which 64% were women, and an estimated mean age of 83 years. Mean admission rate was 2 admissions per person-year (95% confidence interval (CI): 1.89–2.11). The admission rate varied with age, and hospital incidents rates were higher for men in all age groups. The overall median length of stay was 4 days. The most common reason for hospitalization was the need for further medical assessment (23%). We found associations between increasing age and hospitalizations due to physical general decline, and associations between male gender and hospitalizations due to infections (e.g., airways infections, urinary tract infections).

Conclusions: We found the main reasons for hospitalizations to be related to falls, infections and general decline/pain/unspecified dyspnea. Men were especially at risk for hospitalization as they age. Our study have identified some clinically relevant factors that are vital in understanding what health care personnel in community care need to be especially aware of in order to prevent hospitalizations for this population.

Keywords: Hospitalizations, Elderly, Community care, Assistive living technology, Prevention

* Correspondence: martha.therese.gjestsen@sus.no
[1]Centre for age-related medicine (SESAM), Stavanger University Hospital, Stavanger, Norway
[2]University of Stavanger, Faculty of Health Sciences, Centre for Resilience in Healthcare (SHARE), Stavanger, Norway
Full list of author information is available at the end of the article

Background

The global phenomena of ageing populations (> 65 years) [1] alongside reduced number of personnel available for both formal and informal care [2], may threaten the sustainability of the health care systems [3, 4]. Persons over 65 years of age are substantial consumers of both hospital- and primary care [5, 6], and a peak in hospitalization rates for both men and women can be seen in all European countries through the age group 80 and over [1]. In Norway, 35% of all individuals over 80 years were hospitalized in 2013 and 68% of these also received community health- and care services [6]. Also, older persons over 65 years accounted for nearly 27% of all overnight stays, while only comprising 11% of the population, and an increase in over-night stays from 17.8% in 2003, to 19.6% in 2013 were shown within this population [5]. The proportion of increasing age is thus associated with an increasing demand for specialized health care [7, 8], and this rising demand for acute hospital beds leads to a strong policy interest in identifying interventions which are effective in reducing avoidable hospital admissions [9–13].

Previous studies on factors predicting hospitalizations of older persons have reported different findings, but there is a discrepancy in findings regarding risk factors associated with hospitalizations for older persons. Whereas quite a few studies have found that a previous hospital admission were associated with a higher risk to be re-hospitalized [12, 14, 15], Roland and colleagues [16] found that having two or more admissions one year, proved to have a low sensitivity in detecting older patients who will have high admissions in the following year. Several studies underline that the severity of disease and the burden of comorbidity are strong predictors of hospitalizations [11, 12, 15, 17], and also that functional disability, cognitive impairment, as well as factors related to living conditions (i.e., low socio-economic level and social deprivation) also seem to play a part in frequency of hospitalizations for older persons [15, 18, 19].

Gender differences in health care utilization are illustrated in several studies, but are inconclusive as to whether being male or female is a risk factor [12]. Some studies found that men above the age of 80 had approximately 25% more inpatient stays than women in the same age group [20–22] but others find that female sex is associated with multi-morbidity, and consequently have an increased risk of hospitalization [23].

A literature review [24] identified nine predictors which were independently associated with unplanned admissions to hospital in older people aged over 75 years: male gender, history of falls in the previous 12 months, ischaemic heart disease, respiratory disease, atrial fibrillation, cancer, having leg ulceration, living alone without help and having difficulty with mobility. Other studies have identified that emergency hospital admissions often occurs when an older person has reached a point of crisis, due to a combination of circumstances; such as an exacerbation of a chronic condition, change in social setting, or a cascade of symptoms due to multi-morbidity and frailty [12, 17, 25, 26].

The various risk factors related to hospitalizations for older persons, as identified in previous research, are summed up in Table 1.

It is an ongoing discussion whether a proportion of the hospital admissions among older persons could have been prevented in primary treatment and care [7, 27, 28]. Studies from Scandinavia have found that older persons are hospitalized due to lack of an appropriate alternative in primary care [28, 29], however a Norwegian study found no association between the volume of municipality general practitioners provided (in a universally accessible health-care system) and unplanned hospitalizations of the entire elderly population (aged ≥65 years) [8, 30]. The picture concerning the prevention of hospitalizations within this age group is thus not clear; heterogeneity in terms of health status and age-related conditions, as well as numerous contextual factors related to the health care system, represent a challenge for isolating factors concerning the-matter. It is therefore of vital importance to understand the actual clinical reasons for hospitalization in order to develop more timely and appropriate care services interventions [9, 15, 31], as well as the impact of policy efforts to reduce and prevent avoidable hospitalizations [10].

Part of the policy efforts is to shift resources from hospitals to the community care setting, and in this context the use of assistive living technologies is suggested to help monitor and treat degenerative and chronic diseases through the use of sensors, alarms and reminders [32, 33]. In a review by Purdy & Huntley [27], the use of

Table 1 Various risk factors associated with hospitalizations for older persons

Risk domain	Specific risk factors
Age	Increasing age
Frequency of hospitalizations	Previous hospitalization
Gender	Male Female
Health-related conditions	Severity of disease Comorbidity Functional decline/disability Respiratory disease Ischaemic heart disease Atrial fibrillation Cancer Leg ulcers
Living conditions	Low socio-economic level Deprivation Living alone, without help
Behavioral factors	Lack of exercise Falls Poor nutrition

automated vital signs monitoring and telephone follow-up by nurses was promising with regards to preventing and reducing avoidable emergency admissions.

Previous research underlines that more studies are needed to assess outcome and effectiveness related to the use of assistive living technologies in the context of preventing hospitalizations for older persons [34, 35], but there is a potential to do so by providing early warnings of exacerbation events or deterioration. This is a significant issue in regard to both quality and cost [24, 32].

This knowledge can further contribute to develop appropriate assistive living technology interventions, thus focussing on timely interventions in primary care together with understanding the actual clinical reasons for hospitalization.

Therefore, to identify ways to prevent hospitalizations with the use of assistive living technology, the aim of this study is to identify the reason for referral to hospital, and further to describe the prevalence and correlates associated with admissions to hospital for home-dwelling older persons (> 67 years of age) receiving community care in a Norwegian municipality.

More specifically, we will

i.   Describe the frequency related to reasons for referral, and characteristics of hospital admissions of home-dwelling older persons receiving community care.
ii. Describe the associations between demographic characteristics and admission to hospital.

Methods

Study design and setting

This is a descriptive, cohort study of 1531 home-dwelling persons aged ≥67 years, receiving community-based care in a Norwegian municipality. Demographic characterisitics of the study cohort are presented in Table 2. According to the World Health Organization (WHO), the age cut-off is 60+ years to refer to the older or elderly persons [36]. This

study however, has applied the age-cutoff as provided by Statistics Norway, because when extracting information about health service provision in Norway, 67 years of age is the standard age-distinction. The study was carried out in a municipality where 10.4% of the population is ≥67 years of age [37]. The number of cases in this cohort was determined by the number of hospitalizations during the one-year study period and thus, they are mirroring the influence of ageing on hospital admissions, as they closely match the current age structure of the Norwegian population receiving community care [38]. We retrospectively scrutinized admissions to hospital for the study cohort between April 1st 2012 and March 31st 2013. Data were collected electronically from existing registries. The studied hospitalizations stems from a hospital located in an urban area, it is the only hospital within an 80 km radius and serves approximately 365,000 persons.

Community care

Community care represents the lowest level of care services provided by the municipality and there are few formal demands required in order to receive community care in Norway. The proper instance in the health- and social district one geographically belongs to, defines the need for assistance and/or care, together with the person seeking help. Referrals to hospital are made either from patients' general practitioner, or from an out-of-hours community-based emergency department. The persons included in our study received services from the municipality, including medical care provided by nurses (medication, wound/ulcer dressing, personal hygiene) and practical home care provided by formal carers (not necessarily nurses).

Variables and data analysis

The variables entered into the analysis were selected primarily for their clinical importance, based on previous research to be essential [9, 39–41], and included gender, age and reason for referral. The primary reason for referral to hospital was retrieved through hospital-based patient records, based on the International Classification of Diseases version 10 (ICD-10) main chapters. When reason for referral to hospital was inexplicit (i. e., to clarify whether the patient was referred either for COPD exacerbation or pneumonia), the first author checked the patients' hospital records to identify the most accurate reason for referral. A second rater evaluated the reasons for referral to hospital for 141 randomly selected cases, and then we performed an agreement-testing, using Cohen's Kappa (κ) to test interrater reliability [31]. The coefficient was 0.7, which supports the reliability and validity of the rating procedure. Length of stay (LoS) was calculated from admission to discharge date and

Table 2 Demographic characteristics of study cohort

Selected variables	% of total (N = 1531)		Mean ± sd
Gender:			
Male	32.6		
Female	67.4		
Age:		*Male (% within age group)*	
67–79	27.1	40.7	
80–89	43.3	31.9	
90 +	29.6	24.9	
Mean age			83.7 ± 7.435

Sd standard deviation

presented in days; for persons who had less than 6 hours at the hospital, LoS is calculated to be 0 days.

Continuous variables are described as means and standard deviations, while categorical variables are reported as frequencies.

The hospital admission incidence was calculated by dividing the number of admissions by the number of individuals included in the study cohort, stratified by age and gender (Table 3). Frequency of admissions was evaluated separately for each reason for referral for the age groups 67–79 years, 80–89 years and ≥ 90 year using Z-tests for testing differences of admission proportions in each age group for each reason for referral to hospital. Confidence intervals are also reported for each age group. A multinomial logistic regression analysis was then performed in order to investigate the partial, independent effects of age and gender on the most common reasons for referral to hospital (fall, infections or general decline) The dependent variable was categorical, i.e., fall, infections or general decline using no hospitalizations as a reference group. Age and gender were entered as predictor variables. Alpha level was set at $p < .05$. All statistical analyses were conducted using SPSS Release 23.0.0.0 (IBM, Inc., Chicago, IL, USA).

Results
Demographic and frequencies related to hospitalizations
We identified a total of 1457 admissions, represented by 729 unique individuals from the study cohort ($n = 1531$), out of which 64% were women. The estimated mean age was 83 years. 384 persons (53%) of the hospitalized individuals ($n = 729$) were admitted only once during the study period. 169 individuals (23%) were admitted twice, 78 (11%) were admitted three times, while 98 persons (13%) were admitted more than four times during the one-year study period. The mean admission rate was 2 admissions per person-year (95% confidence interval (CI): 1.89–2.11). The overall median length of stay was 4 days (mean = 7.21, SD ± 9.9, range 1–138, interquartile range (IQR) =7). The most common reason for referral was the need for further medical assessment due to general decline, based on symptoms such as pain/unspecified dyspnea/dehydration/anemia (334 referrals = 23%).

303 referrals related to infections (ICD-10 chapter A J K L N) constituted nearly 21% of overall admissions, while falls caused 13% (191 referrals) of the hospitalizations for the study cohort. The most common reason for referral within infections were related to the respiratory system (e.g., pneumonia), urinary tract infections and skin infections (e.g., erysipelas). These results are depicted in Table 4. Some hospital admissions were associated with age, whilst others were associated with gender.

Age as a predictor for hospitalization
We found a higher admission rate in the lowest age group (67–79 years), compared to the other two age groups; the youngest had a mean admission rate of 1.0, which is slightly higher than the mean annual admission rate for the whole study population (.95) (see Table 3). I. e., the annual admission rate varied with age, but there was a statistically significant negative correlation between age and annual admission rate (Spearman's rho = .-117, CI -.186- -.041, $p = .002$). We investigated this issue further by testing differences in proportions of hospitalizations in the three age groups related to the various reasons for referral to hospital using Z tests. We found that in connection to hospitalizations due to fall and infections, there was a statistically significant difference in proportions between the lowest and the highest age group (Fall $p < .01$; infections $p = .02$), and likewise between the middle age group and the highest age group (Fall $p < .01$; Infections $p = .04$), but not between the lowest and the middle age group (Fall $p = .82$; infections $p = .65$). As for general decline/pain/unspecified dyspnea as a reason for hospitalizations, we found a statistically significant difference in proportions between both the lowest and the middle age group ($p < .01$), as well as between the lowest and the highest age group ($p < .01$), but not between the middle and the highest age group ($p = .08$). The results are depicted in Table 4.

Gender as a predictor for hospitalization
Overall, men had an annual admission rate of 1.1, while the corresponding rate for women was .9. The mean hospital admission rate for the entire study population was .95 (see Table 3). We found that hospital incidents rates were

Table 3 Hospital incidence rate for the study cohort, stratified on gender

Total			Men			Women		
Persons Total cohort	Admissions (n)	Mean annual admission rate	Persons - age	Admissions (n)	Mean annual admission rate	Persons - age	Admissions (n)	Mean annual admission rate
1531	1457	0.95	494	566	1.1	1038	891	0.9
67–79 years 415	426	1.0	169	210	1.2	246	216	0.9
80–89 years 664	655	0.98	212	254	1.2	452	401	0.9
90+ years 453	377	0.83	113	102	0.9	340	274	0.8

Table 4 Differences in age groups for different reasons for referral to hospital

Reason for referral		A: 67–79 years	B: 80–89 years	C: 90+ years	p-value*
	Frequency of admissions (%)	426 (29.2)	655 (45.0)	376 (25.8)	
Fall/accident	191 (13.1)	36 (8.5)	77 (11.8)	78 (20.7)	
Z-score (C.I.)		0.083 (0.062–0.115)	0.118 (0.095–0.144)	0.207 (0.169–0.251)	A vs B = .82; A vs C < .01; B vs C < .01
Infection	303 (20.8)	98 (23.0)	143 (21.8)	62 (16.5)	
Z-score (C.I.)		0.23 (0.193–0.272)	0.218 (0.188–0.252)	0.165 (0.131–0.206)	A vs B = .65; A vs C = .02; B vs C = .04
General decline/pain/ unspecified dyspnea	334 (22.9)	65 (15.3)	159 (24.3)	110 (29.3)	
Z-score (C.I.)		0.153 (0.122–0.189)	0.243 (0.211–0.277)	0.293 (0.248–0.340)	A vs B < .01; A vs C < .01; B vs C = .08
Unspecified chest pain	90 (6.2)	29 (6.8)	41 (6.3)	20 (5.3)	
Z-score (C.I)		0.068 (0.048–0.096)	0.063 (0.046–0.084)	0.053 (0.035–0.081)	A vs B = .72; A vs C = .38; B vs C = .54
Heart attack	43 (3)	8 (1.9)	22 (3.4)	13 (3.5)	
Z-score		0.019 (0.009–0.037)	0.034 (0.022–0.050)	0.035 (0.020–0.058)	A vs B = .15; A vs C = .16; B vs C = .94
Congestive heart failure	58 (4)	15 (3.5)	25 (3.8)	18 (4.8)	
Psychiatry	41 (2.8)	38 (8.9)	2 (0.3)	1 (0.3)	
Old age psychiatry	32 (2.2)	7 (1.6)	16 (2.4)	9 (2.2)	
Neurology	91 (6.2)	20 (4.7)	47 (7.2)	24 (6.4)	
Cancer	137 (9.4)	68 (16.0)	56 (8.5)	13 (3.5)	
COPD	37 (2.5)	17 (4.0)	18 (2.7)	2 (0.5)	
GI symptoms	100 (6.9)	25 (5.8)	49 (7.5)	26 (6.9)	
Total (%)	1457 (100)	426 (29.2)	655 (45.0)	376 (25.8)	

higher for men in all age groups, and further a statistically significant negative correlation between female gender and frequency of admission to hospital with a correlation coefficient (Spearman's rho) of −.088 (CI 95%-.157- -.017, $p = .018$). This implies that in our study, being female was not associated with higher hospitalization rate, thus not presenting as a risk factor for admission to hospital.

The final prognostic index included age (categorized as 67–79, 80–89, ≥ 90), gender and reason for referral. We applied a multinomial logistic regression analysis to investigate whether age or gender were associated with admission to hospital (reason for referral) due to falls, infection or general decline (see Table 5). The results depicted in Table 5 shows the odds ratios for hospitalizations due to falls, infection or general decline vs. the reference group of no hospitalizations in the model.

Age was not a statistically significant predictor for hospitalization due to fall or infections, but we found that increasing age was associated with hospitalization due to general decline ($p = .001$). With regards to gender, we found that being male increased the odds for hospitalization when presenting symptoms related to

infections by a factor of .5, being statistically significant ($p < .001$). As for associations between gender (=being male) and hospitalizations due to fall or general decline, the slightly increased odds were not statistically significant in either groups.

We further investigated whether there was a difference in the three age groups related to the various reasons for referral to hospital. In relation to hospitalization due to fall, we found a statistically significant difference ($p = .01$) between the youngest of age (age group A: 67–79 years) and the eldest (age group C: 90+), and also between the eldest (age group C) and age group B (80–89). There was no difference between age group A and B in this matter.

Also for hospitalizations due to an infection we found a statistically significance between the same age groups as for fall as reason for referral to hospital, i. e., between age groups A and C, and B and C.

Hospitalizations due to general decline had a slightly other expression; here we found a difference between age group A and B, and also between A and C, but not between B and C. The first and the latter result differ from the other two reasons for referral.

Table 5 Predictors for hospitalization by multinomial logistic regression; demonstrating whether age or gender were associated with admission to hospital (reason for referral) due to falls, infection or general decline

Fall			Infection			General decline		
	OR (95% CI)	P-value		OR (95% CI)	P-value		OR (95% CI)	P-value
Age	1.03 (1.00–1.05)	.044		0.99 (0.97–1.02)	.469		1.04 (1.02–1.06)	**.001**
Gender	1.2 (0.77–1.86)	.418		0.47 (0.38–0.69)	**.000**		0.65 (0.45–0.93)	.017

OR Odds ratio, CI Confidence Interval. Alpha level 0.05. Bold values indicate variables that reached statistical significance. Reference group: No hospitalizations

Discussion

We found that 50% of the study cohort had at least one hospitalization during a one-year period, and that age and gender were associated with some hospitalizations. The most common reasons for referral were the need for further medical assessment, based on symptoms related to general decline, such as unspecified dyspnea/dehydration/anemia (23%), and referrals related to infections (21%) and falls (13%). More specifically we found that age was a predictor for hospitalization ($p \leq .001$) due to general decline, whereas in relation to falls and infections, we found no association between age and hospitalizations. We found that male gender was a predictor for hospitalizations due to infections ($P \leq .000$), but were not associated with hospitalizations related to falls or general decline. Several findings are noteworthy, especially in the context of current efforts using assistive living technologies to prevent hospitalizations for older persons.

First, the 50% admission rate we found highlight the point that this population is prone to conditions for which a doctor evaluates that a hospitalization is required. This is noteworthy in itself, but previous research have shown that taking only the frequency of admissions for older persons into account when predicting future admissions, have a low sensitivity [16]. We have therefore looked more into for which conditions older persons are hospitalized.

The most frequent reason for referral we identified in our study was general decline/pain/unspecified dyspnoea. This substantiate an already well-known perception that older persons often present general and diffuse symptoms before the doctor, and often may be in a severe state of illness [42]. Symptoms related to general decline/pain/unspecified dyspnoea could be related to non-communicable and chronic diseases, thus potentially preventable. However, these hospitalizations are often appropriate due to the degree of severity and the need for further assessment and examinations which only could be performed, in specialized health care [11, 15, 27]. The line of argument that follows the trajectory that high quality primary care prevents hospitalizations related to the reported symptoms, indicate that vigilant health care personnel in community care is a prerequisite for timely and accurate observations. The potential for preventing hospitalizations for this patient group lies in discovering and addressing the patients' general decline and/or pain

and/or unspecified dyspnea before the state of illness, where hospitalization is the only appropriate option for assessment, treatment and care. According to Fortinsky and colleagues [19], an increase on a dyspnea severity scale conferred an additional 18% greater likelihood of hospitalization, thus there could be a particular potential for preventing hospitalizations due to dyspnea symptoms. Moreover, monitoring such symptoms can be done through the use of assistive living technologies, as they allow a close and continuous monitoring of symptoms, systematic follow-up by health care personnel, and a proper response [43, 44].

The potential for preventing hospitalizations related to the second most frequent reason for referral as identified in the present study is even greater. Referral to hospital due to infections in the respiratory system (e.g., pneumonia), urinary tract infections and skin infections (e.g., erysipelas) is reported to be conditions causing inappropriate hospitalizations, and for which interventions in primary care should prevent such [11, 18]. Diffusion of community care programs and services that aim to strengthen both patients and health care personnel on how to observe early signs of clinical and functional decline on a systematic basis is one potential strategy to reduce hospital use among older persons. In this regard, the use of assistive living technologies can have a potential positive impact, as the aim of such interventions is to both strengthen the self-management of chronic diseases, and for health care personnel to use various sensors and monitors to track changes in a patient's health and vital signs [32, 45]. Lewin and colleagues [33] expect to see a shift from alarm-based telecare systems to systems including more continuous life style monitoring over the next years. This will release a potential for more vigilant and precise follow-up of patients, but the ethics and safety concerning such comprehensive monitoring of persons are a concerns which many stakeholders are addressing now.

In our study cohort, there were substantially fewer men (33%) then women, but men still had a higher annual admission rate; men had an annual admission rate of 1.1, compared to women who had a rate of .9. The mean hospital admission rate for the entire study population was .95. This finding is in accordance with official Norwegian statistics and previous research [21, 22].

However, a study which focused on reduction of inappropriate hospital use, based on analysis of the causes, found no significant differences when comparing the results of inappropriate admission by gender (male/female) [46]. In our study, we found that male gender was a predictor for hospitalizations due to infections, but were not associated with hospitalizations related to falls or general decline. This is supported by a strand of research literature which suggest that men are generally physically stronger and report fewer diseases and have lower levels of primary care use, but higher hospitalization rates and have higher mortality at all ages compared with women: the so-called male-female health-survival paradox [23, 47]. This may suggest that men perhaps disregard early signs of disease and postpone going to the doctor until the later stages of disease development, thus health care personnel in community care must be especially aware of men in the context of prevention of hospitalizations [21].

In our study, we found that age was a predictor for hospitalizations due to general decline, but were not associated with hospitalizations related to falls or infections. This is harmonized with a common understanding that the most problematic expression of an ageing population is the clinical condition of frailty [26]. For this population, it is of vital importance to apply a systematic approach in community care, in order to reduce the use of inappropriate procedures, iatrogenic diseases and nosocomial infections, which are associated with hospitalization [29, 48].

Urgent and emergency services have been the subject of a wide range of policy discourse and decisions over the years, all over Europe. In general, socio-demographic (i.e., age, social deprivation, levels of morbidity, area of residence) factors are associated with increased rates of admissions [18]. These are factors which are highly relevant in understanding other reasons than the clinical conditions for hospitalizations, but in terms of potentially preventing an admission to hospital for the individual patient, it is paramount that personnel in community care are vigilant observers and good clinical practitioners. Proper treatment and care for the most vulnerable, with a view to managing their conditions at home and/or supported by community care, can potentially reduce the risk of hospitalizations, but it also implies to shift resources from hospitals to the community setting, thus reducing the disruptive impact of acute unscheduled hospital admissions [9]. Our study have identified some clinically relevant factors that are vital in this context.

Limitations

We should mention a number of limitations of the present study. First, we cannot draw any gender-specific conclusion in the present study, due to heterogeneity among populations. Second, diseases with no treatment and asymptomatic conditions could be missed by doctors when recording a medical history, as well as the raters in this study. Third, the findings in this study pertain to the studied municipality in Norway, thus limiting the generalizations of the findings, as financing and organization of health care in Norway is different compared to other countries.

Conclusions

The potential for preventing hospitalizations for home-dwelling elderly receiving community care lies in discovering and addressing the patients' symptoms so early that they don't come to a severe state of illness that requires hospitalization. The most common reasons for referral to hospital were the need for further medical assessment, based on symptoms related to general decline, such as unspecified dyspnea/dehydration/anemia, and referrals related to infections and falls. Our study shows that men are especially at risk for hospitalization with increasing age. This information is vital when vigilant health care personnel in community care make timely and accurate observations. The appliance of assistive living technologies in this context can have a positive impact, as they can be used to track changes in the patients' vital signs and health condition, but further investigation is needed in this regard.

Abbreviations

COPD: Chronic Obstructive Pulmonary Disorder; ICD-10: International Classification of Diseases 10th revision; LoS: Length of stay; UN: United Nations

Acknowledgements

The authors would like to thank the other partners in the project.

Funding

The study is part of a larger project; "Development and Implementation of assistive living technologies in Municipalities". It is funded by the Regional Research Fund for Western Norway; Centre for Age-related Medicine, Stavanger University Hospital, Norway; and University of Stavanger, Norway.

Authors' contributions

MTG planned the study design, was responsible for data collection, contributed to data analysis and drafted this manuscript. KB contributed to the study design, data collection, data analysis, and contributed to drafting of the manuscript. IT contributed planning of study design, data analysis and drafting of the manuscript. All authors have read and approved the final version of the manuscript.

Competing interests

The authors declare that they have no competing interests.

Author details

[1]Centre for age-related medicine (SESAM), Stavanger University Hospital, Stavanger, Norway. [2]University of Stavanger, Faculty of Health Sciences, Centre for Resilience in Healthcare (SHARE), Stavanger, Norway. [3]Centre for Clinical Research in Psychosis (TIPS), Stavanger University Hospital, Stavanger, Norway. [4]University of Stavanger, Faculty of Health Sciences, Stavanger, Norway. [5]University of Exeter Medical School, Exeter, Devon, UK.

References

1. Rechel B, Grundy E, Robine J-M, Cylus J, Mackenbach JP, Knai C, McKee M. Ageing in the European union. Lancet. 2013;381(9874):1312–22.

2. Rechel B, Doyle Y, Grundy E, McKee M: How can health sytems respond to population ageing? European Observatory on Health Systems and Policies, Policy Brief 10 2009.

3. Bloom DE, Chatterji S, Kowal P, Lloyd-Sherlock P, McKee M, Rechel B, Rosenberg L, Smith JP. Macroeconomic implications of population ageing and selected policy responses. Lancet. 2015;385(9968):649–57.

4. Christensen K, Doblhammer G, Rau R, Vaupel JW. Ageing populations: the challenges ahead. Lancet. 2009;374

5. Huseby BM. Samdata spesialisthelsetjenesten 2013. In: Edited by Norwegian Directorate of Health, vol. Is 2194; 2014.

6. Huseby BMr: Samhandlingsstatistikk 2013–14. Directorate of Health 2015.

7. Roland M, Abel G. Reducing emergency admissions: are we on the right track? BMJ (Clinical research ed). 2012;345:e6017.

8. Deraas TS, Berntsen GR, Jones AP, Førde OH, Sund ER. Associations between primary healthcare and unplanned medical admissions in Norway: a multilevel analysis of the entire elderly population. BMJ Open. 2014;4(4): e004293.

9. Hippisley-Cox J, Coupland C. Predicting risk of emergency admission to hospital using primary care data: derivation and validation of QAdmissions score. BMJ Open. 2013;3(8)

10. Department of Health. Supporting people with long term conditions. An NHS and Social Care Model to support local innovation and integration 2005. http://webarchive.nationalarchives.gov.uk/20130105013243/http://www.dh.gov.uk/prod_consum_dh/groups/dh_digitalassets/@dh/@en/documents/digitalasset/dh_4122574.pdf

11. Soria-Aledo V, Carrillo-Alcaraz A, Campillo-Soto A, Flores-Pastor B, Leal-Llopis J, Fernandez-Martin MP, Carrasco-Prats M, Aguayo-Albasini JL. Associated factors and cost of inappropriate hospital admissions and stays in a second-level hospital. Am J Med Qual. 2009;24(4):321–32.

12. Crane SJ, Tung EE, Hanson GJ, Cha S, Chaudhry R, Takahashi PY. Use of an electronic administrative database to identify older community dwelling adults at high-risk for hospitalization or emergency department visits: the elders risk assessment index. BMC Health Serv Res. 2010;10:338.

13. Sinclair HSA, Furey A. Reducing unplanned hospital admissions in older people with high needs: a review of local practice in a small sample of primary care patients in an inner London borough. Int J Pers Cent Med. 2016;6(2):11.

14. Epstein AM, Jha AK, Orav EJ. The relationship between hospital admission rates and Rehospitalizations. N Engl J Med. 2011;365(24):2287–95.

15. Landi F, Onder G, Cesari M, Barillaro C, Lattanzio F, Carbonin PU, Bernabei R. Comorbidity and social factors predicted hospitalization in frail elderly patients. J Clin Epidemiol. 2004;57(8):832–6.

16. Roland M, Dusheiko M, Gravelle H, Parker S. Follow up of people aged 65 and over with a history of emergency admissions: analysis of routine admission data. BMJ. 2005;330(7486):289–92.

17. Gamper G, Wiedermann W, Barisonzo R, Stockner I, Wiedermann C. Inappropriate hospital admission: interaction between patient age and co-morbidity. Intern Emerg Med. 2011;6(4):361–7.

18. Purdy S, Griffin T, Salisbury C, Sharp D. Prioritizing ambulatory care sensitive hospital admissions in England for research and intervention: a Delphi exercise. Prim Health Care Res Dev. 2010;11(01):41–50.

19. Fortinsky RH, Madigan EA, Sheehan TJ, Tullai-McGuinness S, Kleppinger A. Risk factors for hospitalization in a National Sample of Medicare home health care patients. J Appl Gerontol. 2014;33(4):474–93.

20. Norway S. Health and health care utilization - gender differences. Report. 2007/37; ISSN 0806-2056

21. Galdas PM, Cheater F, Marshall P. Men and health help-seeking behaviour: literature review. J Adv Nurs. 2005;49(6):616–23.

22. Juel K, Christensen K. Are men seeking medical advice too late? Contacts to general practitioners and hospital admissions in Denmark 2005. J Public Health (Oxf). 2008;30(1):111–3.

23. Corrao S, Santalucia P, Argano C, Djade CD, Barone E, Tettamanti M, Pasina L, Franchi C, Kamal Eldin T, Marengoni A, et al. Gender-differences in disease distribution and outcome in hospitalized elderly: data from the REPOSI study. Eur J Intern Med. 2014;25(7):617–23.

24. Lyon D, Lancaster GA, Taylor S, Dowrick C, Chellaswamy H. Predicting the likelihood of emergency admission to hospital of older people: development and validation of the emergency admission risk likelihood index (EARLI). Fam Pract. 2007;24(2):158–67.

25. Philp I, Mills KA, Thanvi B, Ghosh K, Long JF. Reducing hospital bed use by frail older people: results from a systematic review of the literature. Int J Integr Care. 2013;13:e048.

26. Clegg A, Young J, Iliffe S, Rikkert MO, Rockwood K. Frailty in elderly people. Lancet. 2013;381(9868):752–62.

27. Purdy S, Huntley A: Predicting and preventing hospital admissions. A review. . J R Coll Physicians Edinb 2013; 43:340–4 2013(3443):4.

28. Lillebo B, Dyrstad B, Grimsmo A. Avoidable emergency admissions? Emerg Med J. 2012;

29. Strømgaard S, Rasmussen SW, Schmidt TA. Brief hospitalizations of elderly patients: a retrospective, observational study. Scand J Trauma Resusc Emerg Med. 2014;22:17.

30. Deraas TS, Berntsen GR, Jones AP, Forde OH, Sund ER. Associations between primary healthcare and unplanned medical admissions in Norway: a multilevel analysis of the entire elderly population. BMJ Open. 2014;4(4):e004293.

31. Mytton OT, Oliver D, Mirza N, Lippett J, Chatterjee A, Ramcharitar K, Maxwell J. Avoidable acute hospital admissions in older people. Br J Healthc Manag. 2012;18(11):597–603.

32. May C, Finch T, Cornford J, Exley C, Gately C, Kirk S, Jenkings K, Osbourne J, Robinson A, Rogers A. Integrating telecare for chronic disease management in the community: what needs to be done? BMC Health Serv Res. 2011; 11(1):131.

33. Lewin D, Adshead S, Glennon B. Assisted living technologies for older and disabled people in 2030. In: A final report to Ofcom; 2010.

34. Khosravi P, Ghapanchi AH. Investigating the effectiveness of technologies applied to assist seniors: A systematic literature review. Int J Med Inform. 85(1):17–26.

35. Wootton R. Twenty years of telemedicine in chronic disease management – an evidence synthesis. J Telemed Telecare. 2012;18(4):211–20.

36. World Health Organization: Health situation and trend assessment. http://www.searo.who.int/entity/health_situation_trends/data/chi/elderly-population/en/].

37. Statistics Norway. Table 09503 statistics Norway. In: January 1st; 2015.

38. Statistics Norway. Table 04467. In: Accessed march 15th; 2012.

39. Regitz-Zagrosek V. Sex and gender differences in health: Science & Society Series on sex and science. EMBO Rep. 2012;13(7):596–603.

40. Damush TM, Smith DM, Perkins AJ, Dexter PR, Smith F. Risk factors for nonelective hospitalization in frail and older adult, Inner-City outpatients. Gerontologist. 2004;44(1):68–75.

41. Chandra A, Crane SJ, Tung EE, Hanson GJ, North F, Cha SS, Takahashi PY. Patient-reported geriatric symptoms as risk factors for hospitalization and emergency department visits. Aging Dis. 2015;6(3):188–95.

42. Rashidi F, Mowinckel P, Ranhoff AH. Severity of disease in patients admitted for acute care to a general hospital: age and gender differences. Aging Clin Exp Res. 2010;22(4):340–4.

43. Eron L. Telemedicine: the future of outpatient therapy? Clin Infect Dis. 2010; 51(Supplement 2):S224–30.

44. Kang HG, Mahoney DF, Hoenig H, Hirth VA, Bonato P, Hajjar I, Lipsitz LA. For the Center for Integration of M, innovative technology working group on advanced approaches to physiologic monitoring for the a: in situ monitoring of health in older adults: technologies and issues. J Am Geriatr Soc. 2010;58(8):1579–86.

45. McLean S, Protti D, Sheikh A. Telehealthcare for long term conditions. BMJ. 2011;342

11

Anti-hypertensive medications and injurious falls in an older population of low socioeconomic status: a nested case-control study

Zafirah Banu[1†], Ka Keat Lim[2†] [iD], Yu Heng Kwan[2], Kai Zhen Yap[1], Hui Ting Ang[1], Chuen Seng Tan[3], Warren Fong[5,6,7], Julian Thumboo[2,5], Kheng Hock Lee[4,6], Truls Ostbye[2] and Lian Leng Low[4,6*]

Abstract

Background: This study aimed to determine whether the number of anti-hypertensive medication classes or any change in anti-hypertensive medication were associated with injurious fall among the community-dwelling older population of low socioeconomic status.

Methods: Using data from electronic medical records, we performed a nested case-control study among older Singapore residents (≥60) of low socioeconomic status ($N = 210$). Controls ($n = 162$) were matched to each case ($n = 48$) by age and gender. Variables with $p < 0.10$ in univariate analysis were included in multivariate analysis. We used conditional logistic regression to assess the associations of the number of anti-hypertensive medication classes and change in anti-hypertensive medication with injurious falls. We also performed stepwise regressions as sensitivity analyses. $p < 0.05$ was considered statistically significant.

Results: The mean (±SD) age of participants was 78.1 (± 8.33) years; 127 (60.4%) were female, 189 (90.0%) were Chinese. Those on ≥2 anti-hypertensive medication classes had an increased risk of experiencing an injurious fall compared to those not on any anti-hypertensive medication (OR = 5.45; CI:1.49–19.93; $p = 0.01$). Among those who were taking anti-hypertensive medication, those who had a change in the medication 180-day prior to injurious fall had a significantly increased risk of experiencing an injurious fall compared to those that did not report any change in anti-hypertensive medication (OR = 3.88; CI:1.23–12.19; $p = 0.02$). Sensitivity analyses generated consistent findings.

Conclusion: Both ≥2 anti-hypertensive medication classes and change in anti-hypertensive medication were associated with an increased risk of experiencing an injurious fall among the older population of low socioeconomic status. Our findings could guide prescribers to exercise caution in the initiation of anti-hypertensive medications or in making medication changes, especially among the older population of low socioeconomic status.

Keywords: Aged, Antihypertensive agents, Falls, Socio-economic status

* Correspondence: low.lian.leng@singhealth.com.sg
†Zafirah Banu and Ka Keat Lim contributed equally to this work.
4Department of Family Medicine and Continuing Care, Singapore General Hospital, Singapore, Republic of Singapore
6Duke-NUS Medical School, Singapore, Republic of Singapore
Full list of author information is available at the end of the article

Background

Falling is a common and severe problem faced by the older population worldwide with 28–35% of community-dwelling older adults > 64 years and 32–42% of those > 70 years estimated to experience at least one fall each year [1]. This has significant social, economic and health implications. Falls result in increased morbidity and mortality, with approximately 10% of falls leading to serious injuries, such as fractures, intracranial bleeding, serious lacerations and even death [2]. Besides higher healthcare utilization due to falls-related injuries [3], older adults may also experience psychological damages that result in self-imposed limitation in mobility, increased dependency on others for activities of daily living, depression and anxiety [4]. This leads to higher psychological and economic burden for the caregivers and the country [5].

While numerous studies have examined the association between anti-hypertensive medications and falls, most studies only focused on specific classes of anti-hypertensive. Existing systematic reviews and meta- analyses of these studies found weak or no association between the different anti-hypertensive classes and falls [6–8].

Recent evidence suggests that intensity of treatment [9, 10] or changes in anti-hypertensive medication [11] may be associated with falls. This is plausible as anti-hypertensive treatment intensity and changes in anti-hypertensive medication have been associated with orthostatic hypotension [12] and neurological side effects [11] which could lead to falls.

Our study aimed to examine whether a higher number of anti-hypertensive medication classes or a recent change in anti-hypertensive medication was associated with injurious falls, defined as falls that required medical services. The focus on injurious falls is due to its direct implication on healthcare utilization, compared to any fall occurrence commonly examined in previous studies [13]. We were interested in studying the older adults of low socioeconomic status (SES) because they are at higher risk of falls [14] and suffer from a higher burden of hypertension [15, 16]. As such, our findings could guide prescribers to exercise extra precaution in the initiation of anti-hypertensive medications or in making medication changes, especially among the older adults of low SES.

Methods
Study design

We conducted a nested case-control study involving participants ($N = 264$) taking part in the Integrated Community of Care (ICoC) programme [17], a novel care model in Singapore General Hospital (SGH) that integrates hospital-based transitional care with health and social care in the community. This ongoing programme targets older adults (≥ 60 years old) living in public rental flats, which offer heavily subsidized rents for the underprivileged population, among whom 88% earn less than S$670/month (USD498.12 based on SGD1: USD0.74 conversion) [18]. Participants were included in the ICoC programme if they had at least one inpatient and/or outpatient encounter with SGH 3 years prior to entry into the ICoC programme. For those with dementia, they were included if they were capable of independent living or had a caregiver. This study was reviewed and approved by the SingHealth Centralized Institutional Review Board. Written informed consent was obtained for every participant.

We defined cases as participants who experienced any injurious falls from August 2014 to August 2017. For those with multiple injurious falls, we collected information on their baseline characteristics from the most recent injurious fall. For each case, up to 8 controls who had no recorded injurious falls within the same time period were matched on age (±5 years) and gender. For each control, the fall date of their matched case was taken as the baseline to obtain the relevant independent variables (e.g., medications) 180-day prior to the fall date.

To examine the association between the number of anti-hypertensive medication classes and injurious falls, we identified 48 participants who experienced an injurious fall and 162 matched controls who did not experience any injurious falls during the 3-year period. An average of 3 controls (minimum = 1; maximum = 8) were matched to each case on age (±5 years) and gender.

To examine the association between a change in anti-hypertensive medication and injurious fall, we used the same matching but restricted our sample to include only those who took anti-hypertensive medication. In total, 38 cases and 101 controls were included in this analysis ($N = 139$). An average of 2 controls (minimum = 1; maximum = 8) were matched to each case on age ± 5 years) and gender.

Dependent variable of interest

We defined an injurious fall as a fall that required medical services either in the emergency department or inpatient hospitalisation in SGH. This could be minor injuries such as those that required only dressing and wound cleaning or major injuries such as those that required surgery, casting or resulted in neurological or internal injury.

Exposure variables of interest

We categorized the number of anti-hypertensive medication classes consumed during the 180-day prior to the fall date into 3 categories: None, 1 class and ≥ 2 classes of anti-hypertensive medications.

We considered any anti-hypertensive medications from the following classes – angiotensin converting enzyme inhibitors (ACEI), angiotensin receptor blockers (ARB), beta blockers (BB), calcium channel blockers (CCB) and diuretics. Specifically, the older adults in our sample took enalapril, captopril or lisinopril as ACEI; losartan, valsartan, telmisartan or irbesartan as ARB; atenolol or bisoprolol as BB. amlodipine or slow-release nifedipine as CCB; hydrochlorothiazide, frusemide or spironolactone as diuretics.

We defined a change in anti-hypertensive medication as an addition of a new class of anti-hypertensive medication, an increase in the dosage of the existing medication or a switch to a new class of anti-hypertensive medication. No participants in our study experienced a reduction in dosage or in number of anti-hypertensive medications. Participants who reported no change in anti-hypertensive medication were those who had the same anti-hypertensive medications throughout the 180-day period prior to the fall date or matched fall date.

Data collection

We reviewed existing literature to determine the information to be collected. All data were collected from SGH medical records for patients, in accordance to the consent provided by the ICoC participants.

For each participant, we collected information on age, gender, body mass index, race, blood pressure and Morse Fall Scale score at the time of the fall. All other baseline characteristics of participants were based on the 180-day prior to the fall date or matched fall date. Information on visual or hearing impairment, prior smoking and alcohol history was also obtained. Cognitive impairment was measured using the Abbreviated Mental Status Test [19] or the Short Portable Mental Status Questionnaire [20]. Both tests consist of 10 items appraising orientation, memory, calculation and facial recognition. The cut-offs for these 2 tests were adjusted according to age and education. Our measure of co-morbidity was the Charlson's Comorbidity Index (CCI) [21], an indicator based on diagnoses of 17 diseases, including myocardial infarction, diabetes and cerebrovascular disease.

Fall risk was assessed using the Morse Fall Scale based on a patient's history of falling, presence of > 1 medical diagnosis, use of ambulatory aids such as a cane, wheelchair, or walking frame, insertion of intravenous/heparin lock, types of gait and mental status. The scale was validated in Singapore [22] with participants scoring ≥55 considered to be at a high risk of falling. As such, we categorised participants into 2 categories: with and without a high fall risk.

Lastly, we recorded prescription drug name, class, dose, frequency and any change in anti-hypertensive medications during the 180-day period prior to the most recent fall date. Besides antihypertensive medications, falls could also be attributed to other medications such as psychotropic medications and statins. Psychotropic medications could lead to falls by causing sedation, orthostatic hypotension, confusion, slow reaction times and impaired balance [23] whereas statin therapy could result in a decline in muscle strength [24]. Thus, we also recorded the use of statin and psychotropic medication 180-day prior to the fall date. Psychotropic medications included antidepressant, antipsychotic, sedative-hypnotic, antiepileptic, anti-Parkinson's medication, or narcotic.

We defined polypharmacy as the use of ≥4 chronic medications [25]. We recorded details of all medications dispensed for a period of ≥3 months. This included prescription, non-prescription and over-the-counter (OTC) medication but excluded anti-hypertensive medication to avoid double-counting. We considered fixed-dose combinations (multiple active ingredients in one preparation) as a single medication because we were interested in looking at the pill count rather than the total classes of medication. A higher pill count results in poorer medication adherence which has been associated with an increased rate of falls among older adults [26].

Statistical analysis

We first summarized the baseline characteristics of participants using means and standard deviations (SDs) or frequencies and percentages. We compared participants who did with those who did not experience any injurious fall using t-tests or Wilcoxon rank-sum tests for continuous variables and Chi-squared or Fisher's exact tests for categorical variables.

Subsequently, we performed conditional logistic regression, using injurious fall as the dependent variable. We began with univariate regression and independent variables with $p < 0.10$ were included in the multivariate regression models. We performed two multivariate conditional logistic regressions, using the number of anti-hypertensive medication classes or any change in anti-hypertensive medication as the exposure variables respectively. Associations with $p < 0.05$ in the multivariate regressions were regarded as statistically significant. To examine whether the results were consistent in parsimonious models, we also performed sensitivity analyses by including variables with $p < 0.10$ into both forward and backward stepwise regressions. We specified $p > 0.10$ for removal from the model and $p < 0.05$ for addition to the model. We examined all final models for collinearity using variance inflation factor (VIF). All analyses were performed using STATA SE version 14.0 (StataCorp College Station, Texas).

Results

Participant characteristics

Table 1 presents the demographic and clinical characteristics of both cases and controls. The mean (±SD) age of the 210 participants was 78.1 (± 8.33) years; 127 (60.4%) were female, 189 (90.0%) were Chinese. Of the 48 participants who experienced an injurious fall, 44 (91.2%) experienced minor injuries and 4 (8.33%) experienced major injuries.

Majority of the participants (*n* = 148, 70.4%) were on anti-hypertensive medication. Among anti-hypertensive medication users, 76 (51.3%) took 1 class of medication and 72 (48.6%) took ≥2 classes of medications. No participants in our study took fixed-dose combinations of anti-hypertensive medication. In addition, 41 (27.7%) participants had a change in anti-hypertensive medication within the 180-day period prior to the fall.

Participants who experienced an injurious fall reported a higher risk of fall, greater use of psychotropic medication, a higher rate of previous falls and a higher proportion with polypharmacy. They were more likely to use walking aids and have a higher mean CCI compared to those that did not experience any injurious fall. In addition, they reported greater use of ACEI, ARB, BB and diuretics.

Association between the number of anti-hypertensive medication classes and injurious falls

In univariate analysis (Table 2), five variables were associated *(p < 0.10)* with the occurrence of injurious falls: Charlson's Comorbidity Index (OR:1.33; 95% CI:1.14–1.56; *p* < 0.001), high fall risk (OR:5.69; 95% CI:2.42–13.36; *p* < 0.001), visual impairment (OR:2.48; 95% CI:1.01–6.08; *p* = 0.05), exposure to psychotropic medication (OR:2.21; 95% CI:0.97–5.06; *p* = 0.06) and polypharmacy (OR:2.22; 95% CI:1.08–4.54; *p* = 0.03). These variables were included as predictors in the multivariate model (Table 2), which showed a significant association between the number of anti-hypertensive medication classes and the odds of experiencing an injurious fall (OR = 5.45; 95% CI:1.49–19.93; *p* = 0.01). VIF for each independent variable in the final model was < 5. While walking aid and prior history of falls had *p* < 0.10 in the univariate analyses, they were not included in the multivariate model as they were part of the high fall risk, which we had already adjusted for.

Apart from the exposure variable, the only other variables that reached statistical significance in the multivariate model were Charlson's Comorbidity Index (OR:1.26; 95% CI:1.04–1.54; *p* = 0.02) and high fall risk (OR:7.21; 95% CI:2.37–21.94; *p* = 0.001). However, the odds ratio of those taking only 1 class of anti-hypertensive medication (OR:2.10; 95 CI:0.48–

9.18; *p* = 0.33) was not significantly associated with experiencing an injurious fall.

In sensitivity analyses, both forward and backward stepwise regressions yielded identical models (Additional file 1: Table S1). Those on ≥2 anti-hypertensive medication classes had increased odds of experiencing an injurious fall compared to those with no anti-hypertensive medication. The odds ratio was consistent with the main analyses, indicating that our findings were robust. VIF for each independent variable in stepwise regression model was < 5.

Association between a change in anti-hypertensive medication and injurious falls

In our univariate analysis (Table 3), 3 variables were associated *(p < 0.10)* with the occurrence of injurious falls: Charlson's Comorbidity Index (OR:1.28; 95% CI:1.08–1.51; *p* = 0.004), high fall risk (OR:6.32; 95% CI:2.16–18.46; *p* = 0.001) and a history of hypertension (OR:0.28; 95 95% CI:0.07–1.21; *p* = 0.09). After adjusting for Charlson's Comorbidity Index, high fall risk and history of hypertension, any change in anti-hypertensive medication within the 180-day period prior was associated with higher odds of experiencing an injurious fall (OR = 3.88; 95%CI:1.23–12.19; *p* = 0.02). VIF for each independent variable in the final model was < 5.

In our sensitivity analyses, both the forward and backward stepwise regressions yielded identical models (Additional file 1: Table S2). Those who had a recent change in anti-hypertensive medication had higher odds of experiencing an injurious fall compared to those with no change in anti-hypertensive medication (OR:3.66; 95 CI:1.19–11.23; *p* = 0.01). The odds ratio was consistent with that our main analyses, implying that our findings were robust. VIF for each independent variable in the stepwise regression model was < 5.

Discussion

We found that older adults with low SES on ≥2 anti-hypertensive medication classes had higher odds of experiencing an injurious fall compared to those without any anti-hypertensive medication. Among older adults with anti-hypertensive medication, those with a recent change in anti-hypertensive medication also had increased odds of experiencing an injurious fall. These findings contribute to the literature as most existing studies examined the association between anti-hypertensive classes and falls among general community dwelling older adults [13].

Our findings were consistent with an earlier study [9] which quantified treatment intensity using defined daily dose (DDD) and examined any falls as the outcome. Meanwhile, Tinetti et al. that also examined the number of anti-hypertensive medication classes [10] like our study

Table 1 Baseline characteristics of study participants

Characteristics	Total sample (n = 210)	Cases (n = 48)	Controls (n = 162)	P-value
Age, years, mean ± SD	78.1 ± 8.3	79.5 ± 8.4	77.7 ± 8.3	0.18
Female, n (%)	127 (60.4)	32 (66.7)	95 (58.6)	0.32
Body mass index, kg/m², mean ± SD	23.9 ± 5.2	24.8 ± 6.0	23.7 ± 4.8	0.40
Chinese[c], n (%)	189 (90.0)	46 (95.3)	143 (88.3)	0.17
SBP on admission, mmHg, mean ± SD	133.1 ± 19.2	137.7 ± 23.7	131.7 ± 17.7	0.07
DBP on admission, mmHg, mean ± SD	68.3 ± 10.3	69.3 ± 11.8	67.9 ± 9.9	0.78
Visual impairment, n (%)	29 (13.8)	10 (20.8)	19 (11.7)	0.15
Hearing impairment, n (%)	18 (8.6)	5 (10.4)	13 (8.02)	0.57
Use of walking aid, n (%)	84 (40.0)	37 (77.1)	47 (29.0)	< 0.01
High risk of fall[a], n (%)	42 (20.0)	21 (43.8)	21 (13.0)	< 0.01
Smoking history, n (%)	48 (22.9)	10 (20.8)	38 (23.4)	0.70
Alcohol history, n (%)	23 (11.0)	5 (10.4)	18 (11.1)	0.90
Medical history, n (%)				
Hypertension	162 (77.1)	37 (77.1)	125 (77.2)	0.88
Cerebrovascular accident or transient ischaemic attack	39 (18.6)	12 (25.0)	27 (16.7)	0.19
Ischaemic heart disease	52 (24.8)	12 (25.0)	40 (24.7)	0.97
Diabetes mellitus	75 (35.7)	18 (37.5)	57 (35.2)	0.79
Hyperlipidaemia	147 (70.0)	33 (68.8)	114 (70.4)	0.83
Osteoporosis	20 (9.5)	5 (10.4)	15 (9.3)	0.78
Cancer	26 (12.4)	7 (14.5)	19 (11.7)	0.60
Cognitive impairment	21 (10.0)	6 (12.5)	15 (9.3)	0.59
Prior history of falls, n (%)	49 (23.3)	18 (37.5)	31 (19.1)	0.01
Charlson Comorbidity Index, mean ± SD	5.1 ± 2.3	6.3 ± 2.5	4.7 ± 2.1	< 0.01
Medication use, n (%)				
Statin	124 (59.0)	29 (60.4)	95 (58.6)	0.83
Psychotropic medication	36 (17.1)	13 (27.1)	23 (14.2)	0.04
Anti-hypertensive medication	148 (70.4)	40 (83.3)	108 (66.7)	0.03
≥ 2 anti-hypertensive medication	72 (34.3)	31 (64.6)	41 (25.3)	< 0.01
Any change in anti-hypertensive medication[b]	41 (19.5)	20 (41.7)	21 (13.0)	< 0.01
Type of anti-hypertensive, n (%)				
Angiotensin-converting enzyme inhibitor	43 (20.5)	15 (31.3)	28 (17.3)	0.04
Angiotensin II receptor blocker	41 (19.5)	15 (31.3)	26 (16.0)	0.02
Beta-blocker	56 (26.7)	21 (43.8)	35 (21.6)	< 0.01
Calcium channel blocker	75 (35.7)	17 (35.4)	58 (35.8)	0.94
Diuretic	24 (11.4)	12 (25.0)	12 (7.41)	< 0.01
Polypharmacy, n (%)	109 (51.9)	32 (66.7)	77 (47.5)	0.02

SD Standard deviation, SBP Systolic blood pressure, DBP Diastolic blood pressure

[a]High risk of fall = Defined using Morse Fall Scale risk score of 55 or more

[b]Any change in anti-hypertensive medication = An addition of a new class of anti-hypertensive medication or an increase in the dosage of the existing medication or a switch to a new class of anti-hypertensive medication; Polypharmacy = Use of 4 or more chronic medication

Reference group:

[c]Non-Chinese

found no association between it and injurious falls. This difference in results may be attributable to different study samples as our study examined older adults of low SES who are at higher risk of falls whereas Tinetti et al. examined general community-dwelling older adults [10]. To illustrate it in local context, the proportion of those with hypertension (162/210 = 77.1%) and those who experienced falls (48/210 = 22.9%) were higher in our study

Table 2 Association between number of anti-hypertensive medication and injurious falls (N = 210)

	Unadjusted OR (95% CI)	P-value	Adjusted OR (95% CI)	P-value
Number of anti-hypertensive medication				
0	1.00		1.00	
1	0.92 (0.30–2.87)	0.89	2.10 (0.48–9.18)	0.33
≥ 2	4.75 (1.77–12.72)	< 0.01	5.45 (1.49–19.93)	0.01
Charlson comorbidity index	1.33 (1.14–1.56)	< 0.01	1.26 (1.04–1.54)	0.02
High risk of fall[a]	5.69 (2.42–13.36)	< 0.01	7.21 (2.37–21.94)	< 0.01
Visual impairment	2.48 (1.01–6.08)	0.05	2.02 (0.70–5.86)	0.19
Exposure to psychotropic medication	2.21 (0.97–5.06)	0.06	1.12 (0.38–3.37)	0.83
Polypharmacy	2.22 (1.08–4.54)	0.03	1.29 (0.49–3.43)	0.61
Age (years)	0.92 (0.82–1.04)	0.19		
BMI (kg/m^2)	1.06 (0.98–1.13)	0.13		
Chinese[c]	2.99 (0.62–14.34)	0.17		
SBP on admission (mmHg)	1.01 (0.99–1.03)	0.13		
DBP on admission (mmHg)	1.01 (0.98–1.04)	0.52		
Hearing impairment	1.27 (0.41–3.92)	0.67		
Use of walking aid[b]	8.18 (3.29–20.31)	< 0.01		
Smoking history	1.06 (0.42–2.67)	0.90		
Alcohol history	1.13 (0.34–3.74)	0.84		
Medical history				
Hypertension	1.05 (0.47–2.38)	0.90		
Cerebrovascular accident or transient ischaemic attack	1.97 (0.87–4.49)	0.11		
Ischaemic heart disease	1.26 (0.57–2.76)	0.56		
Diabetes mellitus	1.17 (0.60–2.28)	0.65		
Hyperlipidaemia	0.91 (0.44–1.89)	0.81		
Osteoporosis	1.05 (0.33–3.32)	0.93		
Cancer	1.28 (0.48–3.46)	0.62		
Cognitive impairment	1.33 (0.47–3.80)	0.59		
Prior history of falls[b]	2.51 (1.18–5.37)	0.02		
Statin use	0.88 (0.45–1.71)	0.71		

OR Odds ratio, CI 95% confidence interval, SBP Systolic blood pressure, DBP Diastolic blood pressure

[a]High risk of fall = Defined using Morse Fall Scale risk score of 55 or more; Polypharmacy = Use of 4 or more chronic medication

[b]Even though these variables had p < 0.10 in univariate analysis, they were not included in the multivariate analysis as these variables were part of the high fall risk, which we had already adjusted for

Reference group:

[c]Non-Chinese

cohort compared to the general older population (73.9%, 8.2% respectively) in Singapore [27, 28]. Concurrent administration of ≥2 anti-hypertensive medication classes may increase risk of experiencing an injurious fall by exacerbating postural hypotension or symptoms of dizziness and fatigue [12].

Our literature search only retrieved one study examining the association between a change in anti-hypertensive medication and the risk of experiencing an injurious fall [11]. The study found that long term addition or titration of anti-hypertensive medication was not associated with

serious fall injuries. We also included those who switched to a different class of anti-hypertensive medication in our analysis and this might have contributed to the increased risk of experiencing an injurious fall in our study. A change in medication may induce electrolyte disturbances which consequently impairs balance and gait [11] and makes older adults more susceptible to falls.

Our findings have several clinical implications. It is important to be wary of the number of anti-hypertensive medications prescribed to the older population as some older people may be taking more anti-hypertensive

Table 3 Association between change in anti-hypertensive medication and injurious fall (N = 139)

	Unadjusted OR (95% CI)	P-value	Adjusted OR (95% CI)	P-value
Any change in anti-hypertensive medication[a]				
No	1.00		1.00	
Yes	5.66 (2.12–15.15)	< 0.01	3.88 (1.23–12.19)	0.02
Charlson comorbidity index	1.28 (1.08–1.51)	< 0.01	1.28 (1.04–1.58)	0.02
High risk of fall[b]	6.32 (2.16–18.46)	< 0.01	5.73 (1.60–20.51)	0.01
Visual impairment	2.10 (0.74–6.01)	0.17		
Exposure to psychotropic medication	2.07 (0.78–5.49)	0.14		
Polypharmacy	1.83 (0.80–4.19)	0.15		
Age (years)	0.90 (0.78–1.04)	0.16		
BMI (kg/m^2)	1.05 (0.97–1.14)	0.21		
Chinese[d]	2.10 (0.43–10.42)	0.36		
SBP on admission (mmHg)	1.00 (0.99–1.03)	0.99		
DBP on admission (mmHg)	1.00 (0.96–1.04)	0.36		
Hearing impairment	0.55 (0.65–4.75)	0.59		
Use of walking aid[c]	18.07 (4.15–78.65)	< 0.01		
Smoking history	1.31 (0.45–3.76)	0.62		
Alcohol history	0.85 (0.17–4.31)	0.85		
Medical history				
Hypertension	0.28 (0.07–1.21)	0.09	0.30 (0.05–1.75)	0.18
Cerebrovascular accident or transient ischaemic attack	1.50 (0.63–3.59)	0.36		
Ischaemic heart disease	0.89 (0.39–2.07)	0.79		
Diabetes mellitus	0.99 (0.46–2.17)	0.99		
Hyperlipidaemia	0.77 (0.27–2.19)	0.62		
Osteoporosis	1.52 (0.44–5.20)	0.50		
Cancer	1.76 (0.61–5.09)	0.30		
Cognitive impairment	1.00 (0.29–3.45)	1.00		
Prior history of falls	1.84 (0.79–4.30)	0.16		
Statin use	0.50 (0.21–1.18)	0.12		

OR Odds ratio, *CI* 95% confidence interval, *SBP* Systolic blood pressure, *DBP* Diastolic blood pressure

[a]Any change in anti-hypertensive medication = An addition of a new class of anti-hypertensive medication or an increase in the dosage of the existing medication or a switch to a new class of anti-hypertensive medication

[b]High risk of fall = Defined using Morse Fall Scale risk score of 55 or more.; Polypharmacy = Use of 4 or more chronic medication

[c]Even though this variable had p < 0.10 in univariate analysis, it was not included in the multivariate analysis as these variables were part of the high fall risk, which we had already adjusted for

Reference group:

[d]Non-Chinese

medication than needed [29]. Prescribers should develop patient-specific treatment goals and avoid "over-treatment" of hypertension, particularly among older population of low SES. A recent study by Zia et al. [30] showed that the consumption of two or more fall risk increasing drugs (FRID) is a significant predictor for falls. Anti-hypertensive medication was identified to be one of the many FRIDs. As such, it is imperative that healthcare providers discuss risk and preventative strategies for falls with patients when commencing anti-hypertensive medications or when

adding, switching or increasing the dose of anti-hypertensive medications.

The findings from this study should be interpreted within the context of the following limitations. We defined "injurious falls" based on healthcare use [31], specifically falls requiring medical services as we were concerned about healthcare utilization resulting from falls. We acknowledge that there are other definitions of "injurious falls" in literature [31] such as those based on symptoms only (e.g. fractures) or a combination of symptoms and healthcare use. Therefore, our findings may not be generalizable to other definitions of "injurious falls". We checked for confounding for a wide array of conditions and medications associated with falls and adjusted for the appropriate variables in multivariate analyses. However, we acknowledge there is still a possibility of residual confounding as our study lacked information on important variables such as frailty and blood pressure. Previous study [32] found substantial differences in the associations between cardiovascular medication use and fall risk in frail and robust older adults. In addition, as blood pressure measurements immediately prior to falls were not available, we were unable to ascertain whether the falls were due to orthostatic hypotension resulting from anti-hypertensive medications.

We also did not collect any measures of adherence to anti-hypertensive medication. Nevertheless, we note that non-adherence would result in underestimation of a true effect. We did not consider the dose of each anti-hypertensive medication. As such, we could not attribute our findings to the dose intensity of each medication. Due to the small samples, our analyses were unable to account for specific type and class of anti-hypertensive medications. Lastly, although the small sample size and the small number of injurious fallers in our study may have posed some challenges, such as imprecise estimates and potentially the sample is not representative of the population, our findings from both the main and sensitivity analyses were consistent.

Conclusion

In a nutshell, our study demonstrated that ≥2 anti-hypertensive medication classes and a change in anti-hypertensive medication were associated with an increased risk of injurious falls among older adults of low SES. Prescribers should design patient-specific treatment goals to prevent the "over-treatment" of hypertension. In addition, the risk of and preventative strategies for falls should be discussed with patients when commencing anti-hypertensive medications or when adding, switching or increasing the dose of anti-hypertensive medications, especially among older adults of low SES who are more prone to falling.

Abbreviations

ACEi: Angiotensin converting enzyme inhibitors; ARB: Angiotensin receptor blockers; BB: Beta blockers; CCB: Calcium channel blockers; CCI: Charlson's co-morbidity index; DDD: Defined-daily dose; FRID: Fall risk increasing drugs; ICoC: Integrated Community of Care programme; OR: Odds ratio; OTC: Over-the-counter; SD: Standard deviation; SES: Socio-economic status; SGD: Singapore Dollar; SGH: Singapore General Hospital; USD: United States Dollar; VIF: Variance inflation factor

Acknowledgements
We would like to acknowledge the Integrated Community of Care project team for their effort in recruiting participants.

Funding
There was no external funding for this study. The ICoC study was originally supported by the SingHealth Regional Health System and Duke-NUS Medical School Centre for Aging Research and Education.

Authors' contributions
LLL is the principal investigator of the study. LLL and KZY conceptualized the study. TO, KHL, JT and WF advised the study design. ZB and HTA collected the data, supervised by KKL, YHK and KZY. CST and YHK advised the statistical analyses. ZB and KKL performed the analyses. TO, KHL, JT and WF assisted in the interpretations of the findings. ZB and KKL prepared the first draft of the manuscript. All co-authors critically reviewed and agreed to the final content of the manuscript before submission. All authors read and approved the final manuscript.

Competing interests
The authors declare that they have no competing interests.

Author details
[1]Department of Pharmacy, Faculty of Science, National University of Singapore, Singapore, Republic of Singapore. [2]Program in Health Services and Systems Research, Duke-NUS Medical School, Singapore, Republic of Singapore. [3]Saw Swee Hock School of Public Health, National University of Singapore and National University Health System, Singapore, Republic of Singapore. [4]Department of Family Medicine and Continuing Care, Singapore General Hospital, Singapore, Republic of Singapore. [5]Department of Rheumatology and Immunology, Singapore General Hospital, Singapore, Republic of Singapore. [6]Duke-NUS Medical School, Singapore, Republic of Singapore. [7]Department of Medicine, Yong Loo Lin School of Medicine, National University of Singapore, Singapore, Republic of Singapore.

References
1. World Health Organization. WHO Global Report on Falls Prevention in Older Age. Geneva: World Health Organization; 2007.
2. Tinetti ME, Doucette J, Claus E, Marottoli R. Risk factors for serious injury during falls by older persons in the community. J Am Geriatr Soc. 1995; 43(11):1214–21.
3. Chan K, Pang W, Ee CH, Ding Y, Choo P. Epidemiology of falls among the elderly community dwellers in Singapore. Singap Med J. 1997;38(10):427–31.
4. Cumming RG, Salkeld G, Thomas M, Szonyi G. Prospective study of the impact of fear of falling on activities of daily living, SF-36 scores, and nursing home admission. J Gerontol A Biol Sci Med Sci. 2000;55(5):M299–305.
5. Hartholt KA, Polinder S, Van der Cammen TJ, Panneman MJ, Van der Velde N, Van Lieshout EM, et al. Costs of falls in an ageing population: a nationwide study from the Netherlands (2007-2009). Injury. 2012;43(7): 1199–203.
6. Wiens M, Etminan M, Gill SS, Takkouche B. Effects of antihypertensive drug treatments on fracture outcomes: a meta-analysis of observational studies. J Intern Med. 2006;260(4):350–62.
7. Leipzig RM, Cumming RG, Tinetti ME. Drugs and falls in older people: a systematic review and meta-analysis: II. Cardiac and analgesic drugs. J Am Geriatr Soc. 1999;47(1):40–50.
8. Zang G. Antihypertensive drugs and the risk of fall injuries: a systematic review and meta-analysis. J Int Med Res. 2013;41(5):1408–17.
9. Callisaya ML, Sharman JE, Close J, Lord SR, Srikanth VK. Greater daily defined dose of antihypertensive medication increases the risk of falls in older people-- a population-based study. J Am Geriatr Soc. 2014;62(8):1527–33.
10. Tinetti ME, Han L, Lee DS, McAvay GJ, Peduzzi P, Gross CP, et al. Antihypertensive medications and serious fall injuries in a nationally representative sample of older adults. JAMA Intern Med. 2014;174(4):588–95.
11. Shimbo D, Barrett Bowling C, Levitan EB, Deng L, Sim JJ, Huang L, et al. Short-term risk of serious fall injuries in older adults initiating and

intensifying treatment with antihypertensive medication. Circ Cardiovasc Qual Outcomes. 2016;9(3):222–9.

12. Milazzo VSC, Servo S, Crudo V, Fulcheri C. Drugs and Orthostatic Hypotension: Evidence from Literature. J Hypertens. 2012;1(104). https://www.omicsonline.org/open-access/drugs-and-orthostatic-hypotension-evidence-from-literature-2167-1095.1000104.php?aid=6762.

13. Ang HT, Lim KK, Kwan YH, Tan PS, Yap KZ, Banu Z, et al. A Systematic Review and Meta-Analyses of the Association Between Anti-Hypertensive Classes and the Risk of Falls Among Older Adults. Drugs Aging. 2018;35(7):625–35. https://link.springer.com/article/10.1007%2Fs40266-018-0561-3.

14. Gill T, Taylor AW, Pengelly A. A population-based survey of factors relating to the prevalence of falls in older people. Gerontology. 2005;51(5):340–5.

15. Beverly H, Brummett MAB, Ilene C, Siegler MS, Harris KM, Elder GH, Williams RB. Systolic blood pressure, socioeconomic status, and biobehavioral risk factors in a nationally representative US young adult sample. Hypertension. 2011;58:161–6.

16. Lam CSP. The socioeconomics of hypertension. Hypertension. 2011;58:140–1.

17. Low LL, Maulod A, Lee KH. Evaluating a novel Integrated Community of Care (ICoC) for patients from an urbanised low-income community in Singapore using the participatory action research (PAR) methodology: a study protocol. BMJ Open. 2017;7(10):e017839. https://bmjopen.bmj.com/content/7/10/e017839.info.

18. Housing & Development Board. Public housing in Singapore: residents' profile, hosuing satisfaction and preferences: HDB sample household survey 2013. Published by: Housing & Development Board. Year published: 2014. Country: Singapore. https://www.hdb.gov.sg/cs/infoweb/monograph-1-29-dec-2014.

19. Sahadevan S, Lim PP, Tan NJ, Chan SP. Diagnostic performance of two mental status tests in the older chinese: influence of education and age on cut-off values. Int J Geriatr Psychiatry. 2000;15(3):234–41.

20. Malhotra C, Chan A, Matchar D, Seow D, Chuo A, Do YK. Diagnostic performance of short portable mental status questionnaire for screening dementia among patients attending cognitive assessment clinics in Singapore. Ann Acad Med Singap. 2013;42(7):315–9.

21. Charlson's ME, Pompei P, Ales KL, MacKenzie CR. A new method of classifying prognostic comorbidity in longitudinal studies: development and validation. J Chronic Dis. 1987;40(5):373–83.

22. Yuh AS, Perera K, Yunn R. Evidence-based management of patients risk for falls in the inpatient setting. Publisher: Singapore Healthcare Management Conference; 2013. [Accessed 03 March 2018; Last Update 2015]. http://www.singaporehealthcaremanagement.sg/Abstracts/Documents/PDFs/RM0002%20-%20Ang%20Shin%20Yuh.pdf.

23. de Jong MR, Van der Elst M, Hartholt KA. Drug-related falls in older patients: implicated drugs, consequences, and possible prevention strategies. Ther Adv Drug Saf. 2013;4(4):147–54.

24. Scott D, Blizzard L, Fell J, Jones G. Statin therapy, muscle function and falls risk in community-dwelling older adults. QJM. 2009;102(9):625–33.

25. Bor A, Matuz M, Csatordai M, Szalai G, Bálint A, Benkő R, et al. Medication use and risk of falls among nursing home residents: a retrospective cohort study. Int J Clin Pharm. 2017;39(2):408–15.

26. Berry SD, Quach L, Procter-Gray E, Kiel DP, Li W, Samelson EJ, et al. Poor Adherence to Medications May Be Associated with Falls. J Gerontol A Biol Sci Med Sci. 2010;65a(5):553–8.

27. Malhotra R, Chan A, Malhotra C, Ostbye T. Prevalence, awareness, treatment and control of hypertension in the elderly population of Singapore. Hypertens Res. 2010;33(12):1223–31.

28. Yeo YY, Lee SK, Lim CY, Quek LS, Ooi SB. A review of elderly injuries seen in a Singapore emergency department. Singap Med J. 2009;50(3):278–83.

29. Mancia G, Fagard R, Narkiewicz K, Redon J, Zanchetti A, Bohm M, et al. 2013 ESH/ESC guidelines for the management of arterial hypertension: the task force for the management of arterial hypertension of the European Society of Hypertension (ESH) and of the European Society of Cardiology (ESC). J Hypertens. 2013;31(7):1281–357.

30. Zia A, Kamaruzzaman SB, Tan MP. The consumption of two or more fall risk-increasing drugs rather than polypharmacy is associated with falls. Geriatr Gerontol Int. 2017;17(3):463–70.

31. Schwenk M, Lauenroth A, Stock C, Moreno RR, Oster P, McHugh G, et al. Definitions and methods of measuring and reporting on injurious falls in randomised controlled fall prevention trials: a systematic review. BMC Med Res Methodol. 2012;12(1):50.

32. Peeters G, Tett SE, Hollingworth SA, Gnjidic D, Hilmer SN, Dobson AJ, et al. Associations of guideline recommended medications for acute coronary syndromes with fall-related hospitalizations and cardiovascular events in older women with ischemic heart disease. J Gerontol A Biol Sci Med Sci. 2017;72(2):259–65.

12

Effect of cognitive and executive functions on perception of quality of life of cognitively normal elderly people dwelling in residential aged care facilities in Sri Lanka

Madushika Wishvanie Kodagoda Gamage[1]*(iD), Chandana Hewage[2] and Kithsiri Dedduwa Pathirana[3]

Abstract

Background: Although cognitive functions affect the health related quality of life (QoL), the relationship between perceived QoL and cognition including executive functions has not been studied adequately. Available studies show moderate to weak correlations. We evaluated the association of cognition and executive functions, namely working memory (WM) and inhibitory control (IC) with the perceived QoL of a sample of elderly people dwelling in residential aged care facilities (RACFs) in Southern Province of Sri Lanka.

Methods: Cognition was assessed using Mini-Mental State Examination (MMSE), while verbal WM (VWM), visuo-spatial WM (VSWM) and IC (interference control, inhibition of pre potent and ongoing responses) were assessed using VWM, VSWM tasks, colour word Stroop (CWS), go/no-go (GNG) and stop signal (SS) tasks respectively. WHOQoL-Bref (Total score and domain scores) were used to assess QoL. The relationship was analysed using Pearson correlation and hierarchical multiple regression analysis.

Results: Study included 237 elderly people with a mean age of 71.11 ± 6.44 years. Participants scored the highest in the domain of environment (63.48 ± 10.63) and lowest in the domain of social relationships (55.43 ± 21.84) of QoL. Psychological health domain positively correlated with MMSE, VSWM and VWM scores and negatively correlated with CWS, SS and GNG task errors. Both physical health domain and total QoL demonstrated positive correlations with MMSE, VSWM and VWM scores, while negative correlations were observed with CWS task errors. Social relationships domain demonstrated a significant positive correlation with VSWM score. Environment domain positively correlated with MMSE, VSWM and VWM scores and negatively correlated with CWS and SS task errors. All were significant but weak correlations. When controlled for covariates, such as educational status, physical activity and marital status, cognition was a predictor of the domain of environment of QoL, while executive functions were not predictors of total QoL and domains of QoL.

Conclusion: Cognition and executive functions weakly but significantly correlated with different domains of QoL. Only the level of cognition measured by MMSE was a predictor of the domain of environment of QoL and executive functions were not predictors of total QoL and domains of QoL in elderly people with normal cognitive functions dwelling in RACFs.

Keywords: Cognition, Working memory, Inhibitory control, Quality of life, Elderly

* Correspondence: mkgamage@yahoo.com
[1]Department of Nursing, Faculty of Allied Health Sciences, University of Ruhuna, Galle, Sri Lanka
Full list of author information is available at the end of the article

Background

Population ageing is a characteristic of the twenty-first century. It is estimated that the proportion of elderly in the population will reach 16.5% and 7.5% in developed and developing countries respectively by 2025 [1]. Sri Lanka is regarded as one of the fastest ageing countries in the world. Although caring for older people is regarded as a moral obligation of children, socio-demographic changes such as increase in proportion of women who engage in employment, decline in number of offspring due to decline in fertility rate, migration of youth and conversion of extended families into nuclear families have resulted in reduction of elderly care [2]. With this, the number of elderly people moving to residential aged care facilities (RACFs) is increasing [2]. These facilities are available in the country for several decades [2]. Meals, accommodation, recreation, protection and other facilities for the residents are provided free of charge and are sponsored by the government throughout the country. Out of 447 elderly care facilities available in Sri Lanka, only 300 (67.1%) are RACFs, while others provide day care [3]. In Sri Lanka, the reason for the provision of residential care is not due to health problems, such as dementia or disability, but due to the lack of infrastructure and availability of personnel to provide care in the community. Having fewer children, the demands of formal sector employment of their children and changing values are the main reasons for their admissions to care facilities [4].

World Health Organization QoL (WHOQoL) Group [5] defined QoL as "individuals' perceptions of their position in life in the context of the culture and value systems in which they live and in relation to their goals, expectations, standards and concerns". The individuals' perception will be affected via their physical health status, personal beliefs, psychological status, social relationships and interaction with the environment. Perception of their position in life is an important aspect for the well-being of the elderly.

Cognition is a process by which "sensory inputs are transformed, reduced, elaborated, stored, recovered and used" [6]. Cognitive health promotion, that is, maintaining "brain health" with ageing has become increasingly important for the elderly [7]. Identification of specific cognitive processes that may underlie cognitive decline is essential for planning preventive measures. Studies are still inconclusive as to whether all components of the nervous system demonstrate a similar degree of age-related changes or whether the effect selectively affects specific brain regions/systems. One such system that has attracted research is prefrontal cortex area-mediated executive functions [8].

Executive functions (EFs) consist of higher order cognitive processes important for goal directed behavior [9].

Working memory and inhibition are regarded as two core processes in EFs [10]. WM is a cognitive system which allows temporarily maintenance of information and manipulation for generating and executing complex activities [11]. It includes a visuo-spatial sketchpad and an articulatory loop, which holds and manipulates visual images including spatial relationship (visuospatial WM) and speech-based information (verbal WM), respectively [12]. Inhibition is the process which regulates information that enters and leaves the WM [13]. Inhibition consists of the ability to overcome interference (protecting a response from disruption by competing responses or events), suppression of pre-potent responses (a response that is or has been previously associated with reinforcement) or stopping of ongoing responses which allows for a delay in the decision to continue responding [14]. Decline in EFs observed with ageing has been associated with significant limitations of functionality, independent living [15] and impaired health enhancing behaviour [16] leading to reduction in QoL of elderly [17]. Therefore "promotion of successful cognitive and emotional ageing" that minimizes loss of information processing capacity and maintains cognitive reserve for elderly, is an important aspect that has to be addressed with population ageing [18].

Although there is a growing interest on assessing effect of cognition on QoL among elderly, currently only a few studies have focused their attention on the relationship between cognition and QoL [19]. Most of the previous studies have focused their attention on association between health related QoL and cognition [20, 21] but not with perception of QoL. Furthermore, the effect of cognition, including EFs on the QoL dimensions, had been inconsistent among different studies [17, 19]. One study revealed significant correlations between MMSE score and QoL domains as physical, environment and overall QoL and not with psychological and social relationships [19], while another revealed significant correlation only between environment domain of QoL and MMSE score [17]. Although they were significant, they demonstrated weak correlations [17, 19]. This reflects that there would be other strong factors that influence QoL. Previous studies have demonstrated the influence of physical activity [22], educational status [23] and marital status [24] on QoL of elderly people. Hence, we thought to identify the association between cognitive and executive functions and QoL when controlled for the factors as physical activity, educational status and marital status. As elderly population is increasing, it is necessary to have a better understanding of the influence of specific neural sub-systems, like EFs, on cognitive decline and its effect on the QoL among elderly. In Sri Lankan culture elderly care is unique and cannot be compared to similar studies. This will enable planning therapeutic interventions in the future.

Methods

Study design and participants

The study sample consists of 237 elderly people who are 60 years and older, dwelling in residential aged care facilities in Galle and Matara Districts in Sri Lanka, recruited using probability proportional to size sampling method. During the process of recruitment, an aged care facility was selected randomly. All the elderly people were screened and those who fulfilled the selection criteria and who volunteered to participate were recruited as the study sample in the selected institution. Recruitment of subjects was performed as shown in Fig 1.

Previous literature has shown significant declines in QoL in people with mild cognitive impairment [25]. Hence, we investigated the effect of cognitive and executive functions on QoL of those who have apparently normal cognition. For this purpose, subjects with conditions that affect communication ability, physical activity and cognition were excluded as they affect test performance and they themselves will be confounding factors.

We excluded the subjects with severe loss of vision (corrected vision worse than 6/60), loss of hearing (interviewer-rated), loss of communication ability (interviewer-rated), impaired colour vision, impaired ability to read, write and to follow verbal instructions, subjects with major physical disabilities, who scored less than 100 in Barthel's index and subjects with conditions that affect performance of tasks, such as stroke, osteoarthritis, amputation, fractures, neurological disorders, subjects with psychiatric illnesses, developmental disabilities and cognitive impairment (MMSE score less than 24).

Demographic characteristics of the participants were obtained using a questionnaire. Physical activity level was assessed using International Physical Activity Questionnaire (IPAQ) modified for elderly version. It provides continuous scores as well as categorical values. Based on

their physical activity score, they were categorized as inactive, minimally active and as having health enhancing physical activity level [26].

Global cognitive measures- mini mental state examination (MMSE)

It is a brief 30-point scale mental health examination which assessed five areas: orientation, registration, attention and calculation and recall and language.

Core components of EFs- WM and response inhibition

The two core EFs, WM and inhibition were assessed using computerized tasks. Working memory was assessed using verbal WM (VWM) and visuo-spatial WM (VSWM) tasks. Response inhibition was assessed using colour word stroop (CWS), stop signal (SS) and go/no-go (GNG) tasks. All participants were individually tested in a quiet room. The order of task administration was the same for all participants and they received a practice session prior to all the tasks. A period of rest was given between two tasks.

Colour word Stroop task [27, 28]: In this task different colour words appeared on the computer screen one at a time. The task was to name the colour the word was printed, disregarding what the colour word reads. The colour of the word printed was in the same colour as the meaning of the word (congruent trials, eg; "red" is printed in red colour), or it was different from the meaning (incongruent trials, eg; word "green" is printed in blue colour). There were 75 congruent trials and 25 incongruent trials for one test session. Incorrect responses on incongruent trials were taken to assess the level of inhibitory control. The higher the errors the lower the interference control is.

Visuo-spatial WM task: A 4×4 matrix with 16 squares was displayed on the computer screen as a pig house with a pig appearing in each window one at a time. The task was to recall in reverse order the locations where each target (pig) had appeared. The test started with a span length of two, that is, two pigs appeared one after another. Each span consisted of two trials and the test was concluded when the participant failed both trials at that same span length. Each correct location was given one point with a maximum score of 88. The score was taken as the measure of VSWM. At the end of the test, obtained score was automatically displayed on the computer screen.

Stop signal task: It assessed the ability to inhibit ongoing responses. This was like a car game [29] where a car appeared on the computer screen. Every time the car appeared, the participant was supposed to press a designated key as fast as possible to drive the car away. But when a stop-sign board appeared next to the car,

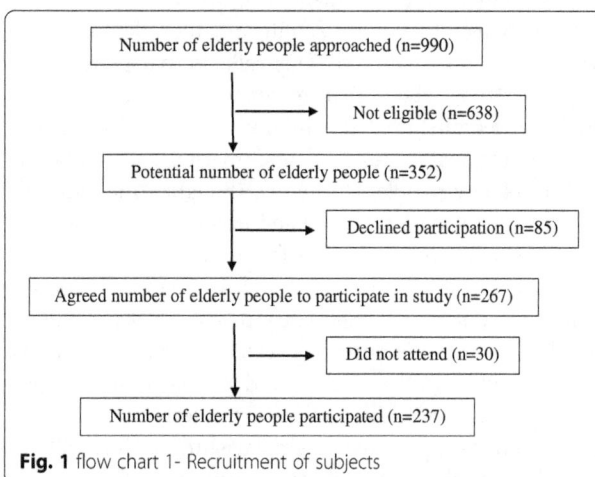

Fig. 1 flow chart 1- Recruitment of subjects

participants had to refrain from pressing for the car to stand still. Each session in this task consisted of 24 trials with six stop-signs-trials. Number of incorrect presses in stop sign (commission errors) was considered as the measure of inhibition and it was automatically displayed on the screen at the end of the task.

Verbal WM task (adapted from [30]): These were power point slides. Each slide had different numbers of red circles with squares as distracters. The task was to count the total number of red circles in each slide, keep total in memory and recall the numbers in the correct order. The test started with a length of memory recall (span) of two, that is, the participant had to recall two slides first. Each level of memory recall consisted of three trials and the test was concluded when the participant failed two trials out of three at that same length of recall. If the participant was successful in 2 out of three trials, he/she was allowed to go to the next span. A total score was calculated after adding a mark for each correct recall [30].

Go/no-go task (two versions: colour and shape): It assessed ability to inhibit pre potent responses. The subject was presented with four different stimuli on the screen, one at a time in random order. There were two squares and two circles in blue and red. In the first session, the subject was instructed to respond by pressing a key each time when a blue figure appeared (go-trials) regardless of the shape, and not to respond when a red figure appeared. In the second session, the subject was instructed to respond each time when a square appeared, regardless of the color, and not to respond when a circle appeared [31]. Together the two consecutive sessions included 60 stimuli with 77% go-trials. The number of incorrect responses (commission errors) was used as a measure of inhibition and it was automatically displayed on the screen at the end of the task.

QoL was assessed using WHOQoL-Bref short version questionnaire. It measured the perception of an individual about his/her QoL. It contained a subset of 26 items taken from the 100 item questionnaire. It produced a profile with four domain scores which were physical, psychological, environment and social relationships and two individually scored items about an individual's overall perception of QoL and health. In the questionnaire, the question "How satisfied are you with your sex life?" was omitted from the analysis as all the participants responded either as no or were reluctant to respond.

Domain score, which is a collection of obtained scores for the questions relevant to one domain, was obtained, and it was transformed to a percentage score using the formula shown below. Additionally, total score was calculated reflecting the total QoL.

$$\text{Transformed scale} = \frac{(\text{Actual raw score-lowest possible raw score}) * 100}{\text{Possible raw score range}}$$

Statistical analysis

Statistical analyses were performed using SPSS 20.0 version. The statistical significance was kept at $p < 0.05$. Descriptive analysis was performed to calculate distribution measures. To assess the correlation among QoL and cognitive variables, Pearson correlation test was used, following the classification of Cohen [32], which considered a correlation as weak if $r < 0.3$; moderate if $0.3 \leq r < 0.5$ and strong if $0.5 \leq r \leq 1.0$. The variables, such as, educational status, physical activity level and marital status were included as covariates in evaluation of the effect of cognitive and executive functions on QoL. For each of the domains, only the significantly correlated variables were considered as covariates. For physical health domain and total QoL, educational status, physical activity level and marital status were considered as covariates. For psychological health domain, educational status and physical activity were considered as covariates. For environment domain, marital status and physical activity were the covariates while for social relationships, only the educational status was considered as a covariate. Hierarchical multiple linear regression analysis was conducted including covariates into Block 1 and cognitive and executive function scores into Block 2. For block 2, only the cognitive and executive function scores that significantly correlated with QoL domain scores were included.

Results

The mean age of the participants was 71.11 ± 6.44 of which 63.7% were females. The socio-demographic characteristics are tabulated in Table 1. Most of them were in the age category of more than 70 years, had obtained upper secondary, advanced level and higher education and were married. The participants had the highest score in the domain of environment of QoL and the least score in the domain of social relationships of QoL. Female participants scored higher than male participants in all the domains of QoL except psychological health.

Male participants performed a higher number of errors in response inhibition tasks and obtained lower scores in VWM and VSWM tasks than female participants. The mean scores of the MMSE, EF tasks and QoL domains in WHOQoL Bref are presented in Table 2. Table 3 indicates the correlation between QoL domains with MMSE score, WM tasks scores and inhibitory tasks errors. Psychological health domain positively correlated with MMSE ($r = 0.18, p = 0.006$), VSWM ($r = 0.17$, $p = 0.007$) and VWM ($r = 0.15$, $p = 0.021$) scores and negatively correlated with CWS ($r = -0.14$, $p = 0.03$), SS ($r = -0.13$, $p = 0.037$) and GNG ($r = -0.13$, $p = 0.048$) task errors.

Table 1 Socio-demographic characteristics and clinical characteristics of the participants

Characteristic	All elderly (n = 237)		Female (n = 151)		Male (n = 86)	
	N	(%)	N	(%)	N	(%)
Age						
≤ 70 years	108	45.6	79	52.3	29	33.7
> 70 years	129	54.4	72	47.7	57	66.3
Education						
Primary and lower secondary education	101	42.6	67	44.4	34	39.5
Upper secondary, advanced level and higher education	136	57.4	84	55.6	52	60.5
Marital status						
Married	96	40.5	57	37.7	39	45.3
Unmarried	88	37.1	56	37.1	32	37.2
Widowed/ Divorced/Separated	53	22.4	38	25.2	15	17.4
Chronic diseases						
No diseases	87	36.7	53	35.1	34	39.5
1	86	36.3	59	39.1	27	31.4
≥ 2	64	27	39	25.8	25	29.1
Physical activity						
Inactive	3	1.3	2	1.3	1	1.2
Minimally active	169	71.3	101	66.9	68	79.1
Health Enhancing physical activity	65	27.4	48	31.8	17	19.8

Both physical health domain and total QoL demonstrated positive correlations with MMSE ($r = 0.27$, $p < 0.001$; $r = 0.25$, $p < 0.001$ respectively), VSWM ($r = 0.27$, $p < 0.001$; $r = 0.25$, $p < 0.001$ respectively) and VWM ($r = 0.21$, $p = 0.001$; $r = 0.19$, $p = 0.004$ respectively) scores while negative correlations were observed with CWS ($r = -0.26$, $p < 0.001$; $r = -0.21$, $p = 0.001$ respectively) task errors. Social relationships domain demonstrated a significant correlation only with VSWM score ($r = 0.15$, $p = 0.023$) and it was a positive correlation. Environment domain positively correlated with MMSE ($r = 0.29$, $p < 0.001$), VSWM ($r = 0.18$, $p = 0.006$) and VWM ($r = 0.22$, $p < 0.001$) scores and negatively correlated with CWS ($r = -0.18$, $p = 0.006$) and SS ($r = -0.19$, $p = 0.003$) task errors. All were weak significant correlations.

Hierarchical multiple linear regression analysis predicting total QoL and QoL domain scores are shown in Table 4. In the domain of physical health, the introduction of cognitive and executive functions explained an additional 5.7% of variance after controlling for covariates (F $(7, 229) = 6.97$; $p < 0.001$). Physical activity level

Table 2 Mean score of the MMSE, EF tasks and QoL domains

Task	All elderly Mean (SD)	Female Mean (SD)	Male Mean (SD)	p
MMSE score	26.81 (± 1.88)	26.95 (± 1.88)	26.57 (± 1.87)	0.13
CWS task incorrect readings	8.62 (± 3.83)	8.13 (± 3.68)	9.49 (± 3.96)	0.008**
SS task incorrect presses	1.83 (± 1.24)	1.76 (± 1.27)	1.95 (± 1.19)	0.24
GNG task incorrect presses	1.11 (± 1.26)	0.98 (± 1.18)	1.32 (± 1.36)	0.053
VSWM task score	12.67 (± 5.44)	12.86 (± 5.52)	12.33 (± 5.33)	0.47
VWM task score	4.29 (± 1.77)	4.39 (± 1.79)	4.13 (± 1.73)	0.27
Physical health domain	62.82 (± 13.94)	63.34 (± 13.21)	61.92 (± 15.16)	0.45
Psychological health domain	59.60 (± 14.08)	59.52 (± 13.86)	59.74 (± 14.54)	0.90
Environment domain	63.48 (± 10.63)	63.80 (± 10.03)	62.90 (±11.65)	0.53
Social relationships domain	55.43 (± 21.84)	55.96 (± 20.51)	54.51 (±22.68)	0.61
Total QoL	59.46 (± 10.54)	59.82 (± 10.56)	58.83 (±10.53)	0.49

SD Standard deviation, Significance value $p < 0.01$; **

Table 3 Correlation between cognitive variables and domain scores of QoL

Task Domain	Physical health	Psychological health	Environment	Social relationships	Total QoL
	R	R	R	R	R
MMSE	0.27**	0.18**	0.29**	0.09	0.25**
VSWM task score	0.27**	0.17**	0.18**	0.15*	0.25**
VWM task score	0.21**	0.15*	0.22**	0.08	0.19**
CWS task errors	−0.26**	−0.14*	−0.18**	−0.02	−0.21**
SS task errors	−0.12	−0.13*	−0.19**	−0.04	−0.11
GNG task errors	−0.01	−0.13*	−0.12	−0.02	−0.07

Significance value $p < 0.05$; *, $p < 0.01$; **

was the statistically significant variable ($p < 0.05$). Introduction of cognitive and executive functions explained only an additional 7.8% of variance after controlling covariates ($F (7, 229) = 5.26$; $p < 0.001$) in the domain of environment of QoL. MMSE score was the statistically significant variable ($p = 0.005$). Introduction of cognitive and executive functions did not make a significant difference in variance in total QoL and in the domains of psychological health and social relationships of QoL.

Discussion

Our study included physically independent participants in RACFs with relatively normal cognitive function. Results revealed that participants scored highest in the domain of environment in QoL and least in the domain of social relationships in QoL. This may be due to elderly people in RACFs in Sri Lanka being mostly satisfied with the surroundings they were living in. It might have provided more opportunity to engage in spiritual and recreational activities away from family responsibilities.

Several studies have been done in different settings using various tools to assess the QoL of elderly people [33–36]. Sri Lanka has no previously published literature which assesses QoL of elderly people living in RACFs. A study conducted to assess QoL among community dwelling elderly people in Sri Lanka [35] has shown "home and neighbourhood" had the highest score which was similar to social relationships in our study that scored the least. These disparate results may be due to the difference in living arrangements, such as elderly people in care facilities being away from their usual relationships.

An Indian study found a difference in QoL domain scores between elderly people in community and institutions. Similar to our findings, they showed elderly people in institutions had scored the least in the domain of social relationships in QoL [36]. Furthermore, studies done with community elderly who had scored the highest in social relationships [37] and physical health [38], with least in psychological health [38] and physical health domains [37] in QoL, were mentioned. Although in our study, the environment domain scored the highest and social relationships domain scored the least in QoL, a study in Brazil

has insisted on contradictory results [17]. Studies done with community elderly in other countries show different levels of QoL experienced by community dwelling elderly as moderate QoL [33] and good QoL [34].

A Brazilian study done with community dwelling elderly has shown a correlation between physical health domain and performance in executive function tasks and MMSE score. Their explanation was that better physical health contributes to better performance of cognitive tasks, whereas, better physical health may contribute to autonomy and independent living which may improve cognitive functioning [19]. However, Schaie and Wills argue that it may be the better cognitive health that plays a protective role against physical loss [39]. Although the Brazilian study has shown a moderate positive correlation between MMSE score and physical health, our study has demonstrated a poor correlation. In our study, each of MMSE, VSWM, VWM scores and SS, GNG and CWS task errors were correlated with psychological health. Beckert et al., [19], reflected a correlation of attention with psychological health which was not assessed in our study. This may be because people with better memory and interference control feel better psychological health.

MMSE, VSWM, VWM scores and SS, CWS task errors correlate with environment domain. This may be because better cognitive abilities perceive the living environment as an enhanced one. Other studies support this finding reflecting a correlation between environment domain and performance of executive function tasks [19] and MMSE score [17, 19], the explanation being that living in an enriched environment helps to maintain higher levels of cognitive abilities [19]. Our study showed weak correlation between MMSE score and environment domain similar to the other studies [17, 19].

Social relationship domain correlated only with VSWM score. This could be explained as those who have better memory perceive better relationships despite arguments with others. Our study did not show a significant correlation between MMSE score and social relations. Perera et al., [17] and Beckert et al., [19] also have not shown a significant correlation between MMSE score and social

Table 4 Hierarchical multiple linear regression predicting total QoL and QoL domain scores

Variable	R	Adjusted R^2	R^2 change	Beta	t	p
Physical Health domain						
Block 1	0.345	0.108				
Physical activity				.263	3.909	< 0.0001***
Marital status				−.035	−.544	0.59
Educational status				.141	2.187	0.03*
Block 2	0.419	0.150	0.057**			
Physical activity				.174	2.503	0.01**
Marital status				.012	0.186	0.85
Educational status				.091	1.420	0.16
MMSE score				.121	1.781	0.08
VSWM task score				.104	1.453	0.15
VWM task score				.042	0.628	0.53
CWS task errors				−.122	−1.842	0.07
Psychological health domain						
Block 1	0.294	0.079				
Physical activity				.244	3.733	< 0.0001***
Educational status				.106	1.611	0.11
Block 2	0.325	0.074	0.019			
Physical activity				.190	2.661	0.008**
Educational status				.085	1.261	0.21
MMSE score				.055	0.773	0.44
VSWM task score				.044	0.606	0.54
VWM task score				.022	0.301	0.76
CWS task errors				−.019	−.279	0.78
SS task errors				−.054	−.805	0.42
GNG task errors				−.055	−.816	0.42
Social relationships domain						
Block 1	0.135	0.014				
Educational status				.135	2.089	0.04*
Block 2	0.180	0.024	0.014			
Educational status				.107	1.611	0.11
VSWM task score				.123	1.853	0.06
Environment domain						
Block 1	0.246	0.052				
Physical activity				.214	3.214	0.001***
Marital status				−.073	−1.106	0.27
Block 2	0.372	0.112	0.078**			
Physical activity				.109	1.567	0.12
Marital status				−.038	−.569	0.58
MMSE score				.197	2.843	0.005**
VSWM task score				.004	.056	0.96
VWM task score				.103	1.478	0.14
CWS task errors				−.026	−.389	0.70
SS task errors				−.110	−1.709	0.09

Table 4 Hierarchical multiple linear regression predicting total QoL and QoL domain scores *(Continued)*

Variable	R	Adjusted R^2	R^2 change	Beta	t	p
Total QoL						
Block 1	0.344	0.107		.272	4.030	< 0.0001***
Physical activity				−.052	−.805	0.42
Marital status				.115	1.787	0.07
Educational status						
Block 2	0.390	0.126	0.034			
Physical activity				.202	2.854	0.005**
Marital status				−.011	−.170	0.86
Educational status				.077	1.175	0.24
MMSE score				.107	1.551	0.12
VSWM task score				.095	1.312	0.19
VWM task score				.034	.495	0.62
CWS task errors				−.067	−1.002	0.32

Significance value *p < 0.05, **p < 0.01 , ***p < 0.001

relations. The total QoL was correlated with MMSE, VSWM, VWM scores and CWS task errors. This finding corroborates a previous study which found correlation with MMSE score and executive functions [19]. Thus, older people with higher cognition may perceive higher life satisfaction and QoL. Moreover, those who have better memory and inhibitory control may perceive higher life satisfaction and QoL due to less interference with others.

Davis et al., [20] has shown an independent association between WM and health related QoL but not with inhibition. They have suggested further research on contribution of response inhibition to health related QoL to understand it better. In our study, interference control was associated with total QoL and three domains of QoL, except social relationships domain. The ability to inhibit ongoing responses with psychological and environment domain and ability to inhibit prepotent responses with psychological health reflect association with perceived QoL.

Although MMSE, WM scores and response inhibition task errors were correlated at statistically significant level with different domains of QoL, they were weak correlations. Hence we thought to control for covariates and to look for the existence of this relationship. For covariates, we selected educational status, marital status and physical activity as previous literature has shown a significant effect of these factors on QoL [22–24]. When controlled for the covariates, among cognitive and executive variables, only MMSE score became a predictor of environment domain of QoL. WM and IC were not predictors of QoL when controlled for covariates. The level of variance was low.

In the domain of physical health, the introduction of cognitive and executive functions only explained an additional 5.7% of variance after controlling for covariates

and in environment domain of QoL, it only explained an additional 7.8% of variance after controlling for covariates. This may be because there might be other factors which affect the QoL of the elderly people dwelling in RACFs which are more important than cognitive and executive functions. Exploring these factors will assist in initiation of measures to improve QoL of elderly people in RACFs. Although physical activity was considered as a covariate, it was a predictor of total QoL and domains of physical and psychological health of QoL, which demands further explanations. Physical activity can have a positive effect on physical function and mental health in elderly people. Confidence in physical function that arises from physical activity could have contributed for this [22].

Obtaining a sample of physically independent elderly people with normal cognitive functioning might be the reason for poor correlations and for cognitive and executive functions not being the predictors of QoL. This might be different if we include elderly people with cognitive impairment in the sample. Hence, we recommend future studies with both samples using appropriate instruments. With population ageing, as there is a demand for increase in long term care of elderly in various forms [40], we suggest future studies to be further focused on the QoL of these populations.

Our study has several limitations. We could not conclude a causal relationship between level of cognition and performance of executive functions with QoL due to cross sectional design. The other limitation is the small sample size, which might affect the strength of true associations. We feel that future studies with larger sample size are needed to confirm the findings.

Conclusion

Cognition and executive functions weakly and significantly correlated with different domains of QoL of elderly people dwelling in RACFs. Only the level of cognition measured by MMSE was a predictor of the domain of environment of QoL and executive functions were not predictors of total QoL and domains of QoL in elderly people with normal cognitive functions dwelling in RACFs.

Abbreviations

CWS: Colour Word Stroop; EFs: Executive Functions; GNG: Go/No-Go; IC: Inhibitory control; IPAQ: International Physical Activity Questionnaire; MMSE: Mini Mental State Examination; QoL: Quality of life; RACFs: Residential aged care facilities; SD: Standard Deviation; SPSS: Statistical Package for Social Sciences; SS: Stop Signal; VSWM: Visuo-spatial Working Memory; VWM: Verbal Working Memory; WHOQoL-Bref: World Health Organization Quality of Life Bref; WM: Working memory

Acknowledgements

I would like to acknowledge, Prof. Bilesha Perera, Department of Community Medicine, Faculty of Medicine, University of Ruhuna for providing me statistical support.

Funding

University of Sri Jayewardenepura research Grant (ASP/01/RE/SCI/2015/36).

Authors' contributions

MWKG involved in designing the study, collection of data, preparing the data base, statistical analysis of data, interpretation of data and writing the first draft of the manuscript. DCH involved in designing the study, obtaining funding, interpretation of data, critical analysis of results, manuscript writing, drafting the manuscript, final proof reading before submission and supervision of progress of the study. KDP involved in designing the study, interpretation of data, critical analysis of results, final proof reading before submission, manuscript writing, drafting the manuscript and supervision of progress of the study. All authors read and approved the final manuscript.

Competing interests

The authors declare that they have no competing interests.

Author details

[1]Department of Nursing, Faculty of Allied Health Sciences, University of Ruhuna, Galle, Sri Lanka. [2]Department of Physiology, Faculty of Medical Sciences, University of Sri Jayewardenepura, Gangodawila, Nugegoda, Sri Lanka. [3]Department of Medicine, Faculty of Medicine, University of Ruhuna, Galle, Sri Lanka.

References

1. Xavier F, Ferraz MPT, Bisol LW, Fernandes DD, Schwanke C, Moriguchi EH. Octogenarians of Veranópolis: the psychological, social and health conditions of a representative group over the age 80 living in the community. Revista da AMRIGS. 2000;44(1/2):25–9.
2. Siddhisena KAP. Socio-economic implications of ageing in Sri Lanka: an overview, working paper WP105. Oxford: Oxford Institute of ageing; 2004.
3. Perera ELSJ. Ageing Population of Sri Lanka; Emerging issues, needs and policy implications; Thematic Report based on Census of Population and Housing 2012, United Nations Population Fund, Sri Lanka; 2017. [Accessed 8 Aug 2018]. Available from: http://srilanka.unfpa.org.
4. World Bank. Addressing the needs of an aging population. Human Development Unit South Asia Region; 2008.
5. World Health Organization. Active ageing: a policy framework. Geneva: WHO; 2002 [Accessed 19 Sept 2017]. Available from: http://www.who.int/ageing/publications/active_ageing/en/
6. Neisser U, Cognitive Psychology. New York: Appleton-century-crofts; 1967. Cited by Posner MI, Bourke P, cognitive psychology. Am J Psychol. 1993; 105(4):621–6.
7. Williams K, Kemper S. Exploring Interventions to reduce cognitive decline in aging. J Psychosoc Nurs Ment Health Serv. 2010;48(5):42–51.
8. Daffner KR. Promoting Successful Cognitive Aging: A Comprehensive Review. J Alzheimers Dis. 2010;19(4):1101–22.
9. Lezak MD. Neuropsychological assessment. New York: Oxford University press; 1995.
10. Stuss DT, Levine B. Adult clinical neuropsychology: lessons from studies of the frontal lobes. Annu Rev Psychol. 2002;53:401–33.
11. Brown LA. Processing speed and visuospatial executive function predict visual working memory ability in older adults. Exp Aging Res. 2012;38:1–19.
12. Miyake A, Shah P. Models of working memory: mechanisms of active maintenance and executive control. Cambridge: Cambridge University Press; 1999.
13. Tun PA, O'Kane G, Wingfield A. Distraction by competing speech in young and older adult listeners. Psychol Aging. 2002;17(3):453–67.
14. Barkley RA. Behavioral inhibition, sustained attention, and executive functions: constructing a unifying theory of ADHD. Psychol Bull. 1997;121(1):65–94.
15. Grisgby J, Kaye K, Baxter J, Shetterly SM, Hamman RF. Executive abilities and functional status among community-dwelling older persons in the San Luis Valley health and aging study. J Am Geriatr Soc. 1998;46(5):590–6.
16. Allan JL, McMinn D, Daly M. A bidirectional relationship between executive function and health behavior: evidence, implications, and future directions. Front Neurosci. 2016;10:386.
17. Pereira RN, Pontes MDLF, Silva AO, Monteiro ED, Da Silva CR, Silva LM, et al. Quality of life and the cognitive condition of elderly served in family health unit. Int Arch Med. 2015;8(225):1–9.
18. Jeste DV, Depp CA, Vahia IV. Successful cognitive and emotional aging. World Psychiatry. 2010;9(2):78–84.
19. Beckert M, Irigaray TQ, Trentini CM. Quality of life, cognition and performance of executive functions in the elderly. Studies Psychol (Campinas). 2012;29(2):155–62.
20. Davis JC, Marra CA, Najafzadeh M, Liu-Ambrose T. The independent contribution of executive functions to health related quality of life in older women. BMC Geriatr. 2010;10(16):1–8.
21. Pan C, Wang X, Ma Q, Sun H, Xu Y, Wang P. Cognitive dysfunction and health related quality of life among older Chinese. Sci Rep. 2015. https://doi.org/10.1038/srep17301.
22. Rejeski WJ, Mihalko SL. Physical activity and quality of life in older adults. J Gerontol Series. 2001;56A(Special Issue II):23–35.
23. Colet CDF, Mayorga P, Amador TA. Educational level, socio-economic status and relationship with quality of life in elderly residents of the city of Porto Alegre/RS, Brazil. Braz J Pharm Sci. 2010;46(4):805810.
24. Han K, Park E, Kim J, Kim SJ, Park S. Is marital status associated with quality of life? Health Qual Life Outcomes. 2014;12:109.
25. Teng E, Tassniyom K, Lu PH. Reduced quality of life ratings in mild cognitive impairment: analyses of subject and informant responses. Am J Geriatr Psychiatry. 2012;20(12):1016–25.
26. International Physical Activity Questionnaire. International Physical Activity Questionnaire – cultural adaptation; 2009. [Accessed 20 June 2018]. Available from: https://sites.google.com/site/theipaq/scoring-protocol.

Effect of cognitive and executive functions on perception of quality of life of cognitively normal elderly...

125

27. Stroop JR. Studies of interference in serial verbal reactions. J Exp Psychol. 1935;18:643–61.

28. Macleod CM. Half a century of research on the Stroop effect: an integrative review. Psychol Bull. 1991;109:163–203.

29. Tillman CM, Thorell LB, Brocki KC, Bohlin G. Motor response inhibition and execution in the stop-signal task: development and relation to ADHD behaviors. Child Neuropsychol. 2007;14(1):42–59.

30. Towse JN, Hitch GJ, Hutton UA. Re-evaluation of working memory capacity in children. J Mem Lang. 1998;39:195–217.

31. Berlin L, Bohlin G. Response inhibition, hyperactivity, and conduct problems among preschool children. J Clin Child Adolesc Psychol. 2002;31:242–51.

32. Cohen J. Statistical power analysis for behavioural sciences. Hillsdale: Lawrence Erlbaum; 1998.

33. Campos ACV, Ferreira EF, Vargas AMD, Albala C. Aging, gender and quality of life (AGEQOL) study: factors associated with good quality of life in older Brazilian community dwelling adults. Health Qual Life Outcomes. 2014; 12(166):1–11.

34. Baernholdt M, Hinton I, Yan G, Rose K, Mattos M. Factors associated with quality of life in older adults in the United States. Qual Life Res. 2012;21(3): 527–34.

35. Rathnayake S, Siop S. Quality of life and its determinants among older people living in rural community in Sri Lanka. Indian J Gerontol. 2015;29(2): 131–53.

36. Kumar P, Udyar SE, Arun D, Sai S. Quality of life of elderly people in institutional and non-institutional setting: a cross sectional comparative study. Nat J Commun Med. 2016;7(7):546–50.

37. Sowmiya KR, Nagarani A. Study on quality of life of elderly population in Mettupalayam, a rural area of Tamilnadu. Nat J Res Com Med. 2012;1(3): 123–77.

38. Thadathil SE, Jose R, Varghese S. Assessment of domain wise quality of life among elderly population using WHOBREF scale and its determinants in a rural setting of Kerala. Intl J Curr Med App Sci. 2015;7(1):43–6.

39. Schaie KW, Willis SL. Psychometric intelligence and aging. In: Blanchard E, Fields & Hess TM, editors. Perspectives on cognitive change and aging in adulthood. New York: McGraw-Hill; 1996. p. 293–322.

40. Böckerman P, Johansson E, Saarni S. Institutionalisation and quality of life for elderly people in Finland, Enepri research report no. 92. In: European network of economic policy research institutes; 2011.

13

Sleep duration and sleep disturbances in association with falls among the middle-aged and older adults in China: a population-based nationwide study

Samuel Kwaku Essien[1], Cindy Xin Feng[1*] (ID), Wenjie Sun[2,3], Marwa Farag[1], Longhai Li[4] and Yongqing Gao[3]

Abstract

Background: Falls pose major health problems to the middle-aged and older adults and may potentially lead to various levels of injuries. Sleep duration and disturbances have been shown to be associated with falls in literature; however, studies of the joint and distinct effects of those sleep problems are still sparse. To fill this gap, we aimed to determine the association between sleep duration, sleep disturbances and falls among middle-aged and older adults in China controlling for psychosocial, lifestyle, socio-demographical factors and comorbidity.

Methods: Data were derived from the China Health and Retirement Longitudinal Study (CHARLS) based on multi-stage sampling designs, with respondents aged 50 and older. Associations were evaluated by using multiple logistic regression adjusting for confounders and complex survey design. To further determine if the association of sleep duration/disturbance and falls depends on age groups, the study data were divided into two samples (age 50–64 vs. age 65+) and comparison was made between the two age groups.

Results: Of the 12,759 respondents, 2172 (17%) had falls within the last 2 years. Our findings indicated that the participants who had nighttime sleep duration ≤5 were more likely to report falls than those who had nighttime sleep duration ≥6 h; whereas no association between nighttime sleep duration > 8 h and falls. Participants having sleep disturbances 1–2 days, or 3–4 days, and 5–7 days per week were also more likely to report falls than those who had no sleep disturbance. The nap sleep duration was not significantly associated with falls. Although the combined sample found both sleep duration and sleep disturbance to be strongly associated with falls after adjusting for various confounders, sleep disturbance was not significantly related to falls among participants aged 65 +.

Conclusions: Our study suggested that there is an independent association between falls and short sleep duration and disturbed sleep among middle-aged and older adults in China. Findings underscore the need for evidence-based prevention and interventions targeting sleep duration and disturbance among this study population.

Keywords: Falls, Sleep duration, Sleep disturbance, Middle-aged and older adults

* Correspondence: cindy.feng@usask.ca
[1]School of Public Health, University of Saskatchewan, Health Sciences Building E-Wing, 104 Clinic Place, Saskatoon, SK S7N 2Z4, Canada
Full list of author information is available at the end of the article

Background

Falls pose major health problems to the middle-aged and older adults and may potentially lead to various levels of injuries, disability [1], death [2], and hospitalizations [3]. Increased prevalence of falls in elderly populations per year has been reported globally, such as 31% in the United States [4], 20–30% in Canada [5], 25.6% in Australia [6] and 27.6% in Brazil [7]. In China, the aging population has increased rapidly over the past two decades [8], contributing to China having the "largest aging population in the world" [9]. Out of over 160 million Chinese aged 60 and above globally, 99% currently reside in China [10]. The annual prevalence of falls among the Chinese elderly has been reported to range from 6 to 31% according to WHO global report on fall [11]. Increased fall rate among middle-aged and older adults comes with high economic repercussions in terms of direct and indirect cost. It was reported that the economic cost associated with fall-related health problems is about 8.7 billion CAD dollars in Canada [12], 19.2 billion US dollars in the United States [13] and 500 million dollars in Australia [14]. In China, an estimated yearly cost of falls in elderly Chinese is projected to be between 1.6–1.8 billion Chinese Yuan Renminbi, which is 1.5 times higher than the projected cost for the adolescent-adult [14].

Despite the evidence, both intrinsic (e.g., depression, impaired vision, gender) and extrinsic (e.g., medication especially polypharmacy, poor lighting, footwear) factors are associated with falls [15], limited research has been conducted focusing on the Chinese middle-aged and older adults. The elderly Chinese represent the population at greatest risk of falls in China [14], who are more vulnerable to the risk factors attributable to falls, such as poor sleep [16, 17], feeling lonely because of "their greater rates of widowhood" [18] and other lifestyles including alcohol consumption and smoking [19]. It has been reported that large proportion of Chinses older persons are prone to sleep inadequacies and poor sleep quality [20, 21]. For instance, Liu et found that almost 53% of Chinese older persons experience "more than one day per week" poor quality sleep [20]. This highlights the vulnerability to poor sleep quality experienced by this group. As such, identifying and understanding the risk factors associated with falls in the Chinese middle-aged and older adults is imperative for designing effective prevention and intervention strategies for falls.

One primary risk factor that has been shown to be associated with falls is sleep duration; however, the evidence in literature is mixed with some agreeing an association between shorter sleep duration ($\leq$ 5 h) and falls [22–25] exists and others suggesting an association between longer sleep duration (> 8 h) and falls [23, 25, 26]. Ascertaining the importance of good sleep (e.g. sleep duration/quantity) especially in larger samples with varied age range and gender, has been encouraged in sleep-related research [27]. Sleep quality might also be characterized as sleep disturbance, which has been shown to be associated with the risk of falling [28, 29]. Sleep disturbance may be attributable to environment factors such as exposure to noise [30, 31]. Other non-environmental factors such as myocardial infarction [32, 33] and obstructive sleep apnea [34] have also been reported to be associated with sleep disturbance/poor sleep. However, these factors were beyond the scope of the data source used for the current study analyses. Investigating sleep duration effect independently in middle-aged and older adults may be ideal, but since the association between sleep duration and sleep disturbance is unclear [35], accounting for both simultaneously is necessary as they may have some distinct features impacting on the risk of falls.

Better understanding of the relationship between sleep duration and disturbance with falls will shed light on designing the evidence-based prevention and interventions targeting this vulnerable population. Therefore, the objective of this study is to investigate association of sleep duration and disturbance with falls using a national-wide representative data focusing on the middle-aged and older adults in China, while adjusting for various psychosocial, lifestyle, socio-demographical factors and comorbidity.

Methods

The national baseline data from the China Health and Retirement Longitudinal Study (CHARLS) was used to investigate the association between sleep duration, sleep disturbances and falls in Chinese middle-aged and older adults adjusting for psychosocial, lifestyle, socio-demographic factors and comorbidity. The CHARLS baseline data collection took place in June 2011 and March 2012 on 17,708 respondents in 10,257 households [36, 37] and the target population was middle-aged and older adults and their spouse aged 45 years and above and currently residing in a household in China [9, 36]. The CHARLS national survey commenced after the Health and Retirement Study have been introduced and conducted in the United States [9, 37]. The survey was pilot tested on a sample of middle-aged and older adults and their spouse from 95 communities in 32 counties [9] to test for face validity. A complex survey structure consisting of a four-stage, stratified, cluster probability sampling design was used to collect the CHARLS data [9, 38]. The data contains information on the socio-demographics, family, health status, health care, employment, and the household economy. Health-related questions included self-reported health status, previous medical history, lifestyle, health behaviors, and activities of daily living. However, for the purpose of the present study, all analyses focused on 13,727 of participants aged 50 and over. Ethical approval for collecting data on human subjects was received at Peking University by their institutional review board (IRB). The CHARLS data are publicly available from the China Health and Retirement Longitudinal Study website: http://charls.pku.edu.cn/en.

Fall
The primary outcome of interest in this study is fall. Participants were asked to respond "yes" or "no" to the question "Have you fallen down in the last two years?"

Sleep duration and sleep disturbance
Sleep duration was assessed with the question "During the past month, how many hours of actual sleep did you get at night?" which was recorded as an integer. The sleep duration question was adapted from the Pittsburgh Sleep Quality Index (PSQI) [20, 39, 40]. The reliability and validity of the questions in the Pittsburgh Sleep Quality Index (PSQI) has been reported elsewhere [39, 41]. Following the literature [22–25], sleep duration was categorized in "≤5 h", "6–7 h", "8 h", "9–10 h" and "≥11" at night in the past month. Sleep disturbance from combined sources of having trouble falling asleep [26], frequently nighttime awakenings and earlier waking [42] was measured in days per week on a scale of four: "none (<1 day)", "little (1-2 days)", "occasionally (3-4 days)" and "most (5-7 days)". Besides sleep duration at night and sleep disturbance, participants were also asked to report time in minutes to the question "During the past month, how long did you take a nap after lunch?"

Psychosocial, lifestyle, sociodemographic factors and comorbidity
Psychological wellbeing was assessed with the self-report question "how you have felt during the last week" for depression and anxiety (fear) with the following options: "none (<1 day per week)", "little (1-2 days per week)", "occasionally (3-4 days per week)" and "most (5-7 days per week)". Marital status was reported as married with spouse present, married not living with spouse, separated divorced and widowed and never married. Participants were classified into individuals who had never exposed to alcohol and participants who had exposed to alcohol at some time in their lives. Frequent smoking was rated as never smoker, past smoker and current smoker. Age of participants were categorized into three levels: "50–64 years", "65–74", and "75 years and over". Body mass index (BMI) was computed as current weight in kilograms according to self-reporting in postal survey divided by the square of height in meters. In addition, fall related comorbidities available in the data including diabetes, stroke [43], visual impairment/problem [44], mental impairment [45] and arthritis [46] were considered. Diabetes, hypertension, stroke and arthritis were accessed as "yes/no" based on the question "Have you been diagnosed with conditions listed below by a doctor?" Visual and

mental impairments were also accessed on the question "Do you have one of the following disabilities?" and participants answered "yes/no" to the question.

To further determine if the association of sleep duration/disturbance and falls depends on age groups, the study data were divided into two samples (age 50–64 vs. age 65+) and comparison was made between the two age groups.

Data analysis
The variables were screened by examining the unconditional association between each risk factor and the outcome using logistic regression. Variables where the p-value < 0.25 based on the type 3 Wald test were retained for consideration in building the final model [47]. The Akaike information criterion (AIC) [48] was then used to decide whether to include a variable as continuous or categorical. Manual backward selection was used to develop a main effects model, retaining only variables where p-value < 0.05. A variable was considered a confounder "if the adjusted estimate is different from the crude estimate" by at least 20% [49]. All possible interactions were tested among all predictors that are significant in the final main effects model. All the analyses were performed using *proc surveylogistic* in SAS 9.4 to properly account for the complex survey sampling structures, including designs, stratification, clustering, and unequal weighting [50]. The associations between covariates and falls in the final model were reported as adjusted odds ratios (AOR) with 95% confidence intervals (95% CI) and p-values.

Results
Of the 12,759 middle-aged and older adults who responded questions on falls, 2172 (17%) had falls within the last 2 years.

The characteristics of the current study sample (see Table 1) revealed almost 32% of the participants had sleep duration no more than 5 h per day, less than half of the participants, about 40% had sleep duration between 6 and 7 h per day and almost 21% had sleep duration 8 h per day. Among those who had sleep duration no more than 5 h, about 22% had falls, whereas only 13% participants had falls for those who had sleep duration of 8 h. For sleep disturbance, almost 20% of the participants had sleep disturbance 5–7 days per week, 15.4% had 3–4 days per week, 16.7% had 1–2 days per week and 47.6% reported less than 1-day sleep disturbance. Among those who had sleep disturbance 5–7 days per week, almost 23% had falls as compared to 13.5% for those who reported less than 1-day sleep disturbance.

A large portion of the participants aged between 50 and 64 years (65.4%). Of the 6533(51.2%) females, 19.4% had falls, which is higher than 14.6% for males. The alcohol use, 8666(68.0%) was more common compared to

Table 1 Descriptive statistics and *p*-values computed from the bivariate analysis

Variables	Total (%)	Fall		*p*-value
		Yes (%)	No (%)	
Sleep duration^a (in hours) (n = 12,629)				
≤ 5	3971 (31.4)	878 (22.1)	3093 (77.9)	< 0.0001
6–7	5008 (39.7)	773 (15.4)	4235 (84.6)	
8 (ref)	2602 (20.6)	338 (13.0)	2264 (87.0)	
9–10	943 (7.5)	138 (14.6)	805 (85.4)	
≥ 11	105 (0.8)	22 (20.9)	83 (79.1)	
Sleep disturbance^b (n = 12,562)				
None (> 1 day) (ref)	5983 (47.6)	810 (13.5)	5173 (86.5)	< 0.0001
Little (1–2 days)	2098 (16.7)	354 (16.9)	1744 (83.1)	
Occasionally (3–4 days)	1932 (15.4)	377 (19.5)	1555 (80.5)	
Most (5–7 days)	2549 (20.3)	595 (23.3)	1954 (76.7)	
Age in years (n = 12,739)				
50–64 (ref)	8331 (65.4)	1271 (15.3)	7060 (84.7)	< 0.0001
65–74	3045 (23.9)	598 (19.6)	2447 (80.4)	
75+	1363 (10.7)	299 (21.9)	1064 (78.1)	
Gender (n = 12,751)				
Female (ref)	6533 (51.2)	1265 (19.4)	5268 (80.6)	< 0.0001
Male	6218 (48.8)	907 (14.6)	5311 (85.4)	
Smoking (n = 12,745)				
Never (ref)	7554 (59.3)	1343 (17.8)	6211 (82.2)	0.0049
Past	1241 (9.7)	218 (17.6)	1023 (82.4)	
Current	3950 (31.0)	610 (15.4)	3340 (84.6)	
Drinking Behaviour (n = 12,747)				
No intake of alcohol	4081 (32.0)	722 (17.7)	3359 (82.3)	0.2380
Exposed to alcohol intake	8666 (68.0)	1449 (16.7)	7217 (83.3)	
Depression^b (n = 12,450)				
None (< 1 day) (ref)	5630 (45.2)	745 (13.2)	4885 (86.8)	< 0.0001
Little (1–2 days)	2830 (22.7)	449 (15.9)	2381 (84.1)	
Occasionally (3–4 days)	2361 (19.0)	483 (20.5)	1878 (79.5)	
Most (5–7 days)	1629 (13.1)	432 (26.5)	1197 (73.5)	
Anxiety ^b (n = 12,544)				
None (> 1 day) (ref)	9905 (78.9)	1569 (15.8)	8336 (84.2)	< 0.0001
Little (1–2 days)	1299 (10.4)	238 (18.3)	1061 (81.7)	
Occasionally (3–4 days)	786 (6.3)	172 (21.9)	614 (78.1)	
Most (5–7 days)	554 (4.4)	151 (27.3)	403 (72.7)	
Loneliness ^b (n = 12,497)				
None (> 1 day) (ref)	8650 (69.2)	1311 (15.2)	7339 (84.8)	< 0.0001
Little (1–2 days)	1598 (12.8)	287 (18.0)	1311 (82.0)	
Occasionally (3–4 days)	1189 (9.5)	258 (21.7)	931 (78.3)	
Most (5–7 days)	1060 (8.5)	264 (24.9)	796 (75.1)	
Marital Status (n = 12,758)				
Never (ref)	116 (0.9)	21 (18.1)	95 (81.9)	0.0101
Married with spouse present	10,367 (81.2)	1731 (16.7)	8636 (83.3)	

Table 1 Descriptive statistics and *p*-values computed from the bivariate analysis *(Continued)*

Variables	Total (%)	Fall		*p*-value
		Yes (%)	No (%)	
Married not living with spouse	478 (3.8)	70 (14.6)	408 (85.4)	
Separated/Divorced/Widowed	65 (0.5)	8 (12.3)	57 (87.7)	
Divorced	102 (0.8)	14 (13.7)	88 (86.3)	
Widowed	1630 (12.8)	328 (20.1)	1302 (79.9)	
Hypertension (n = 12,701)				
No	9228 (72.7)	1482 (16.1)	7746 (60.9)	< 0.0001
Yes	3473 (27.3)	674 (19.4)	2799 (80.6)	
Arthritis (n = 12,731)				
No	8220 (64.6)	1172 (14.3)	7048 (85.7)	< 0.0001
Yes	4511 (35.4)	994 (22.0)	3517 (78.0)	
Stroke (n = 12,725)				
No	12,397 (97.4)	2077 (16.8)	10,320 (83.2)	< 0.0001
Yes	328 (2.6)	90 (27.4)	238 (72.6)	
Diabetes (n = 12,641)				
No	11,826 (93.5)	1960 (16.6)	9866 (83.4)	0.0011
Yes	815 (6.5)	193 (23.7)	622 (76.3)	
Mental Impairment (n = 12,746)				
No	12,421 (97.4)	2063 (16.6)	10,358 (83.4)	< 0.0001
Yes	325 (2.6)	106 (32.6)	219 (67.4)	
Vision Impairment (n = 12,755)				
No	11,835 (92.8)	1927 (16.3)	9908 (83.7)	< 0.0001
Yes	920 (7.2)	244 (26.5)	676 (73.5)	
		MEAN (SE)		
BMI	12,759	23.3 (0.10)	23.3 (0.04)	0.6233
Nap sleep duration/mins	12,759	31.1(0.90)	32.8 (0.42)	0.7519

[a] in hours at night in the past month
[b] in days per week
SE standard error, *ref* reference category

their exposure to smoking 5191 (40.7%) among this study population. Among the psychosocial factors, more than half of the participants reported depression, about 21% reported anxiety and almost 30% reported loneliness. Almost one quarter of the participants who were either depressed, anxious or lonely most of the time (5–7 days) per week reported falls. The comorbidities considered in the present study revealed that almost 27% reported being diagnosed of hypertension, 35% diagnosed of arthritis, 2.6% diagnosed of stroke and 6.5% diagnosed of diabetes. Those who reported having mental and vision impairments constituted 2.6% and 7.2%, respectively.

The results of the bivariate analysis are presented in Table 1. Findings revealed the risk of falls is significantly higher for those who had short sleep duration ≤5 h than those who had long sleep duration ≥6. In addition, middle-aged and older adults who had their sleep disturbed more often were more likely to report falls.

However, duration of nap after lunch did not show significant association with falls. Females were more likely to experience fall than males. The linearity assumption for the continuous covariates (age and BMI) were assessed by comparing the AICs for model with those covariates modeled as continuous variables versus categorical variables. The model with a smaller AIC indicates a better fit to the data. Our results indicated the AIC for the model with age as a categorical variable is smaller than the AIC for the model with age as continuous variable. However, the AIC for the model with BMI as a continuous variable had a smaller AIC when compared with the AIC of BMI modeled as categorical variable, so we proceed the analysis modeling age as categorical variable and BMI as continuous variable for the purpose of parsimony. As age increases, the risk of falls increases; whereas BMI is not significantly associated with falls. Exposure to alcohol did not show significant difference from those not exposed to these factors in relation to falls in the bivariate analysis. In contrast, there was a significant difference between those exposed to smoking and those not exposed in relation to falls. Psychosocial factors including depression, anxiety and number of days of loneliness were significantly associated with falls. The marital status of participants did show significant difference in falls in the bivariate analysis. All comorbidities were found to be significantly associated with falls in our study population.

In the final multivariable model (see Table 2), after adjusting for various psychosocial, lifestyle, socio-demographic characteristics and comorbidities, those participants who had sleep duration of ≤5 were more likely to report falls than those who slept 8 h (≤ 5 h: AOR = 1.34, 95% Cl 1.10–1.62). Those who had their sleep disturbed even as few as a day or two per week were more likely to report falls (AOR = 1.39, 95% Cl 1.09–1.77) and the odds of falls were also higher for those who had sleep mostly or occasionally disturbed (5–7 days per week: AOR = 1.40, 95% CI: 1.16–1.70; 3–4 days per week: AOR = 1.24: 1.02–1.50) than those who had no disturbed sleep. A dose response relationship was found between age and risk of falls. Thus, as age increases, the risk of falls also increases (age 65–74: AOR = 1.49, 95% CI 1.26–1.75; age 75+ years: AOR = 1.67, 95% CI 1.37–2.03). Males were less likely to report falls as compare to females (AOR = 0.71, 95% CI 0.61–0.82). Those who were exposed to alcohol were more likely to report fall than those with no exposure to alcohol (AOR = 1.53, 95% Cl 1.29–1.81). Participants who reported mostly depressed (5–7 days per week) and occasionally depressed (3–4 days per week) had a significantly higher risk of falls than those who had less than one-day depression (mostly depressed: AOR = 1.82, 95% CI 1.52–2.18; occasionally depressed: AOR = 1.41, 95% Cl 1.20–1.67). The participants who were diagnosed with hypertension (AOR = 1.23, 95% CI 1.09–1.50), arthritis (AOR = 1.57, 95% CI 1.36–1.82), and stroke (AOR = 1.64, 95% CI 1.12–2.41) had higher odds of reporting falls. Similarly, participants had elevated risk of falls if they had mental impairment (AOR = 1.95, 95% CI 1.44–2.65) and vision impairment (AOR = 1.48, 95% CI 1.21–1.82).

Tables 3 and 4 summarize the multivariate results of the association between sleep duration and sleep disturbance with falls by age groups (50–64 vs. 65+). After adjustment for psychosocial, lifestyle, socio-demographic characteristics and comorbidities, short sleep (duration of ≤5 h) among both aged 50–64 (AOR = 1.62; 95%CI 1.27–2.07) and aged 65+ (AOR = 1.42; 95%CI 1.09–1.86), were more likely to report falls than those who slept 8 h. In addition, we observed that participants aged 50–64 who had their sleep disturbed for 3–4 days (AOR = 1.30; 95%CI 1.01–1.67) and 5–7 days (AOR = 1.35; 95%CI 1.08–1.68) were more likely to fall. In contrast, sleep disturbance was not associated with falls among participants aged 65+. Figure 1

presents the odds ratio plots for falls in association with sleep duration and sleep disturbance based on the overall multivariate analysis and the stratified multivariate analyses by age groups (50–64 vs. 65+) for visual comparison.

Depression, arthritis, mental impairment and vision impairment were found to be consistently associated with falls, regardless of participants aged 50–64 or 65+, whereas other factors showed varied results depending on age groups. For instance, male gender (AOR = 0.70; 95%CI 0.57–0.87), stroke (AOR = 2.30; 95%CI 1.50–3.52) and past exposure to smoke (AOR = 1.47; 95%CI 1.09–1.98) were significantly associated with falls among participants aged 50–64; among participants aged 65+, hypertension showed a significant association with falls (AOR = 1.30; 95%CI 1.03–1.63).

Discussion

Falls are increasingly recognised as a leading cause of disability and mortality worldwide. There has been limited research focusing on both sleep duration and disturbance as the primary risk factors for falls [51]. To the best our knowledge, few studies have been conducted examining the Chinese middle-aged and older adults. The primary finding in our study revealed that both sleep duration and sleep disturbance are strongly associated with falls after adjusting for various confounders. Further, our stratified analysis revealed that the effects of sleep duration and sleep disturbance on falls depend on age groups.

For sleep duration, our study found that sleep duration ≤5 h is significantly associated with increased risk of falls compared with sleep duration 6–7 h, which is consistent with literature [23, 24]. However, in the current study, long duration of sleep (> 8 h) was found to be not significantly related to falls. The latter finding has consistently been observed in previous studies [22, 24], whereas the other studies found long sleep duration (> 8 h) to be associated with increased risk of falls in older adults [25, 52]. In an attempt to verify the validity and reliability of the sleep duration variable in the present study data (CHARLS) in comparison with some other national data, such as Chinese Longitudinal Healthy Longevity Survey (CLHLS) [53], we made a comparison of the frequency distributions of the sleep duration variable between the CHARLS and CLHLS. In CHARLS, sleep duration variables considered nighttime sleep duration and nap sleep after lunch as separate variables; whereas CLHLS measured everyday sleep duration including napping [53]. Hence, sleep duration reported in CLHLS tends to be longer than those reported in CHARLS; as a result, less percentage of participants is expected to belong to the lower duration categories, but higher percentage of participants belonging to the higher duration categories in CLHLS as compared to CHALRS.

CLHLS focused on older adults of age ≥ 65, so to make the sleep duration variables between the CHARLS and

Table 2 Multivariable analysis assessing the associations of sleep duration and sleep disturbance with falls ($n = 10{,}368$)

Variables	Adjusted Odds Ratios (AOR)	95% CI	p-value
Sleep duration[a] (in hours)			
≤ 5	1.34	(1.10–1.62)	0.0037
6–7	1.17	(0.98–1.40)	0.0924
8 (ref)			
9–10	1.38	(0.86–2.22)	0.1806
≥ 11	1.43	(0.74–2.74)	0.2867
Sleep disturbance[b]			
None (<1 day) (ref)			
Little (1–2 days)	1.39	(1.09–1.77)	0.0091
Occasionally (3–4 days)	1.24	(1.02–1.50)	0.0293
Most (5–7 days)	1.40	(1.16–1.70)	0.0006
Age in years			
50–64 (ref)			
65–74	1.49	(1.26–1.75)	< 0.0001
75+	1.67	(1.37–2.03)	< 0.0001
Gender			
Female (ref)			
Male	0.71	(0.61–0.82)	< 0.0001
Drinking Behaviour			
No intake of alcohol (ref)			
Exposed to alcohol intake	1.53	(1.29–1.81)	< 0.0001
Depression[b]			
None (< 1 day) (ref)			
Little (1–2 days)	1.14	(0.94–1.39)	0.1787
Occasionally (3–4 days)	1.41	(1.20–1.67)	< 0.0001
Most (5–7 days)	1.82	(1.52–2.18)	< 0.0001
Hypertension			
No (ref)			
Yes	1.23	(1.09–1.50)	0.0028
Arthritis			
No (ref)			
Yes	1.57	(1.36–1.82)	< 0.0001
Stroke			
No (ref)			
Yes	1.64	(1.12–2.41)	0.0115
Mental Impairment			
No (ref)			
Yes	1.95	(1.44–2.65)	< 0.0001
Vision Impairment			
No (ref)			
Yes	1.48	(1.21–1.82)	0.0002

[a] in hours at night in the past month
[b] in days per week

Table 3 Multivariable analysis assessing the associations of sleep duration and sleep disturbance with falls (*n* = 8067) based on sample within the aged 50–64

Variables	Adjusted Odds Ratios (AOR)	95% CI	*p*-value
Sleep duration[a] (in hours)			
≤ 5	1.62	(1.27–2.07)	0.0001
6–7	1.40	(1.12–1.75)	0.0030
8 (ref)			
9–10	1.20	(0.79–1.80)	0.3947
≥ 11	2.08	(0.98–4.43)	0.0576
Sleep disturbance[b]			
None (<1 day) (ref)			
Little (1–2 days)	1.21	(0.98–1.50)	0.0827
Occasionally (3–4 days)	1.30	(1.01–1.67)	0.0436
Most (5–7 days)	1.35	(1.08–1.68)	0.0075
Gender			
Female (ref)			
Male	0.70	(0.57–0.87)	0.0009
Depression[b]			
None (< 1 day) (ref)			
Little (1–2 days)	1.16	(0.96–1.42)	0.1340
Occasionally (3–4 days)	1.46	(1.18–1.81)	0.0006
Most (5–7 days)	2.13	(1.71–2.65)	< 0.0001
Arthritis			
No (ref)			
Yes	1.40	(1.21–1.63)	< 0.0001
Stroke			
No (ref)			
Yes	2.30	(1.50–3.52)	0.0001
Mental Impairment			
No (ref)			
Yes	1.74	(1.20–2.53)	0.0035
Vision Impairment			
No (ref)			
Yes	1.43	(1.09–1.89)	0.0115
Smoking			
Never			
Current	1.15	(0.92–1.43)	0.2183
Past	1.47	(1.09–1.98)	0.0122
Marital Status			
Never (ref)			
Married with spouse present	0.78	(0.38–1.59)	0.4863
Married not living with spouse	0.50	(0.22–1.10)	0.0861
Separated	0.22	(0.04–1.14)	0.0705
Divorced	0.23	(0.07–0.75)	0.0151
Widowed	0.65	(0.30–1.40)	0.2695

[a] in hours at night in the past month
[b] in days per week

Table 4 Multivariable analysis assessing the associations of sleep duration and sleep disturbance with falls ($n = 4180$) based sample with the aged 65 +

Variables	Adjusted Odds Ratios (AOR)	95% CI	p-value
Sleep duration[a] (in hours)			
≤ 5	1.42	(1.09–1.86)	0.0107
6–7	1.10	(0.84–1.44)	0.4950
8 (ref)			
9–10	1.80	(0.92–3.49)	0.0853
≥ 11	1.09	(0.47–2.51)	0.8479
Depression[b]			
None (< 1 day) (ref)			
Little (1–2 days)	1.22	(0.87–1.71)	0.2611
Occasionally (3–4 days)	1.50	(1.17–1.92)	0.0012
Most (5–7 days	1.51	(1.14–1.99)	0.0038
Arthritis			
No (ref)			
Yes	1.85	(1.46–2.34)	< 0.0001
Mental Impairment			
No (ref)			
Yes	2.79	(1.70–4.57)	< 0.0001
Vision Impairment			
No (ref)			
Yes	1.48	(1.11–1.97)	0.0071
Hypertension			
No (ref)			
Yes	1.30	(1.03–1.63)	0.0279

[a] in hours at night in the past month
[b] in days per week

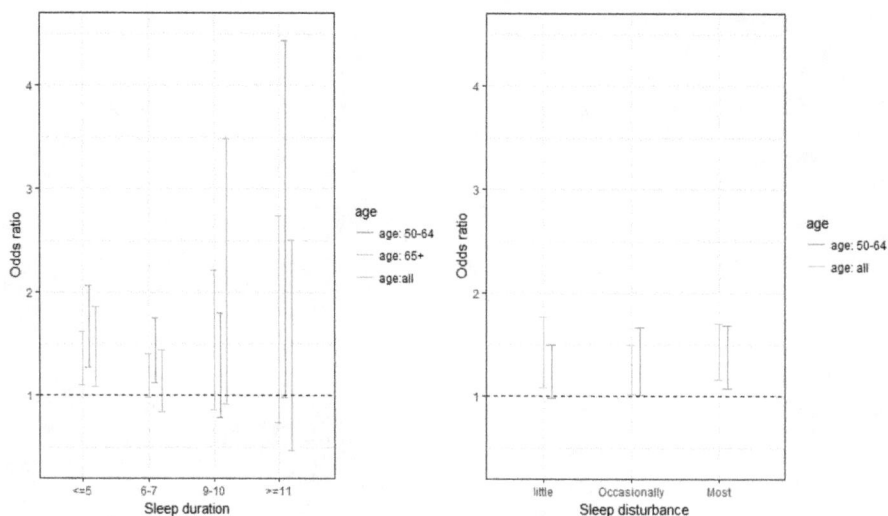

Fig. 1 Odds ratio plots for falls in association with sleep duration and sleep disturbance based on the overall multivariate analysis and the stratified multivariate analyses by age group (age: 50–64 vs. age: 65+)

CLHLS comparable, we considered participants aged ≥65 in CHARLS data and derived total sleep duration variable by combining nighttime sleep and nap sleep. The frequency distributions of sleep duration (Table 5) revealed CHARLS reported more participants (24.6%) who had sleep ≤5 as compared with CLHLS (13.1%), whereas CLHLS reported more participants (24.7%) had sleep duration ≥9 [53] compared with CHARLS (18.2%). The frequency of the rest of the categories were roughly comparable. The differences in the frequency distributions of the sleep duration variable between CHARLS and CLHLS may be due to the differences in the sampling provinces. CHARLS sampled 28 provinces and CLHLS sampled 22 provinces from China. A recent published meta-analysis on Chinese older adults revealed that five studied which reported sleep duration of less than 5 h (< 5 h) had a proportion of 18.8% whereas 15 studies that reported sleep duration less than 6 (< 6 h) had a proportion of 26.7% [21]. The differences observed could be partially attributed to the fact that the CHARLS included those who reported sleep duration of 5 h, which led to the higher proportion compared to studies that reported < 5 h and lower proportion compared to the studies that reported < 6 h. The studies that reported < 6 h might have included those who reported sleep duration more than 5 h but less than 6 h. Other differences could be due to the sample sized used, sampling methods used and where the studies were conducted (urban/rural/mixed). The sleep duration distribution in the CHARLS data therefore may not be the entirely representative of the sleep duration among middle-aged and older adults in China, so further studies are warranted in any attempts to generalize these results to other populations. Nevertheless, these findings contribute to the ongoing knowledge on how the sleep duration is associated with falls among middle-aged and older adults in China.

Despite the potential population difference, sleep disturbances and other sleep-related comorbidities have been proposed as a plausible reason that may cause study findings to differ [25]. In the combined sample of the present study,

sleep disturbance appeared to influence fall incidence, however, after splitting the study data into two samples, this association did not persist among participants aged 65+. The lack of association between sleep disturbance and falls among those aged 65+ could be partly due to sample size limitation, as larger samples would be needed to discover quite small differences [54]. The present study does not rule out the possibility of the association between sleep duration, sleep disturbance and fall being a bidirectional. A recent review on prospective studies ascertaining broadly risk factors for sleep disturbance did not identify fall as a potential risk factor for sleep disturbance [55]. However, sleep disturbance was rather found to be a risk factor of fall in other reviews investigating fall-related risk factors [56, 57]. The later finding suggests that sleep problems are more likely to precede incidence of fall. Napping behaviours may also contribute independently or influence risk of falls [50]. Existing literature therefore urged future studies to consider nap sleeping as part of sleep behaviours [58]. While existing literature found napping to be related to falls in elderly [50], this study found no significant association between napping after lunch and falls.

Our study also showed that falls are related with other factors including psychosocial, lifestyle, socio-demographic characteristics and comorbidity. These factors can either relate to falls independently or act in conjunction with other potential risk factors to impact on fall rates in middle-aged and older adults. For example, depressive symptoms were reported to be the strongest predictor of sleep disturbance [59] and sleep duration was shown to be linearly associated with prevalent and persistent psychological distress [60]. Other studies have also found increased risk of falls in elderly with depressive symptoms [61, 62]. Therefore, existing research evidence demonstrates the importance of controlling for such factors in any sleep-related research. The association between the middle-aged and older adults being depressed for 3 days or more and falls in the current study was consistent with published studies results [63, 64]. Although anxiety is less of a concern in older adult compared to younger people [65], a bivariate association between anxiety and falls was found in the present study. In addition, loneliness [66] has also been reported to be associated with falls in elderly subjects. Despite a crude association found between loneliness and falls in middle-aged and older adults in the present study, after adjusting for other variables, this association did not persist. However, the present study does not rule out the possibility of loneliness being associated with falls in middle-aged and older adults as biological mechanism including motor function decline [67] could play a role and may affect mobility [68]. For instance, Buchman et al. found "feeling alone and being alone" to be associated with "more rapid motor decline" in elderly subjects [67]. In addition, synergistic effect of loneliness and depression may contribute to more fall incidence among

Table 5 Frequency distributions of sleep duration (in hours) in CHARLS vs. CLHLS for older adults of age 65 and above

CHARLS		CLHLS	
Sleep Duration in Hours	(night + nap after lunch)	Sleep Duration in Hours	(night + nap at any time)
≤ 5	24.6%	≤ 5	13.1%
6–7	32.5%	6	16.2%
		7	18.0%
8	24.7%	8	28.0%
9–10	9.1%	9	9.2%
		≥10	15.5%
≥ 11	9.1%		

older adults, as both depression [61] and loneliness [66] have been found to be associated with falls in elderly population.

Lifestyle factors were also accounted for in the current study. Findings revealed that alcohol intake was significantly associated with falls in our study population. This also confirms findings by earlier study that participants without 12 months previous history of exposure to alcohol, after being exposed to small amount of alcohol were more likely to have sleep-related issues including "higher levels of sleep disturbances" [35]; which probably contributed to fall rate in this study population, as 68% of the population under study were exposed to alcohol. Although alcohol may independently relate to fall, there is evidence that alcohol use with other medications like benzodiazepines can rather "heighten the sedative effect of the medication" and hence increased fall rate [69]. Increased in fall rate has consistently been associated with age advancement [70]. The present study results on age and risk of falls was not an exception as a dose-response relationship was demonstrated between age and risk of falls. Similarly, Pearson et al. also found that as age increased both "risk and perceived risk of fall" also increased [71]. Only crude association was found between smoking and falls in the current study. Being female was found to be significantly related to increased risk of falls in older adults [24, 72].

In addition to life style and psychological factors influence on sleep related problems, other chronic conditions including arthritis, diabetes and stroke have been found to be associated with severe sleep problems in individuals 50 years and older [73]. These factors may contribute to sleep problem to increase fall rates in older adults [74, 75]. The present study accounted for several of these variables and found increased risk of fall in middle-aged and older adults with hypertension, stroke, arthritis, vision and mental impairments. The current study findings are consistent with earlier published results. James et al. found in increased risk of fall among older persons with hypertension [76]. Despite a crude association found between diabetes and fall in the current study, falls related to diabetes cannot be deemed as a mere chance. Strong association was found between diabetes and fall among elderly subjects in earlier published studies [76–78], Proposed mechanisms which diabetes mellitus could affect falls include "peripheral neuropathy, impaired vision due to diabetic retinopathy or cataracts and diabetic foot ulcers" [79]. Masil et al. also found increased risk of fall in elderly subjects with visual impairment [44], which highlights the importance of the present study accounting for vision impairment in the primary relationship between sleep related problems and fall in middle-aged and old adults. The present study also adopted the contextual model of elderly fall

risk factors [80]. This model heighted the need for assessing the impact of mental health/cognitive in fall-related research. Hence this study assessed the impact of mental impairment including mental disorders and found that participants with mental impairment were at increased risk of fall. Mental impairment have consistently been found to be related with falls in older adults [45]. The literature also suggested that stroke is a major risk factor for falls. A recent prospective controlled study revealed greater risk of fall in an individual following a stroke when compared to those without stroke [81]. Likewise, increased risk of falling was also shown to be associated with arthritis among the elderly [82]. As such, for stroke survivors and middle-aged and older adults with arthritis, to reduce the risk of falling, interventions such as exercising or receiving physical therapy to improve walking speed, balance, and lower body strength have been recommended.

This study adds to existing evidence on fall by investigating the association of sleep duration and disturbances with fall using a robust procedure adjusting for complex survey design in a large sample [50]. The present study used a sample of the population-based nationwide data [46]. Although sleep variables including sleep duration and disturbance have been encouraged to be considered in sleep-related research as they may affect study results [25], a single study accounting for both variables in relation to fall in middle-aged and older adults is uncommon. Therefore, a notable strength of the present study is that it simultaneously investigates the association of both sleep duration and sleep disturbance with fall.

This study has a number of limitations. The use of cross-sectional design did not allow for causal inference to be drawn on the association between sleep duration and disturbances and fall. Besides, due to the time varying nature of both sleep parameters and fall, the study design used did not permit the ascertainment of which factor occurred first [83], however, paved the way for hypothesis generation which could be tested with rigorous study design. Also, this study assessed sleep disturbance on overall number of days experienced per week and did not allow for factors that led to the disturbance in sleep to be investigated independently. Although this study adjusted for several potential confounding variables, other factors including foot problems [84] and polypharmacy [15], which were reported to be related to fall were not accounted for in the current study, since no such data was collected. In addition, information collected from participants was based on self-report, so this study cannot rule out the possibility of recall bias. Despite the sleep questions were based on Pittsburgh Sleep Quality Index [39] and other questions derived from symptoms of sleep problems highlighted in literature [26, 42] and pilot tested, not all sleep questions stipulated in standardized tools such as Epworth Sleepiness scale [85] or Pittsburgh Sleep Quality Index [39] were considered in the CHARLS questionnaire.

Conclusions

Results of the present study showed that after adjusting for the psychosocial, lifestyle and socio-demographical factors, sleep duration and disturbances were strongly and significantly associated with falls in Chinese middle-aged and older adults. Such significant associations underscore the need for evidence-based prevention and interventions for falls targeting sleep duration and disturbance among the Chinese middle-aged and older adults. Future prospective longitudinal study is warranted to investigate the causal relationship between sleep duration, sleep disturbances and falls.

Abbreviations
AIC: Akaike Information Criterion; AOR: Adjusted Odds Ratios; BMI: Body Mass Index; CHARLS: China Health and Retirement Longitudinal Study; CI: Confidence Intervals; IRB: Institutional Review Board; PSQI: Pittsburgh Sleep Quality Index; WHO: World Health Organization

Acknowledgements
The authors would like to thank the China Health and Retirement Longitudinal Study (CHARLS) for providing the data. CHARLS has received critical support from Peking University, the National Natural Science Foundation of China, the Behavioral and Social Research Division of the National Institute on Aging and the World Bank. We are very grateful for the kind reviewing and very constructive comments of the Editor, the Associate Editor and reviewers, which were extremely helpful for us to improve our work.

Authors' contributions
CF, SE and WJS conceived the research objective. SE conducted the review of the literature, the analyses and took the lead role in writing the manuscript. CF supervised the analysis and interpretation of the findings as well as the writing of the paper. WJS, MF, LL and YQG made substantial contributions to conception and design of the manuscript and revised it critically for important intellectual content. All authors participated in all stages of the preparation of the manuscript and approved its final version for submission.

Competing interests
The authors declare that they have no competing interests.

Author details
[1]School of Public Health, University of Saskatchewan, Health Sciences Building E-Wing, 104 Clinic Place, Saskatoon, SK S7N 2Z4, Canada. [2]Robert Stempel College of Public and Social Work, Florida international University, Miami, FL 33199, USA. [3]School of Food Science, Guangdong Pharmaceutical University, Zhongshan 528458, China. [4]Department of Mathematics and Statistics, University of Saskatchewan, Saskatoon, SK S7N 5E6, Canada.

Reference
1. Kannus P, Sievänen H, Palvanen M, Järvinen T, Parkkari J. Prevention of falls and consequent injuries in elderly people. Lancet. 2005;366(9500):1885–93.
2. Kannus P, Parkkari J, Niemi S, Palvanen M. Fall-induced deaths among elderly people. Am J Public Health. 2005;95(3):422–4.
3. Ravindran RM, Kutty VR. Risk factors for fall-related injuries leading to hospitalization among community-dwelling older persons: a hospital-based case-control study in Thiruvananthapuram, Kerala, India. Asia Pac. J. Public Health. 2016;28(1_suppl):70S–6S.
4. Stevens JA, Mack KA, Paulozzi LJ, Ballesteros MF. Self-reported falls and fall-related injuries among persons aged≥ 65 years–United States, 2006. J Saf Res. 2008;39(3):345–9.
5. Seniors' Falls in Canada Second Report. Public Health Agency of Canada. http://www.phac-aspc.gc.ca/seniors-aines/publications/public/injury-blessure/seniors_falls-chutes_aines/assets/pdf/seniors_falls-chutes_aines-eng.pdf.
6. Milat AJ, Watson WL, Monger C, Barr M, Giffin M, Reid M. Prevalence, circumstances and consequences of falls among community-dwelling older people: results of the 2009 NSW falls prevention baseline survey. N. S. W. Public Health Bull. 2011;22(4):43–8.
7. Siqueira FV, Facchini LA, DSd S, Piccini RX, Tomasi E, Thumé E, Silva SM, Dilélio A. Prevalence of falls in elderly in Brazil: a countrywide analysis. Cadernos de Saúde Pública. 2011;27(9):1819–26.
8. Population Reference Bureau. Today's Research on Aging: China's Rapidly Aging Population. https://assets.prb.org/pdf10/TodaysResearchAging20.pdf.
9. Zhao Y, Strauss J, Yang G, Giles J, Hu P, Hu Y, Lei X, Park A, Smith JP, Wang Y. China health and retirement longitudinal study–2011–2012 national baseline users' guide. Beijing: National School of Development, Peking University; 2013.
10. Kwan MMS, Close JC, Wong AKW, Lord SR. Falls incidence, risk factors, and consequences in Chinese older people: a systematic review. J Am Geriatr Soc. 2011;59(3):536–43.
11. World Health Organization. WHO global report on falls prevention in older age. 2007. In: Geneva (Switzerland); 2007.
12. Parachute. (2015). The Cost of Injury in Canada. Parachute: Toronto, ON. http://www.parachutecanada.org/downloads/research/Cost_of_Injury-2015.pdf.
13. Stevens JA, Corso PS, Finkelstein EA, Miller TR. The costs of fatal and non-fatal falls among older adults. Injury prevention. 2006;12(5):290–5.
14. Hua F, Yoshida S, Junling G, Hui P: Falls prevention in older age in western Pacific Asia region. WHO Background Paper to the Global Report on Falls among Older Persons 2007.
15. Slattum P, Ansello EF. Medications as a risk factor in falls by older adults with and without intellectual disabilities. Age in Action. 2013;28(1):1.
16. Leblanc M-F, Desjardins S, Desgagné A. The relationship between sleep habits, anxiety and depression in the elderly. Nature and science of sleep. 2015;7:33.
17. Foley DJ, Monjan AA, Brown SL, Simonsick EM. Sleep complaints among elderly persons: an epidemiologic study of three communities. Sleep: Journal of Sleep Research Sleep Med. 1995;
18. Ailshire JA, Crimmins EM. Psychosocial factors associated with longevity in the United States: age differences between the old and oldest-old in the health and retirement study. Journal of aging research. 2011;2011
19. Faulkner KA, Cauley JA, Studenski SA, Landsittel DP, Cummings SR, Ensrud KE, Donaldson M, Nevitt M. Group SoOFR: Lifestyle predicts falls independent of physical risk factors. Osteoporos Int. 2009;20(12):2025–34.
20. Liu H, Byles JE, Xu X, Zhang M, Wu X, Hall JJ. Association between nighttime sleep and successful aging among older Chinese people. Sleep Med. 2016;22:18–24.
21. Lu L, Wang S-B, Rao W-W, Ungvari GS, Ng CH, Chiu HF, Zhang J, Kou C, Jia F-J, Xiang Y-T. Sleep duration and patterns in Chinese older adults: a comprehensive meta-analysis. Int J Biol Sci. 2017;13(6):682–9.
22. Stone KL, Ancoli-Israel S, Blackwell T, Ensrud KE, Cauley JA, Redline S, Hillier TA, Schneider J, Claman D, Cummings SR. Actigraphy-measured sleep characteristics and risk of falls in older women. Arch Intern Med. 2008;168(16):1768–75.

23. Mesas AE, LÓPEZ-GARCÍA E, RODRÍGUEZ-ARTALEJO F. Self-reported sleep duration and falls in older adults. J Sleep Res. 2011;20(1pt1):21–7.

24. Kuo H-K, Yang CC, Yu Y-H, Tsai K-T, Chen C-Y. Gender-specific association between self-reported sleep duration and falls in high-functioning older adults. J Gerontol Ser A Biol Med Sci. 2010;65(2):190–6.

25. Kim SY, Kim S-G, Sim S, Park B, Choi HG. Excessive sleep and lack of sleep are associated with slips and falls in the adult Korean population: a population-based cross-sectional study. Medicine. 2016;95(4):e2397.

26. Helbig AK, Döring A, Heier M, Emeny RT, Zimmermann A-K, Autenrieth CS, Ladwig K-H, Grill E, Meisinger C. Association between sleep disturbances and falls among the elderly: results from the German cooperative Health Research in the region of Augsburg-age study. Sleep Med. 2013;14(12):1356–63.

27. ÅKERSTEDT T, Hume K, Minors D, Waterhouse J. The meaning of good sleep: a longitudinal study of polysomnography and subjective sleep quality. J Sleep Res. 1994;3(3):152–8.

28. Latimer Hill E, Cumming RG, Lewis R, Carrington S, Le Couteur DG. Sleep disturbances and falls in older people. J Gerontol A Biol Sci Med Sci. 2007;62(1):62–6.

29. Stone KL, Blackwell TL, Ancoli-Israel S, Cauley JA, Redline S, Marshall LM, Ensrud KE. Sleep disturbances and risk of falls in older community-dwelling men: the outcomes of sleep disorders in older men (MrOS sleep) study. J Am Geriatr Soc. 2014;62(2):299–305.

30. Wallace CJ, Robins J, Alvord LS, Walker JM. The effect of earplugs on sleep measures during exposure to simulated intensive care unit noise. Am J Crit Care. 1999;8(4):210.

31. Aurell J, Elmqvist D. Sleep in the surgical intensive care unit: continuous polygraphic recording of sleep in nine patients receiving postoperative care. Br Med J (Clin Res Ed). 1985;290(6474):1029–32.

32. Broughton R, Baron R. Sleep patterns in the intensive care unit and on the ward after acute myocardial infarction. Electroencephalogr Clin Neurophysiol. 1978;45(3):348–60.

33. Bihari S, McEvoy D, Matheson E, Kim S, Woodman RJ, Bersten AD. Factors affecting sleep quality of patients in intensive care unit. Journal of Clinical Sleep Medicine. 2012;8(3):301–7.

34. Krachman SL, Criner GJ, D'Alonzo GE. Sleep in the intensive care unit. Chest journal. 1995;107(6):1713–20.

35. Kumari M, Green R, Nazroo J. 5. Sleep duration and sleep disturbance. Financial circumstances, health and well-being of the older population in England; 2010. p. 178.

36. Lei X, Sun X, Strauss J, Zhang P, Zhao Y. Depressive symptoms and SES among the mid-aged and elderly in China: evidence from the China health and retirement longitudinal study national baseline. Soc Sci Med. 2014;120:224–32.

37. Lei X, Smith JP, Sun X, Zhao Y: Gender differences in cognition in China and reasons for change over time: evidence from CHARLS. 2013.

38. Zhao Y, Hu Y, Smith JP, Strauss J, Yang G. Cohort profile: the China health and retirement longitudinal study (CHARLS). Int J Epidemiol. 2012:dys203.

39. Buysse DJ, Reynolds CF, Monk TH, Berman SR, Kupfer DJ. The Pittsburgh sleep quality index: a new instrument for psychiatric practice and research. Psychiatry Res. 1989;28(2):193–213.

40. Sleep Quality Assessment (PSQI). Available at: http://uacc.arizona.edu/sites/default/files/psqi_sleep_questionnaire_1_pg.pdf.

41. Spira AP, Beaudreau SA, Stone KL, Kezirian EJ, Lui L-Y, Redline S, Ancoli-Israel S, Ensrud K, Stewart A. Reliability and validity of the Pittsburgh sleep quality index and the Epworth sleepiness scale in older men. J Gerontol Ser A Biol Med Sci. 2011:glr172.

42. Hayward LB, Mant A, Eyland EA, Hewitt H, Pond CD, Saunders NA. Neuropsychological functioning and sleep patterns in the elderly. Med J Aust. 1992;157(1):51–2.

43. Jørgensen TSH, Hansen AH, Sahlberg M, Gislason GH, Torp-Pedersen C, Andersson C, Holm E. Falls and comorbidity: the pathway to fractures. Scand. J. Public Health. 2014:1403494813516831.

44. George M, Azhar G, Kilmer G, Miller S, Bynum L, Balamurugan A. Falls and comorbid conditions among community dwelling Arkansas older adults from a population-based survey. J. Ark. Med. Soc. 2014;111(7):136–9.

45. Bruckner J, Herge EA. Assessing the risk of falls in elders with mental retardation and developmental disabilities. Topics in Geriatric Rehabilitation. 2003;19(3):206–11.

46. Li C, Liu T, Sun W, Wu L, Zou Z-Y. Prevalence and risk factors of arthritis in a middle-aged and older Chinese population: the China health and retirement longitudinal study. Rheumatology. 2014;54(4):697–706.

47. Hosmer DW, Lemeshow S, Cook E. Applied logistic regression. 2nd ed. NY: John Wiley & Sons; 2000.

48. Konishi S, Kitagawa G. Information criteria and statistical modeling: Springer Science & Business Media; 2008.

49. Skelly AC, Dettori JR, Brodt ED. Assessing bias: the importance of considering confounding. Evidence-based spine-care journal. 2012;3(1):9.

50. Agnelli, R., Examples of logistic modeling with the SURVEYLOGISTIC procedure.2014.

51. Brassington GS, King AC, Bliwise DL. Sleep problems as a risk factor for falls in a sample of community-dwelling adults aged 64–99 years. J Am Geriatr Soc. 2000;48(10):1234–40.

52. Stone KL, Ewing SK, Lui LY, Ensrud KE, Ancoli-Israel S, Bauer DC, Cauley JA, Hillier TA, Cummings SR. Self-reported sleep and nap habits and risk of falls and fractures in older women: the study of osteoporotic fractures. J Am Geriatr Soc. 2006;54(8):1177–83.

53. Gu D, Sautter J, Pipkin R, Zeng Y. Sociodemographic and health correlates of sleep quality and duration among very old Chinese. Sleep. 2010;33(5):601–10.

54. Sullivan GM, Feinn R. Using effect size—or why the p value is not enough. J. Grad. Med. Educ. 2012;4(3):279–82.

55. Smagula SF, Stone KL, Fabio A, Cauley JA. Risk factors for sleep disturbances in older adults: evidence from prospective studies. Sleep Med Rev. 2016;25:21–30.

56. Vieira ER, Freund-Heritage R, da Costa BR. Risk factors for geriatric patient falls in rehabilitation hospital settings: a systematic review. Clin Rehabil. 2011;25(9):788–99.

57. Lin S-I. Risk of falls in community-dwelling older adults: a review of evidence and Taiwan experiences. education. 2013;23:26.

58. Picarsic JL, Glynn NW, Taylor CA, Katula JA, Goldman SE, Studenski SA, Newman AB. Self-reported napping and duration and quality of sleep in the lifestyle interventions and independence for elders pilot study. J Am Geriatr Soc. 2008;56(9):1674–80.

59. Matsuda R, Kohno T, Fukuoka R, Kondo M, Maekawa Y, Sano M, Fukuda K. The prevalence of sleep disturbance and its strong impact on depression symptom in patients hospitalized with cardiovascular diseases. Circulation. 2015;132(Suppl 3):A14835.

60. Glozier N, Martiniuk A, Patton G, Ivers R, Li Q, Hickie I, Senserrick T, Woodward M, Norton R, Stevenson M. Short sleep duration in prevalent and persistent psychological distress in young adults: the DRIVE study. Sleep. 2010;33(9):1139–45.

61. Tanaka M, Kusaga M, Ushijima K, Watanabe C. Association between depression and fall risk among elderly community residents. Nihon Ronen Igakkai zasshi Jpn. J. Geriatr. 2011;49(6):760–6.

62. Biderman A, Cwikel J, Fried A, Galinsky D. Depression and falls among community dwelling elderly people: a search for common risk factors. J Epidemiol Community Health. 2002;56(8):631–6.

63. Qader MAA, Amin RM, Shah SA, Isa ZM, Latif KA, Ghazi HF. Psychological risk factors associated with falls among elderly people in Baghdad city Iraq. Open Am. J. Prev. Med. 2013;3(07):441.

64. Whooley MA, Kip KE, Cauley JA, Ensrud KE, Nevitt MC, Browner WS. Depression, falls, and risk of fracture in older women. Arch Intern Med. 1999;159(5):484–90.

65. Gellis Z, Kim E, McCraeken S. Master's advanced curriculum (MAC) project mental health and aging resource review 2014 revision: chapter 2: anxiety disorders in older adults literature review. Council On Social Network Education. 2014;

66. El Fakiri F. Gender differences in risk factors for single and recurrent falls among the community-dwelling elderly. SAGE Open. 2015;5(3): 2158244015602045.

67. Buchman AS, Boyle PA, Wilson RS, James BD, Leurgans SE, Arnold SE, Bennett DA. Loneliness and the rate of motor decline in old age: the rush memory and aging project, a community-based cohort study. BMC Geriatr. 2010;10(1):1.

68. Meyer RP, Schuyler D. Old age and loneliness. The primary care companion for CNS disorders. 2011;13(2):e1.

69. Alcohol and Seniors: The Éduc'alcool Board of Directors. http://educalcool. qc.ca/wp-content/uploads/2011/12/Alcohol_and_health_3.pdf.

70. Rubenstein LZ, Josephson KR. Falls and their prevention in elderly people: what does the evidence show? Med Clin N Am. 2006;90(5):807–24.

71. Pearson C, St-Arnaud J, Geran L: Understanding Seniors' risk of falling and their perception of risk: Citeseer; 2014.

72. Lin C-H, Liao K-C, Pu S-J, Chen Y-C, Liu M-S. Associated factors for falls among the community-dwelling older people assessed by annual geriatric health examinations. PLoS One. 2011;6(4):e18976.

73. Koyanagi A, Garin N, Olaya B, Ayuso-Mateos JL, Chatterji S, Leonardi M, Koskinen S, Tobiasz-Adamczyk B, Haro JM. Chronic conditions and sleep

problems among adults aged 50 years or over in nine countries: a multi-country study. PLoS One. 2014;9(12):e114742.

74. Lyford J: Disturbed sleep linked to falls in elderly. Available at: http://www.news-medical.net/news/20131118/Disturbed-sleep-linked-to-falls-in-elderly.aspx.

75. Sibley KM, Voth J, Munce SE, Straus SE, Jaglal SB. Chronic disease and falls in community-dwelling Canadians over 65 years old: a population-based study exploring associations with number and pattern of chronic conditions. BMC Geriatr. 2014;14(1):22.

76. James K, Gouldbourne J, Morris C, Eldemire-Shearer D, Mona J: Falls and fall prevention in the elderly: insights from Jamaica. In.: Mona, Department of Community Health and Psychiatry, Mona Ageing and Wellness Centre, University of the West Indies, undated; 2009.

77. Schwartz AV, Hillier TA, Sellmeyer DE, Resnick HE, Gregg E, Ensrud KE, Schreiner PJ, Margolis KL, Cauley JA, Nevitt MC. Older women with diabetes have a higher risk of falls a prospective study. Diabetes Care. 2002;25(10):1749–54.

78. De Mettelinge TR, Cambier D, Calders P, Van Den Noortgate N, Delbaere K. Understanding the relationship between type 2 diabetes mellitus and falls in older adults: a prospective cohort study. PLoS One. 2013;8(6):e67055.

79. Malabu UH, Vangaveti VN, Kennedy RL. Disease burden evaluation of fall-related events in the elderly due to hypoglycemia and other diabetic complications: a clinical review. Clinical epidemiology. 2014;6:287.

80. Anantharama N, Rumantir G, Jomon B, Ananda-Rajah M, Gilbert A: Understanding Risk Factors Of Elderly Inpatient Falls Using Contextual Model. 2016.

81. Simpson LA, Miller WC, Eng JJ. Effect of stroke on fall rate, location and predictors: a prospective comparison of older adults with and without stroke. PLoS One. 2011;6(4):e19431.

82. Lawlor DA, Patel R, Ebrahim S. Association between falls in elderly women and chronic diseases and drug use: cross sectional study. Bmj. 2003; 327(7417):712–7.

83. Dohoo IR, Martin SW, Stryhn H: Methods in epidemiologic research; 2012.

84. Yoshida-Intern S. A global report on falls prevention epidemiology of falls. Geneva: WHO; 2007.

85. Johns MW. A new method for measuring daytime sleepiness: the Epworth sleepiness scale. Sleep. 1991;14(6):540–5.

14

The contrasting role of technology as both supportive and hindering in the everyday lives of people with mild cognitive deficits: a focus group study

Eva Lindqvist[1], Annika PerssonVasiliou[1], Amy S. Hwang[2], Alex Mihailidis[2], Arlene Astelle[3], Andrew Sixsmith[4] and Louise Nygård[1*] ⓘ

Abstract

Background: It is well known that people with mild cognitive deficits face challenges when performing complex everyday activities, and that the use of technology has become increasingly interwoven with everyday activities. However, less is known of *how* technology might be involved, either as a support or hindrance, in different areas of everyday life and of the environments where challenges appear. The aim of this study was to investigate the areas of concern where persons with cognitive deficits meet challenges in everyday life, in what environments these challenges appear and how technology might be involved as part of the challenge and/or the solution to the challenge.

Methods: Data were gathered through four focus group interviews with participants that live with cognitive deficits or cohabit with a person with cognitive deficits, plus health professionals and researchers in the field. Data were transcribed, coded and categorized, and finally synthesized to trace out the involvement of technology.

Results: Five areas of concern in everyday life were identified as offering challenges to persons with cognitive deficits: A) Managing personal finances, B) Getting around, C) Meeting family and friends, D) Engaging with culture and media and, E) Doing everyday chores. Findings showed that the involvement of technology in everyday activities was often contrastive. It could be hindering and evoke stress, or it could bring about feelings of control; that is, being a part of the solution. The involvement of technology was especially obvious in challenges linked to Managing personal finances, which is a crucial necessity in many everyday activities. In contrast, technology was least obviously involved in the area Socializing with family and friends.

Conclusions: The findings imply that technology used for orientation and managing finances, often used outside home, would benefit from being further developed in order to be more supportive; i.e. accessible and usable. To make a positive change for many people, the ideas of inclusive design fit well for this purpose and would contribute to an age-friendly society.

Keywords: Older adults, Mild cognitive impairment, Dementia, Technology, Environment, Support

* Correspondence: louise.nygard@ki.se
[1]Department of Neurobiology, Care Sciences and Society (NVS), Division of Occupational Therapy, Karolinska Institutet, Fack 23 200, SE-141 83 Huddinge, Sweden
Full list of author information is available at the end of the article

Background

This study is part of the Ambient Assistive Living Technologies for Wellness, Engagement, and Long Life project (AAL-WELL) [1], aiming at exploring how innovative technologies could support daily activities among older people with mild cognitive deficits. It is well known that people with mild cognitive deficits face challenges when performing complex everyday activities, both inside and outside the home, for example, when managing finances [2, 3], remembering appointments [3, 4], or reading books [3]. Yet, the role of technology in everyday activities is not equally well explored when it comes to users with mild cognitive deficits. Research has however shown that these people have to handle more explicit obstacles related to maintaining activities that include everyday technology than healthy older adults, and that they take on different approaches for that, for examples downsizing by ceasing to use technology or downsizing activities, which could include incorporation of new technology for support [5]. Increasing the knowledge of the role of technology is of great need as mild cognitive deficits are common in the ageing population. These deficits can be due to a minor stroke [6], early stage dementia [7], or mild cognitive impairment (MCI), sometimes described as a condition between normal aging and early Alzheimer's disease [8], although a large proportion of those with MCI do not develop dementia [9]. Hereafter, the abbreviation CD will be used as an overarching term for mild cognitive deficits due to these conditions.

This study has its focus on everyday technologies, that is; electronic, technical and mechanical artefacts that exist in people's lives at home and in the community [10], with the focus on electronic everyday technology, from now on referred to as technology. Even if technology has been a natural part in most people's lives for many decades – for example, washing machines, television – it is obvious that it has become more integrated in everyday activities both in domestic and public life today. It has also become more expected in society, that everyone can manage technology competently and independently, both at home, e.g., remote controls, microwave ovens and personal computers, and in public space, e.g., ticket vending machines or parking meters. The challenges encountered by persons with CD when using technologies have been well described (see for example [5, 11, 12]) although not in relation to the role of technology or to the environments where challenges occur. It is also recognized that to maintain engagement and independence in activities in everyday life, persons with CD have to tackle situations linked to technology, and how these situations are met have shown to be of crucial value for retaining the ability to use technology [13–15]. At the same time, it is also important to keep in mind the positive outcomes from using the technology,

since it can be regarded as a facilitator in everyday life for persons with CD [5, 16], and avoiding technology is neither possible nor desired. This suggests that more in-depth inquiry is needed into the interactions between challenges in everyday activities, technology's role and how persons with CD try to meet and find solutions to these challenges.

There are great expectations in society that technology will provide solutions to a variety of challenges. The hopes are particularly high that so called ambient assisted living (AAL) technologies and services (i.e. technologies that can sense a person's activity or behavior and provide tailored support as needed [17]) will increase autonomy, self-confidence and mobility, and, further, prevent social isolation, enhance security and continued living in an individual's preferred environment [17]. Using technology as support is also a common answer to the question how to afford the expected costs linked to an aging population [18], and many local and international initiatives have been launched to encourage research and development in this field [17]. However, the everyday priorities as expressed by persons with CD, and how these priorities link to technology use, have commonly received less attention. To guide the development of relevant technological support, be it ambient assisted living technologies and services or common everyday technologies, a literature review was first conducted in the AAL-WELL project [19] to identify important but challenging daily activities that persons with CD wanted to continue mastering and why. Although it is well known that the physical environment, e.g. the home or public space, is of major importance for activities of daily living, and also for competent use of technology [20], this literature review [19] pointed out that the empirical information concerning the physical environment involved when persons with CD do their challenging everyday activities is sparse. The findings described reasons for why the challenging activities were desired, and relationships of dependence between activities were found; some activities were prerequisites for other activities. The most difficult activities seemed to hinder outdoor life, but beside that, environmental aspects did not come to the fore although evidently of importance. This led us to continue exploring this topic in the present focus group study.

Having insights into the types of activities that persons with CD prioritize and where they take place, the nature of the challenges that occur and how challenges are met is paramount for developing any support, including technologies for cognitive support that can lead to positive changes for these individuals. The importance of considering environmental factors when designing and developing technological support for people with various needs has been stated previously [21–23]. The Person-

Environment-Occupation Model [24] highlights the strong relationship between a person's activities and the environment, also pointing out how the transactional dynamics between a person's roles, self-concept, abilities, culture and background, the environment – the technology being part of the environment - and the clusters of activities that meet intrinsic needs, together form the outcome of activity performance. This model also supports the importance of placing the activity in focus when examining the relationship between persons and their environments, a feature that is critical for designing appropriate technology [25]. Based on the identified knowledge gap, this study set out to investigate the areas of concern where persons with CD meet challenges in everyday life, in what environments these challenges appear and how technology might be involved as part of the challenge and/or solution to challenges. Our intention is to provide knowledge to facilitate the development of support, particularly the utilization and creation of technological solutions that are relevant to the expected users' priorities, taking the environmental aspects as well as the kind of solutions people with CD might have chosen into consideration.

Methods
Design
This study is a qualitative study in which data were gathered through focus group interviews [26, 27] conducted with the purpose of deepening the understanding and widening the view of the topic; that is the areas of concern where persons with CD meet challenges in everyday life, in what environments these challenges appear and how technology might be involved as part of the challenges and/or solution to challenges [27]. Using focus groups can provide valuable information for developing new solutions [27]. We chose to invite a variety of participants as informants to the focus group interviews. The assumption was that having different backgrounds, prior understandings and perspectives among the participants would enrich the data gathered. Ethical approval was obtained from the ethical board in Stockholm; protocol 2013/833–31/3.

Recruitment and participants
In order to gather as extensive data as possible, three types of stakeholders with different perspectives were recruited with a convenient sampling approach:

1) *Health professionals at memory investigation clinics,* (*n* = 4; Licensed Occupational Therapists [*n* = 3], Licensed Psychologist [*n* = 1]). These health professionals were experienced in conducting clinical interviews with persons with CD about their priorities as well as difficulties in everyday lives,

both at the clinic and during home visits. Among their clients were people who might not typically be interested in being involved in research and whose views would therefore not ordinarily be available to researchers. This group was a 'naturally occurring' group, that is, colleagues at the same clinic, which can be beneficial because they can relate to each other's comments, according to Kitzinger [26].

2) *Researchers in the area of MCI/early stage dementia and public environment/technology (n = 5).* These researchers had a background in occupational therapy and had conducted extensive interviews with persons with CD and their significant others in a variety of studies focusing on understanding the person's situation, but not on assessing their abilities or doing interventions, unlike the health professionals' purposes. This was also a 'naturally occurring' group.

3) *Members of volunteer health organizations.* For the recruitment of the participants from volunteer health organizations the term "mild cognitive deficits" was defined in an everyday language by the following words: *A person who manages relatively well in daily life, but due to cognitive deficits can use a little support now and then from others or from technology; a person who does things a bit more slowly or is in need of paying more attention to detail than others.* The participants had experiences of living with the consequences of cognitive deficits in their everyday lives derived from having mild cognitive deficits themselves (*n* = 5), or from cohabiting with someone with mild cognitive deficits (n = 5). They were divided into two mixed groups, both including persons with CD and spouses of persons with CD as they all volunteered to participate as equal members of volunteer health organizations; i.e. the voices of the persons with CD were given equal weight as the voices of their spouses. The purpose of the mixed groups was to get different perspectives and the reflections on the perceived challenges that persons with CD meet in everyday life and thereby get a more comprehensive understanding of them. In one case, a couple was participating in a focus group; in all other cases there were no close relationships between the participants. The participants with CD and their spouses were considered the most important ones in terms of giving their perspective on data from the other two focus groups. Hence, these focus groups were conducted after the other two groups, in order to allow more in-depth discussions on topics that had emerged (Table 1).

Participants in the first two groups had already been identified by the research team and were contacted

Table 1 Demographics of participants in focus groups

Focus group 1: Professionals at a memory investigation clinic

Sex	35–50 years	51–60 years	61–70 years	Years in the field	Profession
F		X		3	Leg. Occupational Therapist (OT)
F	X			11	Leg. OT
F			X	13	Leg. OT
M	X			2	Leg. Psychologist

Focus group 2: Researchers in MCI/Dementia, technology and public space

Sex	35–50 years	51–60 years	61–70 years	Years in the field	Profession
F	X			16	Doctoral student, Leg. OT
F	X			20	Doctoral student, Leg. OT
F	X			20	Ph. D./Lecturer, Leg. OT
F	X			14	Ph. D./Lecturer, Leg. OT
F	X			20	Doctoral student, Leg. OT

Focus group 3 and 4: Members of volunteer Health Organizations

Sex	35–50 years	51–60 years	61–70 years	Years of membership	Member in:
F			X	2	Alzheimer association and Dementia association
F			X	1	Dementia association
M			X	1	Dementia association
F		X		0	Spouse
F			X	4	Alzheimer association and Dementia association
F			X	2	Alzheimer association and Dementia association
F		X		13	Brain Injury association
F			X	4	Alzheimer association and Dementia association
F			X	4	Alzheimer association and Dementia association
F			X	3	Dementia association

directly for the interviews. With this approach, it was made certain that participants had an interest in and insight into the matter. They were considered able to be "good informants" [26], that is, they were able to reflect on a range of issues relating to the population of interest; that is people experiencing mild cognitive deficits. For recruitment of members of volunteer health organizations, three organizations whose aim was to support people with cognitive deficits were contacted. Their central administrations then either sent a request by e-mail to their members about the study and/or recommended that the researchers visit their social gatherings. Each local organization was then contacted, and they approved and invited the researchers to introduce the study at social gatherings. Interested members contacted the researchers via e-mail, telephone, or in person (at the social gathering) to approve participation. In total, one participant was recruited via the e-mail request, and nine participants were recruited via the social gatherings.

Data collection

The first focus group (health professionals) was conducted at the memory investigation clinic where the participants worked. The session lasted for 90 min. The second focus group (researchers) was conducted at the university just outside Stockholm, and lasted for 2 h. The third and fourth focus groups (members of health organizations) gathered at a geriatric clinic in a central part of Stockholm, and each of the group sessions lasted for 2 h. The clinic was chosen for its central location, as recommended by Murphy [27]. At every focus group session, there were two persons from the research team present. One was a facilitator (EL) who led the discussion based on the topics in the interview guide [26]. The other one (APV) took notes in order to keep a record of whether all topics were covered and if topics discussed in previous groups were mentioned. Refreshments were served and there were opportunities for presentations and some small talk before the discussions, with the purpose of creating a non-threatening atmosphere [27]. In the focus group introduction, the facilitator encouraged the participants to actively take part in the discussions and to ask each other questions during the session. It was also underscored that consensus was not of importance, but that all opinions were of interest. An interview guide (See the Additional file 1 Topics guide) was prepared and used as a flexible support with the purpose of ensuring that all main topics had been covered by the end of each session [27]. The facilitator led and followed the discussion and asked clarifying questions when needed.

The specific questions in the guide were only asked if the participants did not bring up the subject in the discussion. The questions focused on experienced or observed challenges in everyday life due to cognitive deficits, on challenging activities that were important to master, as well as on environmental aspects related to these challenges and priorities. In case participants only described observed challenges among persons with CD, the facilitator tried to encourage descriptions of how the persons with CD in those particular cases had expressed their experiences of these challenges, as one purpose of the focus group discussions was to capture possible priorities of persons with CD. In the last part of each focus group, questions were raised about issues that had been identified in the previous focus groups or in the literature, and that had not been mentioned in the current focus group. Examples of questions were: *The previous group mentioned that xx (xx representing an issue from an earlier focus group). Have you any experiences of that? What do you think of xx, is it a problem? How important do you think xx in general is to persons with CD?* In this way, it was possible to get a variation of perspectives and to enrich the previous data. A final question before wrapping up was posed about whether something was important to add. The interviews were audio-recorded in order to capture the conversation fully.

Data analysis

The focus group discussions were transcribed verbatim and entered into NVivo 10 (QSR International). First, the analysis focused on identifying the activities that, according to focus group participants, were perceived as challenging and important by persons with CD. It was considered fruitful to view the different groups' perspectives as complementary to each other instead of using their different contributions for comparisons, which led to all data being treated as one set [28]. All data that could be of interest for the aim of the study were labeled with concrete and explanatory codes. Examples of codes are: "risk of losing the credit card at the ATM", "difficult to handle stress related to trips abroad". These codes were inductively categorized into five *areas of concern* that emerged from the data [29]. Discussions that were not relevant to the aim, such as challenges related to being a spouse of a person with CD, were not coded regardless of their importance to the individual.

In a next step, each *area of concern* was searched through in order to find the various environmental factors related to challenges that had been reported by the participants. In order to more thoroughly analyze the challenges and the involvement of technology in these challenges, the extracts of data where challenges and their relation to technology came to the fore were categorized for each challenge in a matrix with given codes based upon the aim. These data were examined and questions were posed in order to find similarities, differences and patterns by continuous comparisons within and across areas of concerns.

Finally, the findings were synthesized into written text, using the areas of concern as category headings, describing the challenges, the environments, the role of technology, and the solutions found, as well as the eventual consequences of all these for each area of concern. These are summarized in separate tables within each of the five areas of concern. The order of the areas of concern in the presentations was based upon the degree of urgency for solutions as interpreted from the data. To further clarify the involvement of technology as part of the problem and/or the solution, a summary is presented in the end of the result section.

Results

In the findings, the challenges and how they were met according to the participants is presented in the five inductively created areas of concern; A) Managing personal finances, B) Getting around, C) Meeting family and friends, D) Engaging with culture and media, and (E) Doing everyday chores. In each area, the synthesised text under each area's heading presents where the challenges mostly appeared, with a specific focus on how the technology was involved when meeting the challenges. Also, the approaches used by persons with CD when meeting the challenges are described. Tables 2, 3, 4, 5 and 6 provide an overview of the results for each area of concern.

A) Managing personal finances: Technology adds stress to an already stressful activity but can also bring control

Managing personal finances, an activity performed regularly, stood out from other activities due to its profound influence on the everyday lives of persons with CD. Challenges related to managing personal finances were primarily met at home, but also in public space and in shops. Many of the challenges were linked to online activities.

Worries, stress or insecurity were particularly reported when paying bills with Internet banking services. Challenges linked to using the computer for online purchases were also described, mostly related to finding and making use of online information and instructions when making the transactions, inputting the right digits and finding the right item. Because of these challenges, some people reported returning to using paper forms again instead of Internet banking to ensure accuracy. However, some individuals with CD preferred the Internet bank as there were certain control functions in the system, such as viewing the transaction information afterwards, and because it also allowed a direct debit system. There were also challenges related to remembering to pay the household bills and keeping track of whether they had been paid, which could lead to repeated checking of payments. To avoid that, inserting automatic reminders in their smartphones and PDAs (Personal Digital Assistants),

Table 2 Reported challenges, environments, technology involvement and approaches related to Managing personal finances

Challenge	Physical environment	Technology - part of problem	Technology - part of solution	Approach to meet the challenge
Manage Internet banking	At home	Bank website		Use paper forms again
Make safe online purchase	At home	On-line shopping website		
Keep track whether bills are paid	At home		Internet bank on online computer	Check paid invoices at bank account online
Pay bills on time	At home		Mobile phone/PDA	Insert reminders in mobile phone
Avoid being fooled by telemarketing sales-persons and door-to-door salespersons/imposters	At home	(Telephone)		
Withdraw money from ATM	Public space	ATM		Use ATM when less crowded
Manage ticket vending machines	Public space	Vending machine		
Manage payment	E.g., grocery store	Payment terminal Automated checkout station		Choose familiar cashier, pay with notes instead of coins, use invoice instead of cash
Keep track on expenses	Grocery store		Self scanning	Check expenses on self scanning display when shopping

was one solution people used to handle the problem. Another solution participants described was to develop structures for how to store bills before payment to maintain control. One challenge related to managing finances at home was the risk of being fooled by telemarketing salespersons or by door-to-door salespersons. These salespersons - and there were even experiences of imposters - had to be handled, but no solutions were mentioned in this area, neither with nor without the support of technology.

Outside of the home, challenges in managing finances were linked to online technology in terms of withdrawing money from ATMs or buying tickets for public transportation in ticket vending machines, which both demand the user to understand and input information. Feelings of exposure and being an "easy victim" for criminals at the ATM were common. Withdrawing money from an ATM when there were fewer people around was one solution used to avoid such stressful situations.

Most of the focus in the discussions about managing finances was on money transactions in stores. There were perceptions of vulnerability, exposure and fear of being taken advantage of by dishonest people while paying for things. Challenges in, for example, handing over the right amount of money or remembering the pin code to the credit card, were related to stress and worries. The awareness of a need to be cautious was evident, and one participant (a researcher) cited a person with CD that she had met: " They (other people) can tell that I don't behave like others, that dementia is sort of imprinted in my eyes'...".

Automated checkout stations in stores were often avoided and using technology as support in these cases was very rare. One participant (a person with CD), however, stated that using self-scanning when shopping helped her to keep track of expenses and to avoid the stress at the cashier. Overall, the solutions were often related to avoiding challenging situations, for example,

Table 3 Reported challenges, environments, technology involvement and approaches related to Getting around

Challenge	Physical environment	Technology - part of problem	Technology - part of solution	Approach to meet the challenge
Leave home safely	At home	Stove/coffee machine	Mobile/smart phone, PDA	Set reminders to allow sufficient time for leave safely
Find one's way	Outside home, various areas		Mobile/smart phone (with GPS)	Use app-lications in smart phones for GPS, choose known areas, ask someone, take a taxi, have a companion or companion dog, visit places when less crowded
Remain together with companion	Outside home, various areas		Mobile/smart phone, PDA	Call each other
Find one's way in public transport	Public transport		Website of own on line computer	Print the planned trip ahead via website
Use GPS for orientation	Outside home, various areas	GPS app	Mobile phone/PDA	

Table 4 Reported challenges, environments, technology involvement and approaches related to Meeting family and friends

Challenge	Physical environment	Technology - part of problem	Technology - part of solution	Approach to meet the challenge
Attend to birthdays	At home		Mobile phone/PDA	Use paper calendar and reminders in mobile phone/PDA
Be on time for appointments	At home/at family and friends'		Mobile phone/PDA	Use paper calendar and reminders in mobile phone/PDA
Engage in conversations in the social setting at hand	At family and friends', associations			Withdraw in conversations, avoid social gatherings

to only pay with notes and never with coins in order to conceal difficulties in counting, to choose a familiar cashier to avoid being fooled or to ask for an invoice in the local store to completely avoid using money. If possible, some also brought a companion as support when shopping.

B) Getting around: Technology brings hope for reducing risk and fear of losing orientation

Being able to get around to places came to the fore as a prerequisite for having access to most activities, including those presented in the other areas of concern. The challenges to getting around were mostly identified outside home, although some challenges also occurred at home. Leaving home in a safe and controlled manner was described as crucial and difficult for persons with CD, and common challenges were, for example, to find needed belongings and to check that appliances, especially the stove, were turned off and all doors were locked before leaving home. The perceived risk of not leaving the home safely was related to fears of break-ins or fire accidents. Also, the risk of being delayed or even missing appointments if one could not find the key, and of leaving the home unlocked was a cause of worry, which is shown in this conversation:

A participant with CD said: *I have a balcony, and I have the door locked. The other day, when I was about to leave for my grandchild's first birthday party, I couldn't find the key.*

Another participant with CD asked: *To the balcony door?*

First participant replied: *To the balcony door, yes. And I looked for it, and looked for it. But then I had to leave,* so I left. Otherwise, I would have missed the whole birthday party. Then I searched through (the home) when I came back, and I hadn't had a break-in anyway. You see, I have had two break-ins in the apartment before (someone: oh dear!) so I was so worried.

Reported solutions were described both without and with support from technology; for example to attach valuables to strings in one's purse in order not to lose them and to set reminders about time to leave in the smartphone in order to allow sufficient time for preparations.

Getting around outside home was viewed on the one hand as crucial for maintaining valuable activities, and related to increased confidence and self-esteem, and on the other hand closely related to feelings of fear. One common challenge was to find one's way when going for a stroll in the neighborhood, woods, and fields. Getting lost was viewed as very possible and described as a very traumatic experience. It influenced people's self-image and confidence negatively, which was expressed by one participant with CD as *"One does not trust oneself any longer"*. Another participant with CD said: *But ... I get... because it happened to me once that I lost my way, but it is the only time. Once when I went into... I live in [village]. I went to [the small town] where I've been lots of times, and suddenly, I didn't know where I was. It was so awful. I walked around. I remember that, that I walked around, looked and didn't understand a thing, I didn't understand. I think I went into some stores and asked. And I still don't know how I got home, actually. So it was really... that's why I am a bit afraid when I go out.*

It was not unusual that persons with CD had stopped going for walks in the vicinity because of the fear of getting lost, and this was described as a loss since daily

Table 5 Reported challenges, environments, technology involvement and approaches related to Engaging with culture and media

Challenge	Physical environment	Technology- part of problem	Technology- part of solution	Approach to meet the challenge
Turn on media for watching a program	At home	TV, DVD, remote control		Stop using
Enjoy or take in the content in e.g. film or newspaper	At home			Choose less complex books, re-read books, solve crosswords intended for children
Handle media items	At home/at family and friends'	Smart phones, tablets		

Table 6 Reported challenges, environments, technology involvement and approaches related to Doing everyday chores

Challenge	Physical environment	Technology- part of problem	Technology- part of solution	Approach to meet the challenge
Turn off kitchen equipment after use	At home/kitchen	Stove/coffee machine		
Follow recipes and instructions	At home/kitchen	E.g. Coffee machine		Cook known meals, write own instructions
Adhere to routines; e.g. Take medicine, or eat regularly	At home		Mobile phone/PDA	Insert reminders in mobile phone
Handling online booking system for common laundry room	At home	The landlord's website		Get help from relative for booking
Buy the planned items in shop	In grocery store		Mobile phone	Call relative with mobile phone for recalling shopping list

walks were highly valued as recreation and for social values. Many solutions in order to continue these walks without support from any technology were described, for example, choosing known areas, asking someone in the street for help. Having the spouse or a friend as a companion was one common solution, but some persons with CD instead emphasized the importance of independence. Another more unusual solution was to have a trained companion dog for the purpose of orientation, which gave the owner hope to continue being able to get around outside independently.

Not surprisingly, the mobile or smart phone was viewed as very important for orientation. It was used for instructions from family members on how to find one's way, and the family also felt assured, knowing that they could reach each other. Since retrieving information from ordinary maps was perceived as difficult, some used applications for GPS orientation in order to get information about their position and directions to their planned targets. The participants had met contradictory feelings about the GPS in persons with CD. On the one hand, a need for the GPS service was expressed and the GPS was described as being *"great"* by some persons with CD, and on the other hand, there was a hesitation whether they would make use of it in a stressful situation. One said: *"I won't recall how I will know which buttons to push and know precisely..." (Person with CD).* It was difficult to remember or understand how to provide correct information required to receive support from the GPS, as well as how to use the information given from the GPS about directions, especially when difficulties in distinguishing right from left were present. The efforts that were made to make it work, despite all difficulties, indicated that this service still lent hope to the participants that it would be possible to get around outside.

Traveling by public transportation was a challenging activity and a prerequisite for visiting valued places, such as sports clubs. Apart from the earlier mentioned difficulties related to using vending machines for payments,

the challenges were linked to the need to attend to important details in the environment, both in the streets and underground, especially in traffic in order to orientate. The difficulties in orientation could be seen in losing orientation in the subway or not finding one's parked car.

Traveling was overall challenging to persons with CD according to the participants. At vacation spots new challenges occurred, as neither the hotel room nor the surroundings were familiar, which increased the risk of getting lost, and getting lost could convey feelings of panic. This was described by one participant with CD: *We were traveling somewhere (by train) and I don't remember where we were...and it was in the evening. When we arrived at a station, I thought we should get off there, because we had stood up and were standing there. But in fact we weren't to get off there, but I thought so and I am always in a hurry, so I took my bag and got off there, and then I saw the others (friends) standing there (in the train), staring at me. And I was standing alone on the platform. I understood that I shouldn't have gotten off, and I tried to get on the train again, but it left the platform... the panic I felt there on the railway station... (traveling with friends in Italy).*

The cell phone was described as a necessity if they lost their companions when traveling and some could not imagine how to manage without it. Since traveling had become relatively demanding, it was described as not always worth the effort, and some persons with CD had decided not to travel alone any longer or even stopped traveling completely.

C) Meeting family and friends: Technology can facilitate socializing but not solve the stress of socializing

Socializing with family and friends was mainly related to positive perceptions. It was, however, also challenging. Technology was not part of the socialization, but was important as an enabler, in terms of e.g. reminding of coming appointments. According to the participants, challenges related to socializing mostly appeared outside home, at family and friends' homes, and to some extent at home in terms of attending to birthdays or being on time for appointments, for example, deciding when to leave home. Being on time was described as a prerequisite for many social activities, and being late for an appointment or not being at home when visitors were expected could be perceived as very stressful by persons with CD. In order to avoid such mistakes, support from technology in the form of calendars or reminders in smartphones was used, and some also had access to different types of time aids; for example a PDA with reminders or features that enabled them to stay aware of the time. Family members were often supportive in managing appointments, which enabled persons with CD to meet with friends and acquaintances or attend meetings.

Not surprisingly, socializing with others was described as very meaningful, important, and appreciated. However, socializing was also closely related to stress and embarrassment, and the stress was mainly related to having conversations in the social setting at hand. This meant having to manage complex information in terms of finding subjects to talk about, describing thoughts and remembering earlier events or situations, saying socially appropriate things, finding the right words, and dealing with the intensity in loudness and tempo in conversations. One person with CD said: *"I think it's tough (mm), I think it's tough. HERE, it works really well, because I've met you and you know who we are and so on. But among others, I think it's really tough. I feel so excluded. I'm afraid of talking, I might get stuck on some words, or say something wrong (sigh) so that's what I think ..."*.

Meeting people was described as very demanding and tiresome. It often implied the risk of embarrassment and also feelings of shame due to the consequences of the cognitive deficits, and even small family gatherings could be perceived as hardly worth the effort. This perception was also related to the feelings of not being able to contribute to the group, and some told of becoming increasingly quiet when meeting people, while others withdrew and avoided social gatherings altogether. For some, the only solution was to exclude themselves from valuable social relations. In some cases, however, it was not the persons' choice to withdraw, instead, it was reported that friends had withdrawn after the cognitive deficits had been noticeable. In one case, a participant (wife of a person with CD) described how her husband left his hearing aid at home when visiting his children and thereby could blame his bad hearing when he could not follow the conversation, rather than tell his family about his cognitive deficits. No examples were found in which

technology was used to support socialization – just reminders and time aids. In contrast, the findings show that the need of appearing as no different from others and saving face could make persons with CD hide such assistive technologies for cognitive support, e.g. time aids in PDAs.

D) Engaging with culture and media: Technology impacts the use, but enjoying the actual content could be the biggest challenge

When engaging with culture and media, the challenging activities appeared mostly at home and often related to technology. The challenges could involve attending to specific points in time for TV programs, as well as managing the interaction with the technology, e.g. the TV, the DVD, and the variety of remote controls. Not being able to handle technologies that were used ubiquitously by people in one's surroundings, such as smartphones or tablets, could convey feelings of irritation, sadness, disappointment, and loss. In one specific case, a participant described how her husband with CD became very disappointed when he wanted to learn to use a tablet for watching fun film clips but could not manage it, although he had been very competent in using similar things before. She said he told her: *"Well, I'm not allowed to drive any longer and I can't manage this either"*. The tablet was thereafter not used, since it made him so sad.

However, the challenge in engaging with culture was not always related to the use of technology, but rather to the requirements of the valued activity itself, such as the need to concentrate to be able to enjoy different types of media, or to remember the plot in films and books. Cultural activities and their value had previously been taken for granted, and not being able to take part in them any longer conveyed feelings of sadness, irritation, or anger. This was described by a participant with CD:

"... when I worked, I always read the paper in the morning and that was like (zzip), and it was done. Now, I have to sit half the day if I were to read the whole (morning paper). And then, when I have come to the last page, I can't remember anyway what I've read. (Laughter). It doesn't stick in the same way any longer ... I would never be able to do that anymore. Those things make me sad, actually. I think that's a bit sad."

The main strategy described by the participants was to adapt activities with the purpose of maintaining them in some sense. For example, some persons with CD decided to read less complex books, re-read books that they had read before, or solve crosswords intended for children. In some cases, family members had to take over the handling of the media technology, and when the computer or the DVD became too complicated, it had in some cases been phased out without any feelings of loss.

The technology could also be viewed as supportive to enable enjoying culture, if it was possible to use it in other ways than before, for example, using computers or tablets for enjoyable or stimulating tasks such as reading, playing games, or solving crossword puzzles. Especially media in the form of computers or tablets could provide means for training cognition, and this was generally perceived as positive. As an example, some people with CD played a popular computer game for enjoyment but also for training their cognitive skills.

E) Doing everyday chores: Technology can threaten home safety and independence yet afford reliable reminders

Everyday chores that were described as challenging were by their nature performed frequently, and they were primarily performed at home, except for shopping. Most technology linked to the challenges in this area of concern was offline, which differed from most other areas.

When performing everyday chores at home, in terms of cooking and baking, there was a high risk of forgetting to turn off household equipment, which made technology part of the challenge. However, a more frequently mentioned challenge in this area was using recipes in terms of keeping the procedures in mind when cooking, which led to repeated reading. Cooking and baking was hence time-consuming, and not being able to prepare the food as timely and organized as before was related to sadness, irritation, and anger. One participant with CD said: *"Yes, I get irritated by it, because I had been used to having my hands full. I have done that kind of work. And now, everything goes so slowly for me, and I think that's tiresome. It almost makes me feel a little depressed instead. I don't get angry, instead I think I am so slow because it takes such a long time when I'm about to prepare food, which has been easy before. It took me a whole day to prepare a lasagna! Well, It would have taken an hour, because it is a bit complicated, but, but ... (sigh). It took me a whole day to prepare that darned lasagna and that's insane!"* Stories were told of when persons with CD wrote down instructions for their own use or started preparing less complicated or well-known meals to reduce the need to read recipes. Unsurprisingly, some cohabiting persons with CD had given up cooking. Technology was not mentioned as means to support the persons with CD when cooking and baking. Other challenging everyday chores performed at home included remembering small everyday tasks related to health, such as taking medicine, brushing teeth or eating. Contradictory to the challenges perceived while cooking, using technology as a support in health management was not uncommon. For example, persons with CD inserted reminders in a mobile phone, smartphone or a PDA with the intention to avoid forgetting to take medicine or brushing teeth.

Outside the apartment, in the common laundry room in the housing complex, a relatively new challenging chore had emerged; handling the online booking system for the public laundry room, a common facility in Swedish housing. For this activity, there was a need to quickly navigate on a screen to set one's preferred date and time for the laundry before being logged out and also to understand unfamiliar symbols. In one reported case, the high demands from the technology, i.e. the booking system, had become a severe hindrance; doing the laundry was no longer an activity performed independently.

Outside of the home, the only challenge mentioned in relation to everyday chores, apart from payment, was to remember what items to buy when grocery shopping. Mobile phones and smartphones were very useful for calling a partner in order to be reminded about what to buy in the store. This exemplifies how the combination of using the technology and having support from a person at a distance to get correct information was a supportive solution.

The involvement of technology on challenges in everyday activities

The involvement of technology in the five areas of concern was very contrasting. Technology as hindering and evoking stress, and therefore challenging, was particularly found in areas of concern linked to Managing personal finances, Engaging with culture and media and Doing everyday chores. When the challenges appeared at home, they were linked to managing finances on the computer and handling household equipment or media. When challenges linked to technology appeared outside home, they occurred when making payments or withdrawing money in stores, other public places or when using public transport.

Interestingly, there were also examples of technology being a part of the solution in the same three areas of concern as those where technology was hindering and evoking stress. Solutions were often linked to using mobile phone functions as reminders or checking online status reports for expenses and invoices. Not surprisingly, reminders set in the mobile phone were highly used and could meet some challenges, thereby enhancing control when Managing personal finances, Meeting family and friends and Doing everyday chores. However, the support from the technology could be too limited; for example, in the area Getting around, the GPS function could fail to support the completion of an activity due to its complexity. It was evident, however, that the technology was neither a part of the problem nor the solution for challenges when the expectation was to take in and enjoy the content in a film or to have a social conversation. In those cases, the more common approach to meet the challenge was to stop doing the activity.

Discussion

In this study, five areas of concern in everyday life were identified as offering challenges to persons with CD: A) Managing personal finances, B) Getting around C) Meeting family and friends, D) Engaging with culture and media and, E) Doing everyday chores. Not surprisingly, the challenging activities identified in these areas were to a great extent similar to the challenging activities that persons with CD wanted to continue mastering according to a previous literature study [19], thus empirically verifying former findings. As the challenging activities were found to be of great and existentially profound importance to people with CD [19], enabling these people to come to terms with the identified challenges in the equivalent areas of concern found in the present study may be decisive for success when striving to make a positive impact on everyday life for people with CD. The results of the present study add to previous findings by identifying the contrasting role of technology both as part of the challenge as well as the solution within these five areas of concern, taking the environments in which the challenge occur into account. In addition, a broad variety of approaches to meet the challenges utilized by persons with CD were identified. These approaches span from simplifications (e.g. use of paper forms/paper calendars, choosing less complex activities) to use of smart technology (e.g. GPS). The overview presented in Tables 2, 3, 4, 5 and 6 shows that technology being part of the problem was as common as technology being part of the solution, with variations between the areas of concern. The insights into the role of technology in activities that persons with CD value yet find challenging provided by the concrete examples in the findings will hopefully clarify and suggest new ideas on how and for what purpose to design technological support. For example, when the goal is to design support for the identified challenges, knowledge about the part that technologies and environments might play in the challenge can be used in the development process together with knowledge of how persons with CD have met the challenge. How technology can be involved in challenging activities in different environments will be further elaborated in this discussion.

The area of concern in which technology was found to be most problematic was Managing personal finances. Considering the importance of financial activities for everyday life, as well as the common difficulties in financial ability shown early after onset of CD that previous research has underscored (e.g. [30]), there is a need to emphasize the urgency of this problem. It was evident in our findings that one technological obstacle in this area

was the user interfaces of digital financial services. These had a crucial influence on the outcome when managing personal finances, regardless of whether the activity was conducted at home or in public places. The findings show how persons with CD, as we all do, meet a variety of technological payment or withdrawal systems, including Internet banking and on-line shopping websites, or payment terminals at the local shop, either at the cashier or at the automated check-out station, and, further, at vending machines and ATMs. Considering the difficulties commonly related to memory and new learning in persons with CD (for example, MCI [9, 14]), the variation and lack of congruence between user interfaces may be an important obstacle to the possibility of persons with CD to use these services. The need not only for web access but also increased usability of the web has been stressed as necessary for the full and equal enjoyment of web content by people with cognitive disabilities [31]. Further, the fear of financial abuse also appeared in our findings as well as in others' [32], and this must not be neglected. Being victims of financial crime is not uncommon among older people with cognitive deficits [33] and the feeling of vulnerability might negatively influence the wish to continue engaging in certain everyday activities and to be involved in society, resulting in withdrawal.

In our findings, there were many examples of technology being a part of the solution when meeting challenges in different areas of concern, but the solutions were in most cases limited to services linked to the mobile phone or specific websites. Reminders in the smart phone could support a person with CD to initiate important activities, keep appointments or remember medicine intake, and personal account information on the bank website was regularly checked to confirm whether bills were paid. In these particular cases, it is important to point out that even if the technology did not support the activity per se (e.g. taking medicine or paying bills), it showed to be supportive enough to enable some persons to initiate the activity and to maintain control. It should, however, not be taken for granted that because a person can initiate a challenging activity, they can perform and complete it. Moreover, only addressing a part of the challenge might not make the expected positive change for a person with CD. This was evident in the area of concern Getting around, where technology offered potential support, but at the same time created challenges. It has been stated previously that persons with CD often stop going on outings and traveling due to the demands linked to it [5, 35] and that GPS applications could support continued outdoor activities [23], thereby supporting wellness, enjoyment [36] and even social encounters [37]. Being able of finding one's way comprised many stressful challenges and the supportive technology – the GPS service – was, on the one hand, described by participants as highly needed for persons with CD for location and directions and consequently enabling valued activities outside home. On the other hand, however, using the GPS on a smartphone was described as too complicated to handle. Thus, the GPS technology was not perceived as being able to fully support the person in activities linked to orientation. This illustrates how one group with obvious needs for GPS - support, i.e., persons with CD with well-documented orientation deficits [34], is at risk of being excluded from the use of this vital service, and consequently from valuable activities outside home, due to an interface and functional demands that do not meet their specific needs. It is further important to take into account that, according to these findings, challenges related to handling household equipment at home was mostly linked to leaving the home safely. Providing technology that ensures that the home is secure when leaving it has shown to decrease perceived stress when persons with CD perform activities outside home [23]. Further development of services in this area would be beneficial.

In the area of concern Meeting family and friends, the findings showed that - apart from reminders - technology was neither part of the problem nor the solution when meeting challenges in socializing. One approach to meet challenges related to socializing was instead to withdraw from social gatherings completely since the gains did not outweigh the challenges. Withdrawal from social contact has been reported also in previous studies [38, 39] and could be a consequence of embarrassment and stress [40, 41]. However, it is well known that social engagement is crucial for wellbeing [42] and that loneliness has a negative influence on cognitive capacities and may speed up the rate of cognitive decline [43, 44]. As previously mentioned, the participants in this study did not describe technology as supportive when socializing. Other studies [45] have shown that e.g. smart phones have been beneficial for socializing, for example, for sharing photos and more frequent contacts. The importance of significant others as support in technology use for socializing has been underscored [45]. However, the goal of using technology might differ between significant others and persons with CD, and if a conflict arises, the person with CD is more likely to have the weakest voice [46]. Even if technology for social engagement as a means to decrease the speed of cognitive decline is important, it should not overshadow the role of technology as means to maintain valued social contacts; they are of crucial value in their own right. Yet, it is important to acknowledge that the challenges identified in our findings often were related to the perceived quality of conversations, a much more complex matter than just being able to stay in contact.

One goal of this study was to identify approaches that were used by persons with CD to meet challenges, because paying attention to individuals' self-initiated approaches may reveal their resources and be useful for guiding the development and provision of support [38]. However, such approaches may also pose new problems to the person with CD. Even if individual approaches to manage challenges are necessary, it is plausible that changes in the environment offer more possibilities. According to the Person-Environment-Occupation Model [24], the *environment is considered to be more amenable to change than the person* (p. 17) and changing aspects of the environment can support a compatible fit and thereby increase the person's performance of an activity. When aiming at supporting persons with CD to remain engaged in activities at home and in society, it is important not to neglect the technological environment as one target for change, since most complex challenges were linked to this environment both at home and outside home in our findings. Since technology was shown to be involved in many challenges that occur outside home, often in public spaces and shops where individual support might be less applicable, there are reasons to explore how technologies in public space could be designed to diminish known key challenges and thereby support persons with CD. This is also in line with the WHO initiative for Age-friendly environments [47], which intends to provide accessible public spaces and transportation that enable independence and participation in community life. An age-friendly environment provides services and support to compensate for the loss of function so that people can continue to do valued activities. To accomplish this, it would be beneficial if decision makers would request as well as facilitate that technological services in public space are designed to enable persons with CD to access and use them. Not considering the functional requirements of technology on persons with CD when designing services for e.g. buying tickets or withdrawing money will hinder their continued engagement in society [31]. The technological solutions that persons with CD would benefit from would very likely be supportive also to other people, in line with the guidelines of inclusive design, defined as "the design of mainstream products and/or services that are accessible to, and usable by, as many people as reasonably possible ... without the need for special adaptation or specialized design". [48].

Methodological considerations

It is important to bear in mind that the areas of concern are inductively developed representations of the areas where challenges are experienced and how persons with CD interact with technologies in everyday life, according to the participants in this study. This means that research involving other participants might result in other or additional representations. Most participants in the two focus groups representing voluntary health organisations were females, which might have led to a gender bias. Moreover, the focus group discussions were conducted in 2013. The fast development in technology has probably made especially social activities on the Internet more common. Technological support has also become more accessible and usable. On the other hand, we do not know if people with CD have adopted new technologies and services. Consequently, it is possible that new technologies have become part of new problems, just as well as they might be part of new solutions. Anyway, our findings should be interpreted with the presented limitations in mind.

Conclusion

This study focuses on the involvement of technology in those areas of concern where persons with CD encounter challenges. Findings showed that the involvement of technology in everyday activities was very contrasting, both in public spaces and within the home. It could be hindering and evoke stress or, in contrast, bring about feelings of control – that is, being a part of the solution. The involvement of technology was especially obvious in challenges linked to managing personal finances, which is a crucial necessity in many everyday activities. In contrast, technology was neither a part of the problem nor the solution for challenges when socializing with family and friends, suggesting that technology itself is not the solution to socialization problems, but rather one medium to facilitate staying in touch. Findings imply that technology used for getting around and managing finances, often outside home, would particularly benefit from being further developed in order to be more supportive; i.e. accessible and usable. In order to make a positive change for many people who face challenges in getting around and managing finances, the ideas of inclusive design seem fruitful, as does the WHO initiative of age-friendly societies. As two areas representing public rather than domestic life; getting around and managing finances, came to the fore in our findings, this implies redistributing the balance between designing for the individual and redesigning the environment, especially the public environment and the Internet.

Abbreviations

AAL: Ambient Assisted Living, or Active and Assisted Living; CD: (Mild) cognitive deficits; GPS: Global positioning system; MCI: Mild Cognitive Impairment; PDA: Personal digital assistant

Acknowledgements

The authors are very grateful to all participants in the focus groups, and to the funders.

Funding

The study is a part of the AAL-WELL project (Ambient Assistive Living Technologies for Wellness, Engagement, and Long Life) within the ERA-AGE2 framework, including research groups from Sweden, the UK and Canada. The project is funded by The Swedish Research Council for Health, Working Life and Welfare (FORTE) and the Strategic Research Programme in Care Sciences at Karolinska Institutet, Canadian Institutes of Health Research (CIHR) through the ERA-AGE2 program, and the Economic and Social Research Council (ESRC) in the UK.

Authors' contributions

The study was designed by the first (EL) and last (LN) authors, inn communication with the other authors. Participants were recruited and data was collected by EL and APV. Data analysis was carried out by EL and continuously discussed with APV and LN. The paper was drafted by EL in collaboration with LN, and with input from the others. All authors have read and approved the final manuscript.

Competing interests

As authors, we have no financial or non-financial competing interest.

Author details

[1]Department of Neurobiology, Care Sciences and Society (NVS), Division of Occupational Therapy, Karolinska Institutet, Fack 23 200, SE-141 83 Huddinge, Sweden. [2]University of Toronto and Toronto Rehab Institute-UHN, Toronto, Canada. [3]University of Sheffield, Sheffield, UK. [4]Simon Fraser University, Vancouver, Canada.

References

1. AAL-WELL. Ambient assistive living technologies for wellness engagement and long life. [Retrieved 2013 January 13]. Available from: www.aal-well.org
2. Allaire JC, Gamaldo A, Ayotte BJ, Sims R, Whitfield K. Mild cognitive impairment and objective instrumental everyday functioning: the everyday cognition battery memory test. J Am Geriatr Soc. 2009;57(1):120–5.
3. Farias ST, Mungas D, Reed BR, Harvey D, Cahn-Weiner D, Decarli C. MCI is associated with deficits in everyday functioning. Alzheimer Dis Assoc Disord. 2006;20(4):217–23.
4. Aretouli E, Brandt J. Everyday functioning in mild cognitive impairment and its relationship with executive cognition. Int J Geriatr Psych. 2010;25(3):224–33.
5. Hedman A, Lindqvist E, Nygård L. How older adults with mild cognitive impairment relate to technology as part of and potential support in everyday life. BMC Geriatr. 2016;73. https://doi.org/10.1186/s12877-016-0245-y.
6. Lesniak M, Bak T, Czepiel W, Seniow J, Czlonkowska A. Frequency and prognostic value of cognitive disorders in stroke patients. Dement Geriatr Cogn Disord. 2008;26:356–63.
7. World Health Organisation. The ICD-10 classification of mental and behavioural disorders: Clinical descriptions and diagnostic guidelines. Geneva: World Health Organisation; 2008.
8. Albert MS, DeKosky ST, Dickson D, Dubois B, Feldman HH, Fox NC, et al. The diagnosis of mild cognitive impairment due to Alzheimer's disease: recommendations from the National Institute on Aging-Alzheimer's association workgroups on diagnostic guidelines for Alzheimer's disease. Alzheimers Dement. 2011;7:270–9.
9. Roberts R, Knopman DS. Classification and epidemiology of MCI. Clin Geriatr Med. 2013;29:753–72. https://doi.org/10.1016/j.cger.2013.07.003.
10. Rosenberg L, Kottorp A, Winblad B, Nygård L. Perceived difficulty in everyday technology use among older adults with or without cognitive deficits. Scand J Occup Ther. 2009;16:216–26.
11. Linden A, Lexell J, Lund ML. Perceived difficulties using everyday technology after acquired brain injury: influence on activity and participation. Scand J Occup Ther. 2010;17:267–75.
12. Hedman A, Nygård L, Kottorp A. Everyday technology use related to activity involvement among people in cognitive decline. Am J Occup Ther. 2017;71 https://doi.org/10.5014/ajot.2017.027003.
13. Larsson Lund M, Lövgren Engström A-L, Lexell J. Response actions to

difficulties in using everyday technology after acquired brain injury. Scand J Occup Ther. 2012;19:164–75. https://doi.org/10.3109/11038128.2011.582651.

14. Rosenberg L, Nygård L. Learning and using technology in intertwined processes: a study of people with MCI/AD. Dementia. 2014;13:662–77.

15. Rosenberg L, Nygård L. Learning and knowing technology as lived experience in people with Alzheimer's disease: a phenomenological study. Aging Ment Health. 2017;21:1272–9.

16. Linden A, Lexell J, Lund ML. Improvements of task performance in daily life after acquired brain injury using commonly available everyday technology. Disabil Rehabil Assist Technol. 2011;6:214–24. https://doi.org/10.3109/17483107.2010.528142.

17. AAL-Europe. AAL-Active and assisted living programme. [Retrieved 2016 January 20]. Available from: http://www.aal-europe.eu/about/objectives/

18. Sixsmith A. Technology and the Challenge of Aging. In: Sixsmith A, Gutman G, editors. Technologies for Active Aging. New York: Springer Science & Business Media; 2013. p.7–25.

19. Lindqvist E, Persson Vasiliou A, Gomersall T, Astell A, Mihailidis A, Sixsmith A, Nygård L. Activities people with cognitive deficits want to continue mastering - a scoping study. Br J Occup Ther. 2016;79:399–408. https://doi.org/10.1177/0308022616638689513.

20. Malinowsky C, Almkvist O, Nygård L, Kottorp A. Individual variability and environmental characteristics influence older adults' abilities to manage everyday technology. Int Psychogeriatr. 2012;24:484–95.

21. Blackburn SJ, Cudd PA. A discussion of systematic user requirements gathering from a population who require assistive technology. Technol Disabil. 2012;24:193–204.

22. Eftring H. The Useworthiness of robots for people with physical disabilities. Lund University: Department of Design Sciences, Lund; 1999.

23. Lindqvist E, Nygård L, Borell L. Significant junctures on the way towards becoming a user of assistive technology in Alzheimer's disease. Scand J Occup Ther. 2013;20(5):386–96.

24. Law M, Cooper B, Strong S, Stewart D, Rigby P, Letts L. The person-environment-occupation model: a transactive approach to occupational performance. Can J Occup Ther. 1996;63(1):9–23.

25. Norman D. Human-Centered Design Considered Harmful. Interactions. 2005; (july +august):14–19.

26. Kitzinger J. Qualitative research. Introducing focus groups. BMJ. 1995; 311(7000):299–302.

27. Murphy J, Cockburn M. Murphy; focus groups in healthresearch. Health Promot J. 1992;2(2):37–40.

28. Dahlin Ivanoff S, Hultberg J. Understanding the multiple realities of everyday life: basic assumptions in focus-group methodology. Scand J Occup Ther. 2006;13:125–32.

29. Krippendorff K. Content analysis – an introduction to its methodology. Thousand Oaks: Sage Publications Inc; 2004.

30. Jekel K, Damian M, Wattmo C, Hausner L, Bullock R, Connelly PJ, Dubois B, Eriksdotter M, Ewers M, Graessel E, Kramberger MG, Law E, Mecocci P, Molinuevo JL, Nygård L, Olde-Rikkert MGM, Orgogozo J-M, Pasquier F, Peres K, Salmon E, Sikkes SAM, Sobow T, Spiegel R, Tsolaki M, Winblad B, Froelich L. Mild cognitive impairment and deficits in instrumental activities of daily living - a systematic review. Alzheimers Res Ther. 2015;7:1–20.

31. Blanck P. eQuality: web accessibility by people with cognitive disabilities. Inclusion. 2015;3:75–91. https://doi.org/10.1352/2326-6988-3.2.75.

32. Brorsson A, Öhman A, Cutchin M, Nygård L. Managing critical incidents in grocery shopping as perceived by people with Alzheimer's disease. Scand J Occup Ther. 2013;20:292–301. https://doi.org/10.3109/11038128.2012.752031.

33. Alzheimer's Society: Short Changed - Protecting people with dementia from financial abuse; 2011. [Retrieved 2017, 11 nov] Accessible at http://www.alzheimers.org.uk/shortchanged.

34. Rusconi ML, Suardi A, Zanetti M, Rozzini L. Spatial navigation in elderly healthy subjects, amnestic and non amnestic MCI patients. J Neurol Sci. 2015;359:430–7.

35. Berg AI, Wallin A, Nordlund A, Johansson B. Living with stable MCI: experiences among 17individuals evaluated at a memory clinic. Aging Ment Health. 2013;17(3):293–9.

36. Cedervall C, Torres S, Åberg AC. Maintaining wellbeing and selfhood through physical activity: experiences of people with mild Alzheimer's disease. Aging Ment Health. 2015;19:679–88. https://doi.org/10.1080/13607863.2014.962004.

37. Brorsson A, Öhman A, Lundberg S, Nygård L. Accessibility in public space as perceived by people with Alzheimer's disease. Dementia. 2011;10:587–602.

38. Nygård L, Kottorp A. Engagement in IADLs, social activities and use of everyday technology in older adults with and without cognitive impairment. Br J Occup Ther. 2014;77(11):565–73.

39. Hedman A, Nygård L, Malinowsky C, Almkvist O, Kottorp A. Changing everyday activities and technology use in mild cognitive impairment. Br J of Occup Ther. 2016;79(2):111–9.

40. Caddell LS, Clare L. I'm still the same person: the impact of early-stage dementia on identity. Dementia. 2011;10:379–98.

41. Karlsson E, Axelsson K, Zingmark K, et al. The challenge of coming to terms with the use of a new digital assistive device: a case study of two persons with mild dementia. Open Nurs J. 2011;5:102–10.

42. Adams KB, Leibrandt S, Moon H. A critical review of the literature on social and leisure activity and wellbeing in later life. Ageing & Society. 2011;31: 683–712. DOI:https://doi.org/10.1017/S0144686X10001091

43. Hughes TF, Flatt JD, Fu B, Chang CH, Ganguli M. Engagement in Social Activities and Progression from Mild to Severe Cognitive Impairment: The MYHAT Study. Int Psychogeriatr. 2013;25:587–95. https://doi.org/10.1017/S1041610212002086.

44. Kivipelto M, Mangialasche F, Ngandu T. Can lifestyle changes prevent cognitive impairment? Lancet Neurol. 2017;16:338–9. https://doi.org/10.1016/S1474-4422(17)30080-7.

45. Piper AM, Cornejo R, Hurwitz L, Unumb C. Technological caregiving: Supporting online activity for adults with cognitive impairments. Proceedings of the 2016 CHI Conference on Human Factors in Computing Systems. San Jose, California, USA. 2016: p 5311–5323 DOI: https://doi.org/10.1145/2858036.2858260.

46. Rosenberg L, Nygård L. Persons with dementia become users of assistive technology: a study of the process. Dementia. 2012;11:135–54.

47. World Health Organisation. Age-friendly environments. [Retrieved 2017 oct 29] Available from: http://www.who.int/ageing/projects/age-friendly-environments/en/

48. The British Standards Institute (2005) standard BS 7000–6:2005: 'Design management systems - Managing inclusive design - Guide' defines inclusive design and provides guidance on managing it.

15

Impact of a nurse-based intervention on medication outcomes in vulnerable older adults

Michael A. Steinman[1,2,3,4]* (iD), Marcelo Low[3,4], Ran D. Balicer[3] and Efrat Shadmi[3,4]

Abstract

Background: Medication-related problems are common in older adults with multiple chronic conditions. We evaluated the impact of a nurse-based primary care intervention, based on the Guided Care model of care, on patient-centered aspects of medication use.

Methods: Controlled clinical trial of the Comprehensive Care for Multimorbid Adults Project (CC-MAP), conducted among 1218 participants in 7 intervention clinics and 6 control (usual care) clinics. Inclusion criteria included age 45–94, presence of ≥3 chronic conditions, and Adjusted Clinical Groups (ACG) score > 0.19. The co-primary outcomes were number of changes to the medication regimen between baseline and 9 month followup, and number of changes to symptom-focused medications, markers of attentiveness to medication-related issues.

Results: Mean age in the intervention group was 72 years, 59% were women, and participants used a mean of 6.6 medications at baseline. The control group was slightly older (73 years) and used more medications (mean 7.1). Between baseline and 9 months, intervention subjects had more changes to their medication regimen than control subjects (mean 4.04 vs. 3.62 medication changes; adjusted difference 0.55, $p = 0.001$). Similarly, intervention subjects had more changes to their symptomatic medications (mean 1.38 vs. 1.26 changes, adjusted difference 0.20, $p = 0.003$). The total number of medications in use remained stable between baseline and follow-up in both groups ($p > 0.18$).

Conclusion: This nurse-based, primary care intervention resulted in substantially more changes to patients' medication regimens than usual care, without increasing the total number of medications used. This enhanced rate of change likely reflects greater attentiveness to the medication-related needs of patients.

Keywords: Polypharmacy, Medication management, Primary care, Israel, Aged, Multimorbidity, Quality of care

Background

Prescribing for older adults with multiple chronic conditions often leads to medication regimens that are overly complicated, difficult to adhere to, and contain multiple drug-drug and drug-disease interactions [1, 2]. In addition, prescribing decisions often do not attend to patient preferences, abilities, and goals of care [3]. This leaves patients feeling sidelined and disengaged from their care, with medication regimens that are not tailored to their needs and preferences [4].

Addressing these patient-centered issues requires patient-centered approaches to improving medication use. Such strategies use an understanding of patients' needs and abilities to inform treatment decisions [5]. In addition, these strategies can help patients adhere to and properly use medications to maximally benefit their health and achieve their goals [6]. Yet, this is easier said than done. Programs such as patient-centered medical homes are promising but have shown mixed results, and

* Correspondence: mike.steinman@ucsf.edu
Prior presentation: 6th International Jerusalem Conference on Health Policy, Jerusalem, Israel, May 2016; International Association of Geriatrics and Gerontology quadrennial meeting, San Francisco, CA, USA, July 2017.
[1]University of California, 3333 California St, San Francisco, CA 94118, USA
[2]San Francisco VA Health Care System, 4150 Clement St, Box 181G, San Francisco, CA 94121, USA
Full list of author information is available at the end of the article

there are few models of care that consistently achieve these ends and are practical for widespread use [7].

In recent years, a promising new model called Guided Care has been proposed that is well suited to address these needs [8]. Guided Care is a system of comprehensive, interdisciplinary care that is tailored to the needs of older adults with multiple chronic conditions [9]. In this model, a registered nurse based in a primary care clinic works with a panel of vulnerable older patients. The nurse interfaces with these patients via home visits, over the telephone, and in the clinic. These interactions include elements of case management, support for patient self-management, and help with transitions of care. The nurse also works with patients' clinicians to help coordinate care and bring patients' needs, abilities, and preferences to clinical decision-making. Although it was not designed specifically to improve medication use, and does not incorporate any structured elements that focus explicitly on medications (such as medication review or reconciliation), its philosophy and processes are tightly aligned with the pharmaceutical care needs of older adults [10].

Previous studies have evaluated the impact of Guided Care on several outcomes such as mortality, mental and physical health, and caregiver burden [11–16]. However, little work has been done on how Guided Care impacts medication use and outcomes in vulnerable older adults. To fill this important evidence gap, we evaluated the effect of an intervention based on the Guided Care model on several aspects of medication prescribing for older adults in Israel. We hypothesized that older adults receiving this intervention would have improved markers of patient-centered prescribing – namely, more changes to their overall medication regimens, and more changes to their symptom-focused medications, representing greater attentiveness to adjusting medication regimens in response to patient symptoms, challenges with existing medications, and goals of care.

Methods
Intervention and study population
This study uses data from the Comprehensive Care for Multimorbid Adults Project (CC-MAP), a controlled clinical trial of a nurse-based intervention that was conducted within primary care clinics of Clalit Health Systems [17]. Clalit is Israel's largest integrated health care provider and insurer, serving approximately half the country's population.

In the CC-MAP study, representative (but not randomized) primary care clinics within 2 regions of Israel were selected as intervention and control sites. In the 7 intervention sites, nurses trained in the CC-MAP model were embedded in a clinic, which typically comprised 3 to 4 physicians plus support staff. CC-MAP nurses

followed a panel of vulnerable adults who met the inclusion/exclusion criteria outlined below. Six control clinics were selected with similar demographic and health system characteristics as the intervention clinics. In the control clinics, patients received usual care.

Intervention patients met with the CC-MAP nurse monthly in person or by phone, and in person at least once per quarter, to review their care plan, make adjustments and receive counseling as needed, and follow up. When a patient was hospitalized, the CC-MAP nurse contacted the patient immediately after discharge to review changes in treatment recommendations, and as needed alert the primary care physician to implement treatment changes described in discharge recommendations. As this complex intervention was tailored to the needs and preferences of each participant, some subjects received more intensive services and contacts than others, although all intervention subjects enrolled had a minimum of 3 contacts (in person or by telephone) with CC-MAP nurses per year, with most having substantially more. There was no specific medication reconciliation or pharmacy component to the intervention, although since the nurse was part of a nurse-primary care physician team, part of her role was to periodically assess the patient's status, including adherence to the care plan. Thus, when the nurse identified that the patient had side effects from medications, or that he/she was not adhering to the treatment, she notified the primary care physician. This provided an opportunity to be able to tailor care to patients' evolving status and needs.

Inclusion criteria included community-dwelling adults age 45–94 years and the presence of 3 or more chronic conditions. In addition, we employed a Johns Hopkins Adjusted Clinical Group® (ACG) system predictive modeling score using diagnosis and pharmacy data (the DxRxPM model), restricting enrollment to people with a score > 0.19, indicating high risk of poor clinical outcomes [18]. Exclusion criteria included inability to speak Hebrew or Russian, current participation in a disease management program, use of dialysis or chemotherapy, advanced dementia, or severe mental illness such as schizophrenia (see Fig. 1). Over 70% of the study population was age 65 and older. Intervention subjects were enrolled between April 2013 and June 2014, and control subjects between November 2013 and March 2015.

Measures
The pre-specified primary outcome of the CC-MAP trial was hospital admissions for ambulatory-sensitive conditions, which the trial was powered to detect with an effect size of 0.3 and a type I error of 0.05. After the trial commenced but prior to reviewing outcomes data, we selected 2 new outcomes of interest related to medications,

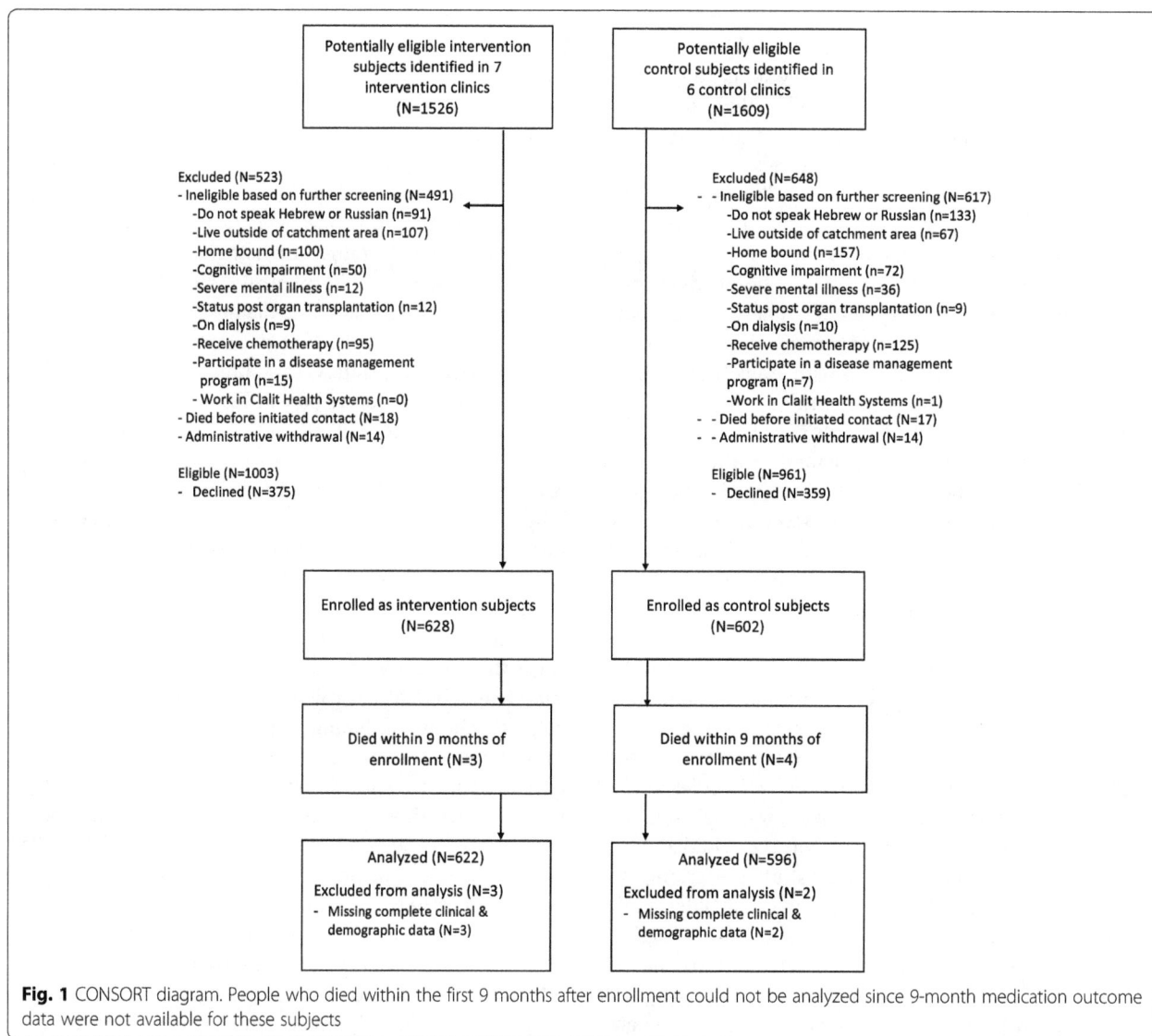

Fig. 1 CONSORT diagram. People who died within the first 9 months after enrollment could not be analyzed since 9-month medication outcome data were not available for these subjects

listed below. We chose these outcomes based on domains where we hypothesized the CC-MAP intervention could have particularly beneficial impacts on medication use. We considered these 2 outcomes co-primary for purposes of this study.

Medication use was assessed using pharmacy dispensing data from Clalit pharmacies and from non-Clalit pharmacies where Clalit insurance was billed. Together these account for the strong majority of prescription medications filled by Clalit members, who have powerful financial incentives to fill their medications using their Clalit benefits [19, 20]. We employed a variant of methods recommended by Lund et al. to identify prevalent medication use at time points of interest [21]. Because it can be difficult to ascertain dose and duration of medications that are delivered topically or locally, we restricted our analyses to medication classes that are delivered systemically and/or have systemic effects.

Outcome #1 - Number of changes in medication regimen

We hypothesized that the CC-MAP intervention would lead to more changes in medication regimens by improving communication about patient symptoms, goals, and problems with existing treatment regimens. Based on prior work, we defined medication changes as the sum of medication additions (medications present at 9 months that were not present at baseline), medication discontinuations (medications present at baseline that were no longer present at 9 months), therapeutic substitutions (a switch from one medication to another within the same drug class, defined at the 4th level of the Anatomic Therapeutic Classification [ATC] system), and dose changes (the same medication given at different daily doses at baseline vs. 9 months) [22].

Outcome #2 – Change in use of symptom-focused medications

We hypothesized that improved communication about patient symptoms would lead to more fine-tuning of symptom-focused medications. Our co-primary outcome was the number of changes in symptom-focused medications between baseline and 9 months. A secondary outcome was the total number of symptom-focused medications in use at 9 months. Methods for defining symptom-focused medications are described in Additional file 1: Appendix S1.

Other variables

Patient demographics were collected from Clalit data systems. Comorbid conditions were assessed using algorithms developed for Clalit clinical and claims data, for example using inpatient and outpatient diagnoses, pharmacy records, and laboratory test results. The unweighted sum of 27 chronic conditions defined a patient-level comorbidity score. ACG scores were calculated using clinical and claims data using standard methods employed by Clalit and validated for CC-MAP patient selection [23, 24]. Higher ACG scores predict a variety of poor clinical outcomes [24].

Main analyses

Our analyses used an intention to treat framework. Overall, 45 intervention subjects and 1 control subject withdrew from participation in the intervention and/or followup assessments between baseline and 9 months, and 3 intervention subjects moved to a different clinic. (The differential drop-out rate is likely explained by burden and/or dislike of the intervention by intervention subjects, whereas control subjects had only usual care.) Although these subjects withdrew from participation or moved, we were able to assess their medication outcomes as medication use was measured using pharmacy claims data, which were generated irrespective of trial participation. Thus, these subjects were included in the final analysis according to their original treatment assignment.

All analyses employed mixed effects regression, using random effects to adjust for clustering of study subjects within physicians, and fixed effects to adjust for region. Clinic-level random effects were negligible after accounting for physician random effects. Outcomes analyses controlled for potential confounders including age, sex, comorbidity count, ACG DxRxPM score, number of medications present at baseline, and the number of medication changes that had occurred between 9 months before baseline and baseline (to account each subject's

pre-baseline rate of medication changes). We used interaction terms to evaluate potential effect modification among pre-specified subgroups defined by age, ACG predictive modeling score, and number of medications used at baseline.

The enrollment period for intervention subjects began and ended earlier than the enrollment period for control subjects, with only partial overlap. To evaluate if secular trends could have impacted our results, we assessed the impact of enrollment time on our medication outcomes in each treatment group. In these analyses, enrollment time was not associated with outcomes in either group ($p > .15$ for all).

Exploratory analyses

We conducted an exploratory analysis to understand the relationship between our primary outcome measure (number of medication changes) and patient-centeredness. We hypothesized that a greater number of medication changes over time would be associated with greater patient-centeredness, reflecting increased attention to patients' medication-related needs and challenges. This analysis used data from the Patient Assessment of Chronic Illness Care (PACIC) questionnaire, which was completed by control subjects at baseline. (Accurate baseline data were not available for intervention subjects). Our predictor variable was the number of medication changes in the 9 months prior to the time the PACIC was administered. Our outcome variable was the sum of scores for the first 3 items on the PACIC questionnaire, which address the patient-centeredness of treatment planning, and which have been validated to have strong psychometric properties (Cronbach's alpha 0.82, standardized factor loadings > 0.75) [25]. Answers to these items were summed into a score ranging from 3 (never involved in treatment planning) to 15 (always involved in treatment planning). We used Poisson regression to evaluate the predictor-outcome relationship, while controlling for potential confounders including number of medications in the pre-baseline period, number of chronic conditions, ACG predictive modeling score, age, race, and sex, and adjusting for clinician as a random effect (see Additional file 1: Appendix S5).

This study adheres to CONSORT guidelines and was approved by the institutional review boards of Clalit Health Services and the University of California, San Francisco.

Results

Subject enrollment and follow-up data are shown in Fig. 1. Of 1230 subjects enrolled, 1218 had full data available for analysis at 9 month follow-up. The 622 intervention patients in the final analytic sample received care in 7 intervention clinics by 21 primary care physicians. The 598 control patients received care in 6 control clinics predominantly by 17 primary care physicians.

Baseline characteristics of intervention control patients are shown in Table 1. Compared with control patients, intervention patients were slightly younger, had fewer chronic conditions, and received fewer medications.

Effect of CC-MAP intervention on changes in medication use

Between baseline and 9 months, intervention patients had a mean of 4.04 changes to their medication regimens (Table 2). Control patients had a mean of 3.62 changes. After adjusting for baseline characteristics, intervention patients had a mean of 0.55 more medication changes than control subjects ($p = .001$; see Additional file 1: Appendix S3 for additional information).

A similar pattern was observed for changes in the use of symptom-focused medications. Between baseline and 9 month followup, intervention patients had more changes to their regimen of symptom-focused medications than control patients (mean 1.38 vs. 1.27 changes, adjusted mean difference 0.20 changes, $p = .003$).

As a sensitivity analysis, we expanded our definition of symptom-focused medications to include drugs used to treat intermittent but highly symptomatic conditions, and medications with mixed symptom-focused and non-symptom-focused uses. Results were similar using this expanded definition: intervention patients had more changes to the regimen of symptom-focused medications than control patients (mean 1.89 vs 1.81 changes, adjusted mean difference 0.20 changes, $p = .01$).

Characteristics of medication changes

In both the intervention and control groups, there was little difference in the total number of medications subjects used at baseline and at 9 months. The intervention group used a mean of 0.09 more medications at 9 months compared with baseline ($p = 0.32$ for change). The control group used a mean of 0.12 fewer medications at 9 months compared with baseline ($p = 0.18$ for change; $p = .12$ for difference in change between intervention and control groups).

The total number of symptom-focused medications also remained generally stable from baseline to 9 months, although there was a small, statistically significant increase in the intervention group. The intervention group used a mean of 0.13 more symptom-focused medications at 9 months compared with baseline ($p = 0.02$ for change). The control group used 0.03 fewer symptom-focused medications at 9 months ($p = 0.59$ for change; $p = 0.06$ for difference in number of changes between groups).

The distribution of types of medication changes (e.g. additions, discontinuations, therapeutic substitutions, and dose changes) were generally similar across groups (Table 3). The distribution of which classes of drugs were changed was also similar in the two groups. The most commonly changed medication class was cardiovascular medications, which accounted for 30% of changes in the intervention group and 29% in the control group ($p = 0.31$ for difference; see Additional file 1: Appendix S4 for additional information).

Subgroup effects

The impact of the intervention on both medication change outcomes did not vary between patients of different age (under 75 vs. 75 or more years), ACG score

Table 1 Baseline characteristics of intervention and control subjects

	Intervention $N = 622$	Control $N = 596$
Age (mean, SD)	71.6 (10.2)	73.4 (9.9)
Female sex	365 (59)	329 (55)
No. of chronic conditions (mean, SD)[a]	4.1 (2.1)	4.8 (2.3)
ACG score (median, IQR)[b]	0.29 (0.22–0.42)	0.25 (0.18–0.39)
Number of medications at baseline (mean, SD)	6.6 (3.3)	7.1 (3.2)
Number of changes in medications in the 9 months prior to baseline	3.9 (2.7)	3.9 (2.8)
Number of symptom-focused medications at baseline		
0	203 (33)	150 (25)
1	161 (26)	165 (28)
2 or more	258 (41)	281 (47)

p value < 0.05 for difference between groups for age, number of chronic conditions, ACG score, and number of medications (overall and symptom-focused) at baseline

[a] From a list of 27 chronic conditions

[b] ACG scores for some subjects are below the enrollment threshold because these scores shifted between the time these subjects were identified as eligible to participate to the time they were enrolled

Table 2 Number of medication changes between baseline and 9 months, intervention vs. control group

	Intervention $N = 622$	Control $N = 596$	Adjusted difference in number of medication changes[a]	p value
Total number of changes to medication regimen (mean, SD)	4.04 (2.8)	3.62 (2.7)	0.55	.001
Total number of changes of symptom-focused medications (mean, SD)	1.38 (1.5)	1.27 (1.5)	0.20	.003

[a] Adjusted for baseline subject characteristics and clustering

(under 0.27 vs. 0.27 or greater), number of medications at baseline (under 7 vs 7 or more), and number of symptom-focused medications at baseline (0 to 1 vs. 2 or more), with p values for interaction > 0.37 in each comparison.

Exploratory analyses

In an exploratory analysis, we used data from the control group to evaluate the relationship between number of medication changes and the patient-centeredness of treatment planning. On a scale of 3–15 (with 15 being best), the median 3-item PACIC score was 6 (interquartile range, 3–9). There was a non-linear relationship between number of medication changes and 3-item PACIC scores. Compared to subjects with 0–2 medication changes, 3-item PACIC scores were a mean of 0.30 points higher in subjects with 3–5 medication changes, but 0.44 points lower in subjects with 6 or more changes ($p = 0.003$ for difference in scores between categories). After controlling for several potential confounders, the differences remained ($p = .03$; see Additional file 1: Appendix S5 for details).

Discussion

In this controlled clinical trial, the CC-MAP intervention – a nurse based, primary care intervention based on the Guided Care model of care – improved several aspects of prescribing in vulnerable Israeli adults. Compared with usual care, patients receiving the CC-MAP intervention had more changes to their medication

regimens in general, and more changes in their symptom-focused medications. This increased rate of changes may reflect more attentive management to patients' medication-related needs.

Our findings build on prior research on the Guided Care model of care. Past studies have shown that Guided Care improves patient-centered processes of care, including goal-setting, coordination of care, decision support, and patient activation [11–14]. This study adds a new dimension to these findings by improving markers of patient-centered medication management. However, despite benefits in processes of care, a large trial of Guided Care did not demonstrate significantly beneficial effects on health outcomes including self-reported measures of physical and mental health, mortality, and several forms of health services utilization [15, 16]. Although these findings are disappointing, they are not the last word. The trial was underpowered to detect small but clinically meaningful differences in these outcomes, and provided lessons about potential future improvements in this care model [15, 16]. Subsequent work testing refined models of Guided Care are underway, including the CC-MAP trial, which is showing promise for improving these hard outcomes.

One noteworthy aspect of our findings is that improving medication use was not a primary goal of the intervention, and in fact the CC-MAP program had no structured elements that focused explicitly on medications. Rather, the improved markers of medication use that we observed appear to be a beneficial "side effect"

Table 3 Types of medication changes between baseline and 9 months, intervention vs. control group

Types of medication change	Intervention $N = 622$ Mean # of changes (% of total)[a]	Control $N = 596$ Mean # of changes (% of total)[a]	Adjusted difference[b]	p value
Medication additions	1.79 (44%)	1.51 (42%)	2%	0.37
Medication discontinuations	1.70 (42%)	1.63 (45%)	3%	0.09
Therapeutic substitutions	0.15 (4%)	0.15 (4%)	0%	0.91
Dose increases	0.18 (5%)	0.19 (6%)	1%	0.39
Dose reductions	0.21 (6%)	0.15 (4%)	2%	0.007
TOTAL NUMBER OF CHANGES	4.04 (100%)	3.62 (100%)	–	–

[a] Results show the mean number of each type of medication change within each group, and the percent of all changes attributable to each type of change
[b] Difference between intervention and control group in the percent of changes attributable to each type of change. Adjusted for baseline subject characteristics and clustering

of the more general goals of the CC-MAP program such as improving communication and care coordination. Vulnerable older adults require support in many areas, for example improving pharmacotherapy, assessing and maintaining functional and cognitive abilities, and much more [26]. Yet, it is impractical to offer multiple discrete interventions, each targeted to only one area [27]. In being able to improve a domain of care that was not an explicit focus of the intervention, CC-MAP and Guided Care show promise as a single intervention which that can favorably affect multiple domains.

The first two measures of prescribing that we evaluated – the number of changes in medications overall, and the number of changes in symptom-focused medications – are not standard measures of prescribing quality, and have not been validated as markers of this construct. Thus, we cannot be sure that the higher number of changes observed in the intervention group represents better care. Our analyses between number of medication changes and treatment-planning components of the PACIC score suggest there may be a threshold effect: a moderate number of changes are associated with more patient-centered care, but a large volume of changes has the opposite effect. However, this finding should be considered preliminary, since it used only a subset of the PACIC score and was unable to control for potentially important confounders.

Although these caveats are important, these markers nonetheless have potential to be valuable [22]. Many commonly used markers of prescribing quality, such as prescribing of drugs to avoid in older adults (e.g. the Beers and STOPP criteria) are not particularly patient-centered [28, 29]. What often matters most for patients is individualizing their medication regimen to suit their particular circumstance, yet studies have shown that clinical inertia and competing demands often prevent appropriate modification of regimens to meet changing patient needs [30–32]. Although more changes are not always better, in this context they may reflect more attention to individual patient circumstances [33].

Additional findings also shed light on the meaning of the increased rate of medication changes observed in the intervention group. The total number of medications used by intervention subjects remained stable despite the higher number of medication changes. The intervention thus appears to have enhanced "fine-tuning" of medications rather than adding to the already-large numbers of medications used by study subjects. It is also noteworthy that the intervention did not preferentially affect one type of medication change or one class of medications. This appears to reflect a generalized effect of the intervention rather than focused changes in one specific area.

Our study has several limitations. Due to practical considerations the selection of intervention and control clinics was not random. However, we were able to control for multiple baseline characteristics of subjects, including their pre-baseline rate of medication changes, which substantially reduces potential for bias in our results. Medication use was ascertained using pharmacy dispensing records. As a result, our measures of medication use are affected both by what medications the physician(s) ordered and patients' adherence to obtaining those medications; we are unable to distinguish the relative contribution of each. Nonetheless, this does not affect our conclusions since both physician prescribing and patient adherence are important facets of medication use that may be improved by the intervention. In addition, we were unable to account for medications not captured in Clalit databases. However, this likely accounts for only a small fraction of medications filled, given strong incentives to fill medications using Clalit insurance benefits, and is unlikely to differ between intervention and control subjects. Finally, we did not evaluate the impact of the intervention on clinical outcomes such as medication errors, hospitalizations, or symptom control; these will be important avenues for future research.

Conclusions
The CC-MAP intervention, a nurse-based primary care program based on the Guided Care model of care, improved markers of patient-centered prescribing in vulnerable adults. With further attention to medication-related issues, this program – which had little explicit focus on medication use – might further improve prescribing and improve medication-related outcomes in vulnerable older adults.

Abbreviations
ACG: Adjusted Clinical Group; CC-MAP: Comprehensive Care for Multimorbid Adults Project; PACIC: Patient Assessment of Chronic Illness Care

Acknowledgements
The authors thank W. John Boscardin, PhD for guidance on statistical issues and Alexander Smith, MD, MPH for his help adjudicating drug classification decisions.

Funding
This work was supported by the Gertner Institute, Clalit Health Services, and by the University of California San Francisco Research Allocation Program. The sponsors had no role in the study design, methods, subject recruitment, data collection, analysis, preparation of manuscripts, or the decision to publish.

Authors' contributions
Study concept and design: MAS, ML, RDB, ES. Subject recruitment and data collection: RDB, ES. Analysis and interpretation of data: MAS, ML, RDB, ES. Drafting of initial version of the manuscript: MAS. Review of manuscript for critical intellectual content: ML, RDB, ES. All authors read and approved the final manuscript.

Competing interests
Dr. Steinman has served as a consultant for iodine.com. Mr. Low and Drs Balicer and Shadmi report no conflicts.

Author details
[1]University of California, 3333 California St, San Francisco, CA 94118, USA. [2]San Francisco VA Health Care System, 4150 Clement St, Box 181G, San Francisco, CA 94121, USA. [3]Clalit Research Institute, Tel Aviv, Israel. [4]University of Haifa, Haifa, Israel.

References
1. Steinman MA, Hanlon JT. Managing medications in clinically complex elders: "There's got to be a happy medium". JAMA. 2010;304(14):1592–601.
2. Osterberg L, Blaschke T. Adherence to medication. N Engl J Med. 2005; 353(5):487–97.
3. Boyd CM, Darer J, Boult C, Fried LP, Boult L, Wu AW. Clinical practice guidelines and quality of care for older patients with multiple comorbid diseases: implications for pay for performance. JAMA. 2005;294(6):716–24.
4. Fried TR, Tinetti ME, Iannone L, O'Leary JR, Towle V, Van Ness PH. Health outcome prioritization as a tool for decision making among older persons with multiple chronic conditions. Arch Intern Med. 2011;171(20):1854–6.
5. McMullen CK, Safford MM, Bosworth HB, et al. Patient-centered priorities for improving medication management and adherence. Patient Educ Couns. 2015;98(1):102–10.
6. Viswanathan M, Golin CE, Jones CD, Ashok M, Blalock SJ, Wines RC, Coker-Schwimmer EJ, Rosen DL, Sista P, Lohr KN. Interventions to improve adherence to self-administered medications for chronic diseases in the United States: a systematic review. Ann Intern Med. 2012;157(11):785–95.
7. Jackson GL, Powers BJ, Chatterjee R, et al. Improving patient care. The patient centered medical home. A systematic review. Ann Intern Med. 2013; 158(3):169–78.
8. Boyd CM, Boult C, Shadmi E, et al. Guided care for multimorbid older adults. Gerontologist. 2007;47(5):697–704.
9. Boult C, Reider L, Frey K, et al. Early effects of "guided care" on the quality of health care for multimorbid older persons: a cluster-randomized controlled trial. J Gerontol A Biol Sci Med Sci. 2008;63(3):321–7.
10. Kuntz JL, Safford MM, Singh JA, et al. Patient-centered interventions to improve medication management and adherence: a qualitative review of research findings. Patient Educ Couns. 2014;97(3):310–26.
11. Boyd CM, Reider L, Frey K, et al. The effects of guided care on the perceived quality of health care for multi-morbid older persons: 18-month outcomes from a cluster-randomized controlled trial. J Gen Intern Med. 2010;25(3): 235–42.
12. Wolff JL, Giovannetti ER, Boyd CM, et al. Effects of guided care on family caregivers. Gerontologist. 2010;50(4):459–70.
13. Marsteller JA, Hsu YJ, Reider L, et al. Physician satisfaction with chronic care processes: a cluster-randomized trial of guided care. Ann Fam Med. 2010; 8(4):308–15.
14. Marsteller JA, Hsu YJ, Wen M, et al. Effects of guided care on providers' satisfaction with care: a three-year matched-pair cluster-randomized trial. Popul Health Manag. 2013;16(5):317–25.
15. Boult C, Reider L, Leff B, et al. The effect of guided care teams on the use of health services: results from a cluster-randomized controlled trial. Arch Intern Med. 2011;171(5):460–6.
16. Boult C, Leff B, Boyd CM, et al. A matched-pair cluster-randomized trial of guided care for high-risk older patients. J Gen Intern Med. 2013;28(5): 612–21.
17. Clalit Research Institute: Multimorbidity Care Management (CC-MAP). http://clalitresearch.org/research-areas/areas/multimorbidity/. Accessed 29 May 2016.
18. Forrest CB, Lemke KW, Bodycombe DP, Weiner JP. Medication, diagnostic, and cost information as predictors of high-risk patients in need of care management. Am J Manag Care. 2009;15(1):41–8.
19. Singer SR, Hoshen M, Shadmi E, et al. EMR-based medication adherence metric markedly enhances identification of nonadherent patients. Am J Manag Care. 2012;18(10):e372–7.
20. Marom O, Rennert G, Stein N, Landsman K, Pillar G. Characteristics and trends in hypnotics consumption in the largest health care system in Israel. Sleep Disord. 2016;2016:8032528.
21. Lund BC, Chrischilles EA, Carter BL, Ernst ME, Perry PJ. Development of a computer algorithm for defining an active drug list using an automated pharmacy database. J Clin Epidemiol. 2003;56(8):802–6.
22. Lam KD, Miao Y, Steinman MA. Cumulative changes in the use of long-term medications: a measure of prescribing complexity. JAMA Intern Med. 2013; 173(16):1546–7.
23. Cohen CJ, Flaks-Manov N, Low M, Balicer RD, Shadmi E. High-risk case identification for use in comprehensive complex care management. Popul Health Manag. 2015;18(1):15–22.
24. Shadmi E, Balicer RD, Kinder K, Abrams C, Weiner JP. Assessing socioeconomic health care utilization inequity in Israel: impact of alternative approaches to morbidity adjustment. BMC Public Health. 2011;11:609.
25. Glasgow RE, Wagner EH, Schaefer J, Mahoney LD, Reid RJ, Greene SM. Development and validation of the patient assessment of chronic illness care (PACIC). Med Care. 2005;43(5):436–44.
26. Wenger NS, Shekelle PG. Assessing care of vulnerable elders: ACOVE project overview. Ann Intern Med. 2001;135(8 Pt 2):642–6.
27. Boult C, Green AF, Boult LB, Pacala JT, Snyder C, Leff B. Successful models of comprehensive care for older adults with chronic conditions: evidence for the Institute of Medicine's "retooling for an aging America" report. J Am Geriatr Soc. 2009;57(12):2328–37.
28. American Geriatrics Society Beers Criteria Update Expert Panel. American Geriatrics Society 2015 updated beers criteria for potentially inappropriate medication use in older adults. J Am Geriatr Soc. 2015; 63(11):2227–46.
29. Gallagher P, Ryan C, Byrne S, Kennedy J, O'Mahony D. STOPP (screening tool of older Person's prescriptions) and START (screening tool to alert doctors to right treatment). Consensus validation. Int J Clin Pharmacol Ther. 2008;46(2):72–83.
30. Kerr EA, Lucatorto MA, Holleman R, Hogan MM, Klamerus ML, Hofer TP. Monitoring performance for blood pressure management among patients with diabetes mellitus: too much of a good thing? Arch Intern Med. 2012; 172(12):938–45.
31. Sussman JB, Kerr EA, Saini SD, et al. Rates of Deintensification of blood pressure and glycemic medication treatment based on levels of control and life expectancy in older patients with diabetes mellitus. JAMA Intern Med. 2015;175(12):1942–9.
32. Steinman MA, Patil S, Kamat P, Peterson C, Knight SJ. A taxonomy of reasons for not prescribing guideline-recommended medications for patients with heart failure. Am J Geriatr Pharmacother. 2010;8(6):583–94.
33. Yam FK, Lew T, Eraly SA, Lin HW, Hirsch JD, Devor M. Changes in medication regimen complexity and the risk for 90-day hospital readmission and/or emergency department visits in U.S. veterans with heart failure. Res Social Adm Pharm. 2016;12(5):713–21.

16

Health behaviors influencing depressive symptoms in older Koreans living alone: secondary data analysis of the 2014 Korean longitudinal study of aging

Heejung Kim[1,2], Sooyoung Kwon[1*] iD, Soyun Hong[1] and Sangeun Lee[1]

Abstract

Background: Geriatric depression is a societal problem, specifically in those living alone in Korea. This study aims are to investigate (1) how sociodemographic factors, health status, and health behaviors are differently associated with depressive symptoms in older Koreans living alone compared to those living with others and (2) how living arrangements attenuated or strengthened the associations between four types of health behaviors and depressive symptoms.

Methods: This secondary data analysis was conducted using data from the 2014 Korean Longitudinal Study of Aging. A structured survey assessing sociodemographic factors, health status, and health behaviors was conducted with people aged 65 or older who lived alone ($n = 1359$) and living with others ($n = 2864$). A multiple linear regression with interaction terms was conducted between mean-centered health behaviors and the status of living alone. All statistical analyses were performed using SPSS Statistics 23.0, and the two-tailed level of significance was set at 0.05.

Results: Those living alone reported higher levels of depressive symptoms than those living with others ($M_{diff} = 2.129$, $SE = 0.005$, $p < 0.001$). The variance of depressive symptoms explained by 13 variables was 18.1% for those living alone compared to 23.7% for those living with others. Compared to health behaviors, sociodemographic factors and health status more explained depressive symptoms, specifically with psychiatric disorders, pain, and impaired functionality as risk factors. Smoking, alcohol abstinence, physical inactivity, and social inactivity were associated with more depressive symptoms. Living arrangements moderated the association between depressive symptoms and each health behavior, except for physical inactivity (all p values < 0.001).

Conclusions: Older Koreans living alone were exposed to different risk factors for depressive symptoms compared to those living with others. Non-modifiable sociodemographic and health status factors were highly associated with depressive symptoms relative to health behaviors; thus, it is important to conduct early assessment and classification of vulnerable subgroups regarding geriatric depression. Specific assessment instruments should be prepared in practice according to living arrangements among older Koreans. Targeted interventions are essential to addressing living arrangements and modifying health behaviors to reduce smoking, alcohol consumption, and social inactivity, specifically in those living alone.

Keywords: Older adult, Health behavior, Depressive symptoms, Living arrangement, Moderation, Korean longitudinal study of aging, Secondary data analysis

* Correspondence: soo.kwon97@gmail.com
[1]College of Nursing, Yonsei University, Seoul, South Korea
Full list of author information is available at the end of the article

Background

Depression is one of the most prevalent mental health problems and is associated with general health and quality of life, specifically in late adulthood [1–3]. Most older adults seem to be exposed to a high risk of depression because they experience a series of losses, such as the death of significant others, retirement, or health problems [4–6]. Bereavement of a loved one results in social isolation and loneliness, which are significant risk factors for poor mental health and low quality of life [7, 8]. Some studies have reported that older adults experience a relatively lower socioeconomic status (SES) than that prior to retirement, which negatively affects mental health [3, 6]. Both social support and social strain differently mediate the relationship between increasing loneliness and decreasing well-being in retired older adults [6, 7]. Previous studies have investigated the diverse types of risk factors related to mental health, and living arrangement is one of the most important factors related to the complex nature of multidimensional vulnerability to depression in late adulthood [9–11].

Living alone influences mental health in the older adult population. Compared to those living with others, older adults living alone reported higher levels of depressive symptoms in several countries, such as Japan, Singapore, Taiwan, and the United States [8–10, 12]. In general, 20–30% of older Asians living alone reported significant depressive symptoms, a ratio that is significantly higher than the 12–18% reported among those living with others [8, 9]. In addition, older Americans living alone reported significantly more depressive symptoms (mean = 4.22, standard deviation [SD] = 4.56) than those living with a family member (mean = 3.36, SD = 3.71, $p < 0.05$) [10]. Similarly, up to 41% of older Koreans living alone reported depressive symptoms, which was significantly higher than up to 30% of those living with others [13, 14]. Oh and colleagues also reported that older Koreans living alone had a higher prevalence of depressive symptoms than those with any other type of living arrangement, such as living with or without a spouse in either an extended or a nuclear family [15].

Korean researchers, clinicians, and policy makers have paid attention to the vulnerability to depression in older adults living alone for several reasons. South Korea is the fastest-aging country among the Organization for Economic Cooperation and Development (OECD) countries, and Korea is also experiencing a rapid increase in one-person households [16, 17]. Older adults living alone comprised 23.0% of the aging population in 2014 [18], a dramatic increase from 13.6% in 1994 [18]. The number of people aged at least 65 years old or older living alone was estimated to be approximately 1.38 million in 2015; the number is estimated to increase to 3.43 million over the next 20 years [19]. The absolute and relative proportions of those living alone in the population mean that a new health care system must respond to the aging one-person household, as the family caregiving system has weakened in Korea due to changes of traditional and cultural perspectives on senior care [13].

In addition, older Koreans are less likely to receive appropriate treatment or perform self-management, despite high levels of depressive symptoms and related mental health problems [13]. In general, depression in older adults is under-reported and under-treated because older adults think that depression is part of the aging process [3, 20]. Specifically, older Korean adults have negative and passive views regarding mental health treatment. One study showed that only 20.9% of participants intend to use mental health services, although almost half of the subjects (49.3%) had issues with depression [21]. Because depression is more costly than other chronic physical diseases [3], untreated depression poses an increased individual and societal burden, influencing morbidity in conjunction with other chronic diseases and influencing mortality secondary to suicide [3, 22, 23]. The Global Burden of Disease Study 2010 identified depressive disorders as the second leading cause of long-term disability, designating it a major public health priority [22]. Older Korean adults are one of the most vulnerable populations to suicide; the suicide rate of older adults in South Korea has increased five-fold during the past two decades (approximately 70 people per every 100,000 in 2014), corresponding to the highest rate among the OECD countries [24].

However, there is limited information for understanding geriatric depression in older adults living alone and for developing specific prevention, detection, and treatment plans. Previous studies have shown that individual characteristics, such as being female, having poor self-rated health, and having impairments in both activities of daily living (ADLs) and instrumental activities of daily living (IADLs), are associated with depression in those living alone [10, 12, 14]. Although geriatric depression has great heterogeneity across people's life spans and individual characteristics [3], few studies have conducted subgroup analyses to examine specific risk factors, particularly regarding different living arrangements [9, 12]. Moreover, these identified factors are more likely to be non-modifiable; therefore, it is difficult to improve the situation using individual efforts for the purposes of health promotion.

In this study, we focus on daily lifestyle health behaviors, which are considered the key components of self-management in disease prevention, treatment options, and physical and mental health [25, 26]. Similar to physical health, mental health status is considered to be influenced by health behaviors, such as alcohol consumption, smoking, and physical and social inactivity. It is well established in the literature that exercise is an effective intervention for improving mental health and well-being in later life [27–29]. Social isolation due to living alone and having less frequent contact with significant others is associated with a higher incidence of depression among older adults [9, 12, 14]. However, it is difficult to draw a concrete conclusion about how smoking and alcohol consumption affect depression in older adults. For example, a multisite cohort study showed that older adults with depression were likely to be alcohol abstinent or less-than-moderate drinkers, regardless of smoking status. However, smokers at risk of high alcohol consumption reported a three-fold greater likelihood of being depressed than those who were alcohol abstinent [30]. In contrast, other studies reported non-significant relationships among alcohol consumption, smoking, and depression in older adults [9, 14]. Thus, more research is needed to understand the consistent patterns of multiple health behaviors among depressed older adults in diverse populations, specifically when considering living arrangements [3].

The aim of this study was to examine the differences in the factors associated with depressive symptoms in older Koreans, specifically focusing on health behaviors moderated by living alone. The following research questions were proposed:

(1) What is the difference in the sociodemographic factors, health status, and health behaviors of those living alone compared with those living with others?
(2) How are sociodemographic factors, health status, and health behaviors associated with depressive symptoms in older adults with different living arrangements?
(3) How does living arrangements differently moderate the relationships between depressive symptoms and four specific health behaviors after controlling for sociodemographic factors and health status?

Methods
Design
This was a cross-sectional correlation study with a secondary data analysis.

Description of the primary data source and procedure for data collection
The primary data for this secondary data analysis were the Korean Longitudinal Study of Aging (KLoSA) collected in 2014 and released in 2015 by the Korea Employment Information Service [31]. The KLoSA is a nationally representative longitudinal study aimed at investigating the health and social welfare information of people aged 45 years or older in South Korea. To understand the selected topic with the most current trend, we chose the most recent set of KLoSA data available for public use.

Since 2006, the KLoSA panel survey has been conducted biennially by trained interviewers using a computer-assisted personal interviewing method in which interviewers read questions to respondents from screens and immediately enter their responses. The survey is conducted with identical content for the same respondents from the first to fifth waves to collect observations at multiple times [32]. The survey targeted the middle-aged and older population nationwide, except in island areas. The sample was randomly selected using a multistage, stratified probability sampling design based on geographical areas and housing types across the nation. At the first data collection, 10,254 individuals in 6171 households participated in the interview, and 7029 subjects remained in 2014, which represented 72.8% of the original respondents [31].

Samples of secondary data analysis
Among the 7029 participants in the 2014 KLoSA dataset, 4223 eligible subjects were included in this study after excluding those aged younger than 65 years old (n = 2803) and those with incomplete reports (n = 3) for the Center for Epidemiological Studies-Depression Scale short-form 10 item (CES-D10). Older adults living alone were defined as individuals aged 65 years old or older in 2014 who reported only one member in a single generation household (n = 1359). The other comparison group included older adults who were 65 years old or older in 2014 and who lived with any members in the same house (n = 2864).

Measures
Depressive symptoms were measured using the Boston version of the CES-D10 in the 2014 KLoSA survey. The CES-D, which was developed by Radloff (1977), is a screening tool used to assess the depressive symptoms experienced during the most recent week. Each item was measured on a 4-point Likert scale (0 = *very rarely* or *less than once a day*; 3 = *almost always* or *5–7 days during the past week*). After two items were reversely recoded to calculate a total CES-D10 score, a composite score was generated by summing ten items. Higher scores indicated more depressive symptoms (range: 0–30). In this study, the Cronbach's alpha coefficient for the CES-D10 was 0.848 in total, 0.841 in those living alone, and 0.853 in those living with others. We used CES-D scores as a continuous variable in line with the methodology employed in previous studies [12, 14, 33] because (1) we aimed to compare our findings to the previous studies' findings, (2) CES-D was developed to offer screening rather than as a comprehensive diagnostic test, and (3) inconsistency arises when using a specific cutoff to differentiate depressed and non-depressed groups in different populations [28].

Sociodemographic factors were included as categorical variables: age, gender, education level, and SES. Considering normative information about older Koreans, the three age groups were categorized as young–old (65–74; coded as 0), old–old (75–84), and oldest–old (85 and over). Gender was dichotomized as female and male (coded as 0). Education level was classified into no school education (coded as 0), elementary school, middle school, high school, and college or above. Self-perceived SES was classified into 3 groups: low, middle (coded as 0), and high.

Self-rated pain was dichotomized as 0 = *none* and 1 = *any pain experienced in one or more body parts*. Psychiatric illness was either diagnosed by a physician or self-reported as having any psychiatric symptoms (coded as 1) and was otherwise coded as 0. A self-rated health status was assessed using the following question: "In general, would you say your health is excellent, very good, good, fair, or poor?" Higher scores indicated perceptions of poorer health status, while the good group was coded as 0. Chronic medical conditions were accounted for in the number of self-reported diagnoses, such as hypertension, diabetes mellitus, any type of cancer, chronic lung disease, liver disease, heart disease, cerebral vascular disease, or rheumatoid arthritis, which are the most frequent conditions reported by older Koreans [34]. Each condition was reported based on 0 = *absent* and 1 = *present*, based on symptoms experienced and medical diagnoses. The impaired functionality of older adults was measured based on LaPlante's expanded ADLs and IADLs scales, including grocery shopping, getting to places, performing light housework, preparing meals, bathing, getting outside, walking, dressing, managing money, transferring, managing medications, using the restroom, using the telephone, and eating [35]. Each item was recoded as 0 = *completely independent* or 1 = *partial/completely dependent*, and the sum of the scores for the 14 items was used in the data analysis. Higher scores indicated that older adults were more dependent on others when performing ADLs and IADLs in daily life. In this study, the Cronbach's alpha coefficient for the LaPlante's ADLs and IADLs was 0.963 in total, 0.958 in those living alone, and 0.967 in those living with others.

Smoking and alcohol use were dichotomized as 0 = *non-smoker* or *non-drinker* and 1 = *current smoker* or *active alcohol user*. The physically active group was defined as those who exercised more than once a week (coded as 0); the others were coded as 1. A lack of social participation was coded as 1, while participation in any social activities, such as attending religious gatherings, meeting friends, volunteering, or joining hobby clubs, was coded as 0.

Analysis

We calculated the weighted proportions, means, and SDs of sociodemographic characteristics, health status,

and health behaviors between older Koreans living alone and those living with others. The missing data for all the variables tested were 0.002%. We did not complete missing data imputation because the total amount of missing data was less than 5.0%, and a missing data analysis found that such missing data occurred at random [36]. All analyses were conducted by applying population weights, which were calculated based on the following: (a) a two-staged stratified sampling probability due to the design effect; (b) the non-response-adjusted weight to reduce the non-response bias; and (c) the benchmark weight, reflecting changes in the general distribution of the total population of the Republic of Korea in 2014 [31].

For preliminary comparison, multivariate linear regression models were used to evaluate the relationship of depressive symptoms with sociodemographic characteristics (Block 1), health statuses (Block 2), and health behaviors (Block 3) in older adults living alone and those living with others. Assumptions of the multivariate linear regression analyses (univariate and multivariate normality, linearity, homoscedasticity, and diagnostic testing for multicollinearity and independence of errors) were met [36].

A multiple linear regression with an interaction term was conducted to assess the associations between health behaviors and depressive symptoms moderated by living arrangement. Age, gender, and low SES were included as covariates in Step 1. The four health behaviors were entered in Step 2 to test each main effect on depressive symptoms over and beyond three covariates, while living arrangement was entered in Step 3. Finally, all the interaction terms between each health behavior and living arrangement were entered in Step 4 to examine the moderating effects. We decided not to include health status variables, which have spurious associations simultaneously with both health behaviors and depressive symptoms. Four health behaviors and living arrangements were mean-centered. A significant standardized regression coefficient and change in R^2 for the interaction term indicated a significant moderation effect [37]. All statistical analyses were performed using IBM SPSS Version 23.0, and the two-tailed level of significance was set at 0.05.

Results

Sociodemographic and health-related characteristics of the sample

Table 1 presents the sociodemographic and health-related characteristics (health status and behaviors) of the weighted sample. The mean age of older Koreans in this study was 73.81 (SD = 6.68) years, and 58.1% were females. Half of the respondents had either no education (22.1%) or had only attended elementary school (34.8%). Most of them identified their SES as middle (45.3%) or low (52.4%). Almost half of the respondents rated their health

Table 1 Group differences in sociodemographic and health-related characteristics

Variables	Overall	Those living alone mean (SD) or weighted %	Those living with others mean (SD) or weighted %	p value
Age	73.81 (6.68)	75.12 (6.68)	72.99 (6.54)	< 0.001
LaPlante ADL/IADL impairment	0.98 (2.92)	1.01 (2.87)	0.97 (2.95)	< 0.001
Number of chronic diseases	0.14 (0.41)	0.15 (0.43)	0.14 (0.39)	< 0.001
CES-D10 scores	7.62 (5.60)	8.52 (5.52)	7.05 (5.59)	< 0.001
Gender[a]				
Female	58.1	76.6	46.5	< 0.001
Education				
No school attended	22.1	30.0	17.1	< 0.001
Elementary school	34.8	37.2	33.4	
Middle school	16.7	14.3	18.2	
High school	17.9	12.8	21.1	
College or above	8.5	5.7	10.2	
Socioeconomic status				
High	2.3	1.7	2.7	< 0.001
Middle	45.3	37.7	50.0	
Low	52.4	60.6	47.3	
Self-rated health				
Excellent	0.6	0.4	0.8	< 0.001
Very good	15.8	14.0	16.9	
Good	44.2	39.5	47.2	
Fair	30.5	36.6	26.7	
Poor	8.9	9.4	8.5	
Pain[a]				
Present	71.3	74.9	69.0	< 0.001
Psychiatric illness[a]				
Diagnosed	5.6	6.4	5.1	< 0.001
Smoking status[a]				
Current smoker	10.2	7.8	11.7	< 0.001
Alcohol use[a]				
Active drinker	27.2	21.3	30.9	< 0.001
Regular exercise[a]				
More than once a week	32.2	31.4	32.7	< 0.001
Social activity [a]				
Participating	71.1	73.0	68.1	< 0.001

SD Standard deviation; *CES-D10* the Center for Epidemiologic Studies Depression Scale-10 items, *ADL/IADL* Activities of daily living/Instrumental activities of daily living
[a], the variable was dichotomized

as good (44.2%), followed by fair (30.5%), very good (15.8%), poor (8.9%), and excellent (0.6%). On average, they experienced 0.98 functional impairments based on LaPlante's ADL/IADL (SD = 2.92), 0.14 chronic diseases (SD = 0.41), and a score of 7.62 on the CES-D10 (SD = 5.60). Approximately 5.6% of them were diagnosed with or self-recognized a psychiatric illness. The percentage of those experiencing any pain was 71.3%. The percentage of people who smoked or drank alcohol was 10.2% and 27.2%, respectively, while 32.2% of the participants regularly exercised more than once a week. More than 70% of them participated in some type of social activities.

Group comparison of characteristics by living arrangements

Most of the characteristics of participants living alone were significantly different from the characteristics of those living with others. Those who lived alone were slightly older (mean difference [M_{diff}] = 2.129, standard error [SE] = 0.005), had more functional impairments (M_{diff} = 0.036, SE = 0.002), had higher CES-D10 scores (M_{diff} = 1.473, SE = 0.005), and lived with more diagnosed diseases than those living with others (all p values < 0.001). Compared to those living with others, the majority of those living alone were female, educated at a less than middle school level, had a lower SES or poorer health status, and experienced more pain (all p values < 0.001). People who lived alone were less likely to smoke, drink alcohol, and exercise regularly than those living with others (all p values < 0.001). However, those living alone participated in more social activities (73.0%) than those living with others (68.1% and 43.4%, respectively; all p values < 0.001).

Multivariate linear regression analyses in two groups
The results of the multivariate linear regression using the CES-D10 score as the dependent variable and the 13 factors in three blocks are shown in Table 2. The

separate models between older adults living alone and those living with others were statistically significant and explained 18.1% and 23.7% of the variance in the depressive symptoms, respectively. In the model of those living alone, the block of health status explained 10.12% of the variance, followed by the sociodemographic block (7.12%) and the block of health behaviors (0.82%; $F = 28,354.14$, p < 0.001). In the model of those living with others, the block of health status explained 16.91%, followed by 5.69% for the sociodemographic block and 1.06% for the block of health behaviors ($F = 64,147.47$, $p < 0.001$).

Table 2 shows significant factors associated with depressive symptoms in both models. Specifically,

Table 2 Comparison of multivariate linear regression models between two groups

Variables	Those who live alone				Those who live with others			
	B	SE	β	Δ R² change	B	SE	β	Δ R² change
Constant	5.454	0.015			4.204	0.012		
Block 1: Sociodemographic factors				0.071***				0.057***
Age (ref., 65–74)								
75–84	0.496***	0.007	0.044		0.144***	0.006	0.012	
Over 85	0.741***	0.013	0.039		−0.195***	0.011	−0.009	
Gender (ref., male)								
Female	0.073***	0.009	0.006		−0.489***	0.006	−0.044	
Education level (ref., no school)								
Elementary school	−0.008	0.008	−0.001		−0.015*	0.008	−0.001	
Middle school	−0.430***	0.011	−0.027		0.066***	0.009	0.005	
High school	0.904***	0.012	0.055		−0.110***	0.009	−0.008	
College and above	−0.465***	0.017	−0.020		−0.066***	0.011	−0.004	
Socioeconomic status (ref., middle)								
High	0.822***	0.025	0.019		0.990***	0.016	0.029	
Low	1.139***	0.007	0.101		0.808***	0.005	0.072	
Block 2: Health status				0.101***				0.169***
Self-rated health status (ref. good)								
Excellent/Very good	−0.762***	0.010	−0.049		1.037***	0.007	0.071	
Fair/Poor	2.214***	0.008	0.201		2.395***	0.006	0.205	
Numbers of current chronic diseases	−0.234***	0.008	−0.018		−0.173***	0.006	−0.012	
Psychiatric illness	2.463***	0.013	0.109		3.431***	0.012	0.136	
Active pain	0.787***	0.008	0.062		1.545***	0.006	0.128	
LaPlante ADL/IADL impairment	0.221***	0.001	0.114		0.383***	0.001	0.202	
Block 3: Health behaviors				0.008***				0.011***
Active smoking	1.337***	0.013	0.065		−0.070***	0.008	−0.004	
Alcohol drinking	−0.672***	0.009	−0.050		−0.958***	0.006	−0.079	
Physical inactivity	−0.023**	0.007	−0.002		0.103***	0.006	0.009	
Social inactivity	0.678***	0.007	0.057		1.015***	0.006	0.081	
Total adjusted R²				0.181***				0.237***

Dependent variable = Total score of the Center for Epidemiologic Studies Depression Scale-10
ADL/IADL Activities of daily living/Instrumental activities of daily living
* $p < 0.05$, ** $p < 0.01$, *** $p < 0.001$

psychiatric illness, active pain, and impaired functionality of ADL/IADL consistently increased depressive symptoms in both groups; however, a stronger impact was observed in those living with others than in those living alone. The levels of education showed a U-shaped relationship with depressive symptoms in both groups; however, greater variability among educational subgroups was observed in those living alone than in those living with others. In the group living alone, those older than 85, women, and those currently smoking reported increased CES-D10 scores compared to the opposite result being found in those younger than 85, males, and non-smokers. In addition, the excellent health status of those living with others was associated with higher CES-D10 scores, while the reverse relationship was found in those living alone.

Moderation effects of living arrangement on the relationship between depressive symptoms and health behaviors

The main and interaction effects of living arrangement on the relationship between depressive symptoms and four health behaviors are presented in Table 3. Smoking, alcohol abstinence, physical inactivity, and social inactivity were associated with higher levels of depressive symptoms, controlling for age, gender, and low SES. Living arrangement was positively associated with depressive symptoms, indicating a main effect on depressive symptoms. Adding interaction variables during the final stage of the analysis revealed different patterns for each health behavior.

Living arrangement showed significant interaction with smoking, alcohol consumption, and social activity, while there was non-significant interaction with physical activity. The association between active smoking and depressive symptoms was attenuated by taking living arrangement into consideration. However, the association of depressive symptoms with alcohol drinking and social isolation became stronger when considering living arrangement, specifically regarding living alone. The mean level of depressive symptoms for each significant moderator stratified by the living arrangement is illustrated in Fig. 1.

Discussion

This study provides important information about the unique factors of geriatric depression identified among older adults living alone and those living with others, specifically focusing on the moderating effects of health behaviors. In general, older Koreans living alone reported higher levels of depressive symptoms than those living with others, which were similar to the findings of previous reports [12, 15, 38]. Our findings confirmed significant similarities and differences among factors influencing depressive symptoms between the two groups.

Our study findings showed inconsistent directions between smoking and depressive symptoms, depending on living arrangements. Older smokers living alone reported more depressive symptoms; however, older smokers living with others had fewer depressive symptoms. In contrast, alcohol abstinence was consistently associated with more depressive symptoms, similar to previous reports [14, 30]. Smoking and drinking alcohol are considered stress-reducing behaviors in adults [26]. Some studies in Western countries reported smoking and heavy drinking as being positively associated with depression [30, 39, 40]. However, some studies have reported a non-significant relationship between geriatric depression and drinking alcohol and smoking in different populations [9, 38, 41]. Interestingly, smoking and alcohol consumption show an inverse association with depressive symptoms in some Asian countries [14, 41, 42]. In Asian culture, smoking and alcohol consumption play a role in media when participating in social interaction. For example, 27.17% of older men and 4.63% of older women reported social drinking, which was associated with a decreased risk for depression [43]. Thus, this finding implies that health-promoting behavior should be understood in the context of culture to understand different patterns of risk factors reported by diverse types of cultural populations [44].

Physical inactivity was associated with more depressive symptoms, regardless of living arrangements. Several studies reported engaging in physical activity as being effective in reducing depressive symptoms among diverse types of older adults [28, 29, 45]. Exercise may provide opportunities to (1) alter or reduce negative thoughts in daily life, (2) learn a new skill dealing with stress responses, and (3) increase social contact outside of family systems [46]. Some previous studies have shown that older adults reported increased levels of cognition, quality of life, and well-being after receiving physically active interventions [27, 29]. In addition, older adults believe that physical activity could be a non-pharmacological treatment that is alternative to antidepressants for reducing depressive symptoms [26, 47]. A Cochrane Database of Systematic Review [48] reported that exercise moderately reduced depressive symptoms compared to no treatment, antidepressants, and psychological therapies. Thus, increasing physical activity for older adults is recommended due to high levels of acceptability, the prevention of polypharmacy, and the reduction of medication-adherence concerns, specifically for mild to moderate depression [49].

Social inactivity was associated with more depressive symptoms in general, similar to previous reports [14, 38]. In our study, socially inactive individuals do not participate in any activities during social gatherings,

Table 3 Result of multiple linear regression with interaction term

	Variables	Adj. R²	Δ R²	B	SE	β	p value
Step 1	Sociodemographic factors	0.068***	0.068***				
	Aged at 75-84[a]			0.807	0.005	0.068	< 0.001
	Aged over 85[a]			1.629	0.008	0.076	< 0.001
	Gender[b]			0.053	0.005	0.005	< 0.001
	Low socioeconomic status[c]			1.427	0.004	0.127	< 0.001
Step 2	Health behaviors	0.104***	0.035***				
	Active smoking			0.371	0.007	0.020	< 0.001
	Alcohol drinking			−1.307	0.005	−0.104	< 0.001
	Physical inactivity			0.614	0.005	0.051	< 0.001
	Social inactivity			1.957	0.005	0.158	< 0.001
Step 3	Living arrangement	0.109***	0.005***	0.916	0.005	0.080	< 0.001
Step 4	Active smoking × Living arrangement	0.112***	0.003***	0.199	0.002	0.035	< 0.001
	Alcohol drinking × Living arrangement			0.081	0.002	0.015	< 0.001
	Physical inactivity × Living arrangement			−0.001	0.002	0.000	0.678
	Social inactivity × Living arrangement			−0.180	0.002	−0.034	< 0.001

[a]Referent group = aged at 65–74; [b]Referent group = male; [c]Referent group = middle level of socioeconomic status; *** p < 0.001

supportive groups, or organizational meetings. Social support is considered to be a protective factor for dealing with stressful life events experienced by older adults [9, 11]. Inadequate levels of perceived social interaction and support result in loneliness and in a lower quality of life, as well as poor mental health [11]. However, our study added more findings, indicating that the difference within groups was more notable in those living with others than those living alone. Providing adequate levels of social support may critically decrease depressive

symptoms in older adults living with others [9, 11], although grown children are expected to live with their aging parents or to provide support through frequent visits in Asian countries [12]. When older adults living alone have less frequent contact with their family, they seek alternative sources of support from their neighborhood, religious group, or community [11, 12]. Thus, the Korean government operates senior centers that are specialized in caring for those living alone in the community. Community nurses working with those living alone

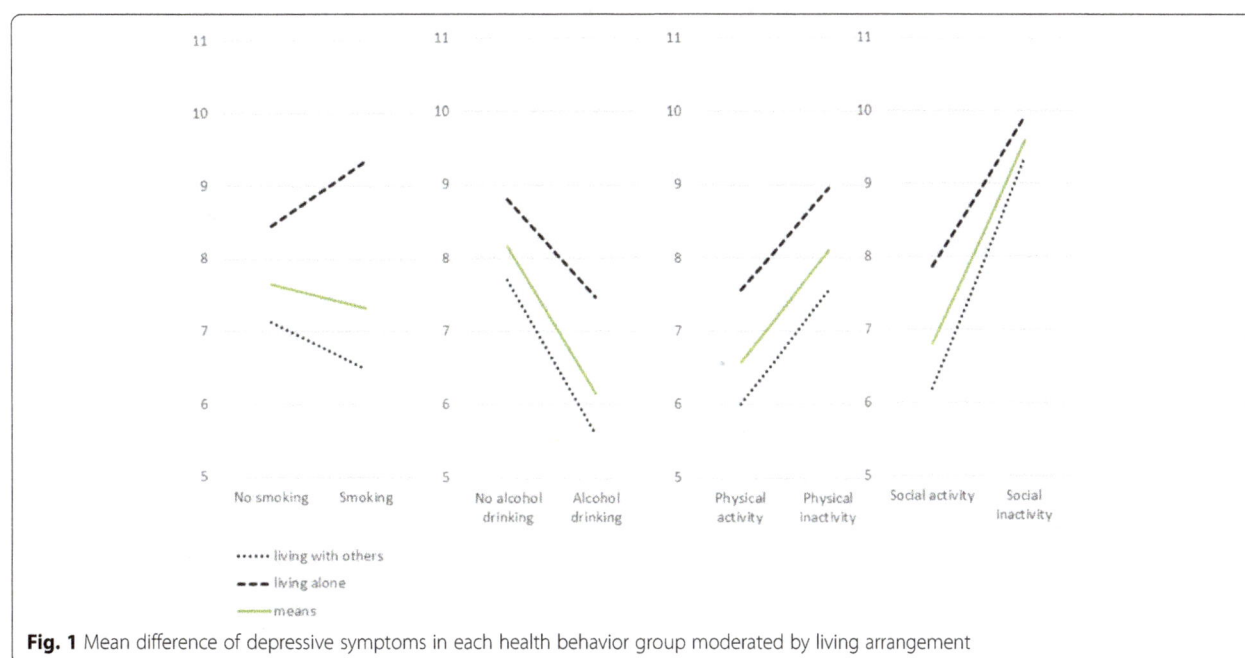

Fig. 1 Mean difference of depressive symptoms in each health behavior group moderated by living arrangement

provide a wide range of interventions or programs to enhance these clients' social connectedness.

The group of older adults living alone showed some expected factors that were associated with more depressive symptoms, such as gender (i.e., women) [3, 14, 15] and advanced age [9, 15, 38], in this study. However, unexpected findings were observed in the group of older adults living with others; namely, men and those aged 75–84 years reported higher scores of depressive symptoms than those younger than 85 years, men, and non-smokers. It is difficult to make a directional conclusion because few studies have reported gender differences in factors associated with depressive symptoms among older Koreans [14, 50]. In general, older men showed lower levels of help-seeking behaviors for informal support than older women when dealing with depressive symptoms [47]. However, both perceived that depression and help-seeking behaviors are greatly influenced by culture; therefore, caution is required when interpreting this finding, and more evidence is necessary to understand older men's depression in Korea.

Similar to previous studies, our findings confirmed that more depressive symptoms were reported in older adults with low SES [1, 38, 51]. In addition, a significant association between education and depressive symptoms was observed in educated individuals in both groups [1, 15]. Because of the high correlation between education levels and income levels, those factors simultaneously affect the levels of SES among Koreans. Those with low SES have a higher chance of depression due to repeated stress from negative life experiences, such as helplessness, poor living conditions, and lack of coping resources [52]. In our study, when we compared subgroups based on education level, those with more depressive symptoms were most likely to have a mid-level education, followed by the lowest and then the highest education. Although educational attainment is associated with stress appraisal when dealing with psychological distress and physical illness [52], this U-shaped relationship between education level and depressive symptoms was not fully explained in previous reports about Korean populations [13–15]. Further investigation is required to develop tailored interventions based on different levels of education.

Unexpectedly, the number of chronic diseases was weakly associated with depressive symptoms, dissimilar to previous studies [1, 3, 15, 38, 51, 53]. Previous studies showed that a combination of multiple chronic disease diagnoses has a limited ability to predict depressive symptoms, although each diagnosis, such as diabetes, stroke, heart disease, and head trauma, uniquely increases depression scores [14, 38]. Instead, psychiatric illness is a consistent factor that increases depressive symptoms, regardless of living arrangements, similar to

the previous report [54]. The status of psychiatric illness may affect the age of onset, the number of lifetime episodes, somatic symptoms, and comorbidities contributing to or resulting from the psychopathology of geriatric depression [3]. Thus, future studies should focus on a specific disease group to differentiate the impacts of various diseases on depressive symptoms among older adults, given that each medical condition has a unique disease trajectory and socio-demographic characteristics [14, 38].

Poor health status, pain, and functional impairments were common factors that increased the depressive symptoms in both groups, similar to previous reports [3, 14, 53]. Those conditions are considered to be age-related factors necessary for maintaining independent living, which is highly associated with increased depressive symptoms [3, 55]. A nationwide survey of the Taiwan Longitudinal Study suggested that those living alone are sufficiently competent to handle their own daily living and manage their medical conditions [12]. However, as functionality decreases with age, an individual's capacity of self-management and self-care mechanisms of health highly depends on impaired function that individual has suffered from chronic diseases [51]. In addition, those factors influence an individual's presentation of atypical symptoms resulting from depression at different levels, which increase the likelihood of being under-detected and underestimated in depressed adults [38]. Thus, the early detection of those factors to differentiate risk factors and atypical symptoms is critically important to provide symptom-based interventions when co-residents are absent.

In clinical implication, depressive symptoms in older Koreans were mostly associated with sociodemographic factors and health status rather than health behaviors, regardless of living arrangement. It is important to assess both the depressive mood and relevant characteristics of older adults in general and to classify the vulnerable subgroups based on predisposing factors of depression. The screening instrument, such as the geriatric depression screening scale [56], is associated with symptoms rather than risk factors. Thus, identification of even non-modifiable factors is important to clearly define the most vulnerable group. In addition, targeted interventions should be designed to consider the unique characteristics and situations of older adults living alone when simultaneously modifying multiple health behaviors differently.

Study limitations and future research

Most of the study's limitations resulted from the study's design, which consisted of a secondary data analysis with cross-sectional data. First, we were unable to include any variables that reflected the influence of the duration of living alone or any recent changes in living arrangements on depressive symptoms. Some research has shown that the impact of living alone is attenuated over time [14]; thus, further research should include variables differentiating between the short- and long-term effects of living alone to maximize the advantage of repeated measures in longitudinal surveys. Second, self-report instruments have limitations in terms of diagnosing major depressive disorder, requiring instant medical attention. Thus, further research must examine the proportion of those diagnosed with major depressive disorder medically to determine the appropriate clinical action for the most vulnerable subgroups of older adults. Third, we included limited numbers of variables associated with health behaviors, namely those available in the primary data. Previous research has shown significant relationships between geriatric depression and other variables, such as diet and sleep [9, 14]. Hence, we suggest that further studies include more extensive information on health behaviors associated with this topic. Health-lifestyle theories have emphasized integrated strategies to simultaneously modify multiple health behaviors for more effective and sustainable health promotion relative to single-behavior modification [26]. The distinct impact of each health behavior on depression is not identical to the cumulative effect of a combination of multiple activities [14]. Further research is required to confirm the best combination of health behaviors to reduce depression in older Koreans living alone, targeting both common and situation-specific depression components.

Conclusion

Health behaviors were weakly associated with depressive symptoms relative to non-modifiable sociodemographic and health-status factors. However, different patterns between each health behavior and depressive symptoms were found in this study. Smoking, alcohol abstinence, and social inactivity were associated with more depressive symptoms moderated by living arrangements; however, physical inactivity was associated with depressive symptoms but was not moderated by living arrangements. Further research should focus on the different patterns of geriatric depression among diverse sociodemographic subgroups and specific types of health behaviors. Policy makers and clinicians should better prepare to understand sociodemographic and health-related characteristics to improve the mental health and quality of life of emerging older adults who live alone.

Abbreviations
ADLs: Activities of daily living; CES-D10: the Center for Epidemiological Studies-Depression Scale short-form 10 items; IADLs: Instrumental activities of daily living; KLoSA: Korean Longitudinal Study of Aging; OECD: Organization for Economic Cooperation and Development; SES: Socioeconomic status

Funding
This research was supported by Basic Science Research Program through the National Research Foundation of Korea (NRF) funded by the Ministry of Education (NRF-2016R1D1A1B03932013) and Mo-Im Kim Nursing Institute, College of Nursing, Yonsei University.

Authors' contributions
All authors critically reviewed the manuscript, provided significant editing of the article and approved the final manuscript. Each author uniquely contributes in the specific research processes: HK, design and concept of analyses, supervision during preparing the data, statistical analysis and interpretation of data, preparing of the manuscript; SK, preparation of data, assisting of statistical analysis and preparing of the manuscript; SH, design and concept of analyses and preparing of the manuscript; and SL, searching for the literature and preparing of the manuscript.

Competing interests
The authors declare that they have no competing interests.

Author details
[1]College of Nursing, Yonsei University, Seoul, South Korea. [2]Mo-Im Kim Nursing Research Institute, Yonsei University, Seoul, South Korea.

References
1. Jia H, Lubetkin EI. Incremental decreases in quality-adjusted life years (QALY) associated with higher levels of depressive symptoms for US adults aged 65 years and older. Health Qual Life Outcomes. 2013;15:9.
2. World Health Organization. Depression and other common mental disorders. Global health estimates. Geneva. Switzerland: WHO Publishing; 2017.
3. Zivin K, Wharton T, Rostant O. The economic, public health, and caregiver burden of late-life depression. Psychiatr Clin North Am. 2013;36:631–49.
4. Lim HJ, Min DK, Thorpe L, Lee CH. Trajectories of life satisfaction and their predictors among Korean older adults. BMC Geriatr. 2017;17:89.
5. Ogle CM, Rubin DC, Siegler IC. Cumulative exposure to traumatic events in older adults. Aging Ment Health. 2014;18:316–25.
6. Wang M, Shi J. Psychological research on retirement. Annu Rev Psychol. 2014;65:209–33.
7. Chen Y, Feeley TH. Social support, social strain, loneliness, and well-being among older adults. J Soc Personal Relat. 2014;31:141–61.
8. Ng TP, Jin A, Feng L, Nyunt MSZ, Chow KY, Feng L, et al. Mortality of older persons living alone: Singapore longitudinal ageing studies. BMC Geriatr. 2015;15:126.
9. Fukunaga R, Abe Y, Nakagawa Y, Koyama A, Fujise N, Ikeda M. Living alone is associated with depression among the elderly in a rural community in Japan. Psychogeriatrics. 2012;12:179–85.
10. Stahl ST, Beach SR, Musa D, Schulz R. Living alone and depression: the modifying role of the perceived neighborhood environment. Aging Ment Health. 2017;21:1065–71.
11. Yi ES, Hwang HJ. A study on the social behavior and social isolation of the elderly Korea. J Exer Rehabil. 2015;11:125–32.
12. Kao YH, Chang LC, Huang WF, Tsai YW, Chen LK. Health characteristics of older people who rotationally live with families: a nationwide survey. J Am Med Dir Assoc. 2013;14:331–5.
13. Korea Institute for Health and Social Affairs, Korean Ministry of Health and Welfare. Living profiles of older-persons-only households and policy implications. Seoul: Korea Institute for Health and Social Affairs Publishing; 2014.
14. Lee J, Ham MJ, Pyeon JY, Oh E, Jeong SH, Sohn EH, et al. Factors affecting cognitive impairment and depression in the elderly who live alone: cases in Daejeon Metropolitan City. Dement Neurocognitive Disord. 2017;16:12–9.
15. Oh DH, Park JH, Lee HY, Kim SA, Choi BY, Nam JH. Association between living arrangements and depressive symptoms among older women and men in South Korea. Soc Psychiatry Psychiatr Epidemiol. 2015;50:133–41.
16. Organization for Economic Cooperation and Development. Economic surveys: Korea. 2016. https://www.oecd.org/eco/surveys/Korea-2016-OECD-economic-survey-overview.pdf. Accessed 5 Sep 2017.
17. Statistics Korea. Complete enumeration results of the 2016 population and housing census. In: Population and Household press release; 2017. http://kostat.go.kr/portal/eng/pressReleases/1/index.board?bmode=read&aSeq=363132. Accessed 5 Sep 2017.
18. Korea Institute for Health and Social Affairs, Korean Ministry of Health and Welfare. The Korean elderly survey. Seoul: Korea Institute for Health and Social Affairs Publishing; 2014.
19. Korea Institute for Health and Social Affairs, Korean Ministry of Health and

Welfare. State of living alone and policy response strategy of old age. Seoul: Korea Institute for Health and Social Affairs Publishing; 2015.

20. World Health Organization. Mental health and older adults fact sheet. 2016. http://www.who.int/mediacentre/factsheets/fs381/en/. Accessed 5 Sep 2017.

21. Lee KY, Choi SS, Park HS, Lim HJ. A Study of factors affecting on the preference of the elderly's mental health services utilization in rural areas-application of Andersen and Newman's model. Korean journal of. Social Welfare. 2010;62:257–78.

22. Ferrari AJ, Charlson FJ, Norman RE, Patten SB, Freedman G, Murray CJL, et al. Burden of depressive disorders by country, sex, age, and year: findings from the global burden of disease study 2010. PLoS Med. 2013;10:e1001547.

23. Kim YS, Byun HS. Effects of pain on memory, physical function, and sleep disturbance in older adults with chronic disease: the mediating role of depression. J Korean Gerontol Nurs. 2014;16:59–67.

24. Organization for Economic Cooperation and Development. Society at a glance 2014: OECD Social Indicators: OECD Publishing; 2014. http://staging.memofin.fr/uploads/library/pdf/8113171e[1].pdf. Accessed 5 Sep 2017

25. Hong SI, Chen LM. Contribution of residential relocation and lifestyle to the structure of health trajectories. J Ment Health Aging. 2009;21:244–65.

26. Saint Onge JM, Krueger PM. Health lifestyle behaviors among U.S. adults. SSM Popul Health. 2017;3:89–98.

27. Langlois F, Vu TTM, Chassé K, Dupuis G, Kergoat MJ, Bherer L. Benefits of physical exercise training on cognition and quality of life in frail older adults. J Gerontol B Psychol Sci Soc Sci. 2013;68:400–4.

28. Mammen G, Faulkner G. Physical activity and the prevention of depression: a systematic review of prospective studies. Am J Prev Med. 2013;45:649–57.

29. Windle G, Hughes D, Linck P, Russell I, Woods B. Is exercise effective in promoting mental well-being in older age? A systematic review. Aging Ment Health. 2010;14:652–69.

30. Van den Berg JF, Kok RM, van Marwijk HW, van der Mast RC, Naarding P, Oude Voshaar RCO, et al. Correlates of alcohol abstinence and at-risk alcohol consumption in older adults with depression: the NESDO study. Am J Geriatr Psychiatry. 2014;22:866–74.

31. Korea Employment Information Service. KLoSA survey overview. 2016. http://survey.keis.or.kr/klosa/klosa01.jsp. Accessed 5 Sep 2017.

32. Kim JH, Park EC, Lee SG, Lee Y, Jang SI. Effects of social integration on depressive symptoms in Korea: analysis from the Korean longitudinal study of aging (2006–12). Aust Health Rev. 2016;41:222–30.

33. Kim JH, Park EC, Lee SG. The impact of age differences in couples on depressive symptoms: evidence from the Korean longitudinal study of aging (2006-2012). BMC Psychiatry. 2015;15:1–10.

34. Korea Institute for Health and Social Affairs, Korean Ministry of Health and Welfare. Analysis of the survey of living conditions and welfare needs of Korean older persons. Seoul: Korea Institute for Health and Social Affairs Publishing; 2012.

35. LaPlante MP. The classic measure of disability in activities of daily living is biased by age but an expanded IADL/ADL measure is not. J Gerontol B Psychol Sci Soc Sci. 2010;65:720–32.

36. Meyers LS, Gamst G, Guarion AJ. Applied multivariate research. London: Sage Publication Inc; 2006.

37. Aiken L, West SG. Multiple regression: testing and interpreting interactions. Newbury Park: Sage; 1991. p. 28.

38. Niti M, Ng TP, Kua EH, Ho RCM, Tan CH. Depression and chronic medical illnesses in Asian older adults: the role of subjective health and functional status. Int J Geriatr Psychiatry. 2007;22:1087-94.

39. An R, Xiang X. Smoking, heavy drinking, and depression among US middle-aged and older adults. Prev Med. 2015;81:295–302.

40. Boden JM, Fergusson DM, Horwood LJ. Cigarette smoking and depression: tests of causal linkages using a longitudinal birth cohort. Br J Psych. 2010;6:440–6.

41. Cheng HG, Chen S, McBride O, Phillips MR. Prospective relationship of depressive symptoms, drinking, and tobacco smoking among middle-aged and elderly community-dwelling adults: results from the China health and retirement longitudinal study (CHARLS). J Affect Disord. 2016;195:136–43.

42. Lee JC, Park JA, Bae NK, Cho YC. Factors related to depressive symptoms among the elderly in urban and rural areas. J agri med commun health. 2008;2:204–20.

43. Cho MJ, Lee JY, Kim BS, Lee HW, Sohn JH. Prevalence of the major mental disorders among the Korean elderly. J Korean Med Sci. 2011;26(1):10.

44. Kreuter MW, Lukwago SN, Bucholtz DC, Clark EM, Sanders-Thompson V. Achieving cultural appropriateness in health promotion programs: targeted and tailored approaches. Health Educ Behav. 2003;30:133–46.

45. Ku PW, Fox KR, Chen LJ. Physical activity and depressive symptoms in Taiwanese older adults: a seven-year follow-up study. Prev Med. 2009;48:250–5.

46. Craft LL. Potential psychological mechanisms underlying the exercise and depression relationship handbook of physical activity and mental health. London: Routledge; 2013.

47. Atkins J, Naismith SL, Luscombe GM, Hickie IB. Elderly care recipients' perceptions of treatment helpfulness for depression and the relationship with help-seeking. Clin Interv Aging. 2015;10:287–95.

48. Cooney GM, Dwan K, Greig CA, Lawlor DA, Rimer J, Waugh FR, et al. Exercise for depression. Cochrane Database Syst Rev. 2013; https://doi.org/10.1002/14651858.CD004366.pub6.

49. Kok RM, Reynolds CF. Management of Depression in older adults: a review. JAMA. 2017;317(20):2114–22.

50. Lim EJ. Gender differences in the relationship between physical functioning and depressive symptoms in low-income older adults living alone. Nurs Health Sci. 2014;16:381–6.

51. Seo HL, Jung YK, Kim HN. The effects of physical diseases on elderly depression and moderate effects of the self-care performance. J Welfare Aged. 2013;61:57–84.

52. Almeida DM, Neupert SD, Banks SR, Serido J. Do daily stress processes account for socioeconomic health disparities? J Gerontol Series B. 2005;60: S34–9. https://doi.org/10.1093/geronb/60.Special_Issue_2.S34.

53. Hairi NN, Bulgiba A, Mudla I, Said MA. Chronic diseases, depressive symptoms and functional limitation amongst older people in rural Malaysia, a middle income developing country. Prev Med. 2011;53:343–6.

54. Lee MY, Kim YS. Factors influencing suicidal ideation in people with mental disorder. Korean J Health Serv Manag. 2014;8:209–20.

55. Ahlqvist A, Nyfors H, Suhonen R. Factors associated with older people's independent living from the viewpoint of health and functional capacity: a register-based study. Nurs Open. 2016;3:79–89.

56. Yesavage JA, Brink TL, Rose TL, Lum O, Huang V, Adey M, Leirer VO. Development and validation of a geriatric depression screening scale: a preliminary report. J Psychiatr Res. 1983;17:37–49.

17

Physical diagnoses in nursing home residents - is dementia or severity of dementia of importance?

Live Bredholt Jørgensen[1†], Berit Marie Thorleifsson[1*†] (ID), Geir Selbæk[2,3,4], Jūratė Šaltytė Benth[3,5,6] and Anne-Sofie Helvik[2,7,8]

Abstract

Background: Dementia and physical morbidity are primary reasons for nursing home admission globally. However, data on physical morbidity in nursing home residents with and without dementia are scarce. The first aim of the present study was to explore whether presence and severity of dementia were related to the number of physical diagnoses in nursing home residents. The second aim was to explore if the severity of dementia was associated with having registered the most frequent complexes of physical diagnoses when controlling for physical health and demographic factors.

Methods: A total of 2983 Norwegian nursing home residents from two cross-sectional samples from 2004/2005 and 2010/2011 were included in the analysis. By the use of assessment scales, the severity of dementia (Clinical Dementia Rating), physical health (General Medical Health Rating), activities of daily living (Physical Self-Maintenance Scale) and neuropsychiatric symptoms (Neuropsychiatric Inventory Nursing Home) were determined. Physical diagnoses and medications were assembled from the medical records. The physical diagnoses were categorized into complexes, using the ICD-10 chapters. Linear mixed models and generalized linear mixed models were estimated.

Results: Residents with dementia were registered with fewer physical diagnoses than residents without dementia. The frequency of physical diagnoses decreased with increasing severity of dementia. Cardiovascular, musculoskeletal and endocrine, nutritional and metabolic diagnoses were the most common complexes of physical diagnoses in individuals with and without dementia. The odds of having cardiovascular and musculoskeletal diagnoses increased for males and decreased for females with increasing severity of dementia, in contrast to endocrine diagnoses where the odds increased for both genders.

Conclusion: Increasing severity of dementia in nursing home residents may complicate the diagnostics of physical disease. This might reflect a need for more attention to the registration of physical diagnoses in nursing home residents with dementia.

Keywords: Dementia, Cognitive impairment, Prevalence, Comorbidity, Multimorbidity, Physical diagnoses, Gender, Nursing home, Institutionalization

* Correspondence: beritmt@stud.ntnu.no
†Live Bredholt Jørgensen and Berit Marie Thorleifsson contributed equally to this work.
[1]Department of Public Health and Nursing, Norwegian University of Science and Technology (NTNU), Trondheim, Norway
Full list of author information is available at the end of the article

Background

Dementia is a common disease in aged populations [1] caused by different brain disorders. It results in a decline in memory, especially evident in the learning of new information. Additionally, dementia involves behavioural changes, functional impairment, and a decrease in other cognitive abilities such as thinking, judgement and processing of information [2]. There is a clear link between severity of dementia, impairment in activities of daily living (ADL) [3], the risk of institutionalization [4] and mortality [5].

Worldwide 46.8 million people live with dementia, and the number will almost double every 20 years [6] due to an aging population [7]. In Norway, with a population of about 5 million [8], the calculated number of older adults with dementia was approximately 80,000 in 2015 [9, 10]. Dementia is not the only disease affecting aging individuals to a great extent, as older adults generally have a higher risk of experiencing multiple chronic conditions, both psychiatric and physical [11].

Management of the rising prevalence of chronic conditions is a main challenge facing governments and health-care systems globally [12]. As multimorbidity is becoming the normal situation rather than an exception in the aging population [13–16], it is crucial to focus on physical diagnoses, as well as decreased functional status [17]. Common physical diagnoses in the aging population are hypertension, lipid metabolism disorders, diabetes, coronary heart disease, heart failure and cancer [18–21]. Several of these diseases represent vascular risk factors, which may contribute to dementia onset and lead to faster progression of dementia [22–24]. Parkinson's disease, congestive heart failure, cerebrovascular disease, cardiac arrhythmia, osteoporosis and retinal disorders [25] are physical comorbidities which seem to be significantly associated with having dementia.

A dementia diagnosis and increasing cognitive impairment are major reasons for nursing home admissions [4, 21]. Residents without dementia are mainly admitted to nursing homes because of severe physical morbidity which makes it difficult for them to continue living at home [26]. Other important factors associated with nursing home admissions are high age, psychosis and increased number of prescriptions [4, 27].

Several international studies have explored the use of psychotropic drugs [28, 29], the prevalence of dementia [30, 31], depression [32, 33] and neuropsychiatric symptoms in nursing homes [33–36]. However, Scandinavian studies exploring physical morbidities in nursing home residents with and without dementia, are to our knowledge missing.

Previous studies have reported a considerable variation in the number of additional diagnoses registered in older adults living with dementia [25, 37, 38]. Studies from primary care found that individuals with dementia had a

higher number of comorbidities than those without dementia [25, 39]. On the contrary, nursing home residents with dementia had fewer comorbidities than residents without cognitive impairment or dementia [40, 41]. This might describe the health situation of nursing home residents, but it may also reflect a lack of diagnostics in nursing home residents with dementia that do not complain, have difficulties in describing their symptoms or do not receive frequent clinical examination [20, 24].

Literature regarding physical morbidity in nursing home residents with and without dementia frequently focuses on the most common ICD-10 diagnoses [24, 40–42], but few studies arrange diagnoses by the main ICD-10 chapters. According to published nursing home studies, the most commonly registered physical diagnoses are linked to cardiovascular, musculoskeletal and endocrine diseases [24, 40–42].

Information about physical diagnoses in nursing home residents with and without dementia, and whether such comorbidity is related to the severity of dementia, is essential for healthcare planners and care professionals [24]. Thus, the first aim of the present study was to explore whether presence and severity of dementia were related to the number of physical diagnoses in nursing home residents. The second aim was to explore if the severity of dementia was associated with having registered the most frequent complexes of physical diagnoses when controlling for physical health and demographic factors.

Methods
Design

The present study includes data collected from two Norwegian cross-sectional samples of nursing home residents. The first collection took place from November 2004 to January 2005 [43] and the second collection took place from June 2010 to November 2011 [30].

Participants

Both samples included nursing home residents with a stay of minimum 2 weeks [30, 43]. In 2004/2005, residents in 26 nursing homes in 18 municipalities participated, and the selection of municipalities reflected small, medium and large municipalities. A total of 1165 residents were eligible for inclusion, and two refused participation. In 2010/2011, residents from 40 other nursing homes in 31 municipalities were approached in addition to 24 of the 26 nursing homes from the previous sample. A total of 2385 residents were eligible for inclusion, but 423 declined to participate either in person or through their next of kin, 33 had a severe physical diagnosis or terminal condition, one left the nursing home prior to the assessment, 17 died prior to the assessment and 53 were not included without any specific reason. As a result, 1858 participants were included in the second study. In total, 3021 nursing home residents participated in the present study. Thirty-eight residents were excluded due to missing important information (Clinical Dementia Rating), leaving a total of 2983 residents in the analysis (Fig. 1).

Measurements
All medical diagnoses assembled from the medical records were classified by the International Statistical Classification of Diseases and Related Health Problems 10th Revision (ICD-10). The diagnoses were collected at assessment, based on what was registered in the charts. The charts were regularly updated, so several diagnoses could have been added after admission. Mental behavioural disorders (F00-F99) and Alzheimer's disease (G30) were omitted to extract only physical diagnoses. The registered physical diagnoses were categorized into complexes of diagnoses, using the ICD-10 chapters. As other authors commonly choose to present single ICD-10 codes, subgroups of the most common ICD-10 codes were included under each complex of physical diagnoses [19, 25, 38, 39]. A minimum of one subgroup was included under each complex.

Dementia and the severity of dementia were determined by using the Clinical Dementia Rating (CDR) scale. The CDR score was determined by healthcare personnel who was the most familiar with the resident, using all available information about the resident. No information was collected directly from their next of kin. CDR assesses six domains of cognitive and functional performing [44]. The categorical score (0, 0.5, 1, 2, 3) is calculated using an algorithm that gives priority to memory [45]. CDR ≥ 1 defines dementia [46, 47]. The

categorical scores indicate normal cognitive function (CDR = 0), mild cognitive impairment (CDR = 0.5), mild dementia (CDR = 1), moderate dementia (CDR = 2) and severe dementia (CDR = 3). The sum-score of the six domains (CDR sum of boxes) ranges from 0 to 18, where a higher score indicates more severe dementia. There is a high correlation (≥0.9) between the categorical CDR score and the CDR sum of boxes (CDR-SOB) [48, 49]. The Spearman correlation in the present study was 0.93 [30]. Many of the residents were too frail or mentally impaired to take part in standardized dementia work-up such as CT or MRI. Therefore CDR ≥ 1 was used as an indication of dementia in both samples.

Physical health was assessed using the General Medical Health Rating (GMHR) scale [50]. GMHR is a 1-item global rating scale with four categories: good, fairly good, poor and very poor. All available information about physical health and drug use formed the basis for the rating. GMHR has previously been used in large studies including older adults with and without dementia [51] and has been translated and used in Norway [52].

The Personal Activities of Daily Living (P-ADL) score was assessed with the Physical Self-Maintenance Scale (PSMS), which includes six items and results in a total score ranging from 6 to 30 [53]. A high score indicates a low level of ADL functioning.

Neuropsychiatric symptoms (NPS) were assessed using a translated and validated Norwegian version [54] of the Neuropsychiatric Inventory Nursing Home version (NPI-NH) [55]. The 10-item inventory covers the following symptoms: delusion, hallucination, euphoria, agitation/aggression, disinhibition, irritability/lability, depression/dysphoria, anxiety, apathy/indifference and aberrant motor

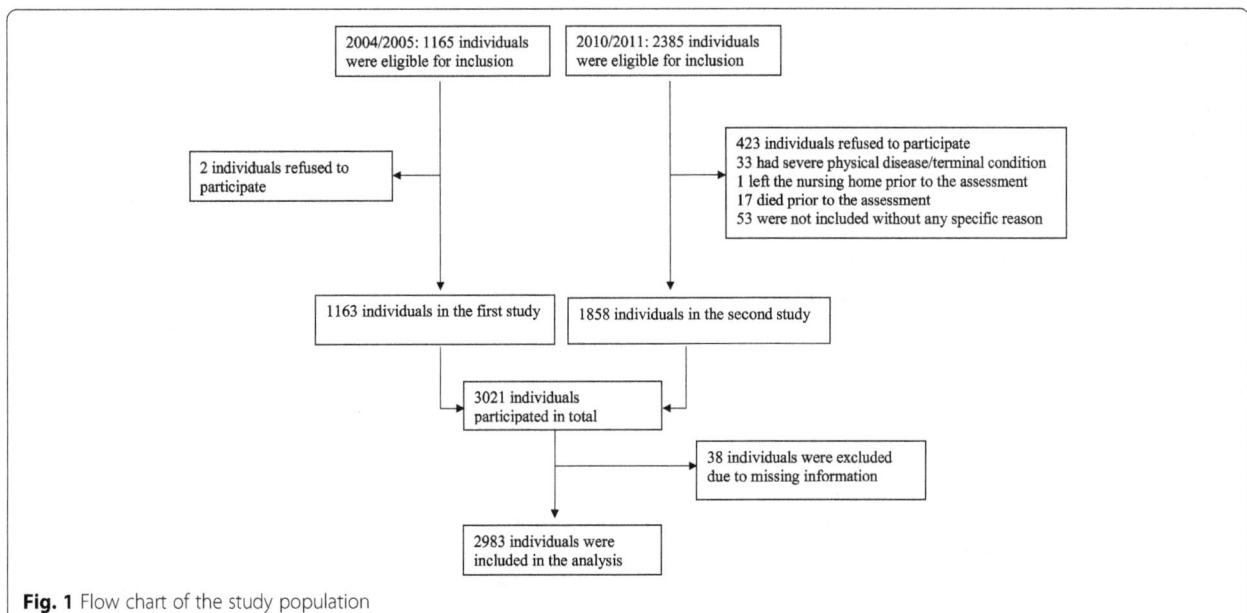
Fig. 1 Flow chart of the study population

behaviour (no/yes). Each symptom is graded by severity (score 0–3) and multiplied by frequency (score 0–4), which provides an item-score from 0 to 12. Based on a previous principal component analysis, subsyndrome scores on psychosis (delusions, hallucination), agitation (agitation/aggression, disinhibition, irritability) and affective symptoms (depression, anxiety) were generated [35, 36, 56]. Apathy/indifference was analysed as a single symptom.

Medications were grouped according to the Anatomical Therapeutic Chemical (ATC) classification system. The ATC-system is a classification of the active ingredients of the drugs and is based on the organ or system they act on, and also their pharmacological, therapeutic and chemical characteristics [57]. The information was collected from the medical record of each resident [43].

Demographic information was determined by use of a standardized questionnaire. The type of unit was recorded from the following: regular unit (RU), special care unit for people with dementia (SCU), rehabilitation unit (REU) and other units (OU), mainly psychogeriatric wards.

Procedure

In both samples, registered nurses with broad clinical experience performed the data collection. All 20 assessors took part in a two-day training course on how to apply the standardized questionnaires prior to the data collection. Data were collected from medical records and a standardized interview with the residents' primary caregivers. Prior to the first study, a pilot study including 41 nursing home residents was conducted to test the inter-rater reliability of the CDR. It was performed between one geriatric psychiatrist (GP) and two assessors, a registered nurse (RN) and a nurse specialized in psychiatry (NP). The kappa values for the global CDR score were 1 (GP vs. NP) and 0.86 (GP vs. RN and NP vs. RN) [43].

Information about the study was given to the residents and to their family members. An explicit consent was not required for enrolment in 2004/2005, but the residents were informed that they could refuse to participate at any stage of the study. In 2010/2011 informed consent was obtained from the resident or their next of kin due to a change in the legislation. The Regional Ethics Committee in the south-east of Norway and the Directorate for Health and Social Affairs recommended and approved the procedures in 2004 and 2010.

Statistical analysis

As data were collected in nursing homes, there might be a hierarchical structure in the data. In addition, some of the participants in the first sample (7.7%) were also included in the second sample. A cluster effect might therefore be present at both the nursing home and participant level, and statistical methods that correctly adjust for such an effect have been used.

Means and standard deviations (SD), or frequencies and percentages, were used to present demographic and clinical characteristics. Linear mixed model for continuous variables and generalized linear mixed model for categorical variables were estimated to compare residents with and without dementia. The models included fixed effects for dementia status, and random effects for either participants or nursing homes or both with participants nested within the nursing home, as appropriate.

To explore whether the severity of dementia was related to the number of physical diagnoses and other factors, a linear mixed model with fixed effects for characteristics and random effects for participants nested within nursing homes was estimated. To assess how certain factors affected the odds of having specific complexes of physical diagnoses, a generalized linear mixed model with the same fixed effects was estimated. The model contained random effects for participants only, as cluster effect on the nursing home level was negligible or not present. Interactions between severity of dementia and gender and age were explored. All multiple models were reduced by applying Akaike Information Criterion (AIC), where the smaller value indicates a better model. In post hoc analysis for factors associated with the number of physical diagnoses and the three most prevalent complexes of physical diagnoses, the GMHR was included to explore whether the level of general medical health influenced an association between level of dementia and the number of physical diagnoses.

Analyses were performed in SPSS v 24 and SAS v 9.4. All statistical tests were two-sided. Results with p-values below 0.05 were considered statistically significant.

Results

Sample characteristics at baseline

The present study included 2983 nursing home residents assessed at two different time-points. In total, 808 residents lived in special care units and 2164 residents lived in other units. Of all participants, 82.8% had dementia (CDR ≥ 1) (Table 1). Among those without dementia (CDR < 1), 81.3% had mild cognitive impairment (CDR = 0.5). Mean (SD) age was 85.1 (7.9) years and 71.5% were females. Individuals with dementia were older than those without dementia. They were also more likely to have a poorer physical health (GMHR), poorer P–ADL functioning (higher PSMS score), higher scores on the NPI subsyndromes agitation, psychosis and affective, and NPI apathy, a longer stay in the nursing home at study inclusion, and to be registered with a lower mean number of drugs.

Factors associated with increasing number of physical diagnoses

Residents without dementia had a higher mean number of physical diagnoses registered than residents with dementia (2.9 versus 2.4) (Table 2). According to the adjusted linear

Table 1 Sample characteristics at baseline

	N (%)	Total	CDR < 1	CDR ≥ 1	P-value[3]
		2983 (100)	513 (17.2)	2470 (82.8)	
Sociodemographics					
Age	Mean (SD)	85.1 (7.9)	84.3 (9.2)	85.3 (7.6)	0.019[1]
Females	N (%)	2132 (71.5)	352 (68.6)	1780 (72.1)	0.137[1]
Education < 10 years	N (%)	2227 (79.7)	376 (78.7)	1851 (80.0)	0.173[2]
Married	N (%)	630 (21.1)	86 (16.9)	544 (22.2)	0.018[2]
Health condition					
GMHR					< 0.001[2]
Good	N (%)	474 (16.1)	101 (20.1)	373 (15.3)	
Fairly good	N (%)	1097 (37.3)	220 (43.7)	877 (36.0)	
Poor	N (%)	1033 (35.1)	142 (28.2)	891 (36.6)	
Very poor	N (%)	335 (11.4)	40 (8.0)	295 (12.1)	
PSMS score	Mean (SD)	18.0 (5.4)	14.9 (5.0)	18.6 (5.2)	< 0.001[1]
NPI Agitation subsyndrome	Mean (SD)	6.0 (8.2)	2.3 (5.1)	6.7 (8.5)	< 0.001[1]
NPI Psychosis subsyndrome	Mean (SD)	2.7 (5.1)	0.9 (3.2)	3.1 (5.3)	< 0.001[1]
NPI Affective subsyndrome	Mean (SD)	3.5 (5.2)	2.4 (4.3)	3.7 (5.3)	< 0.001[1]
NPI Apathy	Mean (SD)	2.0 (3.5)	0.8 (2.3)	2.3 (3.7)	< 0.001[1]
Number of drugs	Mean (SD)	6.6 (3.2)	7.7 (3.6)	6.4 (3.1)	< 0.001[1]
Days in NH[4]	Mean (SD)	931.0 (997.9)	882.5 (1162.8)	941.1 (960.0)	< 0.001[1]

CDR Clinical Dementia Rating, *GMHR* General Medical Health Rating, *PSMS* Physical Self-Maintenance Scale, *NPI* Neuropsychiatric Inventory, *NH* Nursing Home
[1]Adjusted for intra-patient correlations
[2]Adjusted for NH-level
[3]Calculated by estimating linear mixed model for continuous variables and generalized linear mixed model for categorical variables
[4]*p*-value calculated on LN-transformed days in NH

mixed model, residents in special care units were registered with a lower number of physical diagnoses, compared to residents in regular units. Furthermore, lower CDR-SOB, higher age and higher PSMS score were associated with having a higher number of physical diagnoses (Table 3).

Complexes and subgroups of physical diagnoses by dementia (CDR < 1/CDR ≥ 1) and increasing severity of dementia (CDR)

The most frequent complexes of physical diagnoses in individuals with and without dementia were cardiovascular (60.3%), musculoskeletal (23.7%) and endocrine, nutritional and metabolic diagnoses (22.2%) (Table 4). Cardiovascular diagnoses, musculoskeletal diagnoses, respiratory diagnoses and cancer were more frequent in individuals without dementia compared to individuals with dementia. Of the subgroups, cerebrovascular disease, heart failure, inflammatory joint disease and asthma/chronic obstructive pulmonary disease (COPD) were more common in residents without dementia. The prevalence of respiratory diagnoses, and cardiovascular diagnoses such as hypertension, cerebrovascular disease, ischemic heart disease,

Table 2 Number of physical diagnoses

Number of physical diagnoses		Total	CDR < 1	CDR ≥ 1	P-value
0	N (%)	341 (11.4)	24 (4.7)	317 (12.8)	< 0.001[1]
1	N (%)	607 (20.3)	82 (16.0)	525 (21.3)	
2	N (%)	693 (23.2)	127 (24.8)	566 (29.9)	
3	N (%)	601 (20.1)	113 (22.0)	488 (19.8)	
4	N (%)	374 (12.5)	76 (14.8)	298 (12.1)	
5	N (%)	176 (5.9)	50 (9.7)	126 (5.1)	
Over or equal to 6	N (%)	191 (6.4)	41 (8.0)	150 (6.1)	
Mean number of diagnoses	Mean (SD)	2.5 (1.7)	2.9 (1.8)	2.4 (1.7)	

CDR Clinical Dementia Rating
[1]Adjusted for NH-level

Table 3 Factors associated with number of physical diagnoses

Variables	Unadjusted		Adjusted	
	Regression coefficient (95% CI)	p-value	Regression coefficient (95% CI)	p-value
CDR-SOB	−0.06 (− 0.07; − 0.05)	< 0.001	−0.07 (− 0.08; − 0.05)	< 0.001
Males	0.03 (− 0.12; 0.17)	0.720	0.02 (− 0.12; 0.17)	0.734
Age	0.02 (0.01; 0.03)	< 0.001	0.02 (0.01; 0.03)	< 0.001
Education (≥10 years)	−0.18 (− 0.35; − 0.02)	0.025		
PSMS score	−0.001 (− 0.01; 0.01)	0.836	0.03 (0.02; 0.05)	< 0.001
NPI Agitation subsyndrome	−0.02 (− 0.03; − 0.01)	< 0.001		
NPI Psychosis subsyndrome	−0.03 (− 0.04; − 0.02)	< 0.001		
NPI Affective subsyndrome	− 0.01 (− 0.02; 0.005)	0.236		
NPI Apathy	−0.03 (− 0.05; − 0.01)	0.003		
Duration in NH (LN)	−0.04 (− 0.10; 0.01)	0.112		
Type of NH unit				
Regular – ref.	0	–	0	–
Special care	−0.73 (− 0.87; − 0.58)	< 0.001	−0.44 (− 0.59; − 0.28)	< 0.001
Rehabilitation	0.40 (0.01; 0.79)	0.042	0.35 (− 0.04; 0.73)	0.079
Other	−0.12 (− 0.39; 0.14)	0.361	0.07 (− 0.20; 0.34)	0.604

Unadjusted and adjusted analyses using linear mixed model
CDR-SOB Clinical Dementia Rating - Sum of Boxes, *PSMS* Physical Self-Maintenance Scale, *NPI* Neuropsychiatric Inventory, *NH* Nursing Home, *LN* Natural Logarithm

arrhythmia and heart failure, decreased with increasing CDR (Table 4).

Factors associated with the three most prevalent complexes of physical diagnoses

Cardiovascular diagnoses were the most frequently registered complex of physical diagnoses in the present study. According to the adjusted generalized linear mixed model analysis, older age, less severe NPI agitation and a higher total number of physical diagnoses were associated with higher odds of having cardiovascular diagnoses (Table 5). Also, an interaction between gender and CDR-SOB was found. In the unadjusted analysis, the odds for cardiovascular disease were decreasing with increasing values of CDR-SOB for both genders, and the reduction was slightly faster for females (Fig. 2a, b). However, in the adjusted analysis, the odds for cardiovascular disease were decreasing for females and increasing for males with increasing values of CDR-SOB (Fig. 2c). For a 1-unit increase in CDR-SOB, the odds for cardiovascular disease were increasing by 8 % more in males than females (OR = 1.08; 95% CI, 0.98–1.19; *p* = 0.142) (Fig. 2d). The odds became significantly different in males versus females for CDR-SOB values above six.

In the adjusted generalized linear mixed analysis for musculoskeletal diagnoses, factors associated with greater odds were old age, female gender and a higher number of physical diagnoses (Table 6). No interactions were present in the model. The only post hoc analysis being affected by the inclusion of GMHR was post hoc analysis for musculoskeletal diagnoses. Fairly good as

compared to good GMHR, shorter duration in a nursing home, longer education and a higher number of physical diagnoses were associated with higher odds of having musculoskeletal diagnoses (Table 7). Furthermore, an interaction between gender and CDR-SOB was detected. In unadjusted analysis, the odds of having musculoskeletal diagnoses were decreasing with increasing values of CDR-SOB for both genders, but the reduction was more pronounced for females (Fig. 3a, b). In the adjusted model, the odds were slightly decreasing for females and increasing for males with increasing values of CDR-SOB (Fig. 3c). For a 1-unit increase in CDR-SOB, males had 6 % higher odds compared to females (OR = 1.06; 95% CI, 0.98–1.15, *p* = 0.174), but the odds were significantly lower than one for all CDR-SOB values (Fig. 3d).

Factors associated with higher odds of having endocrine, nutritional or metabolic diagnoses in the adjusted generalized linear mixed analysis were a higher score in CDR-SOB, a greater NPI agitation score, younger age and a higher number of physical diagnoses (Table 8).

Discussion
Main findings
In the present study, the mean number of physical diagnoses registered was lower among nursing home residents with dementia than among those without. The number of physical diagnoses registered decreased with increasing severity of dementia. Cardiovascular, musculoskeletal and endocrine, nutritional

Table 4 Frequency of complexes and subgroups of physical diagnoses by dementia and increasing severity of dementia

Physical diagnoses	N (%)	Total	CDR < 1	CDR ≥ 1	P-value	CDR 1	CDR 2	CDR 3	P-value
		2983 (100)	513 (17.2)	2470 (82.8)		543 (22.0)	835 (33.8)	1092 (44.2)	
Cardiovascular diagnoses	N (%)	1798 (60.3)	343 (66.9)	1455 (58.9)	0.001[1]	366 (67.4)	521 (62.4)	568 (52.0)	< 0.001[1]
Hypertension (I10–15)	N (%)	662 (22.2)	121 (23.6)	541 (21.9)	0.315[1]	126 (23.2)	206 (24.7)	209 (19.1)	0.030[1]
Cerebrovascular disease (I60–69)	N (%)	642 (21.5)	130 (25.3)	512 (20.7)	0.026[2]	139 (25.6)	179 (21.4)	194 (17.8)	0.001[2]
Ischemic heart disease (I20–25)	N (%)	466 (15.6)	93 (18.1)	373 (15.1)	0.099[2]	95 (17.5)	137 (16.4)	141 (12.9)	0.011[2]
Arrhythmia (I44–49)	N (%)	404 (13.5)	82 (16.0)	322 (13.0)	0.084[2]	83 (15.3)	111 (13.3)	128 (11.7)	0.049[2]
Heart failure (I50)	N (%)	389 (13.0)	93 (18.1)	296 (12.0)	< 0.001[2]	88 (16.2)	92 (11.0)	116 (10.6)	0.005[2]
Musculoskeletal diagnoses	N (%)	707 (23.7)	153 (29.8)	554 (22.4)	0.001[1]	126 (23.2)	201 (24.1)	227 (20.8)	0.274[1]
Osteoporosis (M80–81)	N (%)	265 (8.9)	57 (11.1)	208 (8.4)	0.077[1]	43 (7.9)	80 (9.6)	85 (7.8)	0.892[1]
Arthrosis (M15–19)	N (%)	237 (7.9)	45 (8.8)	192 (7.8)	0.557[1]	43 (7.9)	62 (7.4)	87 (8.0)	0.815[1]
Inflammatory joint disease (M05–14)	N (%)	137 (4.6)	35 (6.8)	102 (4.1)	0.011[2]	26 (4.8)	38 (4.6)	38 (3.5)	0.181[2]
Endocrine, nutritional and metabolic diagnoses	N (%)	662 (22.2)	112 (21.8)	550 (22.3)	0.838[2]	124 (22.8)	187 (22.4)	239 (21.9)	0.661[2]
Diabetes (E10–14)	N (%)	455 (15.3)	83 (16.2)	372 (15.1)	0.530[2]	86 (15.8)	130 (15.6)	156 (14.3)	0.380[2]
Disorders of the thyroid gland (E00–07)	N (%)	195 (6.5)	30 (5.8)	165 (6.7)	0.494[2]	43 (7.9)	51 (6.1)	71 (6.5)	0.380[2]
Neurological diagnoses	N (%)	464 (15.6)	92 (17.9)	372 (15.1)	0.109[2]	89 (16.4)	108 (12.9)	175 (16.0)	0.810[2]
Parkinson (G20)	N (%)	137 (4.6)	32 (6.2)	105 (4.3)	0.057[1]	25 (4.6)	30 (3.6)	50 (4.6)	0.845[1]
Transient ischemic attack (TIA) (G45.9)	N (%)	119 (4.0)	16 (3.1)	103 (4.2)	0.253[1]	16 (2.9)	36 (4.3)	51 (4.7)	0.107[1]
Respiratory diagnoses	N (%)	271 (9.1)	66 (12.9)	205 (8.3)	0.002[2]	57 (10.5)	77 (9.2)	71 (6.5)	0.006[2]
Asthma/COPD (J40–47)	N (%)	242 (8.1)	60 (11.7)	182 (7.4)	0.002[2]	46 (8.5)	70 (8.4)	66 (6.0)	0.054[2]
Genitourinal diagnoses	N (%)	267 (9.0)	52 (10.1)	215 (8.7)	0.312[2]	42 (7.7)	66 (7.9)	107 (9.8)	0.123[2]
Renal failure (N17–19)	N (%)	95 (3.2)	23 (4.5)	72 (2.9)	0.078[2]	18 (3.3)	24 (2.9)	30 (2.7)	0.552[2]
Malign neoplasms	N (%)	249 (8.3)	62 (12.1)	187 (7.6)	0.001[1]	42 (7.7)	70 (8.4)	75 (6.9)	0.406[1]
Malignant neoplasm of breast (C50)	N (%)	54 (1.8)	9 (1.8)	45 (1.8)	0.920[1]	10 (1.8)	15 (1.8)	20 (1.8)	0.999[1]
Gastrointestinal diagnoses	N (%)	230 (7.7)	36 (7.0)	194 (7.9)	0.379[1]	52 (9.6)	67 (8.0)	75 (6.9)	0.068[1]
Ulcer (oesophagus, stomach and duodenum) (K25–28)	N (%)	65 (2.2)	10 (1.9)	55 (2.2)	0.716[2]	10 (1.8)	21 (2.5)	24 (2.2)	0.781[2]
Other									
Fracture of the femur (S72)	N (%)	261 (8.7)	49 (9.6)	212 (8.6)	0.833[1]	54 (9.9)	65 (7.8)	93 (8.5)	0.651[1]
Cataract (H25–26)	N (%)	138 (4.6)	32 (6.2)	106 (4.3)	0.065[2]	19 (3.5)	35 (4.2)	52 (4.8)	0.238[2]
Glaucoma (H40–42)	N (%)	101 (3.4)	11 (2.1)	90 (3.6)	0.100[2]	25 (4.6)	21 (2.5)	44 (4.0)	0.890[2]

CDR Clinical Dementia Rating, *COPD* Chronic Obstructive Pulmonary Disease
[1]Adjusted for NH-level
[2]Adjusted for intra-patient correlation

and metabolic diagnoses were the three most frequently registered complexes of physical diagnoses.

Cardiovascular diagnoses were more frequently registered in residents without dementia than residents with dementia. Increasing severity of dementia in female residents reduced the odds of having cardiovascular diagnoses, while in male residents the odds increased to some degree. Also, for musculoskeletal diagnoses, the odds slightly decreased for females and increased for males with increasing severity of dementia. For endocrine, nutritional and metabolic diagnoses, the odds increased with severity of dementia for both genders.

Factors associated with the number of physical diagnoses in nursing home residents

Nursing home residents in the present study had a mean number of 2.5 physical diagnoses registered at inclusion. In studies from long-term care facilities, the total number of diagnoses has been reported to be between 3.0 to 6.4, but these studies did not separate physical diagnoses from mental and behavioural diagnoses [40–42]. A comparison is difficult due to differences in the type of diagnoses registered, sample inequalities and the research methods used. We may speculate that inequalities in health care systems can explain some of the differences. For instance, in the U.S., health care facilities may be financed by

Table 5 Factors associated with cardiovascular diagnoses

Variables	Unadjusted		Adjusted	
	OR (95% CI)	p-value	OR (95% CI)	p-value
CDR-SOB	0.92 (0.89; 0.95)	< 0.001	−0.05 (0.03)[1]	0.100
Males	1.64 (1.17; 2.28)	0.005	0.17 (0.62)[1]	0.783
Age	1.06 (1.03; 1.09)	< 0.001	1.07 (1.04; 1.11)	< 0.001
Education (≥10 years)	0.66 (0.46; 0.93)	0.019	0.66 (0.39; 1.14)	0.144
PSMS score	0.98 (0.96; 1.00)	0.094		
NPI Agitation subsyndrome	0.96 (0.94; 0.98)	< 0.001	0.97 (0.94; 0.99)	0.023
NPI Psychosis subsyndrome	0.95 (0.93; 0.98)	0.001		
NPI Affective subsyndrome	0.97 (0.94; 0.99)	0.014		
NPI Apathy	0.93 (0.90; 0.97)	0.001		
Number of physical diagnoses	8.41 (4.63; 15.28)	< 0.001	8.10 (4.56; 14.37)	< 0.001
Duration in NH (LN)	0.88 (0.79; 0.98)	0.022	0.84 (0.70; 1.02)	0.078
Type of NH unit				
Regular – ref.	1	–		
Special care	0.33 (0.21; 0.52)	< 0.001		
Rehabilitation	1.30 (0.59; 2.86)	0.516		
Other	0.88 (0.52; 1.48)	0.620		
CDR-SOB x Females			0.07 (0.05)[1]	0.142

Unadjusted and adjusted analyses using generalized linear mixed model
CDR-SOB Clinical Dementia Rating - Sum of Boxes, PSMS Physical Self-Maintenance Scale, NPI Neuropsychiatric Inventory, NH Nursing Home, LN Natural Logarithm
[1]Regression coefficient (standard error) as the OR has no interpretation for interaction and variables included into interaction term

insurances [58, 59], which links the number of diagnoses registered closely to economy. Conversely, health care in Norway is mostly publicly financed [59], and nursing home cost is related to registered functional needs.

In the present study, a higher number of physical diagnoses was associated with lower severity of dementia, a higher age, poorer physical health and type of nursing home unit. The number of physical diagnoses registered was higher in residents without dementia. This finding could imply that residents without dementia are admitted to nursing homes because of severe physical morbidity, while individuals with dementia are admitted mainly because of cognitive impairment [4, 26]. We can also speculate that residents with cognitive impairment receive less attention to physical symptoms, which may cause undiagnosed physical disease. However, residents with dementia were more likely to have poorer physical health and poorer P-ADL functioning, which have been found to correlate to a higher number of comorbidities [50]. This could imply that residents with dementia have more comorbid conditions than registered.

Furthermore, increasing severity of dementia was associated with a decrease in the number of physical diagnoses registered. Previous literature from nursing homes have similar findings [40]. In individuals with severe dementia, the accompanying neuropsychiatric symptoms may become clinically dominant and detract attention

from other conditions [60]. Moreover, the ability to express physical symptoms and pain is reduced with advanced dementia [61]. Additionally, confusion, agitation and behavioural changes are symptoms that can be interpreted as either symptoms of dementia or physical disease [62]. Finally, the present study also revealed a lower number of physical diagnoses registered in residents in special care units compared to regular care units. The severity of neuropsychiatric symptoms in individuals with dementia is a principal reason for admission to special care units [34]. Thus, careful examination is essential to differentiate between symptoms of delirium, often representing severe underlying physical disease, and neuropsychiatric symptoms associated with dementia [63].

Factors associated with the three most frequent complexes of physical diagnoses

Cardiovascular, musculoskeletal and endocrine, nutritional and metabolic diagnoses were the three most common complexes of diagnoses in the present study. Among the included subgroups, hypertension, cerebrovascular disease, ischemic heart disease and diabetes were found to be the physical diagnoses most frequently registered. These findings are in line with international studies of nursing home residents [40–42].

The odds of having cardiovascular diagnoses decreased in females and increased in males with increasing

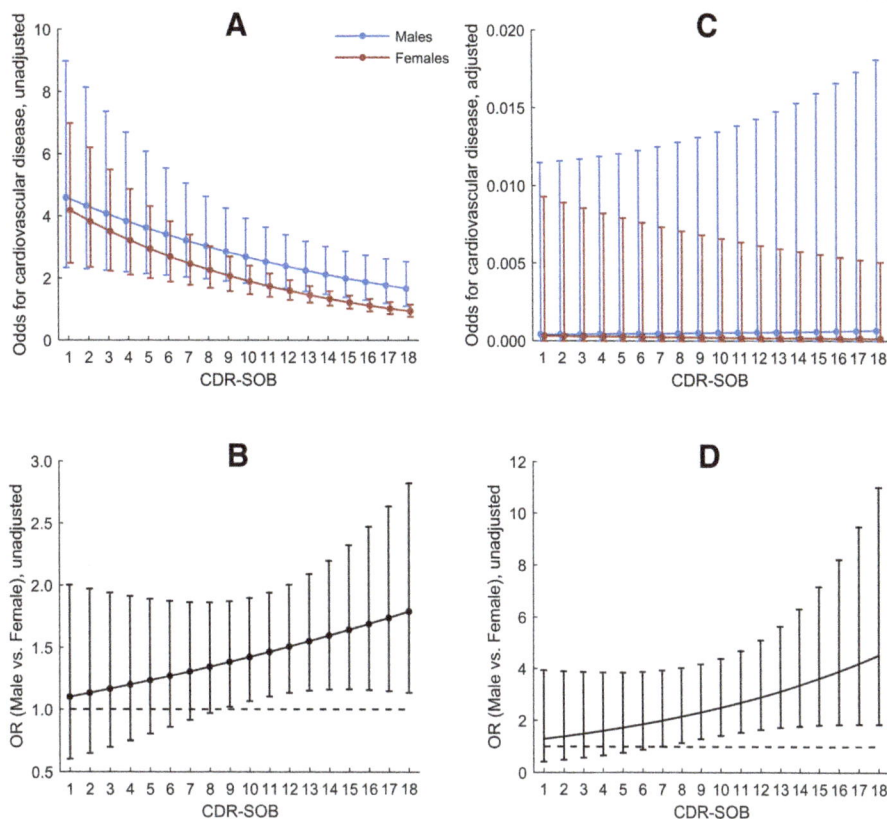

Fig. 2 Interpreting interaction term CDR-SOB x Females in Table 5; unadjusted odds for cardiovascular disease (**a**), adjusted odds for cardiovascular disease (**c**), unadjusted OR for Males vs. Females (**b**), and adjusted OR for Males vs. Females (**d**)

Table 6 Factors associated with musculoskeletal diagnoses

Variables	Unadjusted		Adjusted	
	OR (95% CI)	p-value	OR (95% CI)	p-value
CDR-SOB	0.94 (0.90; 0.97)	0.002	0.97 (0.93; 1.02)	0.220
Males	0.10 (0.04; 0.26)	< 0.001	0.08 (0.02; 0.27)	< 0.001
Age	1.07 (1.03; 1.11)	< 0.001	1.05 (1.01; 1.08)	0.012
Education (≥10 years)	1.04 (0.60; 1.79)	0.888	1.69 (0.99; 2.90)	0.061
PSMS score	0.97 (0.93; 0.99)	0.039		
NPI Agitation subsyndrome	0.97 (0.94; 0.99)	0.006		
NPI Psychosis subsyndrome	0.96 (0.93; 0.99)	0.044		
NPI Affective subsyndrome	1.01 (0.97; 1.05)	0.594		
NPI Apathy	0.93 (0.88; 0.99)	0.018		
Number of physical diagnoses	2.86 (2.15; 3.81)	< 0.001	2.63 (1.66; 4.17)	< 0.001
Duration in NH (LN)	0.88 (0.74; 1.05)	0.165	0.86 (0.71; 1.04)	0.121
Type of NH unit				
Regular – ref.	1	–		
Special care	0.67 (0.44; 1.02)	0.064		
Rehabilitation	1.71 (0.62; 4.73)	0.298		
Other	1.34 (0.67; 2.70)	0.403		

Unadjusted and adjusted analyses using generalized linear mixed model. No significant interactions found in the adjusted model
CDR-SOB Clinical Dementia Rating - Sum of Boxes, *PSMS* Physical Self-Maintenance Scale, *NPI* Neuropsychiatric Inventory, *NH* Nursing Home, *LN* Natural Logarithm

Table 7 Factors associated with musculoskeletal diagnoses

Variables	Unadjusted		Adjusted	
	OR (95% CI)	p-value	OR (95% CI)	p-value
CDR-SOB	0.94 (0.90; 0.97)	0.002	−0.03 (0.02)[1]	0.092
Males	0.10 (0.04; 0.26)	< 0.001	−2.71 (0.50)[1]	< 0.001
Age	1.07 (1.03; 1.11)	< 0.001	1.02 (0.99; 1.04)	0.130
Education (≥10 years)	1.04 (0.60; 1.79)	0.888	1.68 (1.12; 2.52)	0.014
GMHR				
Good – ref.	1	–	1	–
Fairly good	3.18 (1.63; 6.18)	0.001	1.72 (1.05; 2.82)	0.037
Poor	1.95 (1.07; 3.55)	0.030	1.11 (0.66; 1.87)	0.703
Very poor	2.00 (0.94; 4.24)	0.070	1.23 (0.63; 2.40)	0.542
PSMS score	0.97 (0.93; 0.99)	0.039		
NPI Agitation subsyndrome	0.97 (0.94; 0.99)	0.006		
NPI Psychosis subsyndrome	0.96 (0.93; 0.99)	0.044		
NPI Affective subsyndrome	1.01 (0.97; 1.05)	0.594		
NPI Apathy	0.93 (0.88; 0.99)	0.018		
Number of physical diagnoses	2.86 (2.15; 3.81)	< 0.001	2.16 (1.96; 2.38)	< 0.001
Duration in NH (LN)	0.88 (0.74; 1.05)	0.165	0.87 (0.76; 0.99)	0.044
Type of NH unit				
Regular – ref.	1	–		
Special care	0.67 (0.44; 1.02)	0.064		
Rehabilitation	1.71 (0.62; 4.73)	0.298		
Other	1.34 (0.67; 2.70)	0.403		
CDR-SOB x Females			0.06 (0.04)[1]	0.174

Unadjusted and adjusted analyses using generalized linear mixed model. GMHR included as explanatory variable
CDR-SOB Clinical Dementia Rating - Sum of Boxes, GMHR General Medical Health Rating, PSMS Physical Self-Maintenance Scale, NPI Neuropsychiatric Inventory, NH Nursing Home, LN Natural Logarithm
[1]Regression coefficient (standard error) as the OR has no interpretation for interaction and variables included into interaction term

CDR-SOB, and the odds became significantly different for female and male residents when the severity of dementia increased (CDR-SOB > 6). Also, the odds for musculoskeletal diagnoses slightly decreased in females and increased in males with increasing CDR-SOB. Nevertheless, the odds were lower than one for both genders when CDR increased. On the contrary, the odds of having registered endocrine, nutritional and metabolic diagnoses increased with increasing CDR-SOB for both genders. We have no firm explanation for these results, but it may be related to different gender expression of dementia, physical diagnoses and pain, triggering a diagnostic review more often in males. Some cardiovascular disease presentations are commonly undiagnosed in females [64], which might partly explain the decreased odds for cardiovascular diagnoses by increasing CDR-SOB in females. Finally, it is possible that the spouses of males visit or worry more than spouses of females, producing a difference in diagnostics of disease. However, we can only speculate, and further research would be necessary.

Strengths and limitations

The present study has significant strengths. First of all, the study is based on a large sample of individuals in nursing homes (n = 2893). Another strength is the use of well reputed and established scales. Demographic and health variables of potential importance for the outcome of the study were adjusted for. Additionally, GMHR was included in the post hoc analysis to evaluate if the prevalence of physical diagnoses according to the severity of dementia persisted when adjusting for physical health. However, GMHR did not influence the results significantly. Furthermore, both samples benefit from the education of nurses prior to the data collections. Finally, the study includes nursing homes from large parts of the country.

The study also had some limitations. Firstly, dementia and severity of dementia were not based on a standardized dementia investigation with neuropsychological tests. However, CDR assessment is commonly used in nursing home studies as an accepted method to identify and measure dementia [48, 65]. Secondly, a medical examination of the residents was not performed during inclusion.

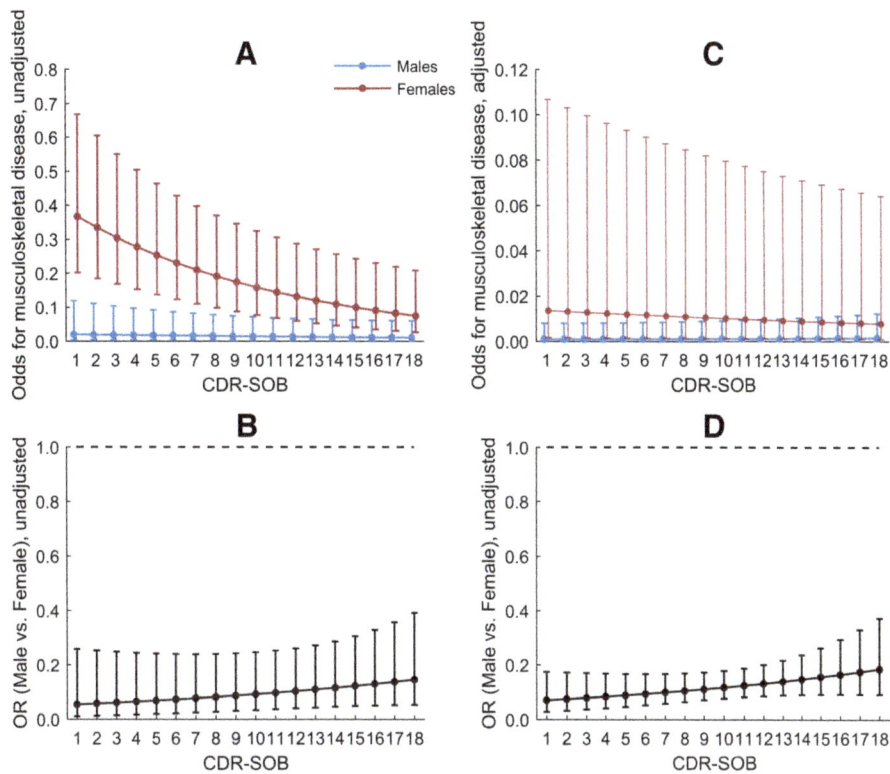

Fig. 3 Interpreting interaction term CDR-SOB x Females in Table 7; unadjusted odds for musculoskeletal disease(**a**), adjusted odds for musculoskeletal disease (**c**), unadjusted OR for Males vs. Females (**b**), and adjusted OR for Males vs. Females (**d**)

Table 8 Factors associated with endocrine, nutritional and metabolic diagnoses

Variables	Unadjusted		Adjusted	
	OR (95% CI)	p-value	OR (95% CI)	p-value
CDR-SOB	0.98 (0.93; 1.02)	0.302	1.07 (1.00; 1.14)	0.049
Males	0.75 (0.42; 1.32)	0.313	0.71 (0.40; 1.26)	0.241
Age	0.99 (0.96; 1.02)	0.588	0.96 (0.92; 0.99)	0.009
Education (≥10 years)	0.54 (0.29; 1.02)	0.056	0.62 (0.33; 1.18)	0.152
PSMS score	0.99 (0.95; 1.04)	0.770	0.94 (0.89; 1.00)	0.053
NPI Agitation subsyndrome	1.02 (0.99; 1.05)	0.334	1.04 (1.00; 1.07)	0.035
NPI Psychosis subsyndrome	0.99 (0.95; 1.04)	0.773		
NPI Affective subsyndrome	1.01 (0.96; 1.06)	0.663		
NPI Apathy	0.99 (0.92; 1.06)	0.663		
Number of physical diagnoses	3.69 (2.82; 4.82)	< 0.001	3.90 (2.95; 5.15)	< 0.001
Duration in NH (LN)	1.07 (0.88; 1.30)	0.509		
Type of NH unit				
Regular – ref.	1	–		
Special care	0.94 (0.53; 1.67)	0.828		
Rehabilitation	2.43 (0.55; 10.77)	0.237		
Other	2.00 (0.73; 5.5)	0.176		

Unadjusted and adjusted analyses using generalized linear mixed model
CDR-SOB Clinical Dementia Rating - Sum of Boxes, *PSMS*: Physical Self-Maintenance Scale, *NPI* Neuropsychiatric Inventory, *NH* Nursing Home, *LN* Natural Logarithm

Diagnoses registered in the medical records were included without any further validation of their exactness [19]. In addition to this, we do not know if the diagnoses were obtained before or after admission to a nursing home. Thirdly, the data material does not distinguish between dementia subtypes, consequently, differences in comorbidity profile of individuals with vascular and neurodegenerative dementia have been left out [19, 37]. Lastly, the inclusion of nursing homes was not based on a random selection, which makes us unable to guarantee that the sample is representative for all nursing homes in Norway.

Implications for clinical practice and future research

The present research contributes to a better understanding of the relationship between dementia and physical comorbidity, which is highly relevant due to a growing elderly population globally [7]. The importance of thoroughly and equal diagnostics among individuals with and without dementia is also emphasised. Specific guidelines for individuals with dementia and comorbid conditions are needed to reduce health care costs and improve quality of care and health outcomes. Future research should focus on physical comorbidity in nursing home residents, and explore if dementia affects the diagnostics of physical disease.

Conclusions

In the present study, the most prevalent complexes of physical diagnoses were cardiovascular, musculoskeletal and endocrine, nutritional and metabolic diagnoses. The number of physical diagnoses registered was lower among residents with dementia than among those without. Furthermore, the odds of having cardiovascular and musculoskeletal diagnoses increased for males and decreased for females with increasing severity of dementia, in contrast to endocrine diagnoses where the odds increased for both genders. In conclusion, comorbidity and increasing severity of dementia may complicate the diagnostics of physical disease. This highlights the importance of more attention to the registration of physical diagnoses in nursing home residents with dementia.

Abbreviations

AIC: Akaike Information Criterion; ATC: Anatomical Therapeutic Chemical; CDR: Clinical Dementia Rating; CDR-SOB: Clinical dementia rating – sum of boxes; CI: Confidence interval; COPD: Chronic obstructive pulmonary disease; CT: Computer tomography; GMHR: General medical health rating; GP: Geriatric psychiatrist; LN: Natural Logarithm; MRI: Magnetic resonance imaging; N: Number; NH: Nursing home; NP: Nurse specialized in psychiatry; NPI: Neuropsychiatric Inventory; NPS: Neuropsychiatric symptoms; OR: Odds ratio; OU: Other units; P-ADL: Personal Activities of Daily Living; PSMS: Physical Self-Maintenance Scale; Ref: Reference; REU: Rehabilitation unit; RN: Registered nurse; RU: Regular unit; SAS: Statistical analysis software; SCU: Special care unit; SD: Standard deviation; SPSS: Statistical package for the social sciences; TIA: Transient ischemic attack

Acknowledgements
Not applicable.

Funding
Unrestricted grants from the Eastern Norway Regional Health authorities and Innlandet Hospital trust funded the data collection. The funding did not influence the collection, analysis or interpretation of any data. In the present study of previously collected data, the analysis and preparation of the manuscript were done without any funding.

Authors' contributions
LBJ and BMT have contributed equally throughout the process of preparing the manuscript. They conducted the first analysis, interpreted the findings and drafted the manuscript. ASH had the research idea and participated in the primary analysis, interpretation of the results and drafting of the manuscript. GS was responsible for the study design and the data collection. JSB conducted the main statistical analyses. All authors participated in the interpretation of the study results and in editing the manuscript, and have read and approved the final manuscript.

Competing interests
The authors declare that they have no competing interests.

Author details
[1]Department of Public Health and Nursing, Norwegian University of Science and Technology (NTNU), Trondheim, Norway. [2]Norwegian National Advisory Unit on Ageing and Health, Vestfold Hospital Trust, Tønsberg, Norway. [3]Centre for Old Age Psychiatric Research, Innlandet Hospital Trust, Ottestad, Norway. [4]Institute of Health and Society, Faculty of Medicine, University of Oslo, Oslo, Norway. [5]Institute of Clinical Medicine, University of Oslo, Oslo, Norway. [6]Health Services Research Unit, Akershus University Hospital, Lørenskog, Norway. [7]Department of Public Health and Nursing, Faculty of Medicine and Health Sciences, Norwegian University of Science and Technology (NTNU), Trondheim, Norway. [8]St Olavs University Hospital, Trondheim, Norway.

References
1. Berr C, Wancata J, Ritchie K. Prevalence of dementia in the elderly in Europe. Eur Neuropsychopharmacol. 2005;15(4):463–71.
2. World Health Organization. International Statistical Classification of Diseases and Related Health Problems 10th Revision (ICD-10) - WHO Version for; 2016 Chapter V Mental and behavioural disorders (F00-F99) Organic, including symptomatic, mental disorders (F00-F09). 2016. http://apps.who.int/classifications/icd10/browse/2016/en#/F00-F09. Accessed 23 Nov 2017.
3. Arling G, Williams AR. Cognitive impairment and resource use of nursing home residents: a structural equation model. Med Care. 2003;41(7):802–12.
4. Luppa M, Luck T, Weyerer S, Konig HH, Brahler E, Riedel-Heller SG. Prediction of institutionalization in the elderly. A systematic review. Age Ageing. 2010;39(1):31–8.
5. Guehne U, Riedel-Heller S, Angermeyer MC. Mortality in dementia. Neuroepidemiology. 2005;25(3):153–62.
6. Alzheimer's Disease International (ADI). World Alzheimer Report 2015. p. 2015. https://www.alz.co.uk/research/WorldAlzheimerReport2015.pdf. Accessed 23 Nov 2017
7. United Nations, Department of Economic and Social Affairs, Population Division. World Population Prospects: The 2015 revision, key findings and advance tables. Working paper no. ESA/P/WP241. 2015. https://esa.un.org/unpd/wpp/publications/files/key_findings_wpp_2015.pdf. Accessed 23 Nov 2017.
8. Statistics Norway. Key figures for the population. 2017. https://wwwssbno/en/befolkning/nokkeltall/population Accessed 23 Nov 2017.
9. Prince M, Bryce R, Albanese E, Wimo A, Ribeiro W, Ferri CP. The global prevalence of dementia: a systematic review and metaanalysis. Alzheimers Dement. 2013;9(1):63–75 e62.

10. Godager GC, Thorjussen CBH. Dementia in Norwegian municipalities 2015–2040: prognoses based on international studies [Demens i norske kommuner 2015–2040: Prognoser basert på internasjonale studier]. 2016. http://healtheconomics.no/rapport2016_1.pdf. Accessed 27 Nov 2017.

11. Ritchie CS, Hearld KR, Gross A, Allman R, Sawyer P, Sheppard K, Salanitro A, Locher J, Brown CJ, Roth DL. Measuring symptoms in community-dwelling older adults: the psychometric properties of a brief symptom screen. Med Care. 2013;51(10):949–55.

12. World Health Organization. Noncommunicable Diseases Progress Monitor. 2017. http://www.who.int/nmh/publications/ncd-progress-monitor-2017/en/. Accessed 23 Nov 2017.

13. Marengoni A, Angleman S, Melis R, Mangialasche F, Karp A, Garmen A, Meinow B, Fratiglioni L. Aging with multimorbidity: a systematic review of the literature. Ageing Res Rev. 2011;10(4):430–9.

14. Fortin M, Stewart M, Poitras M-E, Almirall J, Maddocks H. A systematic review of prevalence studies on multimorbidity: toward a more uniform methodology. Ann Fam Med. 2012;10(2):142–51.

15. Formiga F, Ferrer A, Sanz H, Marengoni A, Alburquerque J, Pujol R. Patterns of comorbidity and multimorbidity in the oldest old: the Octabaix study. Eur J Intern Med. 2013;24(1):40–4.

16. Barnett K, Mercer SW, Norbury M, Watt G, Wyke S, Guthrie B. Epidemiology of multimorbidity and implications for health care, research, and medical education: a cross-sectional study. Lancet. 2012;380(9836):37–43.

17. Gijsen R, Hoeymans N, Schellevis FG, Ruwaard D, Satariano WA, van den Bos GAM. Causes and consequences of comorbidity: A review. J Clin Epidemiol. 2001;54(7):661–74.

18. Jacob L, Breuer J, Kostev K. Prevalence of chronic diseases among older patients in German general practices. GMS Germ Med Sci. 2016;14:Doc03.

19. Bauer K, Schwarzkopf L, Graessel E, Holle R. A claims data-based comparison of comorbidity in individuals with and without dementia. BMC Geriatr. 2014; 14:10.

20. Marengoni A, Rizzuto D, Wang HX, Winblad B, Fratiglioni L. Patterns of chronic multimorbidity in the elderly population. J Am Geriatr Soc. 2009; 57(2):225–30.

21. Eaker ED, Vierkant RA, Mickel SF. Predictors of nursing home admission and/or death in incident Alzheimer's disease and other dementia cases compared to controls: A population-based study. J Clin Epidemiol. 2002; 55(5):462–8.

22. Solfrizzi V, Panza F, Colacicco AM, D'Introno A, Capurso C, Torres F, Grigoletto F, Maggi S, Del Parigi A, Reiman EM, et al. Vascular risk factors, incidence of MCI, and rates of progression to dementia. Neurology. 2004; 63(10):1882–91.

23. Sahathevan R, Brodtmann A, Donnan GA. Dementia, stroke, and vascular risk factors; a review. Int J Stroke. 2012;7(1):61–73.

24. Marques A, Rocha V, Pinto M, Sousa L, Figueiredo D. Comorbidities and medication intake among people with dementia living in long-term care facilities. Rev Port Saúde Pública. 2015;33(1):42–8.

25. Poblador-Plou B, Calderon-Larranaga A, Marta-Moreno J, Hancco-Saavedra J, Sicras-Mainar A, Soljak M, Prados-Torres A. Comorbidity of dementia: a cross-sectional study of primary care older patients. BMC Psychiatry. 2014;14:84.

26. Nygaard HA, Naik M, Ruths S, Straand J. Nursing-home residents and their drug use: a comparison between mentally intact and mentally impaired residents. Eur J Clin Pharmacol. 2003;59(5):463–9.

27. Wergeland JN, Selbæk G, Bergh S, Soederhamn U, Kirkevold Ø. Predictors for nursing home admission and death among community-dwelling people 70 years and older who receive domiciliary care. Dement Geriatr Cogn Dis Extra. 2015;5(3):320–9.

28. Gulla C, Selbaek G, Flo E, Kjome R, Kirkevold O, Husebo BS. Multi-psychotropic drug prescription and the association to neuropsychiatric symptoms in three Norwegian nursing home cohorts between 2004 and 2011. BMC Geriatr. 2016;16:115.

29. Galik E, Resnick B. Psychotropic medication use and association with physical and psychosocial outcomes in nursing home residents. J Psychiatr Ment Health Nurs. 2013;20(3):244–52.

30. Helvik AS, Engedal K, Benth JS, Selbaek G. Prevalence and severity of dementia in nursing home residents. Dement Geriatr Cogn Disord. 2015;40(3–4):166–77.

31. Bergh S, Holmen J, Saltvedt I, Tambs K, Selbæk G. Dementia and neuropsychiatric symptoms in nursing-home patients in Nord-Trøndelag County. Tidsskr Nor Laegeforen. 2012;132(17):1956–9.

32. Borza T, Engedal K, Bergh S, Barca ML, Benth JS, Selbaek G. The course of

33. Tiong WW, Yap P, Huat Koh GC, Phoon Fong N, Luo N. Prevalence and risk factors of depression in the elderly nursing home residents in Singapore. Aging Ment Health. 2013;17(6):724–31.

34. Helvik AS, Engedal K, Wu B, Benth JS, Corazzini K, Roen I, Selbaek G. Severity of neuropsychiatric symptoms in nursing home residents. Dement Geriatr Cogn Dis Extra. 2016;6(1):28–42.

35. Selbaek G, Engedal K, Benth JS, Bergh S. The course of neuropsychiatric symptoms in nursing-home patients with dementia over a 53-month follow-up period. Int Psychogeriatr. 2014;26(1):81–91.

36. Zuidema SU, de Jonghe JF, Verhey FR, Koopmans RT. Neuropsychiatric symptoms in nursing home patients: factor structure invariance of the Dutch nursing home version of the neuropsychiatric inventory in different stages of dementia. Dement Geriatr Cogn Disord. 2007;24(3):169–76.

37. Sanderson M, Wang J, Davis DR, Lane MJ, Cornman CB, Fadden MK. Co-morbidity associated with dementia. Am J Alzheimers Dis Other Demen. 2002;17(2):73–8.

38. Schubert CC, Boustani M, Callahan CM, Perkins AJ, Carney CP, Fox C, Unverzagt F, Hui S, Hendrie HC. Comorbidity profile of dementia patients in primary care: are they sicker? J Am Geriatr Soc. 2006;54(1):104–9.

39. Clague F, Mercer SW, McLean G, Reynish E, Guthrie B. Comorbidity and polypharmacy in people with dementia: insights from a large, population-based cross-sectional analysis of primary care data. Age Ageing. 2017;46(1):33-39.

40. Landi F, Gambassi G, Lapane KL, Sgadari A, Gifford D, Mor V, Bernabei R. Comorbidity and drug use in cognitively impaired elderly living in long-term care. Dement Geriatr Cogn Disord. 1998;9(6):347–56.

41. Martin-Garcia S, Rodriguez-Blazquez C, Martinez-Lopez I, Martinez-Martin P, Forjaz MJ. Comorbidity, health status, and quality of life in institutionalized older people with and without dementia. Int Psychogeriatr. 2013;25(7):1077–84.

42. Moore K, Boscardin W, Steinman M, Schwartz J. Patterns of chronic co-morbid conditions in older residents of U.S. nursing homes: differences between the sexes and across the agespan. J Nutr Health Aging. 2014;18(4):429–36.

43. Selbaek G, Kirkevold O, Engedal K. The prevalence of psychiatric symptoms and behavioural disturbances and the use of psychotropic drugs in Norwegian nursing homes. Int J Geriatr Psychiatry. 2007;22(9):843–9.

44. Knight CF, Knight J. Alzheimer's Disease Research Center: The Clinical Dementia Rating (CDR). 2016. http://alzheimer.wustl.edu/cdr/cdr.htm. Accessed 23 Nov 2017.

45. Hughes CP, Berg L, Danziger WL, Coben LA, Martin RL. A new clinical scale for the staging of dementia. Br J Psychiatry. 1982;140:566–72.

46. Nygaard HA, Naik M, Ruths S. Mental impairment in nursing home residents. Tidsskr Nor Laegeforen. 2000;120(26):3113–6.

47. Waite L, Grayson D, Jorm AF, Creasey H, Cullen J, Bennett H, Casey B, Broe GA. Informant-based staging of dementia using the clinical dementia rating. Alzheimer Dis Assoc Disord. 1999;13(1):34–7.

48. Mjørud M, Kirkevold M, Røsvik J, Selbæk G, Engedal K. Variables associated to quality of life among nursing home patients with dementia. Aging Ment Health. 2014;18(8):1013–21.

49. O'Bryant SE, Waring SC, Cullum CM, Hall J, Lacritz L, Massman PJ, Lupo PJ, Reisch JS, Doody R. Texas Alzheimer's research C: staging dementia using clinical dementia rating scale sum of boxes scores: a Texas Alzheimer's research consortium study. Arch Neurol. 2008;65(8):1091–5.

50. Lyketsos CG, Galik E, Steele C, Steinberg M, Rosenblatt A, Warren A, Sheppard JM, Baker A, Brandt J. The general medical health rating: a bedside global rating of medical comorbidity in patients with dementia. J Am Geriatr Soc. 1999;47(4):487–91.

51. Lyketsos CG, Toone L, Tschanz J, Rabins PV, Steinberg M, Onyike CU, Corcoran C, Norton M, Zandi P, Breitner JC, et al. Population-based study of medical comorbidity in early dementia and "cognitive impairment, no dementia (CIND)": association with functional and cognitive impairment: the Cache County study. Am J Geriatr Psychiatry. 2005;13(8):656–64.

52. Sylliaas H, Selbaek G, Bergland A. Do behavioral disturbances predict falls among nursing home residents? Aging Clin Exp Res. 2012;24(3):251–6.

53. Lawton MP, Brody EM. Assessment of older people: self-maintaining and instrumental activities of daily living. Gerontologist. 1969;9(3):179–86.

54. Selbaek G, Kirkevold O, Sommer OH, Engedal K. The reliability and validity of the Norwegian version of the neuropsychiatric inventory, nursing home version (NPI-NH). Int Psychogeriatr. 2008;20(2):375–82.

55. Cummings JL. The neuropsychiatric inventory: assessing psychopathology in dementia patients. Neurology. 1997;48(5 Suppl 6):S10–6.

56. Selbaek G, Engedal K. Stability of the factor structure of the neuropsychiatric inventory in a 31-month follow-up study of a large sample of nursing-home patients with dementia. Int Psychogeriatr. 2012;24(1):62–73.

57. World Health Organization. The Anatomical Therapeutic Chemical Classification System with Defined Daily Doses. 2003. http://www.who.int/classifications/atcddd/en/. Accessed 23 Nov 2017.

58. Costa-Font J, Courbage C, Swartz K. Financing long-term care: ex ante, ex post or both? Health Econ. 2015;24(Suppl 1):45–57.

59. Mossialos E, Djordjevic A, Osborn R, Sarnak D. International profiles of. Health Care Syst. 2017; http://www.commonwealthfund.org/publications/fund-reports/2017/may/international-profiles. Accessed 24 Nov 2017.

60. Bunn F, Burn A-M, Goodman C, Rait G, Norton S, Robinson L, Schoeman J, Brayne C. Comorbidity and dementia: a scoping review of the literature. BMC Med. 2014;12(1):192.

61. Kovach CR, Logan BR, Simpson MR, Reynolds S. Factors associated with time to identify physical problems of nursing home residents with dementia. Am J Alzheimers Dis Other Demen. 2010;25(4):317–23.

62. Abdelhafiz AH, McNicholas E, Sinclair AJ. Hypoglycemia, frailty and dementia in older people with diabetes: reciprocal relations and clinical implications. J Diabetes Complicat. 2016;30(8):1548–54.

63. Holtta E, Laakkonen ML, Laurila JV, Strandberg TE, Tilvis R, Kautiainen H, Pitkala KH. The overlap of delirium with neuropsychiatric symptoms among patients with dementia. Am J Geriatr Psychiatry. 2011;19(12):1034–41.

64. Garcia M, Mulvagh SL, Merz CNB, Buring JE, Manson JE. Cardiovascular disease in women: clinical perspectives. Circ Res. 2016;118(8):1273–93.

65. Leoutsakos JM, Han D, Mielke MM, Forrester SN, Tschanz JT, Corcoran CD, Green RC, Norton MC, Welsh-Bohmer KA, Lyketsos CG. Effects of general medical health on Alzheimer's progression: the Cache County dementia progression study. Int Psychogeriatr. 2012;24(10):1561–70.

18

Is excess weight a burden for older adults who suffer chronic pain?

Huan-Ji Dong[1]* , Britt Larsson[1], Lars-Åke Levin[2], Lars Bernfort[2] and Björn Gerdle[1]

Abstract

Background: Obesity and chronic pain are common comorbidities and adversely influence each other. Advanced age is associated with more comorbidities and multi-morbidities. In this study, we investigated the burden of overweight/obesity and its comorbidities and their associations with chronic pain in a random population sample of Swedish older adults.

Methods: The cross-sectional analysis involved a random sample of a population ≥ 65 years in south-eastern Sweden ($N = 6243$). Data were collected from a postal questionnaire that addressed pain aspects, body mass index (BMI), and health experiences. Chronic pain was defined as pain during the previous three months. According to the 0–10 Numeric Rating Scale, pain scored ≥7 corresponds to severe pain. Binary logistic regression was used to determine the variables associated to pain aspects.

Results: A total of 2633 (42%) reported chronic pain. More obese older adults (BMI ≥30 kg/m^2) experienced chronic pain (58%) than those who were low-normal weight (BMI < 25 kg/m^2, 39%) or overweight (25 ≤ BMI < 30 kg/m^2, 41%). Obese elderly more frequently had pain in extremities and lower back than their peers. In the multivariate model, obesity (Odds Ratio (OR) 1.59, 95% Confidence Interval (CI) 1.33–1.91) but not overweight (OR 1.08, 95% CI 0.95–1.22) was associated with chronic pain. Obesity (OR 1.53, 95% CI 1.16–2.01) was also significantly related to severe pain. We also found other comorbidities – i.e., traumatic history (OR 2.52, 95% CI 1.99–3.19), rheumatic diseases (OR 5.21, 95% CI 4.54–5.97), age ≥ 85 years (OR 1.66, 95% CI 1.22–2.25), and depression or anxiety diagnosis (OR 1.83, 95% CI 1.32–2.53) – showed stronger associations with pain aspects than weight status. Conclusion: In older adults, excess weight (BMI 30 or above) is a potentially modifiable factor but not the only risk factor that is associated with chronic pain and severe pain. Future studies should investigate the effectiveness of interventions that treat comorbid pain and obesity in older adults.

Keywords: Chronic pain, Older adults, Obesity, Overweight

Background

Chronic pain is common in older adults, but the prevalence varies widely, ranging from 20 to 93% [1]. This wide variation is likely due to the representative population samples used and discrepancies between questionnaires that assess pain. In Sweden, more than 50% of people aged 65 and over report chronic pain [2] and in the future this percentage is likely to increase in the oldest age groups [3].

The prevalence of overweight and obesity in the elderly population is increasing worldwide [4, 5]. Excess weight can affect longevity and disease-specific mortality in old age [5–7]. Rather than just surviving to an old age, more attention is now being paid to healthy aging. Both chronic pain and obesity can be barriers for healthy aging as these factors may affect important domains of life quality such as physical independence, mental well-being, and health [8, 9].

Obesity and chronic pain often occur simultaneously. The two conditions adversely influence each other [10, 11]. Both in the general population and in old age groups, increased Body Mass Index (BMI) is positively related to chronic pain [12, 13], specifically in the lower limbs (i.e., hip, leg, knee, and foot) [12, 14, 15], spine (neck and back)

* Correspondence: huanji.dong@liu.se
[1]Pain and Rehabilitation Medicine, Department of Medicine and Health Sciences (IMH), Faculty of Health Sciences, Linköping University, SE-581 85 Linköping, Sweden
Full list of author information is available at the end of the article

[14, 16], and head as manifested as headaches [13, 17]. Pain can be a barrier to weight reduction. Patients with severe pain lost less weight than those with none-to-moderate pain during a weight management program, suggesting severe pain impeded their weight loss [18, 19]. Unfortunately, current clinical practice is more likely to treat pain and excess weight as separate issues [11, 20]. The complexity of managing each condition independently means that some other factors need to be considered.

Obesity and chronic pain share some co-morbidities (e.g., osteoarthritis, hypertension, depression, and anxiety) [13, 21–23] and poor health-related quality of life [4] as well as being associated with socio-demographic factors such as being female [13], low education [24], and low socio-economic status [25]. Smoking behaviour and alcohol consumption have also been considered as determinants of the relationship between obesity and chronic pain, but the literature is not entirely in agreement [24, 26–29]. However, few studies have examined weight in relation to socio-demographic profiles, comorbidities, and lifestyle habits. Moreover, the increase in life expectancy has resulted in more age-related diseases. The combination of various chronic conditions and diseases were observed frequently in aging populations [30, 31]. A majority of older adults have comorbidities and multi-morbidities [32, 33]. A knowledge gap exists as to whether, and to which extent, multiple comorbidities might substantially contribute to the weight-chronic pain relationship in old age. Using a random population sample of Swedish older adults, this cross-sectional study investigates the weight-chronic pain association with respect to sociodemographic factors, comorbidities, and lifestyle habits.

Methods

Participants and procedure

Using a cross-sectional postal questionnaire, this study collected data from a stratified random sample of 10,000 older adults (≥ 65 years old) based on five age strata (65 to 69 years, 70 to 74 years, 75 to 79 years, 80 to 84 years, and 85 years and older) from the Swedish Total Population Register for the two largest cities (Linköping and Norrköping) of a county (Östergötland) in south-eastern Sweden. The questionnaire was mailed in October 2012 and, if needed, two reminders at two-week intervals were mailed. The collection of questionnaires closed in January 2013.

Measurements

The survey included several validated instruments/ scales. An overview of all parts of the survey has been presented elsewhere [34, 35]. The relevant instruments for this study are described below.

Demographic aspects

Age, sex, educational level, and civil status were recorded from the respondents' answers in the postal survey. Civil status was categorized as single, married, divorced, and widowed. Educational level was classified as high school (elementary/secondary), upper school, or vocational training for more than two years, college or university for one to two years, and college or university for three years or more.

Anthropometric variables

Height and weight were recorded from the respondents' answers in the postal survey and the BMI (kg/m^2) was calculated using these data. Specifically, BMI was calculated as weight (kg)/height (m)^2 and classified according to the criteria developed by the World Health Organization (WHO): < 18.5 = underweight; 18.5–24.9 = normal range; 25.0–29.9 = overweight; and ≥ 30.0 = obesity. Morbid obesity (severely obese) is defined as a BMI category above 35.0.

Several studies have compared the validity of measured weight- and height-calculated BMI and self-reported weight- and height-calculated BMI. High correlations were reported between the two measures (Pearson's $r = 0.89$ to 0.97 for different age groups and gender) [36]. Compared to the measured BMI, self-reported BMI had a sensitivity of 88.1% and specificity of 97.4% for identifying overweight/obesity [37].

Characteristics of pain

Pain intensity over the preceding seven days was assessed using an 11-point numeric rating scale (NRS), ranging from 0 (no pain) to 10 (worst imaginable pain) [38]. The cut-offs of NRS for definitions of mild, moderate, and severe pain vary in the literature [39–42]. In this study, NRS scored 1–3, 4–6, and 7–10 corresponded to mild, moderate, and severe pain, respectively. We selected the cut-offs based on the knowledge that moderate and severe pain make it difficult with an individual's activities of daily living [42, 43]. The duration of pain was registered using one question with three alternatives: no; yes, with less duration than three months; yes, with a duration of more than three months. The present study reports the proportion with chronic pain – i.e., pain with a duration of more than three months.

All the respondents marked their painful site for the previous seven days on a body manikin divided into a total of 45 sections on the front and on the back [44, 45]. From these sections, we identified 23 anatomical pain sites and developed a total index to denote the number of pain sites (NPS), ranging from 0 to 23 [44]. High values indicated higher spreading of pain (multi-site pain).

Co-morbidities

The evaluation of co-morbidities was based on a 12-item self-reported list covering different aspects of common co-morbidities: (1) traumatic accident, (2) rheumatic arthritis and osteoarthritis, (3) cardiovascular diseases (including high blood pressure, angina pectoris, and heart attacks), (4) diseases of airways or lungs, (5) low mood and depression, (6) anxiety, (7) diseases of the gastrointestinal system, (8) diseases of the nervous system, including eyes and ears, (9) diseases of the urogenital organs, (10) diseases of the skin, (11) tumours and cancer, and (12) metabolic diseases such as diabetes, obesity, anorexia, bulimia, and goitre. These co-morbidities were reported on a five-point scale: 1 = no; 2 = yes, according to both my own and my doctor's opinions; 3 = yes, according to my own opinion; 4 = yes, according to my doctor's opinion; and 5 = do not know. We combined the answers for 2 and 4 to increase the robustness of measurements of the presence of a certain comorbidity. Hence, these items were dichotomized as follows: yes, according to both my own and my doctor's opinions plus according to my doctor's opinion and the three other alternatives.

Life style factors

From the instrument "Health Curve" (*Hälsokurvan*) [46], we chose four questions concerning smoking and snuff use that addressed both frequency (from never to daily) and number of cigarettes per day (1 to 9; 10 to 19; and 20 or more) and number of snuff boxes per week (1 to 3 per week and 7 or more per week). Five questions concerned alcohol habits. For those who confirmed alcohol consumption, the four CAGE questions (Cut-down, Annoy, Guilty, and Eye-opener) were used to screen possible alcohol addiction problems [47]; a score of ≥ 2 was considered to indicate potential problems with alcohol abuse.

Statistical analysis

Statistical analysis was performed using the SPSS statistical package (version 22.0 IBM Inc., New York, USA). Data were reported as the mean with standard deviation (SD), the median with interquartile range (IQR), or the number with percentage based on the data distributions. Missing data were excluded from the analysis and calculated percentages were obtained from the number of valid responses. Differences among groups were assessed using the Chi-square, the one-way ANOVA, and the Kruskal-Wallis tests as appropriate. A p-value < 0.05 was considered statistically significant. Binary logistic regression was used to test predictors for chronic pain, moderate pain (NRS 4–6), and severe chronic pain (NRS 7–10). BMI was entered as a categorical predictor using low-normal weight as the reference group. In the univariate analysis,

we examined the effect of each variable on chronic pain, including demographic aspects (age and sex), social economic factors (marital status, education, and yearly income levels), lifestyle habits (smoking and alcohol consumption), and obesity or pain-related comorbidities. In the multivariate logistic regression, a forward (likely ratio, LR) method was used by entering each variable forwardly and removing the least significant variables from the model until all remaining variables were significant ($p < 0.05$ or $p \geq 0.1$ for entry or removal, respectively). Goodness of fit was performed using the Hosmer and Lemeshow test where a p-value greater than 0.05 indicated good fit of the model. Collinearity was tested using a correlation matrix of estimates. Because diagnosis of depression and anxiety showed a high collinearity ($r = 0.608$), we transformed the two variables to a new variable (1 = depression and/or anxiety) and re-tested the correlations. This new variable represents aspects of mental health.

Results

A total of 6243 individuals completed the questionnaire including height and weight variables used to calculate BMI. For the study population, the average BMI was 25.79 ± 4.18 kg/m^2 and 39% (2434) were categorized as overweight and 14% (871) were categorized as obese. In the obesity group, 17.3% (151) were categorized as morbidly obese. Compared with the low-normal weight and the overweight groups, the obesity group was relatively younger (< 75 years old), had a higher proportion of males, lower education, lower yearly income, more smokers, and more suspected high alcohol consumers (Table 1).

As reported elsewhere, chronic pain was reported by 51.3% of the investigated cohort [44]. More than 55% of the obese group had chronic pain, whereas 38.3% of the low-normal weight group and 41.8% of the overweight group had chronic pain ($p < 0.001$). Among the individuals with chronic pain, 32.7% of the obese group, 23.5% of the overweight and 20.6 of the low-normal weight (reported severe pain ($p < 0.001$). Similarly, according to NPS, the spread of chronic pain was more evident in the obese group (median = 4) than in the two other groups (median 3 for both groups) ($p < 0.001$). Pain in extremities and lower back were also more prevalent in the obese group (Fig. 1). A variety of co-morbidities (e.g., rheumatic diseases, cardiovascular diseases, respiratory diseases, gastrointestinal diseases, and metabolic diseases) were more frequently reported by obese individuals than their counterparts (Table 1).

Univariate logistic regression showed that higher BMI, being female, low education (nine-year compulsory school), smoking history, high alcohol consumption, and several comorbidities were positively associated with

Table 1 Demographic characteristics, pain aspects, and prevalence of comorbidities in the three groups of weight status

	Low-normal weight $N = 2938$	Overweight $N = 2448$	Obesity $N = 871$	P-value (F or x^2)
Age, mean ± SD	77.1 ± 7.8	75.6 ± 7.2	74.2 ± 6.5	< 0.001 ($F = 59.5$)
65–74, n (%)	1218 (41.5)	1160 (47.7)	479 (55)	< 0.001 ($x^2 = 111.5$)
75–84, n (%)	1164 (39.6)	982 (40.3)	328 (37.7)	
85+, n (%)	556 (18.9)	292 (12)	64 (7.3)	
Female, n (%)	1675 (57)	1179 (48.2)	481 (55.2)	< 0.001 ($x^2 = 43.5$)
Married, n (%)	1652 (56.2)	1442 (58.9)	497 (57.1)	0.129 ($x^2 = 4.10$)
Education, n (%)[1]				< 0.001 ($x^2 = 31.0$)
9-year Compulsory school	1393 (48.9)	1275 (53.8)	477 (57)	
Upper secondary school	749 (26.3)	614 (25.9)	211 (25.2)	
College/University	705 (24.8)	479 (20.2)	149 (17.8)	
Income (SEK per year), n (%)				< 0.001 ($x^2 = 21.4$)
< 150,000	872 (29.7)	662 (27)	296 (34)	
150,001~ 220,000	982 (33.4)	861 (35)	307 (35.2)	
> 220,000	1084 (36.9)	925 (37.8)	268 (30.8)	
Smoking, n (%)[2]				< 0.001 ($x^2 = 79.7$)
Never smoker	1620 (57.2)	1244 (53.1)	396 (48.2)	
Ex-smoker	917 (32.4)	955 (40.8)	368 (44.8)	
Current smoker	295 (10.4)	143 (6.1)	57 (6.9)	
High alcohol consumption, n (%)	112 (3.8)	118 (4.8)	55 (6.3)	0.006 ($x^2 = 10.3$)
Pain aspects, n (%)				
Chronic pain	1134 (38.6)	1023 (41.8)	482 (55.3)	< 0.001 ($x^2 = 77.5$)
NPS, median (IQR)[a,3]	3 (1–5)	3 (2–5)	4 (2–6)	< 0.001 ($x^2 = 36.1$)
No pain (NRS 0)[a]	17 (1.6)	12 (1.2)	8 (1.8)	< 0.001 ($x^2 = 37.1$)
Mild pain (NRS 1–3)[a]	300 (26.5)	224 (21.9)	79 (16.4)	
Moderate pain (NRS 4–6)[a]	521 (45.9)	501 (49)	217 (45)	
Severe pain (NRS 7–10)[a]	218 (20.6)	226 (23.5)	148 (32.7)	
Comorbidities, n (%)				
History of trauma or injury accident	190 (6.5)	183 (7.5)	64 (7.3)	0.340 ($x^2 = 2.30$)
Rheumatic diseases	638 (21.7)	637 (26)	327 (37.5)	< 0.001 ($x^2 = 88.7$)
Cardiovascular diseases	1242 (42.3)	1301 (53.1)	553 (63.5)	< 0.001 ($x^2 = 142.6$)
Respiratory diseases	317 (10.8)	264 (10.8)	155 (17.8)	< 0.001 ($x^2 = 35.5$)
Gastrointestinal diseases	411 (14)	378 (15.4)	167 (19.2)	0.001 ($x^2 = 14.0$)
Neurological diseases	914 (31.1)	731 (29.9)	228 (26.2)	0.02 ($x^2 = 7.80$)
Urogenital diseases	240 (8.2)	213 (8.7)	87 (10)	0.238 ($x^2 = 2.85$)
Metabolic diseases	290 (9.9)	379 (15.6)	274 (31.5)	< 0.001 ($x^2 = 244.8$)
Cancer diagnosis	230 (7.8)	178 (7.3)	64 (7.3)	0.723 ($x^2 = 0.65$)
Depression	132 (4.5)	105 (4.3)	48 (5.5)	0.337 ($x^2 = 2.18$)
Anxiety	129 (4.4)	97 (4)	47 (5.4)	0.217 ($x^2 = 3.06$)

The far right column shows the result of the omnibus statistical testing (p-value, F and x^2)
NPS number of pain sites; [a]Individuals with chronic pain $N = 2639$
Missing data: [1] = 205; [2] = 262; [3] = 168

chronic pain (Table 2). Most of these positive effects remained in the multivariate regression, except for being overweight, education, yearly income, high alcohol consumption, and having cardiovascular diseases or cancer (Table 2). Being obese (OR 1.59, 95% CI 1.32–1.91, $p < 0.001$) but not overweight (OR 1.08, 95% CI 0.95–

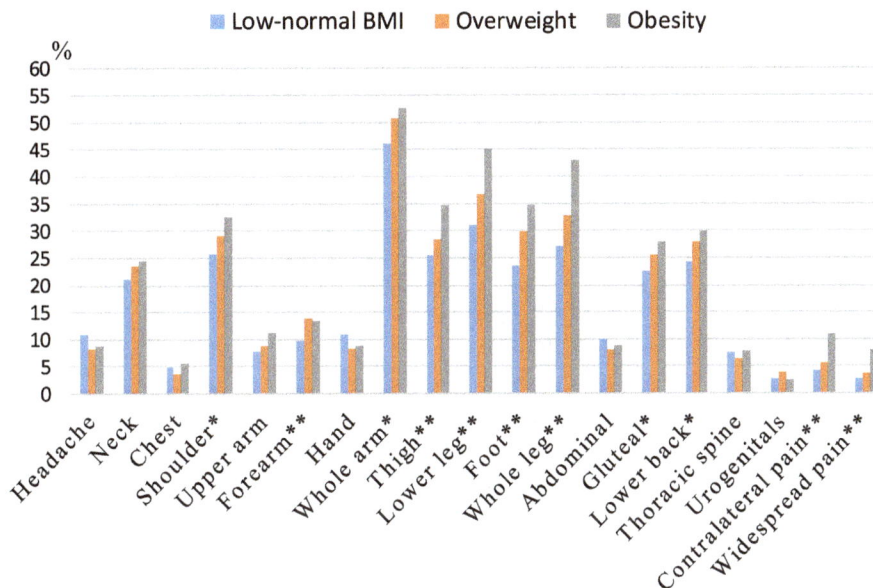

Fig. 1 Prevalence of pain in 23 anatomical regions with BMI stratifications. The regions of head, shoulder, upper arm, forearm, hand, thigh, lower leg, and foot included both right and left sides. *P < 0.05, **P < 0.01

1.21, $p = 0.254$) was more likely associated with chronic pain than low-normal weight. Some factors, such as having trauma or injury accident history (OR 2.52, 95% CI: 1.99–3.19) and rheumatic diseases (OR 5.21, 95% CI: 4.54–5.97), showed higher associations with chronic pain than obesity status.

Within the chronic pain group, obesity and overweight were weakly but significantly associated with moderate pain (OR1.30–1.39, $p < 0.05$, Table 2). In comparison, obesity had stronger impact on severe pain (OR 1.53, 95% CI 1.16–2.01, $p < 0.01$). However, aged 85 and over (OR 1.66, 95% CI 1.22–2.25) and depression and/or anxiety diseases (OR 1.83, 95% CI 1.32–2.53) were more strongly linked to severe pain than being obese. Sociodemographic factors such as age, gender, education, and income levels were also significantly related to having moderate pain. Being an ex-smoker, certain co-morbidities (e.g., rheumatic diseases and cardiovascular diseases), and number of pain sites were also significant regressors of severe pain.

Discussion

Among the older adults in our study cohort, chronic pain was more common in people categorized as obese than in people categorized as overweight or low-normal weight. A distinct difference in anatomical pain distributions to some extent reflected the negative consequence of excess weight. The well-known disparity of pain distributions with respect to sex [13, 48–51] was also found in the cohort, but this was not statistically significant across age stratifications. Our findings contribute to the growing body of evidence that being obese, but not

being overweight, is closely related to chronic pain, including severe chronic pain in the older adults. Furthermore, in our aged sample, having multiple comorbidities was more strongly related to pain-related factors than excess weight.

In the context of the current obesity epidemic, the adverse health consequences of excess weight place older adults at risk for comorbidity, poor physical function, and disability. In later life, chronic pain may show a mediating effect between obesity and these consequences [52]. The literature identifies three dominant aspects that support the relationship between obesity and chronic pain. First, increased mechanical load could explain the connection between excess weight and specific anatomical pain distributions [10, 21]. In our study, this hypothesis was reasonably confirmed by a higher proportion of reported chronic pain in extremities and low back in obese olds than in normal-weight or overweight olds. Second, hyperalgesia can be the result of the gradual development of systematic chronic low-grade inflammation. For example, pain can be modulated by inflammatory processes initiated by altered levels of cytokines (C creative protein, interlukin-6, TNF-α, IL-6, adiponectin, leptin, resistin, and visfatin) in adipose tissue [10, 21, 53, 54]. Furthermore, aging contributes to a pro-inflammatory state by increasing production of cytokines and reducing the capacity to cope with a variety of stressors [55]. Our multivariate models showed that the influence of age on inflammation may contribute to the course of chronic pain and to the increase in pain intensity. Third, obese adults are more likely to suffer poor mental health [56, 57], adding to their inflammation-inducing

Table 2 Univariate and multivariate logistic regression – factors associated with chronic pain and severe pain

	Variables associated with Chronic pain		Variables associated with moderate pain	Variables associated with severe pain
	Univariate [OR (95% CI)]	Multivariate [OR (95% CI)]	Multivariate [OR (95% CI)]	Multivariate [OR (95% CI)]
BMI (Low-normal BMI reference category)	1.0	1.0	1.0	1.0
Overweight	1.14 (1.02–1.27)	1.08 (0.95–1.22)	1.30 (1.04–1.63)*	1.09 (0.87–1.34)
Obesity	1.97 (1.69–2.30)	1.59 (1.33–1.91)**	1.39 (1.02–1.89)*	1.53 (1.17–2.01)**
Age (65–74 y, reference category)	1.0	–	1.0	1.0
75–84 y	1.04 (0.93–1.16)	–	1.11 (0.89–1.40)	1.31 (1.05–1.63)*
85+ y	1.05 (0.90–1.22)	–	1.81 (1.26–2.60)**	1.66 (1.22–2.25)**
Gender (1 = female)	1.66 (1.50–1.84)**	1.40 (1.24–1.58)**	1.33 (1.06–1.67)*	–
Marital status (1 = married)	0.91 (0.83–1.01)	–	–	–
Education (College/university, reference category)	1.0	–	1.0	–
9-year Compulsory school	1.32 (1.16–1.50)**	–	1.47 (1.11–1.94)*	–
Upper secondary school	1.13 (0.98–1.32)	–	1.33 (0.99–1.79)	–
Income per year (< 150,000 SEK, reference category)	1.0	–	1.0	–
150,001~ 220,000	0.83 (0.73–0.94)*	–	0.78 (0.58–1.02)	–
> 220,000	0.64 (0.57–0.73)**	–	0.70 (0.51–0.95)*	–
Smoking (never smoker, reference category)	1.0	1.0	–	1.0
Ex-smoker, n %	1.14 (1.02–1.27)*	1.21 (1.07–1.38)*	–	1.30 (1.05–1.60)*
Current smoker, n %	1.13 (0.93–1.36)	1.29 (1.04–1.59)*	–	1.33 (0.93–1.91)
High alcohol consumption (1 = yes)	1.17 (0.92–1.48)	–	–	–
History of trauma or injury accident	3.2 (2.60–3.94)**	2.52 (1.99–3.19)**	–	–
Rheumatic diseases (1 = yes)	5.92 (5.22–6.72)**	5.21 (4.54–5.97)**	–	1.34 (1.10–1.64)*
Cardiovascular diseases (1 = yes)	1.35 (1.22–1.49)**	–	1.36 (1.10–1.67)**	1.33 (1.10–1.64)*
Respiratory diseases (1 = yes)	1.82 (1.56–2.12)**	1.34 (1.18–1.52)**	–	–
Gastrointestinal diseases (1 = yes)	2.61 (2.35–3.16)**	1.93 (1.64–2.27)**	–	–
Neurological diseases (1 = yes)	1.71 (1.54–1.91)**	1.34 (1.18–1.52)**	–	–
Urogenital diseases (1 = yes)	1.53 (1.36–1.97)**	–	–	–
Metabolic diseases (1 = yes)	1.59 (1.43–1.91)**	1.27 (1.08–1.50)*	–	–
Cancer diagnosis (1 = yes)	1.33 (1.07–1.57)*	–	–	–
Depression and/or anxiety (1 = yes)	1.99 (1.61–2.45)**	1.46 (1.14–1.86)*	–	1.83 (1.32–2.53)**
Number of pain sites (NPS)			1.11 (1.06–1.16)**	1.1 (1.06–1.13)*
Model Nagelkerke R^2		0.236	0.086	0.08
Model Hosmer and Lemeshow test		$x^2 = 7.63, P = 0.47$	$x^2 = 10.40, P = 0.238$	$x^2 = 6.30, P = 0.613$

Note: *$P < 0.05$, **$P < 0.01$

stressors. Previous studies have recognized this co-existence and interactions between mood disorders (depression and/or anxiety) and pain [58–61]. Because the associations between these conditions are bidirectional, it is difficult to ascertain which condition causes or exacerbates the other or indeed if a causal relationship exists.

Smoking history seems to play an important role in the course of chronic pain and severe pain. As with other studies, we found that both current smoking and ex-smoking were associated with chronic pain [62–64]; however, determining the underlying mechanism is difficult as thousands of compounds in cigarette smoke produce physiological effects. Apart from the pharmacological effect of nicotine and other ligands at the nicotinic acetylcholine receptor associated with pain, smoking behaviour to some extent reflects poor mental well-being [65]. Smoking as an unhealthy behaviour is part of negative psychological profiles and it is interconnected with obesity and pain symptoms [26, 27, 65].

In the multivariate model, we found several common comorbidities (e.g., rheumatic diseases) of chronic pain that have a greater impact than obesity. In the logistic regressions, we found that other obesity-related diseases/co-morbidities – e.g., obstructive sleep apnoea (categorized as a respiratory disease), gallbladder disorder (categorized as a gastrointestinal disease), stroke (categorized as a neurological disease), diabetes (categorized as a metabolic disease), and mental illness (depression or anxiety) – exhibited a modest association with chronic pain. These impacts may have been stronger if these diseases/co-morbidities had been asked for specifically and not included in broader categories as in the present study. Therefore, in an aging population with a high prevalence of multiple morbidities, we need to consider the above common comorbidities when evaluating chronic pain and suffering. In addition, these comorbidities are not the same comorbidities younger people experiece when suffering from chronic pain. For example, unlike a chronic pain study of younger people [26], two common obesity-related illnesses, cancer and cardiovascular disease, were not significantly associated with chronic pain in our study population. This difference suggests that the relationship between these conditions and chronic pain in old age are weaker or even absent. It may be that these common comorbidities are also age-related, so they may frequently occur in older adults with or without excess weight and pain suffering.

The analysis of these factors together with weight status provides a subset of the aging population who may be more likely to have chronic pain. To meet the particular needs of pain management for older people (e.g., pharmacological treatment, lifestyle interventions, psychological support, and rehabilitation) [66], health professionals should identify the risk group. Our study results support the growing evidence of the pain-obesity relationship in older adults. The multivariate models strongly indicate the need to have a multifactorial approach to chronic pain when assessing patients with pain. Our results indicate the need to incorporate weight/BMI as one of several factors in such assessments. It is important to be aware that not all risk factors in the models are modifiable – i.e., increased age, female gender, education, income, and having trauma history. Alternatively, the modifiable factors such as obesity, smoking, and certain chronic diseases present the opportunities for intervening. Because more modifiable factors existed in patients with severe pain than in patients with moderate pain, patients with severe pain have more interventions available to them that can relieve their pain. Healthcare professionals need to pay attention to existing multifactorial characteristics so they can identify the people at greatest risk and in most need of interventions. Therefore, pain interventions for older adults should direct their focus on the modifiable risk factors.

One important limitation of this cross-sectional study was the bias from self-reported anthropometric measures. Despite a high correlation between self-reported and measured values, the underestimation of excess weight by self-reported values has been reported [36, 37]. If we consider this bias (men by 1-unit and women by 1.19-unit underestimated BMI) [37], a total of 1117 individuals could be misclassified (28.5% of normal-weight and 14.5% of overweight). When we recalculated the regression analysis using these revised numbers, the estimates in the model did not show significant changes (data not shown).

Another weakness of our study could be the lack of generalizability of the results due to the rate of non-participants in the study population, with a valid response of 62.7% (10,000 subjects selected) [34]. The non-participants may represent a group with severe illness (e.g., admitted in hospital, residing in nursing homes, and unable to answer the questionnaire due to cognitive impairment) or a more healthy group (e.g., without any pain discomforts) so they were not interested in participating in the study [67].

In addition, our cross-sectional analysis did not uncover any causation. We cannot identify a direct cause-and-effect relationship between these factors. The results should be tested longitudinally in future studies. Additionally, although many important co-variates were included in the regression analysis, some potentially meaningful co-variates such as dietary intake and physical activity were not collected in this study. Previous studies demonstrated that unhealthy excess food intake and sedentary living cause weight gain and systemic inflammation [68, 69]. To some extent, this understanding provides for the possibility that interventions could break down the vicious circle of excess weight and chronic pain conditions. A follow-up study or longitudinal studies measuring changes could validate the impacts of changes on comorbid obesity and pain.

Conclusion

Chronic pain affects more obese older adults than their low-normal or overweight peers. Excess weight (BMI 30 or above) is a potentially modifiable factor but not the only risk factor that is associated with chronic pain and severe pain. It is important for healthcare professionals to understand the multiple factors involved in the complex relationship between pain and excess weight. Healthcare professionals and policy makers should address the management of the coexisting modifiable factors instead of focusing on a single achievement (i.e., weight reduction). Future research should investigate the effectiveness of interventions that treat comorbid pain and obesity in older adults.

Abbreviations

BMI: Body Mass Index; CI: Confidence Interval; NPS: Number of Pain Sites; NRS: Numeric Rating Scale; OR: Odds ratio

Acknowledgments

The authors acknowledge and thank the participants.

Funding

The present study was sponsored by a grant from Grünenthal Sweden AB.

Authors' contributions

BL, L-ÅL, LB, and BG made substantial contributions to study conception and design. H-J D and BG performed the data analyses and took part in drafting the manuscript. All authors discussed the results and revised it critically. All authors had full access to all the data in the study and had final responsibility for the decision to submit for publication.

Competing interests

The sponsor of the study had no role in study design, data collection, data analysis, data interpretation, writing of the report, or the decision to submit for publication. The authors had full access to all the data in the study and had final responsibility for the decision to submit for publication. The authors declare that they have no competing interests.

Author details

[1]Pain and Rehabilitation Medicine, Department of Medicine and Health Sciences (IMH), Faculty of Health Sciences, Linköping University, SE-581 85 Linköping, Sweden. [2]Division of Health Care Analysis, Department of Medical and Health Sciences, Linköping University, SE-581 85 Linköping, Sweden.

References

1. Abdulla A, Adams N, Bone M, Elliott AM, Gaffin J, Jones D, Knaggs R, Martin D, Sampson L, Schofield P. Guidance on the management of pain in older people. Age Ageing. 2013;42(Suppl 1):i1–57.
2. Gerdle B, Bjork J, Henriksson C, Bengtsson A. Prevalence of current and chronic pain and their influences upon work and healthcare-seeking: a population study. J Rheumatol. 2004;31(7):1399–406.
3. Ahacic K, Kareholt I. Prevalence of musculoskeletal pain in the general Swedish population from 1968 to 2002: age, period, and cohort patterns. Pain. 2010;151(1):206–14.
4. Salihu HM, Bonnema S, Alio AP. Obesity: what is an elderly population growing into? Maturitas. 2009;63(1):7–12.
5. Chapman IM. Obesity paradox during aging. Interdiscip Top Gerontol. 2010;37:20–36.
6. Zamboni M, Mazzali G, Zoico E, Harris TB, Meigs JB, Di Francesco V, Fantin F, Bissoli L, Bosello O. Health consequences of obesity in the elderly: a review of four unresolved questions. Int J Obes. 2005;29(9):1011–29.
7. Flegal KM, Kit BK, Orpana H, Graubard BI. Association of all-cause mortality with overweight and obesity using standard body mass index categories: a systematic review and meta-analysis. JAMA. 2013;309(1):71–82.
8. Anton SD, Woods AJ, Ashizawa T, Barb D, Buford TW, Carter CS, Clark DJ, Cohen RA, Corbett DB, Cruz-Almeida Y, et al. Successful aging: advancing the science of physical independence in older adults. Ageing Res Rev. 2015;24(Pt B):304–27.
9. Depp CA, Jeste DV. Definitions and predictors of successful aging: a comprehensive review of larger quantitative studies. Am J Geriatr Psychiatry. 2006;14(1):6–20.
10. Okifuji A, Hare BD. The association between chronic pain and obesity. J Pain Res. 2015;8:399–408.
11. Cooper L, Ells L, Ryan C, Martin D. Perceptions of adults with overweight/obesity and chronic musculoskeletal pain: an interpretative phenomenological analysis. J Clin Nurs. 2018;27(5–6):e776–86.
12. Hitt HC, McMillen RC, Thornton-Neaves T, Koch K, Cosby AG. Comorbidity of obesity and pain in a general population: results from the southern pain prevalence study. J Pain. 2007;8(5):430–6.
13. McCarthy LH, Bigal ME, Katz M, Derby C, Lipton RB. Chronic pain and obesity in elderly people: results from the Einstein aging study. J Am Geriatr Soc. 2009;57(1):115–9.
14. Andersen RE, Crespo CJ, Bartlett SJ, Bathon JM, Fontaine KR. Relationship between body weight gain and significant knee, hip, and back pain in older Americans. Obes Res. 2003;11(10):1159–62.
15. Fransen M, Su S, Harmer A, Blyth FM, Naganathan V, Sambrook P, Le Couteur D, Cumming RG. A longitudinal study of knee pain in older men: Concord health and ageing in men project. Age Ageing. 2014;43(2):206–12.
16. Fernandez-de-las-Penas C, Hernandez-Barrera V, Alonso-Blanco C, Palacios-Cena D, Carrasco-Garrido P, Jimenez-Sanchez S, Jimenez-Garcia R. Prevalence of neck and low back pain in community-dwelling adults in Spain: a population-based national study. Spine. 2011;36(3):E213–9.
17. Bigal ME, Rapoport AM. Obesity and chronic daily headache. Curr Pain Headache Rep. 2012;16(1):101–9.
18. Masheb RM, Lutes LD, Kim HM, Holleman RG, Goodrich DE, Janney CA, Kirsh S, Higgins DM, Richardson CR, Damschroder LJ. Weight loss outcomes in patients with pain. Obesity. 2015;23(9):1778–84.
19. Ryan CG, Vijayaraman A, Denny V, Ogier A, Ells L, Wellburn S, Cooper L, Martin DJ, Atkinson G. The association between baseline persistent pain and weight change in patients attending a specialist weight management service. PLoS One. 2017;12(6):e0179227.
20. Cooper L, Ryan CG, Ells LJ, Hamilton S, Atkinson G, Cooper K, Johnson MI, Kirwan JP, Martin D. Weight loss interventions for adults with overweight/obesity and chronic musculoskeletal pain: a mixed methods systematic review. Obes Rev. 2018;19(7):989–1007.
21. Taylor R, Pergolizzi JV, Raffa RB, Nalamachu S, Balestrieri PJ. Pain and obesity in the older adult. Curr Pharm Des. 2014;20(38):6037–41.
22. Wright LJ, Schur E, Noonan C, Ahumada S, Buchwald D, Afari N. Chronic pain, overweight, and obesity: findings from a community-based twin registry. J Pain. 2010;11(7):628–35.
23. Reeuwijk KG, de Rooij M, van Dijk GM, Veenhof C, Steultjens MP, Dekker J. Osteoarthritis of the hip or knee: which coexisting disorders are disabling? Clin Rheumatol. 2010;29(7):739–47.
24. Stone AA, Broderick JE. Obesity and pain are associated in the United States. Obesity. 2012;20(7):1491–5.
25. Ahn S, Huber C, Smith ML, Ory MG, Phillips CD. Predictors of body mass index among low-income community-dwelling older adults. J Health Care Poor Underserved. 2011;22(4):1190–204.
26. Shi Y, Hooten WM, Roberts RO, Warner DO. Modifiable risk factors for incidence of pain in older adults. Pain. 2010;151(2):366–71.
27. van Hecke O, Torrance N, Smith BH. Chronic pain epidemiology - where do lifestyle factors fit in? Br J Pain. 2013;7(4):209–17.
28. Mourao AF, Blyth FM, Branco JC. Generalised musculoskeletal pain syndromes. Best Pract Res Clin Rheumatol. 2010;24(6):829–40.
29. Brennan PL, Schutte KK, Moos RH. Pain and use of alcohol to manage pain: prevalence and 3-year outcomes among older problem and non-problem drinkers. Addiction. 2005;100(6):777–86.
30. Barnett K, Mercer SW, Norbury M, Watt G, Wyke S, Guthrie B. Epidemiology of multimorbidity and implications for health care, research, and medical education: a cross-sectional study. Lancet. 2012;380(9836):37–43.
31. Islam MM, Valderas JM, Yen L, Dawda P, Jowsey T, McRae IS. Multimorbidity and comorbidity of chronic diseases among the senior Australians: prevalence and patterns. PLoS One. 2014;9(1):e83783.
32. Salive ME. Multimorbidity in older adults. Epidemiol Rev. 2013;35:75–83.
33. Marengoni A, Angleman S, Melis R, Mangialasche F, Karp A, Garmen A, Meinow B, Fratiglioni L. Aging with multimorbidity: a systematic review of the literature. Ageing Res Rev. 2011;10(4):430–9.
34. Bernfort L, Gerdle B, Rahmqvist M, Husberg M, Levin LA. Severity of chronic pain in an elderly population in Sweden--impact on costs and quality of life. Pain. 2015;156(3):521–7.
35. Larsson B, Gerdle B, Bernfort L, Levin LA, Dragioti E. Distinctive subgroups derived by cluster analysis based on pain and psychological symptoms in Swedish older adults with chronic pain - a population study (PainS65+). BMC Geriatr. 2017;17(1):200.
36. Kuczmarski MF, Kuczmarski RJ, Najjar M. Effects of age on validity of self-reported height, weight, and body mass index: findings from the third

National Health and nutrition examination survey, 1988-1994. J Am Diet Assoc. 2001;101(1):28–34 quiz 35-26.

37. Vuksanović M, Safer A, Palm F, Stieglbauer G, Grau A, Becher H. Validity of self-reported BMI in older adults and an adjustment model. J Public Health. 2014;22(3):257–63.

38. Ferreira-Valente MA, Pais-Ribeiro JL, Jensen MP. Validity of four pain intensity rating scales. Pain. 2011;152(10):2399–404.

39. Hirschfeld G, Zernikow B. Variability of "optimal" cut points for mild, moderate, and severe pain: neglected problems when comparing groups. Pain. 2013;154(1):154–9.

40. Fejer R, Jordan A, Hartvigsen J. Categorising the severity of neck pain: establishment of cut-points for use in clinical and epidemiological research. Pain. 2005;119(1–3):176–82.

41. Turner JA, Franklin G, Heagerty PJ, Wu R, Egan K, Fulton-Kehoe D, Gluck JV, Wickizer TM. The association between pain and disability. Pain. 2004;112(3):307–14.

42. Jensen M. The pain stethoscope. In: A clinician's guide to measuring pain, vol. IX. London: Springer Healthcare Communications; 2011. p. 53.

43. Breivik H, Collett B, Ventafridda V, Cohen R, Gallacher D. Survey of chronic pain in Europe: prevalence, impact on daily life, and treatment. Eur J Pain. 2006;10(4):287–333.

44. Dragioti E, Larsson B, Bernfort L, Levin LA, Gerdle B. Prevalence of different pain categories based on pain spreading on the bodies of older adults in Sweden: a descriptive-level and multilevel association with demographics, comorbidities, medications, and certain lifestyle factors (PainS65+). J Pain Res. 2016;9:1131–41.

45. Grimby-Ekman A, Gerdle B, Bjork J, Larsson B. Comorbidities, intensity, frequency and duration of pain, daily functioning and health care seeking in local, regional, and widespread pain - a descriptive population-based survey (SwePain). BMC Musculoskelet Disord. 2015;16:165.

46. Persson LG, Lindstrom K, Lingfors H, Bengtsson C. A study of men aged 33-42 in Habo, Sweden with special reference to cardiovascular risk factors. Design, health profile and characteristics of participants and non-participants. Scand J Soc Med. 1994;22(4):264–72.

47. Persson LG, Lindstrom K, Lingfors H, Bengtsson C, Lissner L. Cardiovascular risk during early adult life. Risk markers among participants in "live for life" health promotion programme in Sweden. J Epidemiol Community Health. 1998;52(7):425–32.

48. Rustoen T, Wahl AK, Hanestad BR, Lerdal A, Paul S, Miaskowski C. Gender differences in chronic pain--findings from a population-based study of Norwegian adults. Pain Manag Nurs. 2004;5(3):105–17.

49. Miro J, Paredes S, Rull M, Queral R, Miralles R, Nieto R, Huguet A, Baos J. Pain in older adults: a prevalence study in the Mediterranean region of Catalonia. Eur J Pain. 2007;11(1):83–92.

50. Patel KV, Guralnik JM, Dansie EJ, Turk DC. Prevalence and impact of pain among older adults in the United States: findings from the 2011 National Health and aging trends study. Pain. 2013;154(12):2649–57.

51. Blyth FM, March LM, Brnabic AJ, Jorm LR, Williamson M, Cousins MJ. Chronic pain in Australia: a prevalence study. Pain. 2001;89(2–3):127–34.

52. Fowler-Brown A, Wee CC, Marcantonio E, Ngo L, Leveille S. The mediating effect of chronic pain on the relationship between obesity and physical function and disability in older adults. J Am Geriatr Soc. 2013;61(12):2079–86.

53. Hauner H. Secretory factors from human adipose tissue and their functional role. Proc Nutr Soc. 2005;64(2):163–9.

54. Bas S, Finckh A, Puskas GJ, Suva D, Hoffmeyer P, Gabay C, Lubbeke A. Adipokines correlate with pain in lower limb osteoarthritis: different associations in hip and knee. Int Orthop. 2014;38(12):2577–83.

55. Franceschi C, Bonafe M, Valensin S, Olivieri F, De Luca M, Ottaviani E, De Benedictis G. Inflamm-aging. An evolutionary perspective on immunosenescence. Ann N Y Acad Sci. 2000;908:244–54.

56. Hassan MK, Joshi AV, Madhavan SS, Amonkar MM. Obesity and health-related quality of life: a cross-sectional analysis of the US population. Int J Obes Relat Metab Disord. 2003;27(10):1227–32.

57. Simon GE, Von Korff M, Saunders K, Miglioretti DL, Crane PK, van Belle G, Kessler RC. Association between obesity and psychiatric disorders in the US adult population. Arch Gen Psychiatry. 2006;63(7):824–30.

58. El-Gabalawy R, Mackenzie CS, Shooshtari S, Sareen J. Comorbid physical health conditions and anxiety disorders: a population-based exploration of prevalence and health outcomes among older adults. Gen Hosp Psychiatry. 2011;33(6):556–64.

59. Li JX. Pain and depression comorbidity: a preclinical perspective. Behav Brain Res. 2015;276c:92–8.

60. Okifuji ATD. Chronic pain and depression: vulnerability and resilience. In: aAM FMA, editor. Neuroscience of pain, stress, and emotion. New York: Elsevier; 2015.

61. Aguera-Ortiz L, Failde I, Cervilla JA, Mico JA. Unexplained pain complaints and depression in older people in primary care. J Nutr Health Aging. 2013;17(6):574–7.

62. Jakobsson U. Tobacco use in relation to chronic pain: results from a Swedish population survey. Pain Med. 2008;9(8):1091–7.

63. John U, Hanke M, Meyer C, Volzke H, Baumeister SE, Alte D. Tobacco smoking in relation to pain in a national general population survey. Prev Med. 2006;43(6):477–81.

64. Palmer KT, Syddall H, Cooper C, Coggon D. Smoking and musculoskeletal disorders: findings from a British national survey. Ann Rheum Dis. 2003;62(1):33–6.

65. Shi Y, Weingarten TN, Mantilla CB, Hooten WM, Warner DO. Smoking and pain: pathophysiology and clinical implications. Anesthesiology. 2010;113(4):977–92.

66. Kaye AD, Baluch A, Scott JT. Pain management in the elderly population: a review. Ochsner J. 2010;10(3):179–87.

67. Hardy SE, Allore H, Studenski SA. Missing data: a special challenge in aging research. J Am Geriatr Soc. 2009;57(4):722–9.

68. Arranz LI, Rafecas M, Alegre C. Effects of obesity on function and quality of life in chronic pain conditions. Curr Rheumatol Rep. 2014;16(1):390.

69. Emery CF, Olson KL, Bodine A, Lee V, Habash DL. Dietary intake mediates the relationship of body fat to pain. Pain. 2017;158(2):273–7.

19

Associations between health-related quality of life, physical function and fear of falling in older fallers receiving home care

Maria Bjerk[1]* ⓘ, Therese Brovold[1], Dawn A. Skelton[2] and Astrid Bergland[1]

Abstract

Background: Falls and injuries in older adults have significant consequences and costs, both personal and to society. Although having a high incidence of falls, high prevalence of fear of falling and a lower quality of life, older adults receiving home care are underrepresented in research on older fallers. The objective of this study is to determine the associations between health-related quality of life (HRQOL), fear of falling and physical function in older fallers receiving home care.

Methods: This study employed cross-sectional data from baseline measurements of a randomised controlled trial. 155 participants, aged 67+, with at least one fall in the previous year, from six Norwegian municipalities were included. Data on HRQOL (SF-36), physical function and fear of falling (FES-I) were collected in addition to demographical and other relevant background information. A multivariate regression model was applied.

Results: A higher score on FES-I, denoting increased fear of falling, was significantly associated with a lower score on almost all subscales of SF-36, denoting reduced HRQOL. Higher age was significantly associated with higher scores on physical function, general health, mental health and the mental component summary. This analysis adjusted for sex, education, living alone, being at risk of or malnourished, physical function like balance and walking speed, cognition and number of falls.

Conclusion: Fear of falling is important for HRQOL in older fallers receiving home care. This association is independent of physical measures. Better physical function is significantly associated with higher physical HRQOL. Future research should address interventions that reduce fear of falling and increase HRQOL in this vulnerable population.

Keywords: Health-related quality of life, Falls, Falls-efficacy, Fear of falling, Home care

Background

The increasing number of older adults living longer poses new challenges to health, long-term care and the welfare system [1]. The rising costs of falls and associated injuries are of global concern [2], estimated at 1.5% of health care costs in European countries, both directly from the fall-related injuries and indirectly through loss of mobility, confidence and functional independence [3].

Costs for long-term care are expected to increase substantially in the future. These expenses can be greatly reduced if the older adults are in good health and are able to remain at home [1]. Home care services are important in maintaining independence, contributing to functional health status and improving the quality of life (QOL) among older adults [4].

Home care is here defined as services provided by health professionals to people in their own homes and can cover a wide range of activities, from care related to individual needs to preventative assessments and actions [4]. The population of home care recipients constitutes a

* Correspondence: maria.bjerk@oslomet.no
[1]Department of Physiotherapy, OsloMet – Oslo Metropolitan University, PO Box 4 St. Olavs plass, 0130 Oslo, Norway
Full list of author information is available at the end of the article

transitional group between independent community living older people, and people living in residential care facilities, and their health-related quality of life (HRQOL) and other health outcomes might be different from those [5]. Even though home care could be an important contributor meeting the challenges of an increasing older population, surprisingly few clinical studies have been carried out including this group of older fallers [6, 7]. Falls and disability are strong predictors of institutionalisation. By targeting home care recipients who have experienced falls, the frequency of nursing home admissions could be reduced [8].

In Norway, the municipalities are responsible for providing home care for older adults, and recent governmental guidelines have put more focus on these services to enable older adults to remain at home as long as possible [9]. Home care comprises services like home nursing, practical assistance with daily activities and safety alarm. Home nursing and assistance with personal care are free of charge, while practical assistance and safety alarm services have deductibles. In 2016, 12% of the Norwegian population in the age group 67–79 years received home care services. In the age group 80–90 years, the share was 50%, and 90% for those 90 years or older [10]. Across Europe, health services at home are becoming increasingly important [1]. WHO guidelines point out a change in focus of clinical care for older adults globally, where community and home-based care are emphasised [11].

The literature on falls in the general population of older adults is extensive. Home care receivers and other groups of frailer older adults are still underrepresented in this literature [12]. Older adults receiving home care services have a high incidence of falls, with 10% experiencing multiple falls during the previous 90 days [13]. The level of services provided correlates with the incidence of falls [14]. This group of older adults also report a high prevalence of fear of falling and activity restrictions associated with this fear [15]. In the general population of older adults, fear of falling and its consequences have been identified as important factors influencing HRQOL [16–18]. This relationship has not been established in the population of older home care receivers. It can be expected that receiving care and support could have an impact on the level of fear of falling and on HRQOL. Thus, this group of frailer older adults might be different than the general group of older adults when looking at the relationship between HRQOL and fear of falling.

The general population of fallers scores significantly lower on HRQOL, in particular on the physical component [19]. HRQOL has been shown to be associated with measures of mobility, balance and pain [20]. In the population of older adults receiving home care, studies looking specifically at HRQOL and further associations to physical function is lacking. However, studies exploring a broader concept, QOL, show that it is lower in this population compared to older adults in the same age group [21]. Among home care recipients, higher QOL has been associated with higher age, not living alone, a lower number of complaints like pain or impaired mobility, and managing to be alone at home [22]. Despite finding an association between mobility and QOL, HRQOL was not explored and different factors of physical activity as balance, walking speed or muscle strength were not included.

The complexity of the health challenges in the group of older fallers receiving home care makes it challenging for those delivering primary health care, both to ensure HRQOL for the client and at the same time keeping the costs reasonable [23]. There is a knowledge gap in clinical research on HRQOL and falls including older adults receiving home care [5, 24]. In recent guidelines, both locally in Norway, but also internationally, policy makers are increasingly focusing on the challenges of organising effective and high-quality health care services to meet the needs of the population of older home care recipients [9, 11]. In order to develop services and interventions, thorough information on the health status of this population is needed. The objective of this study is therefore to determine relationships between HRQOL and fear of falling as well as physical function in older fallers receiving home care services.

Method

Study design

The analysis employs cross-sectional data from baseline measurements of a randomised controlled trial conducted in 2016–17 [24]. The trial was registered at ClinicalTrials.gov in February 2015, NCT02374307. First enrolment of participants was in February 2016. The STROBE guidelines are followed to report on the design, analysis and presentation of data [25].

Setting and participants

Participants were recruited in six municipalities in Norway. Recruitment was based on registration lists of older adults receiving home care from primary health care services. The recruitment plan is described elsewhere [24]. The flow of participants at enrolment in the project is illustrated in Fig. 1. Eight hundred sixty five adults receiving home care were initially assessed for eligibility, 320 received an invitation letter and 167 were baseline tested. Data from 155 participants were included in the final sample analysed in this study.

The study was approved by the Regional Committee for Medical Research Ethics in South Norway (Ref. 2014/2051). Participants provided written, informed, consent.

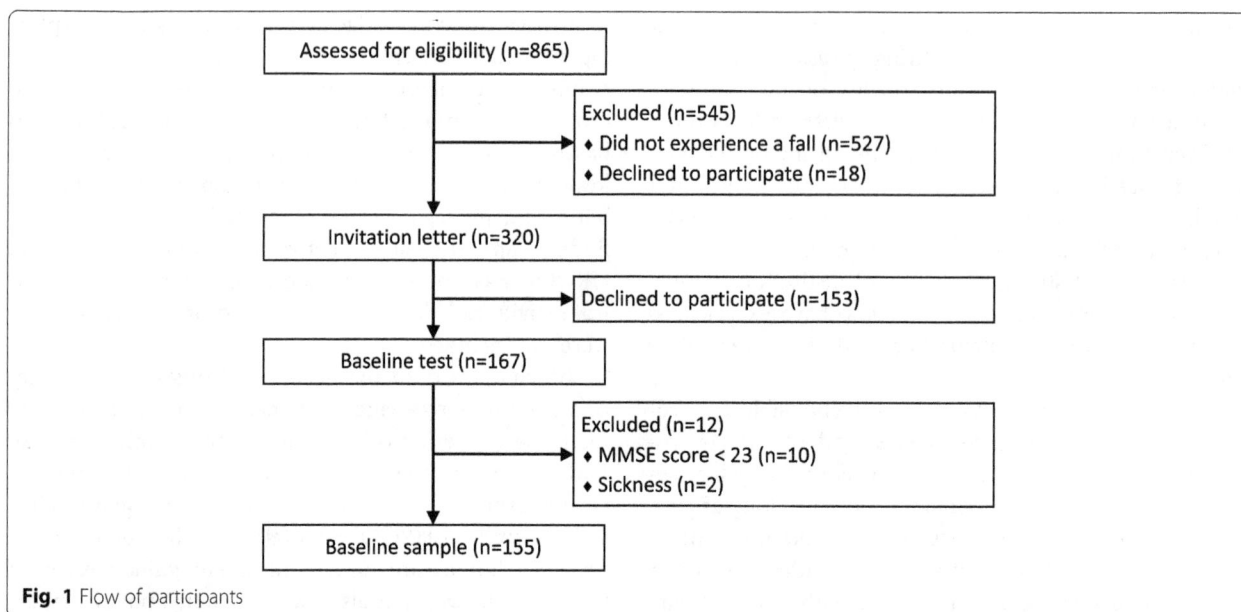

Fig. 1 Flow of participants

Inclusion criteria

Age 67+, receiving home care from the primary health care services, having experienced at least one fall in the last 12 months, able to walk with or without a walking aid and understand Norwegian.

Exclusion criteria

Medical contraindications to exercise, life expectancy less than 1 year, a score below 23 on the Mini Mental State Examination (MMSE) and participating in other falls prevention programmes.

Outcome measures

The outcome measures for this study were selected based on both theoretical and practical reasons [26, 27]. All assessments employed have established reliability and validity, as recommended by the CONSORT guidelines [28]. In addition to improving measurement quality and outcomes, it enables direct comparisons with other studies investigating HRQOL and can possibly contribute to future meta-analyses. The measurements were conducted by physiotherapists in the participants' home in one session, so considerations had to be made both concerning equipment and fatigue of the participants.

Health-related quality of life was assessed using the Short Form 36 Health Survey, version 2 (SF-36). This questionnaire is generic, validated and translated into Norwegian [29]. The 36 items in SF-36 are grouped into eight subscales: physical functioning (PF), role limitations due to physical problems (RP) and due to emotional problems (RE), bodily pain (BP), general health (GH), vitality (VT), social functioning (SF) and mental health (MH). Based on the scores of these eight scales, a physical component summary (PCS) and a mental

component summary (MCS) is calculated. The sum scores range from 0 to 100 (worst-best).

Fear of falling was measured using the Norwegian version of the Falls Efficacy Scale International (FES-I) [30]. In FES-I fear of falling is operationalised as the level of concern about falling when carrying out a range of 16 different physical activities [31]. It has a four-point scale ranging from 1 (not concerned) to 4 (very concerned). A sum score between 16 and 64 is achievable, where 16–19 indicates low concern, 20–27 moderate concern and 28–64 high concern [31].

Physical function was assessed by measurements on balance, gait speed, muscle strength and instrumental activities of daily living (IADL).

The Berg Balance Scale (BBS) assesses balance. The Norwegian version has been shown to have an excellent inter-rater reliability and high internal consistency in the geriatric population [32]. BBS measures performance on a 5-level scale from 0 (cannot perform) to 4 (normal performance) on 14 different tasks. The sum score of the 14 items ranges from 0 to 56, where a score below 45 indicates that the individual has a higher risk of falling.

Gait speed was assessed based on the time required to walk 4 meters, using any usual walking aid, and expressed in meters per second [33].

Muscle strength was measured by using the functional proxy measure of 30 seconds sit-to-stand (STS) test, where the number of rises from a chair within 30 seconds is recorded [34].

IADL was measured using the Norwegian version of the Lawton IADL scale [35]. It assesses a person's self-reported ability to perform complex activities of daily living. There are eight areas of function that are assessed, and the summary scores ranges from 0 (low function) to 8 (high function).

Demographic and background variables were age, sex, living alone, education (primary and lower secondary school/ upper secondary school/university 1–4 years/university more than 4 years), medical history including medications, nutritional status measured by Mini Nutritional Assessment (MNA) [36], walking aid use, type of home care (home help/ home nursing/safety alarm service) and history of falls.

Data analysis
Statistical analyses were conducted using STATA/SE 14. Descriptive characteristics of the study population are reported. Percentages are used to describe categorical data, and mean and standard deviation (SD) are calculated for continuous data. Skewness was examined by comparing mean and median values. Differences between males and females were inspected by t-tests and χ^2 tests. Coefficients with *p*- values ≤0.05 were considered statistically significant.

Pearson correlations coefficients display the association between the subscales of SF-36 and measures of physical function and fear of falling. The strength of correlations was interpreted according to Cohen, where 0.10 to 0.29 is weak, 0.3 to 0.49 is moderate and 0.5 to 1.0 is strong [37].

Explanatory variables for the multivariate regression of the scales of SF-36 were chosen from the available set of variables displayed in Table 1. The regressions adjust for the background variables age, sex, education, living alone, risk of or being malnourished, falls ≥3 during the previous 12 months and the number of different medications. The minimum values from the inclusion criteria were subtracted from age (67) and MMSE (23) to increase interpretability of the coefficients. A dummy variable was created for more than two falls in the last 12 months. Most participants had one or two falls, while some had a large number of falls. Additionally, the regression included as independent variables 4-m walk test (4MWT), BBS, IADL, FES-I and MMSE. STS was highly correlated (> 0.6) with both BBS and 4MWT and this variable was therefore excluded from the regressions. The impact of the variables health care services and walking aid were negligible, and those were also excluded. Four records containing missing observation of medications and 4MWT had to be dropped.

Floor- and ceiling effects were considered when more than 20% of the participants achieved the lowest or highest possible score. For RE, 48.4% reached the top score of 100. In this case, a logistic regression was fitted.

Results
Participants
Table 1 presents the characteristics of the total sample and separately for females and males. The study included 123 females and 32 males. The only statistical significant

difference between sexes was found on the number of falls and if a safety alarm service was provided. Men had a significant higher rate of falls, 4.9, compared to women, 2.1 (*p* < 0.001). Women received a safety alarm more often, 79.7%, than men, 59.4% (*p* = 0.017). Mean (SD) age is 82.7 (6.7). HRQOL, measured by SF-36, shows a better summary score on the mental components (49.4, SD 10.3) than on the physical components (38.3, SD 9.0).

Correlation coefficients
In Table 2, the correlation coefficients between subscales of SF-36 and different measures of physical function and fear of falling are presented. All measures of physical function are highly correlated with the subscale PF (*p* < 0.01). FES-I is moderately negatively correlated with all subscales of SF-36, except from BP and SF, where there is a weaker negative correlation.

Multivariate regressions
Table 3 presents results of multivariate regressions of scales of SF-36 on background variables and measures of physical function and fear of falling. Having a lower score on FES-I is significantly associated with achieving a higher score on all subscales of SF-36 except from BP and SF. Scoring 10 points lower on FES-I, is expected to increase the scores of SF-36 between 0.9 (RE) to 7.3 (RP). The subscale PF is significantly associated with higher scores on the physical measures 4MWT (*p* ≤ 0.05), BBS (*p* ≤ 0.001) and IADL (*p* ≤ 0.01). Higher age is significantly associated with better scores on MCS (*p* ≤ 0.05), PF (*p* ≤ 0.05), GH (*p* ≤ 0.01) and MH (*p* ≤ 0.01). Taking fewer medications is significantly associated with a higher score on PCS (p ≤ 0.001) and GH (*p* ≤ 0.001). Finally, a higher MMSE score is significantly associated with a higher score on MH (*p* ≤ 0.05).

Discussion
The objective of this study was to determine the relationship between HRQOL, fear of falling and physical function in older fallers receiving home care. The results show that a higher level of HRQOL, measured by SF-36, is substantially associated with lower fear of falling, measured by FES-I. The associations are independent of physical measures like BBS and 4MWT, number of falls, cognition and key background characteristics. All associations are statistically significant in almost all scales of SF-36, except BP and SF. On physical function, the results show that a higher score on the subscale PF is significantly associated with better gait speed (4MWT), improved balance (BBS) and better ability in IADL.

The present study extends the results of two previous studies on the association between HRQOL and fear of falling. In a Canadian study of older community-dwelling women, quality-adjusted life years were calculated from the EQ-5D scale and compared to falls-related self-efficacy

Table 1 Characteristics of the study population. Means, standard deviations (SD) and percentages

	Total (N = 155)	Female (N = 123)	Male (N = 32)
Characteristics			
Age, mean (SD)	82.7 (6.7)	83.0 (6.7)	81.3 (6.7)
Living alone, %	84.5	87.0	75.0
Higher education (> 12 years), %	36.1	35.0	40.6
No. of medications weekly, mean (SD)	5.3 (3.4)	5.1 (3.4)	6.0 (3.6)
Primary health care services			
Practical assistance, %	69.7	68.3	75.0
Nursing, %	30.3	27.6	40.6
Safety alarm service, %	75.5	79.7	59.4
Walking aid %	73.5	74.0	71.9
Falls the last 12 months			
No., mean (SD)	2.7 (3.7)	2.1 (2.5)	4.9 (6.0)
Location:			
Indoor, %	47.4	49.6	38.7
Outdoor, %	18.8	19.5	16.1
Both, %	33.8	30.9	45.2
Injuries from falls:			
Minor injuries %	45.5	45.5	45.2
Serious injuries, hospitalisation %	35.1	37.4	25.8
Mini-Mental State Examination			
MMSE, mean (SD)	27.4 (2.2)	27.5 (2.2)	27.2 (2.2)
Falls Efficacy			
FES-I, mean (SD)	30.7 (9.8)	31.0 (9.9)	29.4 (9.5)
Physical function			
IADL, Lawton and Brody. > 6, %	56.1	56.1	56.3
Sit to stand, mean (SD)	5.1 (4.1)	5.1 (4.2)	4.8 (3.7)
4-m walk test m/s, mean (SD)	0.62 (0.21)	0.62 (0.22)	0.61 (0.18)
Berg Balance Scale, mean (SD)	39.1 (11.3)	39.6 (11.4)	37.2 (10.8)
Mini Nutritional Assessment			
Risk of or malnourished %	24.4	27.6	12.5
Health-related quality of life			
SF-36 scores, mean (SD)			
Physical component summary	38.3 (9.0)	38.0 (9.2)	39.4 (8.4)
Mental component summary	49.4 (10.3)	49.0 (10.6)	50.9 (9.1)
Physical function	44.6 (23.1)	44.5 (23.0)	45.2 (23.8)
Role physical	51.7 (29.7)	50.9 (30.1)	54.9 (28.3)
Body pain	53.8 (32.2)	51.8 (32.4)	61.4 (30.7)
General health	57.6 (23.3)	57.6 (23.5)	57.6 (22.7)
Vitality	38.3 (21.5)	36.7 (28.8)	44.2 (19.1)
Social function	66.9 (31.2)	66.1 (31.3)	69.9 (30.8)
Role emotional	75.8 (28.5)	75.6 (28.1)	76.6 (30.6)
Mental health	72.1 (17.4)	71.1 (17.8)	75.6 (15.6)

Table 2 Correlation between HRQOL (SF-36) and different measures on physical function and falls efficacy

SF-36 subscales	Sit to stand	4 Meter Walk Test	Berg Balance Scale	Instrumental ADL	Falls Efficacy Scale - I
Physical Function	0.515***	0.537***	0.585***	0.439***	−0.425***
Role Physical	0.352***	0.275***	0.287***	0.250**	−0.388***
Bodily Pain	0.113	0.146	−0.013	− 0.036	− 0.221**
General Health	0.270***	0.168*	0.175*	0.120	− 0.367***
Vitality	0.193*	0.175*	0.116	0.110	−0.327***
Social Function	0.267***	0.123	0.216**	0.210**	−0.262***
Role Emotional	0.289***	0.120	0.201*	0.134	−0.355***
Mental Health	0.225**	0.100	0.082	0.056	−0.362***

* $p < 0.05$ **$p < 0.01$ ***$p < 0.001$

[17]. This study accounted for similar control variables and found comparable results on their measure of HRQOL. However, the women included did not necessarily experience a fall and it was uncertain whether the results could be generalised to older adults with a lower level of function. Another study from Taiwan reported on the association between HRQOL, measured by summary scores of SF-36, and fear of falling [16]. This larger survey included both fallers and non-fallers and adjusted for some background characteristics. Fear of falling was measured simply by asking a yes/no question. Unlike the study by Davis et al. [17] and this present study, the association was not independent of physical or cognitive function. Here, the results show that fear of falling, measured by a validated and reliable instrument, is independently associated with almost all scales

of SF-36 and thus confirms that it is an important predictor of HRQOL in this group of older fallers with poor function.

All measures of physical function and IADL were significantly associated with the physical subscale of HRQOL. A higher PF was significantly associated with higher scores on the physical measures 4MWT, BBS and IADL. Similar results have been shown in previous studies where lower HRQOL was associated with difficulties with basic and instrumental activities of daily living [38, 39], low maximal gait speed [40] and reduced physical fitness [41]. The present study did not show any significant associations on other subscales, but the sample size could have been too low to detect other associations.

Research on older adults often excludes those who are frailer [7]. In previous studies, participants were younger

Table 3 Regression of SF-36 on measures on demographics, physical measures, cognition and falls efficacy

	Physical Comp. Summary	Mental Comp. Summary	Physical Function	Role Physical	Bodily Pain	General Health	Vitality	Social Function	Role Emotional	Mental Health
Age (years ≥67)	0.19	0.31*	0.49*	0.58	0.80	0.74**	0.04	0.70	0.02	0.64**
	(0.10)	(0.13)	(0.23)	(0.37)	(0.42)	(0.28)	(0.28)	(0.42)	(0.03)	(0.22)
Falls ≥3 last 12 months	2.48	−4.23*	4.57	1.43	3.90	1.06	−4.37	−9.02	−0.27	−4.64
	(1.56)	(1.99)	(3.51)	(5.49)	(6.36)	(4.17)	(4.22)	(6.28)	(0.46)	(3.27)
No. medications weekly	−0.72***	0.16	−0.74	−1.02	−1.10	−2.65***	− 0.58	0.43	0.06	−0.33
	(0.19)	(0.24)	(0.42)	(0.66)	(0.77)	(0.50)	(0.51)	(0.76)	(0.06)	(0.39)
4 Meter Walk Test, m/s	8.28*	− 1.03	21.12*	15.30	23.88	−0.24	16.53	−1.26	0.12	4.37
	(3.84)	(4.88)	(8.61)	(13.47)	(15.62)	(10.24)	(10.35)	(15.43)	(1.18)	(8.03)
Berg Balance Scale	0.14	0.00	0.80***	0.31	−0.12	0.18	−0.23	0.33	0.03	−0.00
	(0.08)	(0.10)	(0.18)	(0.27)	(0.32)	(0.21)	(0.21)	(0.31)	(0.02)	(0.16)
Instrumental Activities of Daily Living	0.50	−0.11	3.16**	2.01	−1.48	−0.96	0.16	2.36	0.02	− 0.85
	(0.51)	(0.65)	(1.15)	(1.80)	(2.08)	(1.37)	(1.38)	(2.06)	(0.15)	(1.07)
Falls Efficacy Scale – International	−0.18*	−0.30**	−0.37*	− 0.73**	−0.55	− 0.55**	−0.63**	− 0.46	−0.09***	− 0.52***
	(0.07)	(0.09)	(0.16)	(0.25)	(0.29)	(0.19)	(0.19)	(0.29)	(0.02)	(0.15)
Mini-Mental State Examination (score ≥ 23)	−0.26	0.45	−0.11	− 0.38	−1.42	0.70	0.78	0.44	−0.03	1.25*
	(0.29)	(0.37)	(0.66)	(1.03)	(1.19)	(0.78)	(0.79)	(1.18)	(0.09)	(0.61)
R^2 adj.	0.32	0.15	0.47	0.21	0.08	0.27	0.10	0.07		0.20

Additionally adjusted for sex, education, living alone, risk of or being malnourished. Ordinary least squares (OLS) regressions, except on role emotional, where a logistic regression is fitted. Unstandardised regression coefficients, standard error (SE) in parentheses. Model fit reported by R^2-adjusted. $N = 151$. * $p < 0.05$ **$p < 0.01$ ***$p < 0.00$

than here, where the mean age is 82.7. Research on older fallers has been carried out, but those who receive home care are underrepresented. Risk factors and incidence of falls in this population have received most attention [13, 14]. Associations between HRQOL and potentially influential factors have not been analysed in this group. QOL among older adults receiving home care has been explored in Sweden [21]. In this study, the extent of help with IADL influenced QOL negatively, while it was positively influenced by the density of the social network. Measures of physical and cognitive function were not included in the Swedish study which was based on a postal questionnaire.

Compared to normative values from a Norwegian sample of adults, aged 70 to 80 years, the sample in the present study has lower values in all subscales of SF-36 [42]. This might be due to better function of older people in the general population, not necessarily requiring home care. Similar findings were demonstrated in a Swedish study, where elderly receiving home care had very low QOL compared to older adults in the same age group [21].

Interestingly, higher age was associated with better scores within the scales MCS, PF, GH and MH. This might be due to what has been described in literature on HRQOL as response shift [43]. It refers to a change in the meaning of one's self-evaluation of HRQOL resulting from changes in internal standards, values and conceptualisation. The oldest of the participants might have lower expectations of their everyday life, what they can manage and their health status, while the younger participants might on average have higher expectations. An earlier Swedish study on QOL of older people living at home found comparable results. High QOL was related to higher age, lower number of complaints and managing to live alone at home [22].

This study has several limitations. First, the sample comprised participants recruited to a controlled trial to potentially perform a falls prevention programme. The participants might be fitter and more motivated for physical activity than the general population of older adults receiving home care. To improve generalisability, recruitment was outreaching, calling from lists of people receiving home care. Half of those who were eligible to participate and sent an invitation letter were also included in the study. This could make self-selection of more active participants less likely. Secondly, the sample was recruited from only six municipalities which are not necessarily representative for Norway in general. However, the six municipalities included both cities and rural areas. Thirdly, performing subgroup analyses on sex is difficult as a low percentage of the sample were males. The descriptive statistics show, however, that males and females in this sample are not significantly different, except for number of falls and if a safety alarm is provided. A further limitation is that the study is cross-sectional and definitive causal relations cannot be established.

Finally, some of the measures like the number of falls are self-reported.

This study contributes new knowledge on the level of HRQOL, physical function and fear of falling in addition to the relationship between these factors in a group of older fallers receiving home care. This population is understudied and more information is needed to be able to improve care and other public services for this group. The results from this study can be of importance for clinicians and health managers for developing interventions and organising clinical services in primary health care. Since this group of older fallers is relatively large in Norway and other developed countries, the information can also be useful for policy makers to set priorities and allocate resources. Future research on interventions on how to modify HRQOL and fear of falling within this group is needed.

Conclusions

Higher HRQOL is substantially associated with a lower level of fear of falling in older fallers receiving home care. This association is independent of physical measures, number of falls, cognition and key background characteristics such as age, sex and education. Better physical function is significantly associated with higher physical HRQOL, independent of the same background characteristics and fear of falling.

Abbreviations

4MWT: 4 Meter Walk Test; BBS: Berg Balance Scale; BP: Bodily Pain; EQ-5D: EuroQol - five dimensions scale; FES-I: Falls Efficacy Scale - International; GH: General Health; HRQOL: Health-related Quality of Life; IADL: Instrumental Activities of Daily Living; MCS: Mental Component Summary; MH: Mental Health; MMSE: Mini Mental State Examination; PCS: Physical Component Summary; PF: Physical Function; QOL: Quality of Life; RE: Role Emotional; RP: Role Physical; SD: Standard Deviation; SF: Social Function; SF-36: Short From 36 Health Survey; STS: Sit to Stand; VT: Vitality

Funding

This study has received no external funding. Internal funding is provided by OsloMet – Oslo Metropolitan University. The institution had no role in the design, conduct of research or decision of publication.

Authors' contributions

MB and AB initiated the study, and all authors contributed to its design. MB managed the data collection, performed the data analysis and wrote the first draft of the manuscript. MB, TB, DS and AB are collectively responsible for interpreting the results, reviewed critically subsequent drafts of the manuscript and approved its final version.

Competing interests

The authors declare that they have no competing interests.

Author details

[1]Department of Physiotherapy, OsloMet – Oslo Metropolitan University, PO Box 4 St. Olavs plass, 0130 Oslo, Norway. [2]School of Health and Life Sciences, Glasgow Caledonian University, Glasgow, UK.

References

1. Rechel B, Grundy E, Robine JM, Cylus J, Mackenbach JP, Knai C, McKee M. Ageing in the European Union. Lancet. 2013;381(9874):1312–22.
2. World Health Organization. WHO global report on falls prevention in older age. Geneva: World Health Organization; 2007.
3. Ambrose AF, Paul G, Hausdorff JM. Risk factors for falls among older adults: a review of the literature. Maturitas. 2013;75(1):51–61.
4. Thome B, Dykes AK, Hallberg IR. Home care with regard to definition, care recipients, content and outcome: systematic literature review. J Clin Nurs. 2003;12(6):860–72.
5. Vikman I. Falls, perceived fall risk and activity curtailment among older people receiving home-help service. PhD thesis. Luleå University of Technology, Luleå, Sweden. Department of Health Sciences; 2011.
6. Genet N, Boerma WG, Kringos DS, Bouman A, Francke AL, Fagerstrom C, Melchiorre MG, Greco C, Deville W. Home care in Europe: a systematic literature review. BMC Health Serv Res. 2011;11:207.
7. Bourgeois FT, Olson KL, Tse T, Ioannidis JP, Mandl KD. Prevalence and characteristics of interventional trials conducted exclusively in elderly persons: a cross-sectional analysis of registered clinical trials. PLoS One. 2016;11(5):e0155948.
8. Brown SH, Abdelhafiz AH. Institutionalization of older people: prediction and prevention. Aging Health. 2011;7(2):187–203.
9. NOU 2011:11. Innovasjon i omsorg. Oslo: Departementenes servicesenter; 2011.
10. Mørk E, Beyrer S, Haugstveit FV, Sundby B, Karlsen H, Wettergreen J. Kommunale helse-og omsorgstjenester 2016. Statistikk om tjenester og tjenestemottakere. In., vol. 2017/26. Oslo: Statistisk sentralbyrå; 2017.
11. Araujo de Carvalho I, Epping-Jordan J, Pot AM, Kelley E, Toro N, Thiyagarajan JA, Beard JR. Organizing integrated health-care services to meet older people's needs. Bull World Health Organ. 2017;95(11):756–63.
12. Sherrington C, Michaleff ZA, Fairhall N, Paul SS, Tiedemann A, Whitney J, Cumming RG, Herbert RD, Close JC, Lord SR. Exercise to prevent falls in older adults: an updated systematic review and meta-analysis. Br J Sports Med. 2016.
13. Fletcher PC, Hirdes JP. Risk factors for falling among community-based seniors using home care services. J Gerontol Ser A Biol Med Sci. 2002;57(8):M504–10.
14. Vikman I, Nordlund A, Näslund A, Nyberg L. Incidence and seasonality of falls amongst old people receiving home help services in a municipality in northern Sweden. Int J Circumpolar Health. 2011;70(2):195.
15. Fletcher PC, Hirdes JP. Restriction in activity associated with fear of falling among community-based seniors using home care services. Age Ageing. 2004;33(3):273–9.
16. Chang NT, Chi LY, Yang NP, Chou P. The impact of falls and fear of falling on health-related quality of life in Taiwanese elderly. J Community Health Nurs. 2010;27(2):84–95.
17. Davis JC, Marra CA, Liu-Ambrose TY. Falls-related self-efficacy is independently associated with quality-adjusted life years in older women. Age Ageing. 2011;40(3):340–6.
18. Cumming RG, Salkeld G, Thomas M, Szonyi G. Prospective study of the impact of fear of falling on activities of daily living, SF-36 scores, and nursing home admission. J Gerontol Ser A Biol Med Sci. 2000;55(5):M299–305.
19. Stenhagen M, Ekstrom H, Nordell E, Elmstahl S. Accidental falls, health-related quality of life and life satisfaction: a prospective study of the general elderly population. Arch Gerontol Geriatr. 2014;58(1):95–100.
20. Davis JC, Bryan S, Li LC, Best JR, Hsu CL, Gomez C, Vertes KA, Liu-Ambrose T. Mobility and cognition are associated with wellbeing and health related quality of life among older adults: a cross-sectional analysis of the Vancouver falls prevention cohort. BMC Geriatr. 2015;15:75.
21. Hellström Y, Andersson M, Hallberg IR. Quality of life among older people in Sweden receiving help from informal and/or formal helpers at home or in special accommodation. Health Soc Care Community. 2004;12(6):504–16.
22. Hellstrom Y, Hallberg IR. Determinants and characteristics of help provision for elderly people living at home and in relation to quality of life. Scand J Caring Sci. 2004;18(4):387–95.
23. Hammar T, Rissanen P, Perälä M-L. Home-care clients' need for help, and use and costs of services. Eur J Ageing. 2008;5(2):147.
24. Bjerk M, Brovold T, Skelton DA, Bergland A. A falls prevention programme to improve quality of life, physical function and falls efficacy in older people receiving home help services: study protocol for a randomised controlled trial. BMC Health Serv Res. 2017;17(1).
25. von Elm E, Altman DG, Egger M, Pocock SJ, Gotzsche PC, Vandenbroucke JP, Initiative S. The strengthening the reporting of observational studies in epidemiology (STROBE) statement: guidelines for reporting observational studies. Lancet. 2007;370(9596):1453–7.
26. Lamb SE, Jørstad-Stein EC, Hauer K, Becker C. Development of a common outcome data set for fall injury prevention trials: the prevention of falls network Europe consensus. J Am Geriatr Soc. 2005;53(9):1618–22.
27. Jørstad EC, Hauer K, Becker C, Lamb SE, Group P. Measuring the psychological outcomes of falling: a systematic review. J Am Geriatr Soc. 2005;53(3):501–10.
28. Schulz KF, Altman DG, Moher D. CONSORT 2010 statement: updated guidelines for reporting parallel group randomised trials. BMC Med. 2010;8(1):1.
29. Loge JH, Kaasa S. Short form 36 (SF-36) health survey: normative data from the general Norwegian population. Scand J Public Health. 1998;26(4):250–8.
30. Helbostad JL, Taraldsen K, Granbo R, Yardley L, Todd CJ, Sletvold O. Validation of the falls efficacy scale-international in fall-prone older persons. Age Ageing. 2010;39(2):259.
31. Delbaere K, Close JC, Mikolaizak AS, Sachdev PS, Brodaty H, Lord SR. The falls efficacy scale international (FES-I). a comprehensive longitudinal validation study. Age Ageing. 2010;39(2):210–6.
32. Halsaa KE, Brovold T, Graver V, Sandvik L, Bergland A. Assessments of interrater reliability and internal consistency of the Norwegian version of the berg balance scale. Arch Phys Med Rehabil. 2007;88(1):94–8.
33. Peters DM, Fritz SL, Krotish DE. Assessing the reliability and validity of a shorter walk test compared with the 10-meter walk test for measurements of gait speed in healthy, older adults. J Geriatr Phys Ther. 2013;36(1):24–30.
34. Jones CJ, Rikli RE, Beam WC. A 30-s chair-stand test as a measure of lower body strength in community-residing older adults. Res Q Exerc Sport. 1999;70(2):113–9.
35. Graf C. The Lawton instrumental activities of daily living scale. Am J Nursing. 2008;108(4):52–62.
36. Vellas B, Villars H, Abellan G, Soto M. Overview of the MNA® - its history and challenges. J Nutr Health Aging. 2006;10(6):456.
37. Cohen J, Cohen P, West SG, Aiken LS. Applied multiple regression/correlation analysis for the behavioral sciences: Routledge; 2013.
38. Lyu W, Wolinsky FD. The onset of ADL difficulties and changes in health-related quality of life. Health Qual Life Outcomes. 2017;15(1):217.
39. Andersson LB, Marcusson J, Wressle E. Health-related quality of life and activities of daily living in 85-year-olds in S weden. Health Soc Care Community. 2014;22(4):368–74.
40. Hörder H, Skoog I, Frändin K. Health-related quality of life in relation to walking habits and fitness: a population-based study of 75-year-olds. Qual Life Res. 2013;22(6):1213–23.
41. Brovold T, Skelton DA, Sylliaas H, Mowe M, Bergland A. Association between health-related quality of life, physical fitness, and physical activity in older adults recently discharged from hospital. J Aging Phys Act. 2014;22(3):405–13.
42. Jacobsen EL, Bye A, Aass N, Fossa SD, Grotmol KS, Kaasa S, Loge JH, Moum T, Hjermstad MJ. Norwegian reference values for the short-form health survey 36: development over time. Qual Life Res. 2017.
43. Sprangers MA, Schwartz CE. Integrating response shift into health-related quality of life research: a theoretical model. Soc Sci Med. 1999;48(11):1507–15.

20

Regional variation in healthcare spending and mortality among senior high-cost healthcare users in Ontario, Canada: a retrospective matched cohort study

Sergei Muratov[1,2]* (iD), Justin Lee[1,3,4,5], Anne Holbrook[1,4], Andrew Costa[1,6,7], J. Michael Paterson[6,11], Jason R. Guertin[8,9], Lawrence Mbuagbaw[1,10], Tara Gomes[6,12,13], Wayne Khuu[6] and Jean-Eric Tarride[1,2,7]

Abstract

Background: Senior high cost health care users (HCU) are a priority for many governments. Little research has addressed regional variation of HCU incidence and outcomes, especially among incident HCU. This study describes the regional variation in healthcare costs and mortality across Ontario's health planning districts [Local Health Integration Networks (LHIN)] among senior incident HCU and non-HCU and explores the relationship between healthcare spending and mortality.

Methods: We conducted a retrospective population-based matched cohort study of incident senior HCU defined as Ontarians aged ≥66 years in the top 5% most costly healthcare users in fiscal year (FY) 2013. We matched HCU to non-HCU (1:3) based on age, sex and LHIN. Primary outcomes were LHIN-based variation in costs (total and 12 cost components) and mortality during FY2013 as measured by variance estimates derived from multi-level models. Outcomes were risk-adjusted for age, sex, ADGs, and low-income status. In a cost-mortality analysis by LHIN, risk-adjusted random effects for total costs and mortality were graphically presented together in a cost-mortality plane to identify low and high performers.

Results: We studied 175,847 incident HCU and 527,541 matched non-HCU. On average, 94 out of 1000 seniors per LHIN were HCU (CV = 4.6%). The mean total costs for HCU in FY2013 were 12 times higher that of non-HCU ($29,779 vs. $2472 respectively), whereas all-cause mortality was 13.6 times greater (103.9 vs. 7.5 per 1000 seniors).
Regional variation in costs and mortality was lower in senior HCU compared with non-HCU. We identified greater variability in accessing the healthcare system, but, once the patient entered the system, variation in costs was low. The traditional drivers of costs and mortality that we adjusted for played little role in driving the observed variation in HCUs' outcomes. We identified LHINs that had high mortality rates despite elevated healthcare expenditures and those that achieved lower mortality at lower costs. Some LHINs achieved low mortality at excessively high costs.

Conclusions: Risk-adjusted allocation of healthcare resources to seniors in Ontario is overall similar across health districts, more so for HCU than non-HCU. Identified important variation in the cost-mortality relationship across LHINs needs to be further explored.

Keywords: Senior high-cost users, Small area variation, Healthcare expenditures, Mortality

* Correspondence: muratos@mcmaster.ca
[1]Department of Health Research Methods, Evidence, and Impact, McMaster University, Hamilton, ON, Canada
[2]Programs for Assessment of Technology in Health (PATH), The Research Institute of St. Joe's Hamilton, St. Joseph's Healthcare, Hamilton, ON, Canada
Full list of author information is available at the end of the article

Background

High-cost health care users (HCU), a minority of individuals who consume a large proportion of health care resources, are a diverse group [1]. Due to their high burden on the healthcare system, a better understanding of various segments of the HCU population is needed to develop evidence-informed health care policy [1, 2]. In particular, seniors (patients 65 years of age and older), who account for about 15% of the population in the province of Ontario, account for approximately 60% of the total costs incurred by all HCU in the province [3–5]. Further, nearly half of senior HCU each year are incident cases [6, 7]. These "new" cases represent a stratum of the HCU population that can potentially be a target of preventative interventions and management, but they have not been adequately studied, especially in the context of regional variation.

Large geographical disparities in health care services have been documented globally [8, 9]. In Canada, marked regional variation has been identified in key healthcare services such as hospitalization [10], surgical procedures [11, 12], and use of prescription drugs [13, 14]. In contrast to this evidence of disparities in individual healthcare services, there is little information on variation in healthcare spending in the Canadian provincial context. While reports on regional variation in healthcare spending, especially the Medicare costs, have dominated the US political debate for more than a decade [15–19], only one Canadian study (British Columbia[BC]) has investigated regional variation in healthcare expenditures and found it to be modest [20]. While very informative, the BC study was not intended to investigate seniors specifically, not to mention senior HCU. Moreover, except for the total healthcare spending, the BC study did not provide information on variation among individual cost components such as hospitalization and physician costs which limits our understanding of the processes of care that contribute to higher or lower variation [21].

Understanding regional variation in health services utilization, costs and health outcomes can inform health services planning for senior patients, including senior HCU, in several ways. First, it allows planners to explore potential drivers of variation that deserve attention by describing the distribution of patient and care characteristics across health districts [22, 23]. Second, evidence suggests that planning and implementing health services with an "equity lens" can improve equity in resources allocation [24] and healthcare services use [25–27], and reduce regional variation in outcome distribution [28]. Third, measuring the relationship between costs and health outcomes among health regions is critical for policy makers to identify geographical "pockets" of efficient care (areas with lower spending and better outcomes). Recent studies have reported the level of inefficiency in Canada at 20% [29] with significant variations across Canadian provinces [30]. Moreover, even though available evidence of

healthcare regional variation and efficiency has led policy makers to entertain the idea of cutting reimbursement rates in higher-spending regions [15, 31] or to establish new provider-physician integrated entities with spending benchmarks (accountable care organizations) [32], there is still a gap in our knowledge as to how regional disparities in healthcare spending affect regional patterns of health outcomes [33]. The lack of evidence on geographical variation in health outcomes seems to have contributed to the gap [34, 35].

To better inform decision and policy making in Ontario and fill a gap in the literature, the objectives of this study were: 1) to estimate regional variation in healthcare costs (total and by cost categories) and mortality among incident senior HCU compared to senior non-HCU; and 2) to examine the relationship between health spending and mortality by health districts for senior incident HCU compared to senior non-HCU.

Methods

Study design

A retrospective population-based matched cohort study was conducted using province-wide linked administrative data. More details on the study population and data sources are published elsewhere but are briefly summarized below [36].

Study population

We generated a cohort of all incident senior HCU in the province of Ontario. This cohort was defined as consisting of seniors (aged ≥66 years) with annual total healthcare expenditures within the top 5% threshold of all Ontarians in the 2013 Ontario government fiscal year (FY2013) (i.e. incident year), and not in the top 5% in the 2012 fiscal year (FY2012).The threshold of 5% to define HCU is aligned with previous Canadian studies of this population [3, 7, 37, 38].The incident HCU cohort was matched to a cohort of non-HCU using a 1:3 matching ratio, without replacement based on age at cohort entry (+/– 1 month), sex and residence (based on Local Health Integration Networks [LHIN]). The "non-HCU" cohort was defined as those whose annual total health care expenditures in the 2012 and 2013 fiscal years were both below the financial threshold of the top 5% of all Ontarians in the respective year.

Data sources

The patient-level dataset was created using 19 health administrative databases [36]. These datasets were linked using unique encoded identifiers and analyzed at the Institute for Clinical Evaluative Sciences (ICES) [39]. Health care expenditures were calculated using a person-level health utilization costing algorithm [40]. Total healthcare expenditures were comprised of 12 separate health service cost categories. Hospital costs were the sum of costs associated with inpatient care and same-day surgery. Physician costs were the sum of fee-for-service billings and capitation payments. Costs reported in this study are based on patients' geographic location of residence. Costs are expressed in 2013 Canadian Dollars.

Geographic unit of analysis

We used LHINs, Ontario's regional health districts, as the geographic unit of analysis. Ontario's 14 LHINs are responsible for the funding, planning and management of hospital- and community-based health services delivered to all residents within their geographic boundaries [41]. Services covered by the LHINs include most of hospital and community care such as inpatient care, long-term and home care, community mental health, rehabilitation and hospices among others [42], but exclude physician services, which are funded from a separate envelope.

Variables

The study population was described at baseline (i.e., the year before HCU incident status), including comparisons of socio-demographic determinants (age, sex, residence, low income), health status (degree of morbidity, proportion of chronic conditions) and health system factors (e.g., number of physicians in the circle of care and whether a geriatrician was visited) between HCU and matched non-HCU. Subjects with low income status were identified based upon net household income reported to receive public drug benefit subsidy in FY2012. Compared to census-based neighborhood income measures, the Ontario Drug Benefit (ODB)-based low income status is a better reflection of personal income, as it relies upon actual net income. For a small proportion of HCU (3%) and non-HCU (13%) who did not fill a prescription in FY2012, low-income status was defined as census neighborhood income quintile 1. Rurality was defined using the Rural Index of Ontario (RIO): an ordinal measure ranging from 0 (urban) to 100 (rural) that considers population density and travel time to the nearest health facility [43].

Several measures were employed to describe health status. Level of morbidity was measured using Johns Hopkins Aggregated Diagnosis Groups (ADGs) that are derived from Johns Hopkins Adjusted Clinical Groups (ACGs): a person-focused, diagnosis-based way to measure patients' illness [44]. In addition, the proportions of patients with prior malignancy and mental health conditions were computed using John Hopkins Expanded Diagnosis Clusters (EDCs). Finally, the proportions of patients with chronic obstructive pulmonary disease, congestive heart failure, diabetes, and rheumatoid arthritis were estimated using ICES-derived, validated chronic disease cohorts [45, 46].

Outcomes

Several outcomes were assessed. HCU rate for each LHIN was defined as the number of senior HCU over the total number of seniors residing in the LHIN per 1000 population. Mean per capita total healthcare expenditures and mean per capita health expenditures for each care category were calculated as the costs incurred in the incident year over the total population in the HCU and non-HCU cohort. Finally, mortality for each cohort was defined as the prevalence of all-cause death within the incident year.

Statistical analysis

Descriptive statistics (counts [%]; mean [SD] or median [Q1, Q3]) were summarized for baseline individual characteristics and outcomes. Characteristics of subjects in both HCU and non-HCU cohorts were compared using absolute standardized differences (SDD). SDDs of more than 0.1 are considered to indicate meaningful differences between the cohorts [47]. To describe the variation between the LHINs in terms of costs and outcomes, the coefficient of variations (CVs) defined as the ratio of the standard deviation to the mean were determined.

Because the calculated intra-class correlation coefficient (ICC) pointed toward statistically significant clustering within the LHINs across most of the cost components and mortality in both cohorts (Additional file 1), we fitted a mixed effects model to estimate between-region variation and risk-adjust for age, sex, the number of ADGs per patient, and low-income status for both costs and mortality. Compared to the CV or other summary statistics characterizing regional variation, these models provide additional information, including the between-LHIN variance estimate and the proportion of the observed variation explained by patient characteristics.

We specified the following general equation (Additional file 2):

$$y_{ij} = (Beta_0 + u_{0j}) + \sum Beta_{ij} \cdot X_{ij} + e_{ij};$$

where yij – the outcome (costs or mortality) in patient i from LHINj; $Beta_0$ - the provincial mean; $u0j$ – the random effect for each LHIN that is assumed $u0j \sim N(0, \sigma2u)$; $Beta_{ij}$ - the fixed effects of individual level characteristics; Xij - the vector of covariates at the individual level; eij - the residual error.

This type of models assumes that the mean outcome value for each LHIN vary randomly according to a normal distribution ($u0j \sim N(0, \sigma2u)$) whereas the effect of the patients' covariates is fixed among the LHINs. The main interest in this type of analyses is the random effect ($u0j$) which characterizes variation between LHINs, where $\sigma2u$ is the direct estimate of the variance.

For the mortality analyses, logistic regression was conducted by fitting generalized linear mixed models (GLMM) according to the general model specification provided above. To model healthcare expenditures, two methods were used based on the proportion of zero costs values in the data. Zero cost values arise when healthcare resources are not consumed (e.g. no contact with healthcare system or no hospitalization). For healthcare categories with no zero costs values GLMM were used. In the presence of zero costs values in the data, Hurdle mixed models were used to account for zeros [48, 49]. Hurdle models, also referred to as a two-part model, assumes that costs are generated by two statistically different processes. A binomial distribution (part 1) was used to determine whether any costs were incurred, and a gamma distribution (part 2) was employed to model positive costs (instances when costs> 0) [49–51]. Expected costs resulting from Hurdle models are then calculated by multiplying the probability of observing a cost by the value of the costs when observed. LHIN-specific random effects were incorporated into each part of the model to estimate between-LHIN variation in the probability of incurring any costs ($\sigma 2u1$) and variation in costs once they were incurred ($\sigma 2u2$), resulting into two random effects values. Similarly, the fixed effects associated with the individual level characteristics were included in each part of the Hurdle model.

Unadjusted and risk adjusted models were compared using both the likelihood ratio test (LRT) that follows a chi-squared distribution (p-value has to be less than 0.05) and information criteria (e.g., Akaike and Bayesian: lower values equal better fit) [52–54]. Statistical significance of coefficients was considered at alpha = 0.05. We also compared the observed data with predicted values by LHIN to investigate model adequacy. The coefficient of determination R^2 was calculated to measure the proportion of the observed regional variation in outcomes explained by the covariate for each model (please see Additional file 2) [55, 56]. To assess uncertainty around the estimates of the random effects, we generated a bootstrap 95% confidence interval (CI) from the bootstrap sample of 1000 by looking at the 2.5th and 97.5th percentiles in this distribution.

To determine whether certain regions are more efficient than others, we examined the relationship between total healthcare spending (positive costs) and mortality in both cohorts. Building on an approach previously employed for hospital profiling [57, 58], the risk-adjusted random effects for total costs and mortality were first ordered from the smallest to the largest and then graphically presented together in a cost-mortality plane, one for each cohort. LHINs located at the left bottom quadrant of the plots (where the X axis represents mortality and the Y axis costs) are more efficient than others provided that the CI of random effects for both total costs and mortality does not cross 0. Analyses were conducted using SAS software version 9.4 (SAS Institute Inc., Cary, NC, USA). The NLMIXED procedure was used to fit all the models. To visualize HCU rates between LHINs, a heat map was created using QGIS (Quantum geographic information system, https://qgis.org).

Results

Baseline characteristics

We included 703,388 subjects (HCU = 175,847, non-HCU = 527,541). The HCU were similar to non-HCU with respect to age, sex, the proportion residing in urban centres, and the number of low-income subjects (Table 1). However, compared to non-HCU, HCU tended to have a higher number of comorbidities, and a larger proportion of subjects with a malignancy, common chronic diseases, and mental health issues. HCU were dispensed a higher number of prescription drugs, had more physicians involved in their circle of care, and were seen by a geriatrician more often. Additional file 3 provides more information on the variation in these characteristics between the 14 LHINs.

HCU rate

Figure 1 shows the distribution of HCU among the 14 health regions. The size of LHINs' senior HCU population ranged from a low of 88.1 per 1000 seniors (Central 08

Table 1 Patient baseline individual and care characteristics, pre-incident year

Characteristic	HCU	Non-HCU	SDD
	Mean (SD)	Mean (SD)	
Age: subgroup (%)			
66–74	39.7 (2.5)	39.7 (2.5)	0.00
75–84	39.9 (0.8)	39.9 (0.8)	0.00
≥ 85	20.5 (2.5)	20.5 (2.5)	0.00
Sex (F, %)	52.7 (1.3)	52.7 (1.3)	0.00
Rurality (urban, %)	61.8 (27.6)	62.7 (28.0)	0.03
Low income senior (%)	17.6 (5.2)	16.8 (5.7)	0.01
Number of ADGs (mean)	10.1 (0.4)	7.9 (0.3)	0.50
Malignant neoplasms (%)	32.2 (2.6)	23.4 (3.2)	0.20
Common chronic conditions* (%)	60.6 (2.4)	44.8 (2.3)	0.30
Mental health# (%)	37.6 (4.1)	26.9 (2.5)	0.20
Number of MDs involved in care (mean)	8.1 (0.5)	5.6 (0.3)	0.50
Seen by a geriatrician (%)	2.8 (1.3)	1.1 (0.5)	0.12
Number of prescription drugs (mean)	8.4 (0.4)	5.6 (0.3)	0.60
Acute inpatient care (%)	3.8 (1.1)	2.1 (0.7)	0.10

ADGs- Aggregated Diagnosis Groups; HCU- high-cost user; *ICES- derived common chronic conditions (either one of the following: CHF-congestive heart failure; COPD- chronic obstructive pulmonary disease; DM- diabetes, MI-myocardial infarction, RA- rheumatoid arthritis); LHIN – Local Health Integrated Network; SD- Standard Deviation; # includes any of mental health conditions among Expanded Diagnosis Clusters (PSY01–12); SDD – absolute standardized difference; SDD ≥ 0.1 indicates a meaningful difference

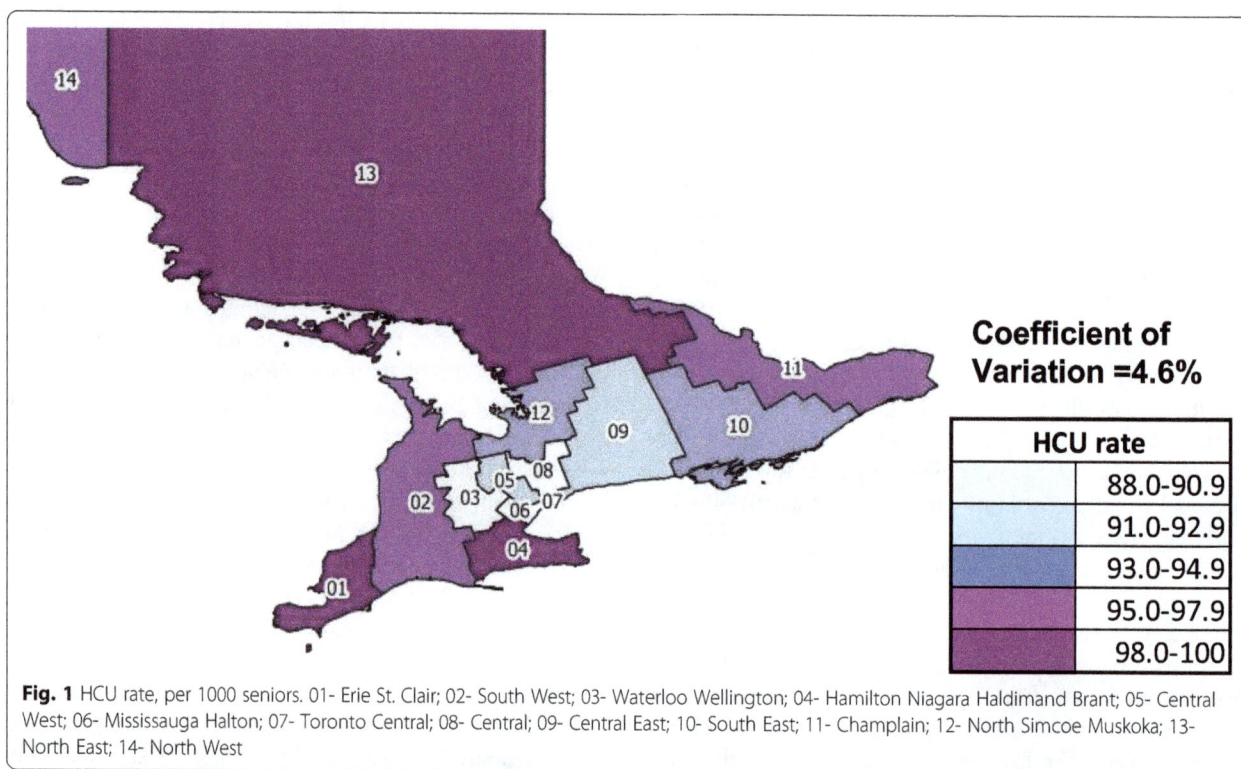

Fig. 1 HCU rate, per 1000 seniors. 01- Erie St. Clair; 02- South West; 03- Waterloo Wellington; 04- Hamilton Niagara Haldimand Brant; 05- Central West; 06- Mississauga Halton; 07- Toronto Central; 08- Central; 09- Central East; 10- South East; 11- Champlain; 12- North Simcoe Muskoka; 13- North East; 14- North West

LHIN) to a high of 100.2 per 1000 seniors (North East 13 LHIN).One of the northernmost regions of Ontario (North East 13 LHIN), and two health regions in the southwest of the province (Erie St. Clair 01 LHIN and Hamilton 04 LHIN) had the highest rates of HCU in the province, whereas health regions in close proximity to Toronto tended to exhibit the lowest rates. Overall variation in HCU rates across the province had a CV of 4.6%.

Unadjusted and adjusted costs and mortality by LHIN
The mean total 1-year observed costs per individual were $29,646 CAD and $2452 CAD for HCU and non-HCU, respectively. Hospital admissions represented the largest cost component among incident HCU accounting for 48.2% of the total costs. In non-HCU, prescription drugs were closely followed by physician costs as the top contributors to the total expenditures at 38.9% and 35.8%, respectively, while hospitalization accounted for 10.2%. All-cause mortality during the incident year among HCU was 13.6 times greater that of non-HCU (104.2 vs. 7.7 per 1000 seniors, respectively). Additional file 4 presents the observed and adjusted mortality and costs (total healthcare expenditures and its components) as well as the associated CVs. As shown in the tables, there was a very good agreement between observed and adjusted mean values across the mortality and cost components in both cohorts suggesting a good fit of the data. CVs for total costs and mortality were 3% and 6.8% for the HCU cohort, indicating little variation between LHINs. Higher CV values were

observed for several cost components such as complex continuing care (CV of 45.1%), rehabilitation (CV of 7.2%), and dialysis (CV of 36.2%), and CVs were higher for the non-HCU matched cohort. In all analyses that converged, the models incorporating patient individual covariates were preferred to the models without covariates as shown by the LRT tests and lower AIC and BIC values. For non-HCU, the two-part mixed effects models did not converge in 4 cost components (mental health, long-term care, complex continuing care, rehabilitation services) due to very low number of patients that incur these costs.

Between-LHIN variation in mortality and costs
Starting with mortality, the results of the mixed models indicate that the LHIN-specific variation in mortality (represented by the variance $\sigma 2u$) was statistically significant and was 10 times as low compared to non-HCU (Table 2). All covariates were statically significant with the expected signs although the impact of the number of ADG was different for HCU and non-HCU. As shown by the values of the coefficient of determination R^2, approximately 9% the observed variation in mortality among HCU is explained by patients' characteristics while this percentage is 18% for non-HCU.

Table 3 presents regression results for total costs among HCU and non-HCU. Since all the HCU had a contact with the healthcare system and incurred a cost, we used a GLMM to fit the data for the HCU. Results indicated that the LHIN-specific variation was small but

Table 2 Regression results: mortality (adjusted, log scale)

Mortality		
Variables	HCU#	Non-HCU#
	Coefficient (SE)	Coefficient (SE)
Variance in mortality, σ2u	0.005 (0.003)*	0.051 (0.021)*
Intercept	−7.154 (0.087)*	−13.883 (0.201)*
Age	0.071 (0.002)*	0.109 (0.003)*
Sex, M	0.346 (0.017)*	0.392 (0.033)*
ADG	−0.04 (0.002)*	0.052 (0.004)*
Low income status	0.091 (0.02)*	0.227 (0.039)*
R^2, %	8.8%	17.9%
LRT (Chi2 dist, $p < 0.05$)	5207.2	2800.21

- Estimated through a mixed effects two-part model; * - estimates were statistically significant at $p < .05$; ADGs- Aggregated Diagnosis Groups; HCU- high-cost user; LHIN – Local Health Integrated Network; LRT- likelihood ratio test; R^2- coefficients of determination; SE- Standard Error

statistically significant ($\sigma2u2$). All covariates were statistically significant too but only 1.6% (i.e. R^2) of the observed regional variation in total costs of senior HCU was due to patient characteristics. Because 9.4% of non-HCU incurred no costs at all, we fitted a mixed effects two-part model to the non-HCU total cost data. Since two distributions generate the data, the model generates two random-effects to estimate between-LHIN variation in the probability of incurring any costs ($\sigma2u1$) and variation in costs once they were incurred ($\sigma2u2$). As shown in this table, the variation ($\sigma2u1$) among HCU in system contacts overall was 65 times as high as $\sigma2u2$, both estimates statistically significant. All covariates were statistically significant in explaining each part of the model. The values of R^2 for the non-HCU cohort indicated that 87% of the LHIN variation related to the probability of incurring a cost was explained by the covariates while only 19.7% of the variation once a cost was incurred was explained by patient characteristics of non-HCU.

In addition to the total costs, Additional file 5A-B presents variance estimates across the cost components in both cohorts ($\sigma2u1$, where available, and $\sigma2u2$, log-scale). With the exception of the analysis of costs associated with physician visits, all cost components were analysed with two-part models. Overall, variation in incurred expenditures across cost components was higher compared with that of the total costs. Similarly, variation in the probability of positive costs was substantially greater. LHIN-specific variation in dialysis costs (both part 1 and part 2 of the model) had the highest significant values in HCU, whereas regional variation in cancer expenditures was an outlier among non-HCU. The covariates traditionally representing health care needs explained much of the observed variation in the probability of accessing healthcare: R^2 for part 1 of the models ranged from 0.5 to 34.5% (HCU) and 6.8% to

Table 3 Regression results: total public healthcare expenditures (adjusted, log scale)

Total costs		
Variables	HCU#	Non-HCU&
	Coefficient (SE)	Coefficient (SE)
Variance in probability of incurring costs, σ2u1		0.065 (0.026)*
Variance in costs once incurred, σ2u2	0.0009 (0.0004)*	0.001 (0.001)*
Covariance between σ2u1 and σ2u2		0.006 (0.003)
Probability (costs≠0)		
Intercept		4.49 (0.16)*
Age		−0.067 (0.002)*
Sex, M		− 0.205 (0.03)*
ADG		1.018 (0.009)*
Low income status		−0.129 (0.035)*
Costs > 0		
Intercept	9.74 (0.02)*	5.946 (0.025)*
Age	0.008 (0.0002)*	0.016 (0.001)*
Sex, M	0.064 (0.003)*	0.044 (0.005)*
ADG	−0.011 (0.0004)*	0.081 (0.001)*
Low income status	0.018 (0.004)*	0.134 (0.006)*
log_theta	0.788 (0.003)*	0.473 (0.004)*
R^2 (part 1), %		87.0%
R^2 (part 2), %	1.6%	19.7%
LRT (Chi2 dist, $p < 0.05$)	2333.0	88,500.57

& - Estimated through GLMM; # - Estimated through a mixed effects two-part model; * - estimates were statistically significant at $p < .05$; ADGs- Aggregated Diagnosis Groups; HCU- high-cost user; LHIN – Local Health Integrated Network; Log-theta- the logarithm of the shape parameter of gamma distribution; LRT- likelihood ratio test; R^2- coefficients of determination; SE- Standard Error

87.0%(non-HCU). In contrast, once the costs were incurred, the role of these covariates greatly diminishes. R^2 for part 2 ranged from 0.3 to 5.1% (HCU) and 2.7% to 19.7% (non-HCU).

Cost-mortality relationship

To identify LHINs that are more efficient than others (e.g. lower spending and mortality), LHINs were ranked by random effects for total costs and mortality (Figs. 2 and 3). As shown in Figs. 2a–c presenting the random effects for each LHIN and the associated 95% CIs among HCU, there were several LHINs in which the random effects were statistically significant for mortality (Fig. 2a) and costs (Fig. 2b). When costs and mortality were combined in a cost-mortality plane (Fig. 2c), only LHINs 1, 3, 4 and 7 had the random effects significant for both

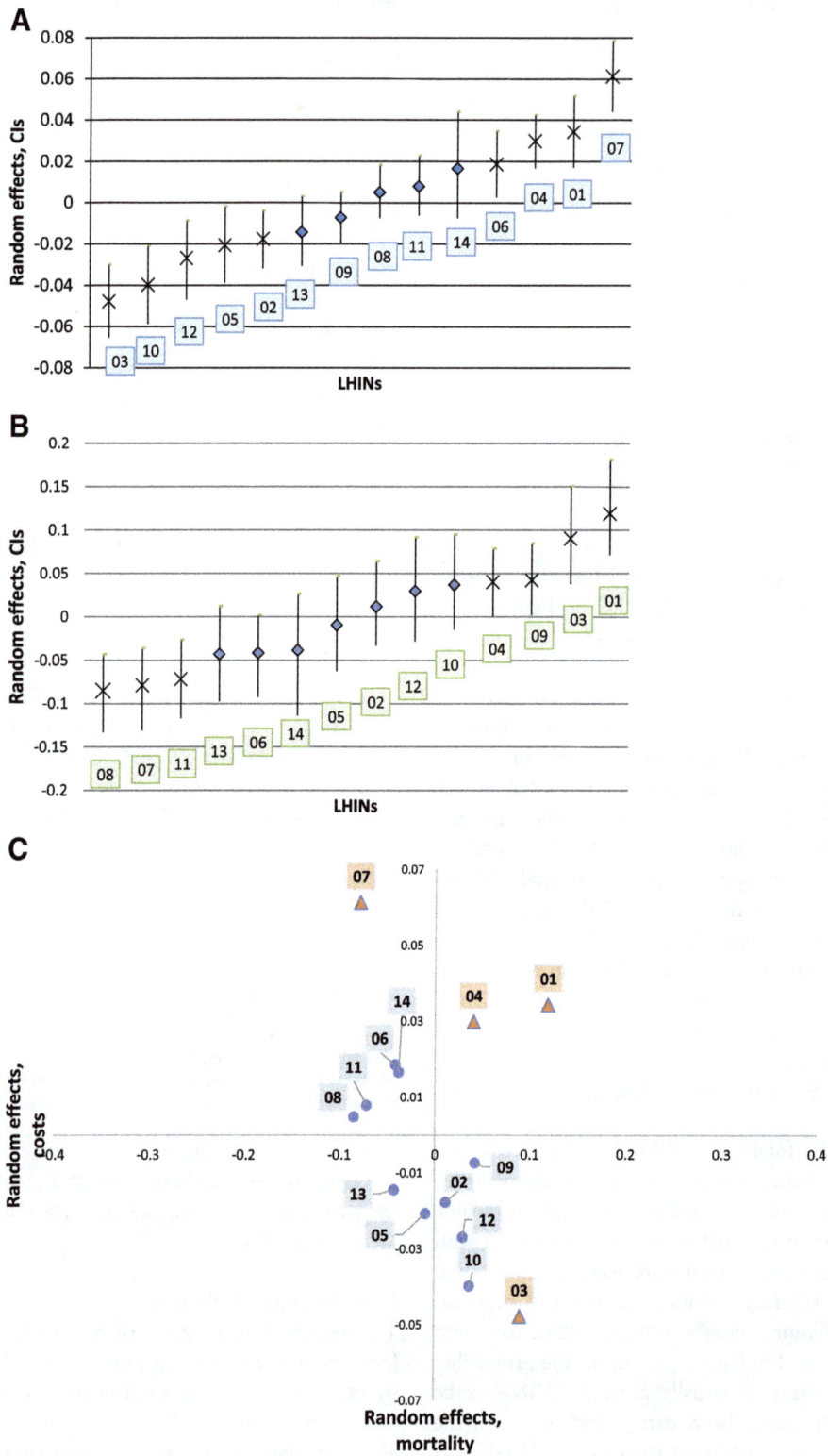

Fig. 2 (See legend on next page.)

total costs and mortality (marked as a triangle). Among those LHINs, none were in the lower bottom quadrant ("higher efficiency" pocket). Erie St. Claire 01 and Hamilton 04 LHINs (right upper) spend more and have a higher risk-adjusted mortality. Toronto Central 07 LHIN (left upper) has one of the lowest mortality rates, but it comes at a higher cost compared to other LHINs. In contrast, LHIN 3 had the lowest costs, but one of the highest mortality rates. For non-HCU (Fig. 3a–c), the list of LHINs with significant random effects for both total costs and mortality is broader and different from HCU. Several LHINs in close proximity to the Toronto area exhibit higher efficiency. On the opposite side, South West 02, South East 10, and North East 13 show signs of lower efficiency.

Discussion

This is the first Canadian study to examine geographic variation in healthcare costs and mortality among senior HCU. We found approximately a 14% difference between the highest (100.2 per 1000 seniors) and lowest (88.1 per 1000 seniors) incident senior HCU rates across the LHINs in Ontario. Overall regional variation in total costs and mortality was low in both cohorts, and lower among HCU compared to non-HCU. Our results indicate that traditional drivers of costs and mortality such as age, sex, comorbidity and income play little role in explaining variation in mortality and costs among HCU. Our analyses of individual cost components revealed greater variability in accessing the healthcare system, but, once the patient enters the system, variation in costs was low. Finally, LHINs vary in their costs per mortality rate, which deserves further analysis to determine whether policies or practices followed in high performing LHINs might be usable in other LHINs.

This study's results are important for several reasons. First, when regional variation is of interest, it is important to account for the regional factor in the model. In the literature on geographic healthcare variation, the authors seem to employ fixed effects models more often to describe variation in observed and predicted values through descriptive statistics (coefficient of variation, extremal quotient or its variations, etc.) [15, 20]. The use of mixed effects models is less frequent but provides richer information when applied. As such, in addition to controlling for the

regional effect, mixed effects models directly measure regional variability by estimating a variance component. In a two-part mixed effects models such as ours, it is also possible to estimate two components of between-LHIN variation: variation in the probability of costs incurred and variation in costs once incurred. Finally, we ran a fixed effects model in parallel (results available upon a request from authors). Comparing the findings with the mixed effects models showed closely matched coefficient estimates but more narrow standard errors which is an expected difference between the fixed effects and models with random effects.

Second, exploration of regional variation across multiple cost categories among seniors has not been reported for Canadian HCU or the general population. Even internationally, this is rarely done likely due to limited availability of such data. This study results indicate that reporting variation in total spending alone hides the contribution of individual cost components. The magnitude of some cost components such as hospitalization (a mean of $13,677 among HCU) absorbs the variation of smaller components (a mean of $181 in lab costs, respectively). It is particularly so among non-HCU where healthcare expenditures are substantially lower compared to HCU. As shown here, examining regional variation as a function of total costs only would present an incomplete picture: e.g., although small regional variation in total costs, there is a much greater variation in dialysis costs among HCU. Also, comparison with non-HCU points to the fact that there is a very small number of non-HCU patients in several cost categories (e.g., mental health, rehabilitation, etc.) suggesting that incurring costs in these categories may convert a patient into an HCU.

Further, our results indicate that after adjustment, allocation of resources to seniors was similar across Ontario LHINs, more so for HCU compared to non-HCU, which is reassuring for healthcare planners. However, whether the allocation is truly equitable is unclear. Judging by the sign and CIs of coefficients in part 2 of the models, for example, the low- income status was associated with greater intensity of healthcare services across most of the cost components in both cohorts. Also, access to services may be an issue: patients with higher income status are more

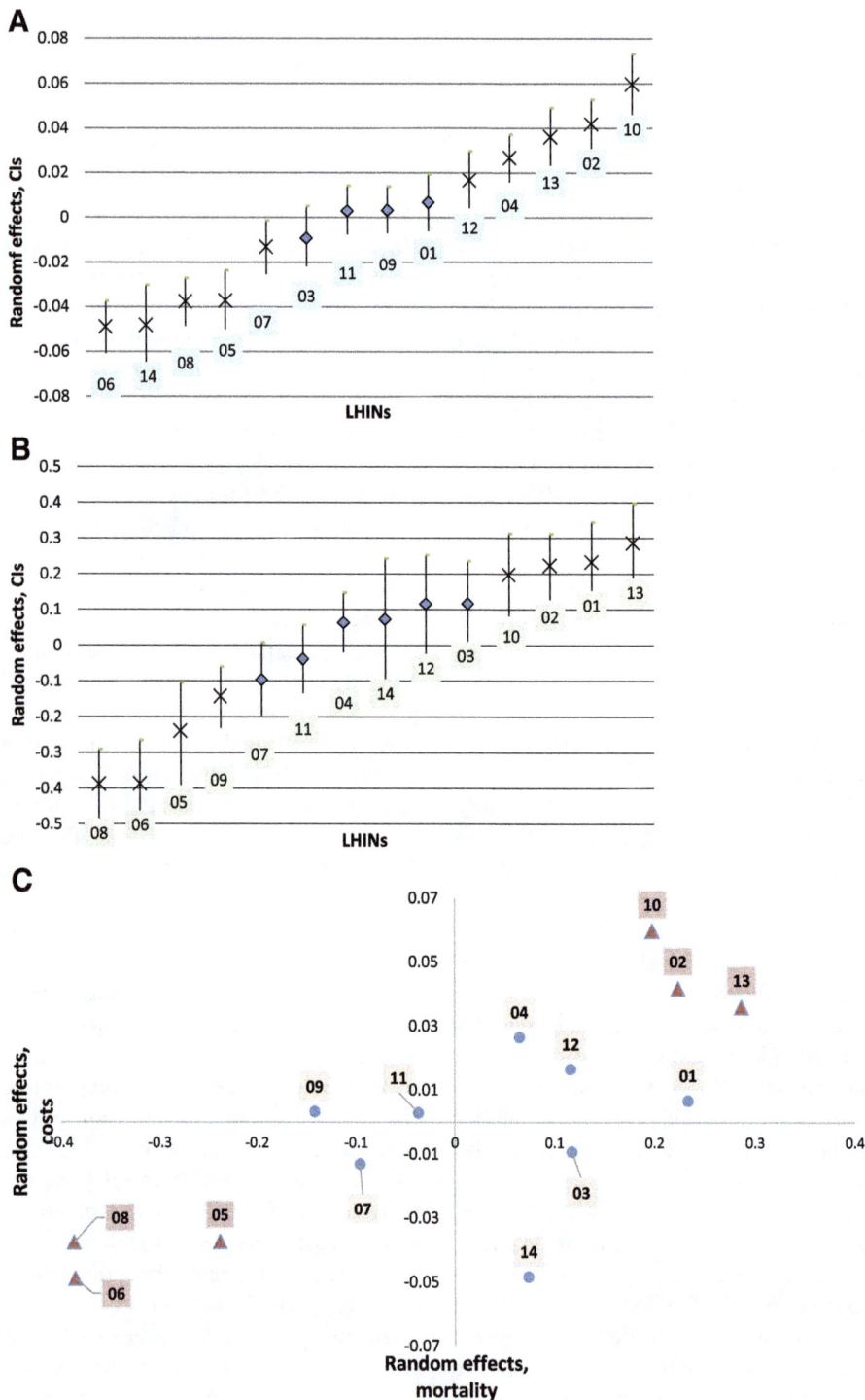

Fig. 3 a: Ranking LHIN-specific random effects in total costs, non-HCU. Marked as X are statistically significant. **b**: Ranking LHIN-specific random effects in mortality, non-HCU. Marked as X are statistically significant. **c**: Cost-mortality relationship, Non-HCU. Both total costs and mortality are adjusted for the regional factor, age, sex, ADGs, and low-income status; colored triangle indicates health district in which variation in both costs and mortality is statistically significant; 01- Erie St. Clair; 02- South West; 03- Waterloo Wellington; 04- Hamilton Niagara Haldimand Brant; 05- Central West; 06- Mississauga Halton; 07- Toronto Central; 08- Central; 09- Central East; 10- South East; 11- Champlain; 12- North Simcoe Muskoka; 13- North East; 14- North West

likely to enter the healthcare system. This is aggravated by much higher LHIN-specific variation in the probability of incurring costs. In particular, higher variation in dialysis and cancer costs may be a concern that requires further elucidation.

Finally, we have studied for the first time the relationship between costs and mortality for HCU and non-HCU across Ontario LHINs to explore health system performance from the efficiency angle. Efforts to examine the relationship between healthcare spending and outcomes, most often mortality, have been made globally applying various approaches [16, 30, 59–65]. The approach taken in our study builds on previous research that conducted hospital profiling [57, 58, 66]. As such, our results provide insight into the distribution of mortality in relation to resources spent across the Ontario LHINs by identifying districts of various cost-mortality performance. Although caution should be applied when interpreting the results of the study, e.g., variation in total costs across LHINs appears quite small, the observed differences in efficiency between health regions merit further examination to determine if health improvement could be achieved without additional healthcare spending.

Strengths and limitations

This study has several strengths. First, the dataset contained information on all incident senior HCU in the province at the time of data collection whereas the matched non-HCU represented approximately 25% of the total senior population in the province. Second, the study examines incident HCU cases which represents a shift in the focus of HCU research dominated by studies of persistent cases (those that retain HCU status over time). Since the two populations are likely to be different, studying incident cases of HCU provides important information to inform health policies and interventions. Third, it directly estimates variation across a number of cost categories using two variance components, which has never been done in the past. Finally, to deal with the large proportion of zero costs in the data (i.e. no healthcare use), we used two part-models which have been shown to provide better estimates than models that ignore the over-representation of zeros [48] .

We note some limitations. While the study's cost data captures public expenditures in the most expensive cost categories such as hospital admissions, physician billings, rehabilitation or home care, cost data for some components may be incomplete. For pharmaceutical care, copayment is not included in the ODB cost and, more importantly, the cost of some chemotherapy not covered by the ODB is not captured by the study, especially the costs incurred in outpatient cancer clinics [40]. The LTC costs do not include accommodation charges unless the patient's stay is subsidized by the government. Another

Canadian-based study into HCU that used the same source of administrative data but examined the entire HCU population across only 5 cost components estimated the extent of unaccounted for cost data at 7% [7]. However, since data on seniors is usually more complete, our conservative estimate is that less than 5% of government expenditures on individual health services to seniors might not have been included in this study, hence their impact on the results is close to negligible. Secondly, this study did not account for the supply side of the examined variation as the data were not available for analysis. That would require access to LHIN-based data on the number of physicians, hospital and LTC beds, HC/CCAC staff. Instead, our approach standardized for the effect of patient needs. Similarly, we did not have access to several variables which could partially explained some of the variation between LHINs (e.g. patient preferences, health behaviors, education, etc). Further, we encountered model convergence and parameter estimation issues when running models for the non-HCU' cost components using the total non-HCU population. To address this, we re-fitted the models on a random sample of the population. Depending on the cost component, the sample size ranged from 30 to 100%.However, convergence issues in mixed effects models run on the entire population are not uncommon with very large datasets [67]. This is a limitation that in our opinion was alleviated by low discrepancy in the estimates generated by RE models compared to FE models run on the full size of the non-HCU population. Not surprisingly, as 30% of the non-HCU population is still a large enough sample (i.e., > 150,000 individuals). Finally, some may argue that a smaller unit of analysis would be preferable to evaluate regional variation. Using a smaller unit (sub-LHINs in our case) could unmask heterogeneity at the more local level. We did not have information on sub-LHINs and therefore we could not conduct these analyses. However, the choice of LHINs as the unit of analysis is supported by the fact that the boundaries of LHINs were developed with local patterns of care provision in mind [68].

Conclusions

Risk-adjusted allocation of healthcare resources to seniors across Ontario is similar across health districts, more so for HCU than non-HCU. However, when analyzed in combination with risk-adjusted mortality, we identified important variation in the cost-mortality relationship among LHINs which needs to be further explored. The traditional drivers of costs and mortality had a weak impact on the observed variation in the outcomes among both HCU and non-HCU, but largely explained the probability of healthcare system access.

Additional files

> **Additional file 1:** Intra-class coefficients (ICC). Provides details on ICC calculation for costs and mortality.
>
> **Additional file 2:** Model specification and other statistical formulas used in statistical analysis. Provides details on model specification and formulas used in calculations.
>
> **Additional file 3:** A-B. Variation (by LHIN) in patient baseline individual and care characteristics, pre-incident year. The files provide information on the variation in individual and care characteristics between the 14 LHINs: for HCU (2A) and non-HCU (2B).
>
> **Additional file 4:** A-C. Observed and adjusted healthcare care expenditures (total and by cost component) and mortality among HCU and non-HCU, incident year. The file provides details observed and adjusted values and model fit.
>
> **Additional file 5:** Estimate coefficients, healthcare care expenditures among HCU and non-HCU, total costs and cost components, incident year. The file provides details on regression coefficients, including the estimates of variance components.

Abbreviations

ACGs: Johns Hopkins Adjusted Clinical Groups; ADGs: Johns Hopkins Aggregated Diagnosis Groups; BC: British Columbia, Canada; CAD: Canadian dollar; CHF: Congestive heart failure; COPD: Chronic obstructive pulmonary disease; CV: Coefficient of variation; DM: Diabetes; EDCs: John Hopkins Expanded Diagnosis Clusters; FY: Fiscal year; GLM: Generalized linear models; HCU: High-cost user; ICC: Intraclass coefficient; ICES: Institute for Clinical Evaluative Sciences; LHIN: Local Health Integration Networks; LRT: Likelihood ratio test; MI: Myocardial infarction; QGIS: Quantum geographic information system; RA: Rheumatoid arthritis; RIO: Rural Index of Ontario; SD: Standard deviation; SDD: Absolute Standardized difference; US: United States

Acknowledgements

Parts of this material are based on data and/or information compiled and provided by the Canadian Institute for Health Information (CIHI). However, the analyses, conclusions, opinions and statements expressed in the material are those of the authors and not necessarily those of CIHI. We thank IMS Brogan Inc. for use of their Drug Information Database.

Funding

This work is supported by personnel funding and in-kind analyst and epidemiologist support from the Ontario Drug Policy Research Network (ODPRN), and personnel awards from the Canadian Institutes of Health Research (CIHR) Drug Safety and Effectiveness Cross-Disciplinary Training (DSECT) Program, the Program for Assessment of Technology in Health (PATH), The Research Institute of St Joe's Hamilton, St Joseph's Healthcare Hamilton, and an Ontario Graduate Scholarship (OGS). The work also is supported by the Institute for Clinical Evaluative Sciences (ICES). ODPRN and ICES are funded by grants from the Ontario Ministry of Health and Long-Term Care (MOHLTC) and the Ontario Strategy for Patient-Orientated Research (SPOR) Support Unit, which is supported by the Canadian Institutes of Health Research and the Province of Ontario. The opinions, results, and conclusions reported in this article are those of the authors and are independent from the funding sources. The funding bodies had no role in the design of the study, the collection, analysis, interpretation of data and in writing the manuscript. No endorsement by the Ontario MOHLTC is intended or should be inferred.

Authors' contributions

SM, JET, AH, JL, JMP, TG, AC, LM, JRG conceptualized the study. SM, JET, AH, JL, AC, JRG, LM, JMP, TG, WK have contributed to its design. JMP, WK, TG were instrumental in creating datasets. SM prepared the initial draft of the manuscript and revised it based on co-authors' feedback: JET, AH, JL, JMP, TG, JRG, LM, AC, WK provided comments to the initial draft, further revisions, read and approved the final manuscript. The responsibility of study implementation lies with the principal investigator (SM) that is supported and supervised primarily by JET.

Competing interests

The authors declare that they have no competing interests.

Author details

[1]Department of Health Research Methods, Evidence, and Impact, McMaster University, Hamilton, ON, Canada. [2]Programs for Assessment of Technology in Health (PATH), The Research Institute of St. Joe's Hamilton, St. Joseph's Healthcare, Hamilton, ON, Canada. [3]Division of Geriatric Medicine, Department of Medicine, McMaster University, Hamilton, ON, Canada. [4]Division of Clinical Pharmacology and Toxicology, Department of Medicine, McMaster University, Hamilton, ON, Canada. [5]Geriatric Education and Research in Aging Sciences Centre, Hamilton Health Sciences, Hamilton, ON, Canada. [6]Institute for Clinical Evaluative Sciences (ICES), Toronto, ON, Canada. [7]Center for Health Economics and Policy Analysis (CHEPA), McMaster University, Hamilton, Canada. [8]Département de Médecine Sociale et Préventive, Faculté de Médecine, Université Laval, Quebec City, QC, Canada. [9]Centre de recherche du CHU de Québec, Université Laval, Axe Santé des Populations et Pratiques Optimales en Santé, Québec City, QC, Canada. [10]Biostatistics Unit, Father Sean O'Sullivan Research Centre, St Joseph's Healthcare, Hamilton, ON, Canada. [11]Institute of Health Policy, Management and Evaluation, University of Toronto, Toronto, ON, Canada. [12]Leslie Dan Faculty of Pharmacy, University of Toronto, Toronto, Canada. [13]Li Ka Shing Knowledge Institute, St. Michael's Hospital, Toronto, ON, Canada.

References

1. Blumenthal D, Chernof B, Fulmer T, Lumpkin J, Selberg J. Caring for high-need, high-cost patients - an urgent priority. N Engl J Med. 2016;375(10):909–11.
2. Hayes SL, Salzberg CA, McCarthy D, et al. High-Need, High-Cost Patients: Who Are They and How Do They Use Health Care? A Population-Based Comparison of Demographics, Health Care Use, and Expenditures. Issue brief (Commonwealth Fund). 2016;26:1–14.
3. Rais S, Nazerian A, Ardal S, Chechulin Y, Bains N, Malikov K. High-cost users of Ontario's healthcare services. Healthcare policy = Politiques de sante. 2013;9(1):44–51.
4. Lee JY, Muratov S, Tarride J-E, Holbrook AM. Managing high-cost healthcare users: the international search for effective evidence-supported strategies. J Am Geriatr Soc. 2018;66(5):1002–8.
5. Statistics Canada: Population by year, by province and territory [http://www.statcan.gc.ca/tables-tableaux/sum-som/l01/cst01/demo02a-eng.htm]. Accessed 25 Jan 2018.
6. Roos NP, Shapiro E, Tate R. Does a small minority of elderly account for a majority of health care expenditures? A sixteen-year perspective. The Milbank Quarterly. 1989;67(3–4):347–69.
7. Wodchis WP, Austin PC, Henry DA. A 3-year study of high-cost users of health care. Cmaj. 2016;188(3):182–8.
8. Geographic Variations in Health Care. Focus on Health- OECD Health Policy Studies [https://www.oecd.org/els/health-systems/FOCUS-on-Geographic-Variations-in-Health-Care.pdf]. Accessed 12 Feb 2018.
9. Kim AM, Park JH, Kang S, Hwang K, Lee T, Kim Y. The effect of geographic units of analysis on measuring geographic variation in medical services utilization. J Prev Med Public Health. 2016;49(4):230–9.
10. Lougheed MD, Garvey N, Chapman KR, Cicutto L, Dales R, Day AG, Hopman WM, Lam M, Sears MR, Szpiro K, et al. The Ontario asthma regional variation study: emergency department visit rates and the relation to hospitalization rates. Chest. 2006;129(4):909–17.
11. Feasby TE, Quan H, Ghali WA. Geographic variation in the rate of carotid endarterectomy in Canada. Stroke. 2001;32(10):2417–22.

12. Feinberg AE, Porter J, Saskin R, Rangrej J, Urbach DR. Regional variation in the use of surgery in Ontario. CMAJ open. 2015;3(3):E310–6.

13. Hogan DB, Maxwell CJ, Fung TS, Ebly EM. Regional variation in the use of medications by older Canadians--a persistent and incompletely understood phenomena. Pharmacoepidemiol Drug Saf. 2003;12(7):575–82.

14. Morgan SG, Cunningham CM, Hanley GE. Individual and contextual determinants of regional variation in prescription drug use: an analysis of administrative data from British Columbia. PLoS One. 2010; 5(12):e15883.

15. Newhouse JP, Garber AM, Graham RP, McCoy MA, Mancher M, Kibria A. Variation in health care spending: target decision making, not geography. In: Committee on geographic variation in health care spending and promotion of high-value care; board on health care services; institute of Medicine; 2013.

16. Elliott S, Fisher M, David E, Wennberg M, Thrse A, Stukel P, Daniel J, Gottlieb MFL, Lucas P, Étoile L, Pinder M. The implications of regional variations in Medicare spending. Part 2: health outcomes and satisfaction with care. Ann Intern Med. 2003;138(4):288–98.

17. Fisher E, Goodman D, Skinner J, Bronner K. Health Care Spending, Quality, and Outcomes. The Dartmouth Insititute for Health Policy Research and Clinical Practice, 2009.

18. Fisher ES, Wennberg DE, Stukel TA, Gottlieb DJ, Lucas FL, Pinder ÉL. The implications of regional variations in Medicare spending. Part 1: the content, quality, and accessibility of care. Ann Intern Med. 2003;138(4):273–87.

19. Zuckerman SWT, Berenson R, Hadle J. Clarifying sources of geographic differences in Medicare spending. N Engl J Med. 2010;363:54–62.

20. Lavergne MR, Barer M, Law MR, Wong ST, Peterson S, McGrail K. Examining regional variation in health care spending in British Columbia, Canada. Health Policy. 2016;120(7):739–48.

21. Brooks GA, Li L, Uno H, Hassett MJ, Landon BE, Schrag D. Acute hospital care is the chief driver of regional spending variation in Medicare patients with advanced cancer. Health affairs (Project Hope). 2014;33(10):1793–800.

22. Ellis RP, Fiebig DG, Johar M, Jones G, Savage E. Explaining health care expenditure variation: large-sample evidence using linked survey and health administrative data. Health Econ. 2013;22(9):1093–110.

23. Bevan G: Using information on variation in rates of supply to questoin professional discretion in public services. 2004.

24. Kephart G, Asada Y. Need-based resource allocation: different need indicators, different results? BMC Health Serv Res. 2009;9:122.

25. O'Neill J, Tabish H, Welch V, Petticrew M, Pottie K, Clarke M, Evans T, Pardo Pardo J, Waters E, White H, et al. Applying an equity lens to interventions: using PROGRESS ensures consideration of socially stratifying factors to illuminate inequities in health. J Clin Epidemiol. 2014;67(1):56–64.

26. Struikmans H, Aarts MJ, Jobsen JJ, Koning CC, Merkus JW, Lybeert ML, Immerzeel J, Poortmans PM, Veerbeek L, Louwman MW, et al. An increased utilisation rate and better compliance to guidelines for primary radiotherapy for breast cancer from 1997 till 2008: a population-based study in the Netherlands. Radiother Oncol. 2011;100(2):320–5.

27. Bierman AS, Shack AR, Johns A, for the POWER Study. Achieving health equity in Ontario: opportunities for intervention and improvement. In: Bierman AS, editor. Project for an Ontario Women's health evidence-based report. Volume 2 ed. Toronto: St. Michael's Hospital and the Institute for Clinical Evaluative Sciences; 2012.

28. Ohinmaa A, Zheng Y, Jeerakathil T, Klarenbach S, Hakkinen U, Nguyen T, Friesen D, Ruseski J, Kaul P, Ariste R, et al. Trends and regional variation in hospital mortality, length of stay and cost in Hospital of Ischemic Stroke Patients in Alberta accompanying the provincial reorganization of stroke care. J Stroke Cerebrovasc Dis. 2016;25(12):2844–50.

29. Joumard, I., André C., Nicq C. "Health Care Systems: Efficiency and Institutions", OECD Economics Department Working Papers, No. 769. Paris: OECD Publishing; 2010. https://doi.org/10.1787/5kmfp51f5f9t-en.

30. Allin S, Veillard J, Wang L, Grignon M. How can health system efficiency be improved in Canada? Healthcare Policy. 2015;11(1):33–45.

31. Zhang Y, Baik SH, Fendrick AM, Baicker K. Comparing local and regional variation in health care spending. N Engl J Med. 2012;367(18):1724–31.

32. Hong YR, Kates F, Song SJ, Lee N, Duncan RP, Marlow NM. Benchmarking implications: analysis of Medicare accountable care organizations spending level and quality of care. J Healthc Qual. 2018. https://doi.org/10.1097/JHQ.0000000000000123. [Epub ahead of print].

33. Skinner J. Causes and consequences of regional variations in health care. In: Handbook of health economics, vol. 2011. Volume 2 ed. p. 45–93.

34. Corallo AN, Croxford R, Goodman DC, Bryan EL, Srivastava D, Stukel TA. A systematic review of medical practice variation in OECD countries. Health Policy. 114(1):5–14.

35. Rosenberg BL, Kellar JA, Labno A, Matheson DH, Ringel M, VonAchen P, Lesser RI, Li Y, Dimick JB, Gawande AA, et al. Quantifying geographic variation in health care outcomes in the United States before and after risk-adjustment. PLoS One. 2016;11(12):e0166762.

36. Muratov S, Lee J, Holbrook A, Paterson JM, Guertin JR, Mbuagbaw L, Gomes T, Khuu W, Pequeno P, Costa AP, et al. Senior high-cost healthcare users' resource utilization and outcomes: a protocol of a retrospective matched cohort study in Canada. BMJ Open. 2017;7(12):e018488.

37. Fitzpatrick T, Rosella LC, Calzavara A, Petch J, Pinto AD, Manson H, Goel V, Wodchis WP. Looking beyond income and education: socioeconomic status gradients among future high-cost users of health care. Am J Prev Med. 2015;49(2):161–71.

38. Rosella LC, Fitzpatrick T, Wodchis WP, Calzavara A, Manson H, Goel V. High-cost health care users in Ontario, Canada: demographic, socio-economic, and health status characteristics. BMC Health Serv Res. 2014;14:532.

39. Institute for Clinical Evaluative Sciences (ICES); www.ices.on.ca . Accessed 10 Dec 2017.

40. Wodchis WP, Bushmeneva K, Nikitovic M, McKillop I. Guidelines on person-level costing using administrative databases in Ontario. In: Working Paper Series, vol. 1. Toronto: Health System Performance Research Network; 2013.

41. Ontario's Local Health Integration Networks. [www.lhins.on.ca]. Accessed 6 Feb 2018.

42. Local Health System Integration Act, 2006, S.O. 2006, c. 4 (amended 2017). [https://www.ontario.ca/laws/statute/06l04]. Accessed 26 Jan 2018.

43. Kralj B. Measuring 'rurality' for purposes of health-care planning: an empirical measure for Ontario. Ont Med Rev. 2000;67(9):33–52.

44. The Johns Hopkins ACG® System Version 10.0 Technical Reference Guide. In.: Department of Health Policy and Management, Johns Hopkins University, Bloomberg School of Public Health; 2014.

45. Gershon AS, Wang C, Guan J, Vasilevska-Ristovska J, Cicutto L, TO T. Identifying individuals with physcian diagnosed COPD in health administrative databases. Copd. 2009;6(5):388–94.

46. Schultz SE, Rothwell DM, Chen Z, Tu K. Identifying cases of congestive heart failure from administrative data: a validation study using primary care patient records. Chronic Dis Inj Can. 2013;33(3):160–6.

47. Austin PC. Balance diagnostics for comparing the distribution of baseline covariates between treatment groups in propensity-score matched samples. Stat Med. 2009;28(25):3083–107.

48. Buntin MB, Zaslavsky AM. Too much ado about two-part models and transformation? Comparing methods of modeling Medicare expenditures. J Health Econ. 2004;23(3):525–42.

49. Liu L, Cowen ME, Strawderman RL, Shih Y-CT. A flexible two-part random effects model for correlated medical costs. J Health Econ. 2010;29(1):110–23.

50. Basu A, Manning WG, Mullahy J. Comparing alternative models: log vs cox proportional hazard? Health Econ. 2004;13(8):749–65.

51. Gregori D, Petrinco M, Bo S, Desideri A, Merletti F, Pagano E. Regression models for analyzing costs and their determinants in health care: an introductory review. Int J Qual Health Care. 2011;23(3):331–41.

52. de Vries EF, Heijink R, Struijs JN, Baan CA. Unraveling the drivers of regional variation in healthcare spending by analyzing prevalent chronic diseases. BMC Health Serv Res. 2018;18(1):323.

53. Liu L, Ma JZ, Johnson BA. A multi-level two-part random effects model, with application to an alcohol-dependence study. Stat Med. 2008;27(18):3528–39.

54. Tooze JA, Grunwald GK, Jones RH. Analysis of repeated measures data with clumping at zero. Stat Methods Med Res. 2002;11(4):341–55.

55. Austin PC, Merlo J. Intermediate and advanced topics in multilevel logistic regression analysis. Stat Med. 2017;36(20):3257–77.

56. Nakagawa S, Johnson PCD, Schielzeth H. The coefficient of determination R2 and intra-class correlation coefficient from generalized linear mixed-effects models revisited and expanded. J R Soc Interface. 2017;14(134):20170213.

57. D'Errigo P, Tosti ME, Fusco D, Perucci CA, Seccareccia F. Use of hierarchical models to evaluate performance of cardiac surgery centres in the Italian CABG outcome study. BMC Med Res Methodol. 2007;7:29.

58. MacKenzie TA, Grunkemeier GL, Grunwald GK, O'Malley AJ, Bohn C, Wu Y, Malenka DJ. A primer on using shrinkage to compare in-hospital mortality between centers. Ann Thorac Surg. 2015;99(3):757–61.

59. Hadley J, Reschovsky JD. Medicare spending, mortality rates, and quality of care. Int J Health Care Finance Econ. 2012;12(1):87–105.

60. Lippi G, Mattiuzzi C, Cervellin G. No correlation between health care expenditure and mortality in the European Union. Eur J Intern Med. 2016;32:e13–4.

61. Gallet CA, Doucouliagos H. The impact of healthcare spending on health outcomes: a meta-regression analysis. Soc Sci Med. 2017;179:9–17.

62. Cohen D, Manuel DG, Tugwell P, Sanmartin C, Ramsay T. Does higher spending improve survival outcomes for myocardial infarction? Examining the cost-outcomes relationship using time-varying covariates. Health Serv Res. 2015;50(5):1589–605.

63. Stargardt T, Schreyogg J, Kondofersky I. Measuring the relationship between costs and outcomes: the example of acute myocardial infarction in German hospitals. Health Econ. 2014;23(6):653–69.

64. Stukel TA, Fisher ES, Alter DA, Guttmann A, Ko DT, Fung K, Wodchis WP, Baxter NN, Earle CC, Lee DS. Association of Hospital Spending Intensity with Mortality and Readmission Rates in Ontario hospitals. Jama. 2012;307(10):1037–45.

65. McKay NL, Deily ME. Comparing high- and low-performing hospitals using risk-adjusted excess mortality and cost inefficiency. Health Care Manag Rev. 2005;30(4):347–60.

66. Zhang M, Strawderman RL, Cowen ME, Wells MT. Bayesian inference for a two-part hierarchical model. J Am Stat Assoc. 2006;101(475):934–45.

67. Gebregziabher M, Egede L, Gilbert GE, Hunt K, Nietert PJ, Mauldin P. Fitting parametric random effects models in very large data sets with application to VHA national data. BMC Med Res Methodol. 2012;12:163.

68. Health Analyst's Toolkit. In.: Health Analytics Branch, Ontario Ministry of Health and Long-Term Care; 2012.

21

Patient-centred access to health care: a framework analysis of the care interface for frail older adults

Donata Kurpas[1,2], Holly Gwyther[3,4*] [iD], Katarzyna Szwamel[1,2], Rachel L. Shaw[4], Barbara D'Avanzo[5], Carol A. Holland[3] and Maria Magdalena Bujnowska-Fedak[1]

Abstract

Background: The objective of this study was to explore the issues surrounding access to health and social care services for frail older adults with Polish stakeholders, including healthy and frail/pre-frail older adults, health care providers, social care providers, and caregivers, in order to determine their views and perspectives on the current system and to present suggestions for the future development of a more accessible and person-centred health and social care system.

Methods: Focus groups were used to gather qualitative data from stakeholders. Data were analysed using framework analysis according to five dimensions of accessibility to care: approachability, acceptability, availability and accommodation, affordability and appropriateness.

Results: Generally services were approachable and acceptable, but unavailable. Poor availability related to high staff turnover, staff shortages and a lack of trained personnel. There were problems of long waiting times for specialist care and rehabilitation services, and geographically remote clinics. Critically, there were shortages of long-term inpatient care places, social care workers and caregivers. The cost of treatments created barriers to care and inequities in the system. Participants described a lack of integration between health and social care systems with differing priorities and disconnected budgets. They described an acute medical system that was inappropriate for patients with complex needs, alongside a low functioning social care system, where bureaucratisation caused delays in providing services to the vulnerable. An integrated system with a care coordinator to improve connections between services and patients was suggested.

Conclusions: There is an immediate need to improve access to health and social care systems for pre-frail and frail patients, as well as their caregivers. Health and social care services need to be integrated to reduce bureaucracy and increase the timeliness of treatment and care.

Keywords: Frailty, Delivery of health care, Health resources, Patient acceptance of health care, Patient preference, Patient satisfaction

* Correspondence: h.gwyther@lancaster.ac.uk
[3]Centre For Ageing Research, Lancaster University, Lancaster, UK
[4]Psychology, School of Life & Health Sciences, Aston University, Birmingham, UK
Full list of author information is available at the end of the article

Background

Equity in health and social care is critical in realising the full health potential of a population. Evidence shows that there are disparities in the quality of health and health care within and between European Union (EU) member states [1]. These disparities can be conceptualised as population-specific differences in the presence of disease, health outcomes, and access to health care, but can also be seen in terms of life expectancy and healthy life years [2]; that is, the number of years lived in good health as an indicator of quality of life rather than longevity.

Health and social care disparities are caused by a range of social determinants including socio-economic policy, environmental characteristics, poverty, unemployment levels, and the organisation and functioning of the health and welfare systems; individual factors such as lifestyle choices, age, and health behaviours are also critical [3] and may also vary between cultures. It is generally accepted that health care inequalities are "unfair and unjust" (p29. [4]) and thus, reducing them is an ethical imperative. In 2005, all EU member states committed to reducing inequalities for access to health care.

Population ageing has many socio-economic and health consequences, but one challenge is the need to build effective and accessible health and social care systems for older adults, as well as appropriate support networks for their families, whilst balancing budgetary constraints [5, 6]. Facilitating access to health and social care is an important step in enabling people to preserve or improve their health but using such services requires effort, and vulnerable groups of people, for example, those who are older or socially deprived, may not have the appropriate range of knowledge-based, social, language or practical skills to mobilise that effort [7].

Within the older adult population, frail people may be particularly vulnerable. Most frail individuals suffer from chronic diseases, with a statistically significant increase in frailty in people with a greater number of co-morbidities [8, 9]. Indeed, the number of chronic diseases is an important constituent part of the calculation of a frailty score, using an accumulation of deficits model of frailty [10]. Such multi-morbidity relates to elevated rates of primary care and multiple specialist visits. Communication between the array of health care providers can be poorly coordinated or lacking, which subsequently affects health care costs, patient outcomes, and experiences of care [11]. In order to formulate effective and enduring care plans for these vulnerable patients, a range of factors must be addressed, including appropriate access to health care, care coordination and improved communication between stakeholders in older adult care, including caregivers [12, 13].

Many caregivers take on all-consuming roles as intermediaries between the health and social care services and their care recipient. In essence, they take on the 'effort' of using services and assume the role of the active participant on behalf of their older relative [14]. However, evidence suggests that these advocates often have poor experiences of the health care system, finding it fragmented, rigid, and difficult to access [13, 15]. In this era of changing health care priorities, an ageing population, and the growing burden of chronic diseases, understanding the challenges faced by caregivers is crucial when designing suitable support services for them within both health care and community settings [16].

It should be emphasised here that treating frailty in older adults is a realistic therapeutic goal [17] and previous interventions have been shown to be effective [18]. One definition suggests that frailty is a dynamic process characterised by frequent transitional stages, which can be modified [19, 20]. This conceptualisation of frailty as a treatable entity may provide new opportunities for prevention, management, and improved care at both the population and clinical level [9] opportunities which are not currently being exploited by all health and social care organisations.

Certainly in Poland, there is a view that the organisation of the health and social care systems are ill-prepared and under-equipped to meet the needs of the growing population of frail older adults. Since 1991, there has been a progressive disintegration of the health and social care systems including division into two separately administered and managed ministries. This division of care has resulted in difficulties in coordinating activities in long term care (LTC: [21]) and reduced collaboration between physicians and social care workers [22]. Further, decentralisation of the previously tax-funded national health service with a social health insurance system in 1999 resulted in a defragmented system, with sixteen regional insurance funds responsible for their own budgets and contractor provision. Although the National Health Fund was established in 2003–04 with overall responsibility for purchasing, responsibility for health is still fragmented with facility ownership, service provision and delivery, and accountability at various regional, county, municipal and national governmental levels [23].

In addition, the profile of social care has changed significantly. It is now delivered by the Ministry of Family, Labour and Social Policy whose responsibilities consist mainly of determining the rights to, and allowances for, caring benefits, rather than solving real social problems [22]. It is well established that poor social support and comorbidities are negatively associated with functional status and mortality, particularly in older patients [24]. Patients who have complex health needs require both medical and social services and support from a wide variety of providers and caregivers, and the patient-centred medical home approach offers promise as a model for providing comprehensive and coordinated care [25].

There is a view that the reintegration of health and social care services for frail older adults would enhance satisfaction, quality of life, efficiency, and health outcomes and would also decrease costs [5]. It is believed that such integrated care delivery would eliminate inefficiency and the duplication of work processes while relieving professionals of their administrative burden in favour of patient-related activities [26]. It is also perceived as the best solution to address health care-related frustrations experienced by patients with chronic conditions [27], to improve their experiences of care [28, 29] and their quality of life [30].

However, there is currently insufficient research to determine whether the current health and social care systems are effective or whether care integration would make a difference to stakeholders in older adult care, in terms of access to services or indeed, the outcomes of those services. Access to health and social care is a complex concept and is dependent on both the provision of adequate services and the absence of financial, organisational, social and cultural barriers to those services [31]. Levesque et al., [32] conceptualise access to health care across five dimensions, along with five corresponding abilities of populations: 1) approachability (ability to perceive); 2) acceptability (ability to seek); 3) availability and accommodation (ability to reach); 4) affordability (ability to pay); and 5) appropriateness (ability to engage).

Previous work with European stakeholders in three countries [12], including Polish nationals, described the need for a new kind of transparent, health and social care system which was integrated and person-centred. This paper also raised awareness of the challenges associated with access to appropriate services in the complex Polish systems and described a need for more accessible care and support for older adults as well as their caregivers.

Therefore, the aim of this study is to explore the issues surrounding access to health and social care services for frail older adults, with Polish stakeholders including frail and robust older adults, health care professionals, social care workers and family caregivers, in order to determine their views and perspectives on the current system and to present stakeholders' suggestions for the future development of more accessible and person-centred health and social care systems.

Method

This study forms part of a wider range of studies known collectively as FOCUS [33, 34]. Qualitative findings from focus groups conducted in three countries: Italy (Milan), Poland (Wroclaw) and the United Kingdom (Birmingham) have previously been reported [12]. This current paper reports a secondary analysis of data from the same study but has the specific purpose of presenting findings relating to access to, and integration of, health and social care from the Polish stakeholders only.

Procedure

Five focus groups were facilitated by two female general practitioners (DK and MBF) with some previous experience of qualitative research. Focus groups were conducted with 44 stakeholders in the care of frail older adults including healthy older adults, frail older adults, health care professionals, social care workers and family caregivers. There were between eight and ten participants in each group. No non-participants were present. Focus groups were conducted in Polish. The sessions lasted between 60 and 90 min. Semi-structured questions, defined in advance through literature review and discussion among partners, were posed (see Table 1), including broadly, experiences and attitudes toward frailty, medical treatment, quality of life and social care. Questions were not pilot tested. The facilitators were known in a professional capacity only to the participants. No personal information was relayed about the researchers to the participants.

Discussions with older adults and caregivers were held in non-medical settings, so that participants could feel more at ease when describing their experiences, expressing their needs and complaints. Sessions were audio-recorded and conversations transcribed verbatim. Transcriptions and preliminary analyses were conducted in Polish.

Recruitment strategy

Older adult participants and their caregivers were recruited purposively from general practice health clinics across the Lower Silesia District. They were invited to take part in the study by their family doctor at their planned practice visit. Older adults were required to be aged 65 years or over and fluent Polish speakers. Healthy older adults had no conditions of frailty or pre-frailty as assessed by a General Practitioner (GP) while frail older adults were assessed as having those conditions. Frailty assessments were undertaken by the general practitioner in the surgery. Frailty was defined as a clinical syndrome in which three or more of the following criteria were present: unintentional weight loss (10lbs in the past year), self-reported exhaustion, weakness (grip strength), slow walking speed, and low physical activity [8]. Caregivers were required to be taking care of a frail older adult on a regular basis, although they did not have to be residing with them. Health professionals were similarly recruited from the general practice health clinics of the Lower Silesia District. They were contacted through professional networks, in person, by telephone and via email. Social workers were all employees of the Regional Social Welfare Centre from Wroclaw. They were

Table 1 Interview schedule

Older adults (frail)	Older adults (healthy)	Health and social care providers	Family caregivers
This project is about frailty. Can you tell me what you think of when you hear that word?			
Do you consider yourself to be frail?		Do you consider the person you are caring for to be frail?	
What does frailty mean to you?			
Taking turns, can you tell me about a typical day?		Taking turns, can you tell me about the patients you care for/work with and how you might consider them frail?	
Does anybody help you with things on a day to day basis (prompts: personal care, shopping, cleaning etc.)?			
Do you receive any formal health or social care services? If so, then what sorts of services are they?		What sorts of services do you offer patients considered to be frail?	Does the person you care for receive any formal health or social care services? If so, then what sorts of services are they?
		Do you provide any support for carers for frail older adults?	Do you receive any support as a carer for a frail older adult?
Do you think there are ways that you could have prevented yourself from becoming frail?	Do you think there's anything you can do to prevent yourself from becoming frail?	Do you think there are ways we could prevent people from becoming frail?	Do you think there are ways that you could have prevented the person you care for becoming frail?
Have you adapted your home so you can move around it more easily?	If it became necessary do you think you would be able to adapt your home so you could move around it more easily if you became frail?		Have you adapted the living space so that the person you care for can move around more easily? Are there other things you would like to do?
Do you think more help with this should be available to you?			Do you think more help with this should be available to you?
Can you think of what led up to you becoming frail?	Do you have any chronic conditions? Do you think there is a time when you might become frail yourself? Do you have friends/relatives you would consider frail?	What do you think are the causes of frailty in the patients you work with?	Can you think of what led up to the person you care for becoming frail?
Can you identify anything you might consider a cause?	What do you think might be the possible causes of frailty?	What would you say are likely causes of frailty?	Can you identify anything you might consider a cause?
Do you need help with personal care? If so, how do you feel about this?	How would you feel if you realised you needed help with personal care?		Do you look after the personal care of the person you care for? If so, did you have experience of this before?
Do you think people providing personal care should receive any guidance or support in how to best do it?		Do you provide support for carers in the provision of personal care? Do you offer any training or guidance on how to do this?	Have you received any training or guidance on how to do it?
Do you feel that your dignity or personal safety is threatened because of your frailty/need for personal care?	Do you think your dignity or personal safety would be threatened if you received help with personal care?	Do you think the dignity or personal safety of frail older adults is threatened?	Do you feel that the dignity or personal safety of the person you care for is threatened because of their frailty?
Do you think anything else could be done to protect your dignity or personal safety?	Do you think anything could be done to protect your dignity or personal safety?	Do you think you could retain a person's dignity more effectively in any way?	Do you think you could retain the person's dignity more effectively with help or support from outside?
		What sorts of treatments are available for frail older adults? Do you expect people to source these themselves or do they require prescription? Do you currently undertake any screening on older adults in standard care?	

Imagine you could assess [your own/a patient's/the person you care for] frailty status via a set of questionnaires on a website. How would you feel about this? Would this be helpful?

Imagine that you could train [your health/a patient's health/the person you care for], in order to reverse frailty or to prevent it via a website. For example, by watching exercise videos on a website that show you how you can train your body to increase your strength. Would this be something

Table 1 Interview schedule *(Continued)*

Older adults (frail)	Older adults (healthy)	Health and social care providers	Family caregivers
you'd be interested in? Where would be the best place to offer these services (prompts: at home, at their local physical therapy centre or somewhere else)?			
What difficulties would you expect if treatments or interventions (such as health or exercise training) for frailty were to be introduced more widely? Do you think that is a good idea? What benefits would that have? What might be the problems with that (prompts: adherence, lack of trust, use of resources, worries about being labelled)?			
Is there anything else you would like to discuss?			

informed about the study by the Director of the Centre and were given time to take part if they wished.

Both health and social care workers were required to have at least two years' experience in their respective fields. Attention was given to balance gender, age, role, and the type of professionals. In total 63 participants were invited and 44 accepted the invitation and took part in the study (response rate 70%). The main reason given for non-participation by all groups was a lack of time.

The final sample size was determined by the research design, a pragmatic outlook and availability of participants. The level of agreement and similarity within and between individual accounts, focus groups and stakeholder groups was very high. We explored individual as well as group perspectives, and the same comments and themes were raised throughout. Six researchers were involved in separately analysing and triangulating translated data. Thus while we cannot conclusively say that saturation was achieved, we are confident that the results are accurate and representative of the various stakeholder groups.

Study duration and schedule
Recruitment started after Ethics approval and took two months. The focus groups were held between October 2015 and January 2016. Separate focus groups for all stakeholders were arranged. The focus groups took place in a non-clinical, seminar room at the University of Wroclaw, except for the meeting with social workers, which took place in a regional welfare centre. Transcriptions were made soon after the last focus group, and were followed by analyses.

Ethical issues
The research was performed in accordance with the Declaration of Helsinki for Human Research of the World Medical Association and was approved by the Bioethics Commission of the Medical University in Wroclaw, Poland; Approval No. KB-502/2015. All participants had the opportunity to review information about the study and gave written informed consent. Information was written in a clear, standardised format. Participants were not reimbursed for their efforts. In order to maintain confidentiality, participants' names and personal information were excluded from the transcripts and all quotations were anonymised.

Data analysis
Interviews were transcribed in Polish by an IT specialist of Wroclaw Medical University, Poland and a GP (DK). Preliminary themes were noted which related to the accessibility of health and social care services. The data were synthesised using framework analysis [35]. This was performed by a psychologist with experience in both qualitative analysis and frailty (HG), a GP (DK) and a nurse (KS). Framework analysis is a five stage process which involves: familiarisation with the data; identifying a thematic framework; indexing responses; reviewing and revising the framework; and mapping and interpretation of themes. Following initial familiarisation with the data, Levesque, Harris, & Russell's [32] theoretical framework was identified as most appropriate to make sense of the data. Data (including relevant participant quotations) were categorised and indexed into an Excel spreadsheet according to five dimensions of accessibility to care: approachability; acceptability; availability and accommodation; affordability; and appropriateness [32]. The framework was reviewed and revised, understanding of the quotations and translations was checked and the framework reordered as necessary. The authors then developed the explanatory account (narrative) for this paper from the revised framework. The Critical Appraisal Skills Programme (CASP: 2017) Qualitative Research Checklist was used to guide the conduct of the methods and to structure the presentation of findings.

Results
The study involved 44 participants: frail patients (FP = 9), non-frail patients (NFP = 11), patients' caregivers (PC = 6), health care professionals (HP = 9 including 6 general practitioners and 3 district nurses) and social care workers (SW = 9).

Five dimensions of accessibility to services are described: *approachability, acceptability, availability and accommodation, affordability,* and *appropriateness* [32]. Each theme is presented with example translated quotations. Quotations are attributed by participant group and participant number.

Approachability

The dimension of approachability relates to the fact that people facing health needs can identify that some form of services exist, can be reached, and have an impact on their health. The corresponding ability required from the population is the ability to perceive that such a service exists.

Participants' perceptions were of an opaque system that was complex and difficult to navigate. Both older adults and caregivers described the effort required to find their way around services and gain advice. They suggested that services should make themselves known and be more transparent, which would contribute to the service becoming more approachable. In particular, there was a strong need for the provision of more detailed information regarding available treatments and services, as well as psychological assistance, specifically for caregivers. During the discussion, one of the participants identified that she was not aware of a particular service, suggesting that this service was not visible, and therefore not approachable.

"I, for example, had no idea that such person existed at all, as you said, a social worker [...] Probably we don't know that such a person exists and that person has no idea of our existence." [NFP11]

Although this person was a non-frail older adult, this lack of knowledge about services was concerning and might have prevented this individual from benefiting from this service in the future. Other caregivers also described the difficulties they faced in navigating the dual health and social care systems and in determining whether the service they required existed. In effect, they described a feeling of 'not knowing what they didn't know', that is, they were unable to determine where the gaps were in their knowledge of the range of health and social care services provided and the type of support they could expect from professionals. This in turn made it difficult to determine how best to fulfill the care needs of older adults.

"all these voluntary services and so on. But we have to know about it all." [PC5]

"It shouldn't be this way that I'm supposed to search, make phone calls and ask for training or something else, we should simply obtain this information." [PC5]

One of the proposed solutions to this lack of transparency was the adoption of a care coordinator as a new position in the health care system. People spoke of the need to create a *"liaison"* [HP6] between the health and social care systems and to be a conduit for information between services and patients.

"this liaison, it should be someone who has knowledge about what kind of people she or he has in her or his area because these ladies from social care are ladies who work in this way that they come, do the shopping, if washing is needed the wash, they cook and they go. [...] Whereas, they don't do an interview, they make no reconnaissance in this area, whether something else is needed when it seems they should do that." [HP1]

For this individual, the coordinator should have a broader responsibility to the older adult than the social carers, they should be perceptive to new needs or requirements and act as a facilitator for, and advocate of care. Other participants also hoped that the coordinator would be able to guide them through the complexities of the legal system, as well as the medical system.

"Yes, it should be exactly as you're saying, a medical coordinator and a legal coordinator. It's because there are some legal matters that need to be taken care of." [PC6]

In summary, this theme suggests that there are challenges associated with the approachability of services in Poland. Stakeholders described issues relating to knowledge of the existence of services and the difficulties they perceive in accessing those services.

Acceptability

This dimension relates to the cultural and social factors affecting services. It examines whether people in a particular population (e.g. age, gender or social group) will accept the service and whether they judge it appropriate. The corresponding ability of the population to seek health or social care also relates to the concept of personal autonomy and the capacity to choose to seek care. Clearly in the case of frail patients, some will have the capacity to seek care while others may require an advocate, perhaps a family member, or a professional social care worker.

Stakeholders raised the idea of the need for psychological care, primarily for caregivers. Culturally, there appeared to be an acceptance of the need for psychological support, notably during caring episodes and also following bereavement. People spoke openly about their need for mental health support. Those who had experienced psychological services, described them as beneficial. One family caregiver described the inability to cope with her emotions, and the adjustment in her lifestyle after taking on the responsibility for caring for her mother:

"Well, sometimes I made serious mistakes in the beginning, I couldn't reconcile myself to it, I reacted, a bit, you know what I mean, emotionally, aggressively

[...] it is [caring for parent] a very big burden for me [...] and I'm already looking for some help for myself... yesterday, I went to a psychologist to talk because I simply can't cope with it." [PC2]

This extract describes the sense of anguish and anger the caregiver felt during the transition period from independent adult to caregiver, and their struggle to create a new sense of self, and to identity as a carer. However, it also demonstrates an adaptive coping strategy in that the participant identified their inability to cope and had the capacity to take positive steps to find help, and found that help acceptable.

Other caregivers also raised the idea of psychological support, specifically following bereavement. One carer, who had taken care of her mother for a long time spoke about her difficulties.

"I want to say that later when you have nobody to care for, the first month you don't even know you're alive or not [...] I am still not completely ok." [PC5]

Although the carer was grieving for her mother, there is an implication here that she is also grieving for her identity as a carer, in that she has lost her sense of purpose, or sense of self. Together, these two extracts address the need for psychological support, suggesting that stakeholders in older adult care and frailty find these types of services both acceptable and appropriate.

In terms of the acceptability of specific health care services, participants focused on their need for specialist health care, in particular, rehabilitation services. Rehabilitation services are a very important element of frailty syndrome prevention and therapy. The demand for such services is high and the participants were aware of the positive and real impact of these services on health, including improving physical fitness and independence. One caregiver who paid privately for a physiotherapist for her mother emphasised the effects of treatment:

"This physiotherapy really came in handy, it was fantastic, it's really hard to believe it. She [the physiotherapist] started to come twice a week, train, do a little massaging and mum is a lot fitter and she even started to exercise with me willingly because when I wanted to exercise with her she didn't believe me and didn't want to." [PC2]

As well as demonstrating a change in physical health, the above extract alludes to a change in beliefs about the acceptability of exercise as well as a change in self-efficacy through the willingness to take ownership of one's health and to take part in additional physical activity.

Other social factors may also affect the capacity of people to choose to access services. Waiting times will be described in the next dimension of access to services - *availability and accommodation*, but long waiting times may place increased social burdens on patients and caregivers. The inconvenience and exasperation of waiting in line for a year for a scheduled doctor's visit while struggling daily with the burdensome symptoms of coexisting chronic illnesses may contribute to loss of wellbeing and quality of life, as well as depleted mood and even the occurrence of depressive symptoms, in both frail older adults and caregivers. Further, the reduced economic status of many Polish older adults and their inability to allocate resources for private treatment may also increase symptoms of frustration and depression.

Availability and accommodation

This dimension examines the ability to reach services, i.e., whether health services are available and can be reached physically and in a timely manner. Despite a common belief amongst participants in the power of physiotherapy and rehabilitation services, according to frail participants, the availability of those services, is difficult.

"I think that rehabilitation would be a great help. Only that receiving rehabilitation is close to being a miracle." [FP3]

"I would like to go to a [rehabilitation] meeting. I would go, because my legs hurt, and maybe I could lose weight, because that's also a problem." [FP7]

Similarly, other services which were perceived as valuable and necessary by stakeholders in terms of effects on their health were also difficult or impossible to access, specifically psychological support and periodic respite care. There was a strong belief that psychological support was 'very important' [HP6] for both older adults and caregivers but an understanding that these services were in very short supply, a view which was confirmed by a health care professional:

"I won't even mention psychological assistance, which, of course, is very important, but in Poland it is practically non-existent." [HP6]

The difficulty of availability here is that there is a limited provision of this specific service - psychological support - which outstrips supply.

Caregivers also indicated a desire for free periodic respite care, specifically to have time for themselves, either to have a chance to relax or devote it to solving other important matters, for instance, their self-care and personal health issues.

> *"Would it be possible to implement a programme so that you could leave such a person but I think you need to pay for that, I don't know if for a week ... So, you could leave that person for weekly rehabilitation and so that the person who cares for her or him could simply have a rest?" [PC6]*

However, one of the greatest difficulties expressed by participants relating to availability of health care services was the waiting time for a doctor's appointment or scheduled surgery. Participants described how the normal waiting time for an appointment with a specialist is a few months, while it may take several years for scheduled surgery.

> *"The Doctor refers me to a specialist. And the man tells me, someone tells me – please come back in 8 months." [NFP 2]*

> *"Today, I talked to my friend, younger than me, I was giving her my best wishes. I asked her how she was feeling because I knew she had had a problem with her hip for a long time. She tells me, I'm OK, you know. I told her I thought she had already been operated on. No, her appointment is in 2020." [NFP7]*

Although participants were pragmatic when describing these long waiting times, there was also an element of frustration associated with the accessibility of specialist medical care, and a view that long waiting times were themselves a contributory factor in ill-health, a view which was described by a participant waiting to see a cardiologist.

> *"I think that [...] one of the principal causes of this frailty of ours is the present day doctor's, medical care. I mean [...] for example registering the patients for the next year." [FP8]*

Certainly, the length of waiting times had an effect on quality of life and independence and was problematic in a number of cases.

> *"I had been making efforts to arrange rehabilitation [for my wife] and when after waiting for a long time the rehabilitation took place my wife was no longer independent." [FP4]*

In this extract, the participant describes an inexorable shift in health and dependency before the rehabilitation treatment could take place. The time lag between the

intervention being suggested and delivered meant that the older adult had transitioned outside the boundaries of that specific intervention treatment window. Preventative medicine in older adults encompasses a range of interventions and some may indeed prevent an individual from tipping over into a more intensive (and consequently expensive) level of treatment or care plan. Unfortunately, the difficulties associated with waiting times were not just limited to health care services. Legal issues were also affected as described by this participant.

> *"The doctor who was supposed to care for my mum said I should arrange my mum's incapacitation.[legal arrangement to appoint a guardian to make decisions on your behalf,] So, we will keep her here for 3 days and you arrange that. It finally took half a year to arrange and then my mum passed away." [PC5]*

In this instance, the participant described how suitable legal provision could not be made for her mother before her death. This participant raised concerns about obtaining the appropriate legal services and the cost implications of those services. They described how difficulties in communication and managing legal matters delayed care. There were other examples of communication issues between departments delaying care. One social worker described how the dissolution of the health and social care system into two separate ministries and the restructuring of care, had resulted in additional bureaucracy and a lack of communication which delayed the onset of social care.

> *"In serious situations when there was a caregiving services division some years ago before it was liquidated, [...] you would find yourself in a situation that for example there was a lady discharged from the hospital, cancer, [...] and I came for the interview and I called them, send me a caregiver because there is this case and she is needed immediately. And they would send her. The decision has not been made yet." [SW1]*

Sadly, there are human and moral costs here, in terms of the quality of life for older adults, as well as issues of availability.

Another issue related to availability and accommodation is the physical availability of clinics and staff. Given staff shortages, health and social care professionals are often located a distance away from their patients.

> *"Whereas these ladies [...] who are supposed to coordinate, they generally sit in the office and it is a great problem to get them to come to a community interview because they don't have money for the lump sum, for gas. And the area is vast, the municipality is very big, so you need drive a lot." [HP8]*

In this instance, we note that dimensions of accessibility to health care are not completely independent constructs. Here, the geographical range of the clinic, shortage of qualified staff and the costs involved for staff to travel long distances, affects the availability of the service.

The theme of availability and accommodation also relates to the characteristics of providers, for example in terms of their qualifications. Some participants spoke about their lack of satisfaction with the availability of doctors, and difficulties in maintaining continuity of care.

"Here the problem is the turnover of the doctors. Since one doctor starts the treatment, grasps everything that is needed, then a year later she/he is gone." [NFP2]

Conversely, when continuity of care was present, it was recognised and greatly appreciated by the patients and caregivers.

The availability and qualifications of social care workers were of particular interest to the stakeholders. The social care system is struggling with the volume of older adults needing assistance and few people are interested in working in this sector. Consequently, care workers are scarce.

"In [the Old Town] we currently have 4 girls who deal with care services and they have 70 persons each. This is a huge number. There are too few caregivers. In [name of city] when I was preparing this map of resources and needs, the thing is that in 2017 in [the Old Town] 25% of the society will be in post-production age.[1]" [SW8]

Critically, the social care professional describes the scale of the problem in a sector of one city and the lack of availability of staff, as well as highlighting an ongoing and escalating crisis in the future. Concerns were also raised about the way in which care workers were recruited to the profession and trained. A professional caregiver should be properly trained and prepared for work with older adults and they should receive appropriate remuneration for it. Currently, this is not the case; participants reported that caregivers are selected and recruited almost randomly and have minimal training.

"They are often unemployed people who we being the social workers send to the Social Welfare Centre: please try to get hired there. They can be completely unprepared for this." [SW8]

"They [the social care workers] are hired through a 'roundup' because there are no caregivers, the caregivers don't want to work." [SW1]

These extracts describe a social care system which has serious issues related to training and competence for care workers and safeguarding for older adults. Participants had a number of sensible suggestions to improve conditions for carers and their patients, including proper training and adopting other good practices.

"I think we should start by educating the workers who are to deal with these problems and care of the elderly and communities." [HP1]

"The UK system, [...] their social care is very much specialised. Here we don't have that at all [...]. There you have social workers for mentally ill patients, there are social workers for patients with cancer. There, if you have some kind of problem with a patient, you call specialist services." [HP8]

Participants described how applying financial incentives, ensuring an employment contract (as compared to the current fee-for-task agreement) and appropriate training (and where appropriate specialist training) of the social care professional, could improve the situation for future cohorts of older adults.

Affordability
This theme relates to the economic capacity of people to spend their time and resources to use health and social care services. Older adults, both frail and robust, relayed their frustration with the inequalities inherent in the current system of health care and their awareness of financial barriers to health, in the first instance relating to access to specialist examinations and doctor's appointments.

"When I am depressed or something else is wrong, I need a referral to a specialist and what? If you don't have a hundred [100 zlotys] you sit [and wait] half a year [for an appointment with a specialist]." [NFP2]

"If it hadn't taken paying 500 zlotys, we would have waited for a year [for an MRI scan after a stroke]. And in this way it is possible in a week's time. Then this is where the problem is." [NFP2]

As illustrated by these quotations, timely access to specialists is perceived as only being available for people with sufficient financial resources. In the latter quotation, the participant described the alternatives of having to wait a significant length of time for a necessary scan after a serious, life threatening medical condition or paying privately to have the scan done immediately. So, it would seem there is capacity within the system to provide resources, they are available, but they are just not accessible to all. This suggests a system of health in-equality. We know that ill health is related to poverty and this is particularly significant here. Given that many frail older adults are in receipt of fixed incomes through pensions and other benefits, these resources may not be sufficient to fund all their health or social care, which suggests that needs or conditions may not be treated at the optimal time, or worse, may be going untreated or unmanaged. Certainly, this was a viewpoint suggested by one of the frail participants in the study.

"if it's a private visit then you have to pay and not all of us can afford that, for example me, I can't afford it." [FP8]

And social workers echoed this viewpoint and con-firmed the inequalities endemic in the system:

"There are no [free] health care centres in [town name]. We have the [name of centre] who charge 100 zlotys a day and another at [name of street] who charge 4,500 zlotys a month. And we have people who get 600 zlotys of their monthly pension. Where should they get the money from? I call the doctor, the head [of one health care institution] and he doesn't ask me about the patient's state, but how much money she/he has. There is no cooperation whatsoever! Because it is all about the money." [SW1]

In this extract, the social worker described a discon-nectedness between the priorities of the stakeholders in-volved in the care of the older adult. On one hand, the social worker is attempting to obtain the most suitable care for their patient, while on the other, the professional in charge of the clinic, ironically a doctor, is 'blocking' treatment and prioritising resources and finances over the individual's health. The extract demonstrates the challenges faced by both professionals in their daily work but also describes an arrangement whereby the social worker is acting as an advocate on behalf of the finan-cially disempowered and potentially vulnerable older adult. A further example of a disconnect between doctor and patient and the social carer as advocate is also evi-dent in the way that this social care worker describes the way in which doctors prescribe medications.

"The doctors are very often unaware of the way in which these patients live. What is their financial situation? There are some medications that are exorbitantly expensive. It is us who tell these patients: please ask the pharmacist, maybe there is a cheaper alternative. These people don't use the medications because they just can't afford them. They come to us and ask for financial assistance. Therefore,

cooperation with the physicians, when it comes to the elderly, is for me the most important thing." [SW8]

This participant details a lack of understanding and awareness on behalf of the doctor of the patients' indi-vidual circumstances and the affordability of prescribed medications. Critically, they describe how financial bar-riers result in cost-related non-adherence to the treat-ment plan which has the potential to affect important health outcomes. Here, this social worker is also advo-cating a closer and more integrated working relationship between the health and social care professionals such that the whole person context is taken into account when developing a treatment regime.

The social carers also drew attention to difficulties and economic barriers in relation to accessing long-term in-patient care.

"There are vacant commercial places, but they cost 4 thousand [zlotys]. Whereas, you need to wait half a year for a subsidy from the National Health Fund." [SW6]

"Half a year up to one year." [SW1]

"Half a year? A year or one and a half years." [SW3]

The key issue here is a shortage of suitable accommo-dation and a lack of institutions that can provide a 'round-the-clock' service for older adults. With limited supply and increasing demand, inevitably the costs asso-ciated with private nursing homes are very high and this is exacerbated by long waiting times for subsidies from the National Health Fund.

One of the key issues within this theme of affordability was that families of frail older adults were willing and prepared to support their loved ones. However, they are not themselves supported to do this through financial means such as a carer's allowance.

"For centuries we have been brought up in a traditional, multi-generation family that took care of the elderly. [...] let's pay, we have these benefits for the caregivers, let's pay for it in some way. Maybe I will be able to choose whether it pays for me to continue working or care for my parents. I will choose one or the other." [SW3]

This participant describes how providing benefits and assuring financial support for family members with caring responsibilities, would provide them with a range of options concerning the most appropriate care for their loved ones; with such support, it would be viable to stay at home and care for their loved ones, rather than relying on social care.

Appropriateness

This dimension relates to the fit between services and the clients' needs. One concern of participants was that the current health care system is 'firefighting', i.e., focusing only on the provision of emergency treatments in urgent cases.

"We only focus on solving emergency problems [...] those patients who require some afterthought and a more integrated care simply slip by. Because there is no chance, there is even no time. Physically there is no time to devote at least some of your attention to them during work. And I also think it is because of the scarcity of funds." [HP8]

Here the health care provider explains how a lack of resourcing means that people with complex health care needs may be ignored in order to concentrate efforts on the most acute cases. This focus on emergency or ad hoc health care was echoed by other participants.

Conversely, participants described how the social care system did not function well in a crisis. Stakeholders described how many older adults are simply allocated a caregiver by default, whoever is available at the time, and described how these personnel are often poorly trained and low paid. Social workers also mentioned that they have no direct influence on matching older adults with their caregiver. Similarly, social workers are unable to change an older adult's caregiver if a relationship breaks down, and are unable to call them off where needs change.

"When we, as social workers, go to implement these services then we no longer have any influence on the choice of the caregivers [...] It is because the entity which realises the services is already another institution." [SW4]

This social worker describes how the allocation of resources from various different bodies and institutions adds layers of unnecessary bureaucracy to the social care system and means that social workers are unable to communicate effectively with caregivers to ensure that the needs of the older adult are properly met. Critically, the social worker participants hoped for a streamlined social care system with a reduced level of bureaucracy. They pointed out that their willingness to assist people is often hampered by complicated and time-consuming bureaucratic procedures.

"Going to see the client and carrying out the community interview is only one tenth of the work. The interview is 16 pages long." [SW5]

"The impression was that someone wanted voluntary services, someone wanted them fast. Two years. I did that in [city district] literally, me and a friend had been thinking for one and a half years how to do that. How to go through personal data protection, the paperwork and all [...] we want to answer people, citizens' needs promptly. It isn't easy, we say that straight away." [SW5]

In these extracts, participants describe how bureaucratic and administrative processes affect the quality and timeliness of care for older adults. However, there was a willingness among participants to improve services and to assist people, and they described working within the regime to try to speed things up. Some participants expressed a desire to return to the caregiving services division, which had existed previously and which participants felt worked well in an emergency situation.

Participants described the need to introduce legislation to enable social workers and caregivers to care for older adults 'around-the-clock' (24 h a day, 7 days a week).

"There is 10% of such people who would require care in the night hours [...] The Act provides for a maximum of 8 hours [...] This is ad hoc care and not 24/7 care." [SW1]

"In fact they [social care workers] work from 8 a.m. to 4 p.m." [SW4]

This statement suggests that current legislation protects employees and workers over vulnerable adults and implies that some vulnerable, dependent older adults are unable to access care for around 16 h per day when residing in their own home. This is a situation which has serious ethical implications and may mean that older adults are placed in nursing homes, which may not be the most appropriate residence for them, and which may be more costly.

The essence of the current functioning of care for frail older adults in Poland could be summarised by the statement of one of the participants.

"There is a seed of a system, there are some nurses, there are some caregivers, but this [system] is still not working, or is unable to work." [NFP5]

In light of the shortcomings of both health and social care systems and the difficulties older adult patients face in satisfying their health and social needs, participants suggested a need for a new type of system, an integrated care system with comprehensive staff training and a multidisciplinary team.

"I think we should start by educating the workers who are dealing with these problems and care of the elderly and communities. And then we could try to create, for example, multidisciplinary groups, medical and social, and I would ask here for a person such as maybe a psychological aid. It would be a cool team, a social and therapeutic team and maybe then we would be able to do something." [HP1]

Participants also expressed an expectation that major legal and organisational changes would be required from the national institutions to manage a welfare state in the face of an ageing population. They recommended the restructuring of the currently disparate health and social care systems, as well as a move towards more comprehensive preventative medicine including more frequent home visits and preventative screening by health practitioners including family doctors and nurses.

Participants asked questions about public finance and resource management, suggesting that these should be reviewed to increase the effectiveness and efficiency of the public sector in order to guarantee appropriate medical and social care to older adults.

"First of all, on our part, withdrawal from the so-called 'radar medicine', which means focusing on ad hoc problem solving in favour of comprehensive care of the patient [..] Second, total reformulation of the social care system, a really deep reformulation." [HP8]

In terms of both health and social care, participants felt that the new system must ensure continuity of care, by more 'permanent' physicians and nurses, as well as caregivers. The aim of this was to ensure that older adults felt secure with their health care provider or caregiver and were able to build a truly cooperative relationship. Within this idea of positive, trusting relationships, people spoke about the importance of assistance from neighbours and the need to formalise some of these necessary but informal caring relationships.

"Within the caregiving services someone from close-by, a neighbour exercised care over a given person and she or he would be paid for that. And it would be great." [SW3]

"That is because that person was close by [SW4]. You didn't even have to look for her or him, she or he was there and could even come along at night." [SW1]

Social workers in these extracts described their suggestions of how neighbourhood carers might be paid for their assistance to older adults, and how well the relationships might work. They noted that there is an element of trust, as the person is local and sometimes known to the older adult, and also how that given that they are located nearby, they could help when required throughout the day, rather than just at set times.

Discussion

Due to their complex and continuously changing health and social care needs, frail older adults require access to a wide range of services over a long period of time [36]. However, in this research participants clearly described the difficulties they had encountered when accessing health and social care. These difficulties included a lack of knowledge regarding the existence of some services, under-supply of services, long waiting times for specialist care and rehabilitation services, geographically remote clinics, staff shortages, a lack of trained and competent social care professionals, high staff turnover, shortages of long-term inpatient care, economic barriers to care and inequity in care standards. In terms of the appropriateness of the current system, participants described issues related to a high functioning emergency health care system which was unsuitable for patients with complex needs and a low functioning emergency social care system, where the bureaucratisation of systems caused serious delays in providing services to the vulnerable. Fundamentally, there were also legislative issues which meant that the most vulnerable older adults were unable to be cared for around-the-clock. In essence, stakeholders conveyed that the Polish system is designed for healthy adults with acute illnesses, not for an ageing population with complex health and social care needs. Certainly, this can be confirmed to some extent by statistical data. In Poland there is a shortage of geriatric medical care (encompassing medical professionals as well as specialist geriatric wards and clinics) for older adults [6]. Moreover the ratio of dependent inpatient care services per 1000 head of capita is one of the lowest in the European Union (25.0 workers in Poland vs. 46.7 in the UE-27 states in 2014) [21].

There were a number of issues relating to availability and accommodation of access to health and social care. Participants in this research placed particular emphasis on staff shortages in both the health care and social care sectors and the scarcity of financial means allocated for care. The high workload of physicians means that resources are directed in an ad hoc manner at urgent and emergency cases. Further, there is a high turnover of family medicine specialists which means that continuity of care is disrupted. In turn, social care workers are under increasing pressure with rising numbers of patients, payment on a fee-for-task agreement (i.e. output work) and low remuneration. All of which contributes to a shortfall in the number of candidates wishing to take on this type of work. Some suggested solutions to these difficulties include introducing appropriate financial incentives for family doctors or 'pay-for-performance' schemes linked to the achievement of specific clinical and organisational targets, similar to the UK model. While these systems may induce this group of professionals to take over the role of the "gatekeeper" and as a consequence prevent offloading the costs to higher levels of care [37], they have also been linked to an increased administrative burden and bureaucracy [38] which the stakeholders in this study were keen to reduce and avoid. We suggest that promotion of social care as a positive career choice with appropriate remuneration, alongside employment contracts and appropriate training would go a long way to solve many of the problems but the mindset of both policy makers and private care providers, as well as potential career carers, would need to change. This would ensure that the quality, competence and professionalism of social care staff would improve, the potential pool of social care candidates would increase, and continuity of care would benefit.

Another critical access issue was the availability of long-term care (LTC) and challenges associated with accessing it. From a public health perspective, a solution to LTC requirements is critical. As yet, Poland has not established comprehensive national LTC programmes, relying on informal caregivers combined with a fragmented mix of formal services that vary in quality and by location [39]. Responsibility for LTC in Poland is divided among the central government, governmental health agency, governmental labour and social agency, and territorial self-government [40]. The decentralisation of the government and public administration has led to a lack of ownership in the development of a strategic LTC plan. Currently, responsibility for organising LTC resides with local governments, while the material responsibility for the form and contents of care and its financing belong to the health care sector, with the consequence of difficulties in action coordination [21]. In addition, the integration of LTC services also face problems from the integration of institutions that operate on the margins of the health care system with institutions that operate within the social assistance scheme, and in the integration of residential care and home care [40]. We suggest that the integration of the health and social care systems could result in better cooperation between the professionals of both sectors. The first stage of integration might consist of multidisciplinary team meetings to share information about the patients' health and social situation and to develop suitable care plans. The introduction of integrated IT systems would also assist in ensuring that all members of the therapeutic team have insight into the treatment history and care of the patient. These are not inconceivable goals, other countries, for example the United Kingdom have implemented similar systems as components of care in an attempt to improve patient outcomes and reduce delays.

In terms of an appropriate system, the need for a coordinated and continued medical and social care system was paramount, and was tangibly expressed by all participants in this study. Some of the proposed solutions to ensuring satisfactory medical and social care for all older adults included the 'new management' of public funds, ensuring around-the-clock care for older adults from a community nurse, reducing the level of bureaucracy in the social care system, formalising assistance from neighbours, ensuring financial assistance to family caregivers and greater cooperation between health and social care staff.

Financial support to informal caregivers was a particular concern to participants. In light of an increasing number of older adults in society, a greater number of caregivers will be required, and therefore it makes sense to develop appropriate 'future-proof' legal and financial mechanisms that will enable caregivers to reconcile professional roles with caring responsibilities. At present, in order to receive a caring allowance, a caregiver must not be in employment [22] but the Polish pension system is such that caring responsibilities are not recognised as reckonable service and thus, informal caregivers are effectively penalised for giving up work to care for loved ones. Further, there is no assistance in helping people re-enter the labour market when their caring duties are over.

Another critical issue for caregivers was the physical and mental toll caring takes on them. In the present study, informal caregivers expressed a need for much greater psychological and informational support as much as periodic relief from performing difficult caring responsibilities. Here there was a suggestion that services were difficult to approach, participants either did not know that they existed, or did not know how to easily navigate them. However, in terms of acceptability, there was an acceptance of the value of such services from participants. The value of psychological services is also borne out in the literature, both for caregivers and older adults. A systematic review [41] described the three main types of support needed by caregivers: respite, psychosocial support and information, and communication technology support. The authors concluded that an integrated support package tailored to the individual caregivers' physical, psychological, and social needs should be preferred when supporting informal caregivers of frail older adults. Further, evidence from eleven randomised controlled trials suggests that supportive interventions may help reduce caregivers' psychological distress [42]. These authors suggested that practitioners should enquire about the concerns of caregivers and should consider that they may benefit from additional support.

In another study [43], caregivers' depression, stress, or burnout increased the risk of institutionalisation for the older adult. While cost-effective caregiver support policies can reduce the demand for expensive institutional care [44]. Thus, we suggest that any health and social care reforms should ensure that caregivers are given appropriate support, both for their own health but also as a potential method of cost saving. Certainly, the cost effectiveness of caregiver support versus ongoing institutionalisation would be worth exploring in future research.

One role which might assist with the approachability and the appropriateness of services was that of the care coordinator. Although the role of a care coordinator was largely dismissed by European health care policymakers as unnecessary [45], the members of all the stakeholder groups in this study indicated the need for a care coordinator as a new, and desirable institution in the Polish care system. The coordinator would be a trusted mediator between the physician and patient and exercise the role of a "liaison" between the health care and social care systems. The envisaged role of the care coordinator would be to assess gaps in health care and to develop a personalised care plan to address the care needs of the participant. Care coordinators might also confer and collaborate with medical providers, review the use and appropriateness of, and adherence with, prescribed medications, accompany individuals to their medical appointments if needed, provide patient and family education, and assist with referral to community resources as appropriate [46]. Certainly, studies have shown that case management is beneficial. For example, in the United States, authors [46] demonstrated that case coordination and subsequent discharge planning reduced hospital admissions in high risk older adults on Medicare (over 70% of whom were aged 75 years and over) and $7.7 million in cost savings, as well as improving the uptake of laboratory tests and surgery visits. Conversely, other authors [47], suggested that the Walcheren Integrated Care Model, which involves care coordination, was not cost-effective, and moreover, the costs per quality-adjusted life year (QALY) were high (an average of 412,450 euros per additional QALY).

Similarly, in another study [48], a 1-year intervention ($n = 150$ frail patients) was carried out by nurses and physiotherapists working as case managers, who undertook home visits at least once a month. Authors showed that there were no significant differences between the intervention group and control group for total cost or two measures of quality-adjusted life years. The results can be explained by the fact that the intervention group had significantly lower levels of informal care and help with instrumental activities of daily living (IADL) both as costs (Euro 3927 vs. Euro 6550, $p = 0.037$) and

provided hours (200 vs. 333 h per year, p = 0.037). However, other studies have demonstrated that care planning and coordination by a case manager resulted in improvements in older persons' subjective well-being. [49] Further, that older people receiving a comprehensive continuum of care intervention, including a care coordinator, perceived statistically significantly higher quality of care on items about care planning compared with those receiving the usual care and had increased their knowledge of whom to contact about care/services, after three and 12 months [50]. Certainly, given the strong desire of the stakeholders to adopt this model of assistance with health and social care, it may be worthwhile exploring in other Polish populations in future research.

Lastly, the affordability of services was a significant issue for participants. Although there is the premise in Poland that health care is free to the most vulnerable in society, in practice, many services are oversubscribed and have long waiting times and so to resolve issues more swiftly, private health care is common. However, in effect this is creating a two-tier system in that health care is only available to those who can afford it. Such a system has human, moral and ethical implications. In order to improve this system, there should be a renewed focus on the integration of health and social care services, investment in preventative measures in primary care, and a change of focus from outmoded bureaucracy to person-centred care which is responsive to the changing needs of the Polish community.

Strengths/limitations

The heterogeneous sample with five groups of stakeholders enabled a comprehensive, multidisciplinary assessment of the accessibility of the health and social care systems in Poland and a broader look at the changes required by stakeholders in the future. Stakeholders demonstrated a significant level of agreement about the key access issues for frail older adults including timely, accessible and affordable care for all; continuity of care; and significant improvements in social care staff recruitment and training. Although this article only concerns access to health and social care in Poland, the results may also be useful in countries with similarly functioning systems, for example decentralised health and social care systems with low health care capacity.

Conclusion

There can be little doubt that a rapidly ageing population generates complex access requirements for health and social care at both the individual and community level. Such changes in age distribution accompany a significant increase in the prevalence of chronic diseases, frailty, and disability, involving greater expenditure of resources and higher utilisation of community services.

Table 2 Recommendations to Improve Access to Health and Social Care Systems in Poland[a]

Access Issue	Recommendations
Approachability	Services should be transparent about what they offer, when and to whom. Where services are not transparent or easily navigated, a care coordinator (liaison or advocate) should be available to help caregivers and older adults to access health and social care services.
Acceptability	Psychological support should be available for caregivers, both during the caregiving activities and after bereavement. Rehabilitation services are in short supply but may result in changed attitudes towards exercise and ownership of individual's health where provided.
Availability and accommodation	Timeliness is critical when developing interventions for older adults. There needs to be a reduction in waiting times for specific treatments for older or frail adults, in order to prevent the need for potentially more intensive (and consequently expensive) treatments or care plans. Bureaucracy should be reduced and administrative systems streamlined to prevent communication failures and significant delays in medical treatment or provision of social care for frail older adults The availability of low or no cost respite care should be investigated. There should be appropriate training and remuneration for professional caregivers.
Affordability	Doctors should recognise the reduced financial situation of some older adults and consider how that situation might affect adherence to (paid for) medical treatment. There is a willingness among some participants to care for older relatives at home with limited financial support. The cost effectiveness of financially supported home care versus existing alternatives should be explored.
Appropriateness	The current health care system provides high functioning emergency provision, which is unsuitable for patients with complex needs. A new model of care should be evaluated which moves away from acute crisis management in older adults and considers a more integrated and holistic health pathway. The current social care system is low functioning in an emergency situation and bureaucratisation causes serious delays in providing services to the vulnerable. There should be a change in legislation in order to provide effective social care for older adults outside normal office hours.

[a]Based on Levesque, Harris, & Russell's [32] theoretical framework of access to health care

This results in an urgent need to build effective care systems for older adults as well as support networks for their families. Based on our findings, we make recommendations (see Table 2) to act as pragmatic guidance for the reader interested in improving their health and social care system. To summarise, for frailty care to be properly accessible to older adults in Poland, health and social care services need to be integrated in order to reduce bureaucracy and increase the timeliness of treatment and care. Further, the recruitment strategy and training of social care professionals should be reviewed to build capacity and competence within the profession.

Endnotes

[1]Post-production age in Poland is over 65 years for men and over 60 years for women.

Abbreviations
CASP: Critical Appraisal Skills Programme; EU: European Union; FP: Frail patients; GP: General Practitioner; HP: Health care professionals; IADL: Instrumental activities of daily living; LTC: Long term care; NFP: Non-frail patients; PC: Patients' caregivers; QALYS: Quality-adjusted life years; SW: Social care workers

Acknowledgements
We acknowledge the contribution of other members of the FOCUS project: A. Cano (University of Valencia), A. Nobili (IRCCS Istituto di Ricerche Farmacologiche Mario Negri IRCCS, Italy), A.González Segura (EVERIS Spain S.L.U, Spain), A. M. Martinez-Arroyo (ESAM Tecnología S.L., Spain), E. Bobrowicz-Campos (Nursing School of Coimbra, Portugal), F. Germini (IRCCS Ca'Granda Maggiore Policlinico Hospital Foundation, Milan, Italy), J. Apostolo (Nursing School of Coimbra, Portugal), L. van Velsen (Roessingh Research and Development, Netherlands), M. Marcucci (McMaster University, formerly IRCCS Ca'Granda Maggiore Policlinico Hospital Foundation, Milan, Italy) and S. Santana (University of Aveiro, Portugal) who were co-responsible for the design and delivery of the FOCUS project.

Funding
This work was supported by the Consumers, Health, Agriculture and Food Executive Agency (CHAFEA) of the European Commission, under the European Union Health Programme (2014-2020). The survey forms part of a larger study, 'Frailty Management Optimisation through FIP-AHA Commitments and Utilisation of Stakeholders Input' [Grant number 664367 FOCUS]. Funding was also received from the Ministry of Science and Higher Education in Poland (funding in years 2015-2018 allocated for the international co-financed project). The Sponsors were not involved in the study design, in the collection, analysis and interpretation of data, in the writing of the report and in the decision to submit the article for publication.

Authors' contributions
CH conceptualised this study. All authors participated in questionnaire design (see Table 1). Participants were recruited by DK and MBF. DK and MBF interviewed participants, and transcribed and/or translated interviews. Analysis and interpretation of the data were conducted by HG, DK and KS with input from RS, CH and BDA. KS prepared the original manuscript. HG revised the manuscript using a framework analysis approach, with all authors contributing to later drafts or critical revision of important intellectual content. DK and MBF managed the local study while CH managed the European study. All authors have approved this version to be published.

Competing interests
The authors declare that they have no competing interests.

Author details
[1]Department of Family Medicine, Wrocław Medical University, ul. Syrokomli 1, 51-141 Wrocław, Poland. [2]Opole Medical School, ul. Katowicka 68, 45-060 Opole, Poland. [3]Centre For Ageing Research, Lancaster University, Lancaster, UK. [4]Psychology, School of Life & Health Sciences, Aston University, Birmingham, UK. [5]Istituto di Ricerche Farmacologiche Mario Negri IRCCS, Milan, Italy.

References

1. Marmot M. Health inequalities in the European Union — final report of a consortium: European Commission Directorate General for Health and Consumers; 2003. https://doi.org/10.2772/34426.

2. European Commission. Reducing health inequalities in the European Union: Directorate General for Employment, Social Affairs and Equal Opportunities; 2003. http://docplayer.net/13894583-Reducing-health-inequalities-in-the-european-union.html. Accessed 17 Jan 2018

3. Dahlgren G, Whitehead M. European strategies for tackling social inequities in health: Levelling up Part 2. Copenhagen: Health October 24 WHO Regional Office for Europe (Studies on social and economic determinants of population health, No. 3); 2007. http://www.euro.who.int/__data/assets/pdf_file/0018/103824/E89384.pdf?ua=1 Accessed 17 Jan 2018

4. Whitehead M. The concepts and principles of equity and health. Int J Health Serv. 1992;22(3):429–45.

5. Fabbricotti IN, Janse B, Looman WM, de Kuijper R, van Wijngaarden JDH, Reiffers A. Integrated care for frail elderly compared to usual care: a study protocol of a quasi-experiment on the effects on the frail elderly, their caregivers, health professionals and health care costs. BMC Geriatr. 2013;13(1):31.

6. Supreme Audit Office. Raport Najwyższej Izby Kontroli (NIK) Opieka medyczna nad osobami w wieku podeszłym. KZD-4101-003/2014 Nr ewid.2/2015/P/14/062/KZD. 2014. https://www.nik.gov.pl/plik/id,8319,vp,10379.pdf. Accessed 14 Apr 2017.

7. Dixon-Woods M, Kirk MD, Agarwal MS, Annandale E, Arthur T, Harvey J, Hsu R, Katbamna S, Olsen R, Smith L and Riley L. Vulnerable groups and access to health care: a critical interpretive review. National Coordinating Centre NHS Service Delivery Organ RD (NCCSDO) 2005: http://www.netscc.ac.uk/hsdr/files/project/SDO_FR_08-1210-025_V01.pdf. Accessed 17 Jan 2018.

8. Fried LP, Tangen C, Walston J, Newman A, Hirsch C, Gottdiener J, Seeman T, Tracy R, Kop W, Burke G, McBurnie M. Frailty in older adults: evidence for a phenotype. J Gerontol A Biol Sci Med Sci. 2001;56(3):M146–57.

9. Bergman H, Ferrucci L, Guralnik J, Hogan DB, Hummel S, Karunananthan S, Wolfson C. Frailty: an emerging research and clinical paradigm–issues and controversies. J Gerontol A Biol Sci Med Sci. 2007;62(7):731–7.

10. Rockwood K, Song X, MacKnight C, Bergman H, Hogan DB, McDowell I. A global clinical measure of fitness and frailty in elderly people. CMAJ. 2005; 173(5):489–95.

11. Hussey PS, Schneider EC, Rudin RS, Fox D, Lai J, Pollack C. Continuity and the costs of care for chronic disease. JAMA Intern Med. 2014;174(5):742–8.

12. Shaw R, Gwyther H, Holland C, Bujinowska-Fedak M, Kurpas D, Cano A, Marcucci M, Riva S, D'Avanzo B. Understanding frailty: meanings and beliefs about screening and prevention across key stakeholder groups in Europe. Ageing Soc. 2017:1–30. https://doi.org/10.1017/S0144686X17000745.

13. D'Avanzo B, Shaw R, Riva S, Apostolo J, Bobrowicz-Campos E, Kurpas D, Bujinowska M, Holland C. Stakeholders' views and experiences of care and interventions for addressing frailty and pre-frailty: a meta-synthesis of qualitative evidence. PLoS One. 2017;12(7):e0180127.

14. Bragstad LK, Kirkevold M, Foss C. The indispensable intermediaries: a qualitative study of informal caregivers' struggle to achieve influence at and after hospital discharge. BMC Health Serv Res. 2014;14(1):331.

15. Sussman T. The influence of service factors on spousal caregivers' perceptions of community services. J Gerontol Soc Work. 2009;52(4):406–22.

16. Vasileiou K, Barnett J, Barreto M, Vines J, Atkinson M, Lawson S, Wilson M. Experiences of loneliness associated with being an informal caregiver: a qualitative investigation. Front Psychol. 2017;8:585. https://doi.org/10.3389/fpsyg.2017.00585.

17. Cameron ID, Fairhall N, Langron C, Lockwood K, Monaghan N, Aggar C, Sherrington C, Lord SR, Kurrle SE. A multifactorial interdisciplinary intervention reduces frailty in older people: randomized trial. BMC Med 2013;11(1):1–10.

18. Boyd CM, McNabney MK, Brandt N, Correa-de-Araujuo R, Daniel M, Epplin J, Fried TR, Goldstein MK, Holmes HM, Ritchie CS, Shega JW. Guiding principles for the care of older adults with multimorbidity: an approach for clinicians: American geriatrics society expert panel on the care of older adults with multimorbidity. J Am Geriatr Soc. 2012;60(10):E1–E25.

19. Freiberger E, Kemmler W, Siegrist M, Sieber C. Frailty and exercise interventions. Z Gerontol Geriatr. 2016;49(7):606–11.

20. Gill TM, Gahbauer EA, Allore HG, Han L. Transitions between frailty states among community-living older persons. Arch Intern Med. 2006; 166(4):418–23.

21. The World Bank. The present and future of long-term care in ageing Poland. 2015 https://das.mpips.gov.pl/source/opiekasenioralna/Long%20term%20care%20in%20ageing%20Poland_ENG_FINAL.pdf. Accessed 17 Jan 2018.

22. Kujawska J. Organisation and management of care for the elderly, University in Szczecin no 855, Finance, Financial Markets, Insurance vol 1, 2015 pp709–722 (Original in Polish: Organizacja i zarządzanie opieką nad osobami starszymi. Zeszyty Naukowe Uniwersytetu Szczecińskiego nr 855 Finanse, Rynki Finansowe, Ubezpieczenia nr 74, t. 1. 2015), http://www.wneiz.pl/nauka_wneiz/frfu/74-2015/FRFU-74-t1-709.pdf. Accessed 17 Jan 2018. doi: https://doi.org/10.18276/frfu.2015.74/1-62 s.709–722.

23. OECD/European Observatory on Health Systems and Policies. Poland: country health profile 2017. State of Health in the EU. Brussels: OECD Publishing, Paris/European Observatory on Health Systems and Policies; 2017.

24. Napolitano F, Napolitano P, Garofalo L, Recupito M, Angelillo IF. Assessment of continuity of care among patients with multiple chronic conditions in Italy. PLoS One. 2016;11(5):e0154940 https://doi.org/10.1371/journal.pone.0154940.

25. Rich E, Lipson D, Libersky J, Parchman M. Coordinating care for adults with complex care needs in the patient-centered medical home: challenges and solutions. In: White paper prepared by Mathematica Policy Research under Contract No. HHSA290200900019I/HHSA29032005T. AHRQ Publication No. 12–0010-EF. Rockville: Agency for Healthcare Research and Quality; 2012.

26. Janse B, Huijsman R, Fabbricotti IN. A quasi-experimental study of the effects of an integrated care intervention for the frail elderly on informal caregivers' satisfaction with care and support. BMC Health Serv Res. 2014;14:140.

27. Smith ML, Bergeron CD, Adler CH, Patel A, Ahn SN, Towne SD, Bien M, Ory MG. Factors associated with healthcare-related frustrations among adults with chronic conditions. Patient Educ Couns. 2017;100(6):1185–93.

28. Stein KV. Integrated care around the world. Examples to help improve (primary) health care in Poland. 2016; http://akademia.nfz.gov.pl/wp-content/uploads/2016/12/Raport_Opieka_koordynowana_ENG.pdf. Accessed 16 Jan 2018.

29. Berwick DM, Nolan TW, Whittington J. The triple aim: care, health, and cost. Health Aff. 2008;27(3):759–69.

30. Looman WM, Fabbricotti IN, de Kuyper R, Huijsman R. The effects of a pro-active integrated care intervention for frail community-dwelling older people: a quasi-experimental study with the GP-practice as single entry point. BMC Geriatr. 2016;16(1):43.

31. Gulliford M, Figueroa-Munoz J, Morgan M, Hughes D, Gibson D, Beech R, Hudson M. What does 'access to health care' mean? J Health Serv Res Policy. 2002;7(3):186–8.

32. Levesque J-F, Harris MF, Russell G. Patient-centred access to health care: conceptualising access at the interface of health systems and populations. Int J Equity Health. 2013;12(1):18.

33. Cano A, Kurpas D, Bujnowska-Fedak M, Santana S, Holland C, Marcucci M, Gonzalez-Segura A, Vollenbroek-Hutten M, D'avanzo B, Nobili A, Apostolo J, Bobrowicz-Campos E, Martinez-Arroyo A. FOCUS: frailty management optimisation through EIPAHA commitments and utilisation of stakeholders' input – an innovative European project in elderly care. Fam Med Prim Care Rev. 2016;18(3):373–6.

34. FOCUS - Frailty management optimization through EIP-AHA commitments and utilization of stakeholders input. 2018. http://focus-aha.eu/en_GB/home. Accessed 25 Jan 2018.

35. Ritchie J, Spencer L, O'Connor W. Carrying out qualitative analysis. In: Qualitative research practice: a guide for social science students and researchers. London: Sage; 2003.

36. Espinoza S, Walston JD. Frailty in older adults: insights and interventions. Cleve Clin J Med. 2005;72.

37. Kowalska K, Kalbarczyk WP. Coordinated health care. International experience, proposals for Poland. Original in Polish: Koordynowana opieka zdrowotna. Doświadczenia międzynarodowe, propozycje dla Polski. 2013 Report accessed on 17 Jan 2018 http://www.ey.com/Publication/vwLUAssets/EY_Sprawne_Pa%C5%84stwo_Raport_Koordynowana_Opieka_Zdrowotna/$FILE/EY_Sprawne_Panstwo_KOZ.pdf.

38. Roland M, Olesen F. Can pay for performance improve the quality of primary care? BMJ. 2016;354:4058.

39. Beck O, Kędziora-Kornatowska K, Kornatowski M. (2014) Opieka długoterminowa domowa w Polsce – ramy, problemy, perspektywy. Long-term home care in Poland – framework, problems, prospects. Hygeia Public Health. 2014;49(2):192–6.

40. Golinowska S. The system of long-term care in Poland. CASE Network Studies & Analyses. Warsaw: Centre for Social and Economic Research; 2010. p. 416:s6.

41. Lopez-Hartmann M, Wens J, Verhoeven V, Remmen R. The effect of caregiver support interventions for informal caregivers of community-dwelling frail elderly: a systematic review. Int J of Integr Care. 2012;12:e133.

42. Candy B, Jones L, Drake R, Leurent B, King M. Interventions for supporting informal caregivers of patients in the terminal phase of a disease. Cochrane Database Syst Rev. 2011;15(6):CD007617.

43. Okamoto K, Hasebe Y, Harasawa Y. Caregiver psychological characteristics predict discontinuation of care for disabled elderly at home. Int J Geriatr Psychiatry. 2007;22(11):1110–4.

44. Colombo F, Llena-Nozal A, Mercier J, Tjadens F. Help wanted? Providing and paying for long-term care. OECD health policy studies, 2011:OECD Publishing, Paris. https://doi.org/10.1787/9789264097759-en. Accessed 25 Jan 2018.

45. Gwyther H, Shaw RL, Jaime Dauden E-A, D'Avanzo B, Kurpas D, Bujnowska-Fedak MM, Kujawa T, Marcucci M, Cano A, Holland C. Understanding frailty: a qualitative study of European healthcare policy-makers' approaches to frailty screening and management. BMJ Open. 2018;8(1).

46. Hawkins K, Parker PM, Hommer CE, Bhattarai GR, Huang J, Wells TS, Ozminkowski RJ, Yeh CS. Evaluation of a high-risk case management pilot program for Medicare beneficiaries with Medigap coverage. Popul Health Manag. 2015;18(2):93–103.

47. Looman WM, Huijsman R, Bouwmans-Frijters CAM, Stolk EA, Fabbricotti IN. Cost-effectiveness of the 'Walcheren integrated care model' intervention for community-dwelling frail elderly. Fam Pract. 2016;33(2):154–60.

48. Sandberg M, Jakobsson U, Midlöv P, Kristensson J. Cost-utility analysis of case management for frail older people: effects of a randomised controlled trial. Health Econ Rev. 2015;5:12.

49. You EC, Dunt D, Doyle C, Hsueh A. Effects of case management in community aged care on client and carer outcomes: a systematic review of randomized trials and comparative observational studies. BMC Health Serv Res. 2012;12(1):395.

50. Berglund H, Wilhelmson K, Blomberg S, Dunér A, Kjellgren K, Hasson H. Older people's views of quality of care: a randomised controlled study of continuum of care. J Clin Nurs. 2013;22(19–20):2934–44.

22

A comparison of perceived uselessness between centenarians and non-centenarians in China

Yuan Zhao[1,2], Hong Fu[3], Aimei Guo[4], Li Qiu[5], Karen S. L. Cheung[6], Bei Wu[7], Daniela Jopp[8] and Danan Gu[9*]

Abstract

Background: Self-perceived uselessness is associated with poorer health in older adults. However, it is unclear whether there is a difference in self-perceived uselessness between centenarians and non-centenarians, and if so, which factors contributed to the difference.

Methods: We used four waves of a nationwide longitudinal dataset from 2005 to 2014 in China to investigate these research goals. We first performed multinomial logit regression models to examine the risk of the high or moderate frequency of self-perceived uselessness relative to the low frequency among centenarians (5778 persons) in comparison with non-centenarians aged 65–99 (20,846 persons). We then conducted a cohort analysis for those born in 1906–1913, examining differences in self-perceived uselessness between those centenarians and those died between ages 91 and 99 during 2005–2014.

Results: Compared to persons aged 65–79, centenarians had 84% (relative risk ratio (RRR) = 1.84, 95% CI:1.69–2.01) and 35% (RRR = 1.35, 95% CI: 1.25–1.46) higher risk to have the high frequency and the moderate frequency of feeling useless versus low frequency, respectively, when only demographic factors were controlled for. However, centenarians had 31% (RRR = 0.69, 95% CI: 0.54–0.88), 43% (RRR = 0.57, 95% CI: 0.49–0.68), and 25% (RRR = 0.75, 95% CI: 0.67–0.83) lower risk, respectively, to have the high frequency of self-perceived uselessness relative to the low frequency when a wide set of study covariates were controlled for. In the case of the moderate versus the low frequency of self-perceived uselessness, the corresponding figures were 18% (RRR = 0.82, 95% CI: 0.66–1.02), 22% (RRR = 0.78, 95%CI: 0.67–0.90), and 13% (RRR = 0.87, 95% CI: 0.79–0.96), respectively. The cohort analysis further indicates that those who became centenarians were 36–39% less likely than those died at ages 91–94 to report the high and the moderate frequencies of self-perceived uselessness versus the low frequency; no difference was found between centenarians and those died at ages 95–99. In both period and cohort analyses, behavioral and health-related factors affected the perception substantially.

Conclusions: Overall, centenarians were less likely to perceive themselves as useless compared to non-centenarians of younger birth cohorts when a wide set of covariates were considered and non-centenarians of the same birth cohort. How centenarians manage to do so remains an open question. Our findings may help improve our understanding about the longevity secrets of centenarians.

Keywords: Centenarians, Self-perceived uselessness, China, Healthy longevity, CLHLS

* Correspondence: gudanan@yahoo.com
[9]United Nations Population Division, Two UN Plaza, DC2-1910, New York, NY 10017, USA
Full list of author information is available at the end of the article

Background

Evidence from various populations has indicated that a strong sense of usefulness to others among older adults plays a crucial role in shaping positive views about their own aging, health behaviors and adequate adaptations that contribute positively to their good health and psychological wellbeing, and even longevity [1–15]. By contrast, perceiving one's life as useless is associated with higher prevalence of chronic diseases [16, 17], poorer cognitive function and mental health status [7, 18–20], poorer self-rated health and life satisfaction [7, 21–24], lower physical functioning [5–7, 11, 25], and higher risk of mortality [6, 8, 10, 15, 26–29]. Perceptions of uselessness are also linked with higher levels of depression and lower levels of social and physical activity engagements, self-efficacy and self-esteem [5, 6, 11]. Although these studies have enriched our understanding about the associations between self-perceived uselessness and health behaviors, psychological wellbeing, and health outcomes [7, 30], most of these studies focused on general populations of older adults. It is less clear whether low levels of perception of uselessness still play a crucial role at very old age in helping long-lived persons reach successful aging and healthy longevity. Given the statistical robustness of self-perceived uselessness in affecting behaviors and in predicting health outcomes in the existing literature [7, 15, 30], it thus may have important implications for public health interventions to study self-perception of uselessness among centenarians and compare it with that of non-centenarian older adults.

Centenarians are often considered as the best age group to study healthy longevity and successful aging [31, 32]. Although centenarians show a poorer physical health and cognitive function compared to younger older adults [31–35], their psychological wellbeing may not be in disadvantage [32, 36]. More importantly, evidence shows that in comparison with their same cohort peers, centenarians are more psychologically resilient and have higher levels of physical and cognitive function than those who died younger [32, 36, 37].

Researchers generally agree that there is a large variation in disease conditions, physical/cognitive functions, and psychological wellbeing among these long-lived individuals [31, 35, 38], and that centenarians may follow a different trajectory of health decline from those non-centenarians [32]. Thus, the significance of comparison of self-perception of uselessness between centenarians and non-centenarians cannot be undervalued. Yet, studies about centenarians' own views on aging or self-perceived usefulness are virtually nonexistent in the literature. Do centenarians have a more positive perception about their usefulness than their younger counterparts? And if so, what are the factors that could explain the differences? To our knowledge, there is currently no

study available to address these research questions, possibly due to unavailability of data. This present study thus aims to investigate these research questions using the largest centenarian sample in the contemporary world from a nationwide longitudinal survey in mainland China.

Methods
Study sample

The four latest waves of datasets conducted in 2005, 2008/2009 (thereafter as 2008), 2011/2012 (thereafter as 2011), and 2014 from the Chinese Longitudinal Healthy Longevity Survey (CLHLS) were used to address our research questions. These four waves of datasets were pooled together to obtain more robust results. The 1998, 2000, and 2002 waves were excluded from our analyses in that some key variables used in the analyses were not available in these first three waves. The CLHLS is an ongoing project. Its samples were randomly selected from the half of the counties/cities in 22 of 31 provinces in mainland China. The proportion of the population of the sampled 22 provinces was about 87% of China in 2010 [7, 8]. The remaining nine provinces were excluded in the CLHLS to avoid age-reporting inaccuracy at oldest-old ages among non-Han minorities [39]. In 2008 and later waves, the CLHLS included an additional county (Chenmai County) with relatively good quality of age reporting quality from Hainan Province, one of these nine provinces. The present study includes 26,624 participants with 48,476 observations in 2005–2014. Among the 26,624 participants, 5778 were centenarians at the time of interview. The detailed sampling procedures and the assessments of data quality of the CLHLS can be found elsewhere and thus are not described here [7, 39].

One of the biggest challenges for centenarian studies is to validate the participants' age for countries where a vital registration system is not well-developed, including China [39]. The CLHLS collected data on the date of birth and age. If the age of a respondent was reported in the lunisolar calendar, the age was converted into the solar calendar. The validation of respondents' (especially centenarians') self-reported ages in the CLHLS involved several rigorous procedures with different sources [39, 40]. These sources included household registration data, date of birth certification, genealogical data if available, marriage certificate if available, birth history, sibling history, and any other records available that could be used for validation [39, 40]. The systematic assessments showed that the accuracy of age reporting was high [39].

Measurements
Self-perceived uselessness

Self-perceived uselessness was measured in the CLHLS by a single question: "As you age, do you feel more useless?" This question was designed based on an item from the Attitude toward Own Aging subscale of the Philadelphia Geriatrics Center Morale Scale [11, 12]. There were six response categories: always, often, sometimes, seldom, almost never or never, and unable to answer. Following previous research [5, 15, 30], we combined "always" and "often" into one category, and "seldom" and "almost never or never" into one category. We then renamed the new categories into *high frequency*, *moderate frequency*, *low frequency*, and unable to answer the question. The purpose of keeping the category "unable to answer" is to have the original information as intact as possible, whereas the purpose of collapsing five categories into three is to obtain more robust results because the sample size of some categories was relatively small. Of the 6207 participants who selected "unable to answer," around 90% of them indicated that their refusal was due to poor health [5]. Although "unable to answer" was modeled, its results were not presented in the main text for a better focus on research objectives and enhanced presentation. These results are available upon request.

Associated factors

One recent study proposed a framework highlighting factors associated with self-perceived useless [30]. The framework, named REHAB, includes resource (R), social environments (E), health (H), demographic attributes (A), and behaviors (B). We relied on this framework to investigate possible factors that affect the difference in self-perceived uselessness between centenarians and non-centenarians. Specifically, we selected few major factors in each abovementioned domain. Demographic attributes included sex (men vs. women), urban-rural residence (urban vs. rural), and ethnicity (Han vs. non-Han). Resource factors consisted of years of schooling (0, 1–6, and 7+), financial independence (yes vs. no), lifetime primary occupation (white-collar occupation vs. others), and whether a participant was covered by a state medical insurance program (yes vs. no). If the respondent had a retirement wage or a pension, he or she was considered as financially independent. The state medical insurance programs included the new rural cooperative medical scheme, urban resident medical scheme, and urban employee medical scheme [41]. The respondents were asked to provide information whether they were covered by any of these three schemes (yes vs. no). Social environmental factors included current marital status (currently married vs. no), co-residence with children (yes vs. no), providing monetary support to children (yes vs. no), receiving monetary support from children (yes vs. no). Behavioral factors were measured by frequency of leisure activities. Levels of leisure activities were represented by the sum of frequencies of six items,

including doing housework, gardening, raising domestic animals or poultry, reading books/newspapers, watching TV/listening to radio, and any other personal outdoor activities. For each item, response category used a five-point Likert-scale from never or almost never (score = 0) to almost daily (score = 4). The reliability coefficient of these six items is 0.66. We split the sample into three levels (low, moderate, and high) of activity engagement on the basis of the sample distribution.

Health status is possibly among the most important elements in affecting self-perception about aging [27]. In this study, we included two functional health measures: basic activities of daily living (ADL) and cognitive functioning. Although those with severe cognitive impairment were unlikely to answer the questions, evidence shows that those with slight or mild cognitive impairment still can answer easy self-report questions [42]. Following the common practice in the field [8], if a respondent needed assistance in performing any one of the six tasks (bathing, dressing, indoor transferring, toileting, eating, and continence), he or she was classified as ADL disabled; otherwise, he or she was considered as having no ADL disability. Cognitive impairment was measured by a validated Chinese version of the Mini-Mental State Examination (MMSE), which included six domains of cognition (i. e., orientation, reaction, calculation, short memory, naming, and language) with a total score of 30 [43]. A respondent was considered as cognitively impaired if his or her MMSE score was less than 24; otherwise, he or she was considered as cognitively normal [43]. An alternative cut-point score of 18 was also examined and yielded very similar results. The selection of factors and our coding of the variables were consistent with one recent study [44].

Analytical strategy

Because the self-perceived uselessness item in the current study was classified into four response categories (i.e., high frequency, moderate frequency, low frequency, and unable to answer), multinomial logistic regression models were employed to investigate whether centenarians were less likely to perceive themselves as useless than non-centenarians, and if so, which factors were associated with high or moderate frequency of self-perceived uselessness relative to the low frequency (the reference group). The results were reported in relative risk ratios (RRRs), which indicate how the risk of the high or moderate frequency of self-perceived uselessness relative to the low frequency in centenarians compared to the risk of the high or moderate frequency of self-perceived uselessness relative to the low frequency in non-centenarians. An RRR > 1 indicates that centenarians are more like to have the high or moderate frequency of self-perceived uselessness rather than to have the low frequency in comparison with non-centenarians, and vice versa. Some alternative approaches were also tested, including generalized ordered logistic regression models and binary logistic regression models. The generalized ordered logit models treated the self-perceived uselessness as an ordinal variable, whereas the logistic regression models treated the self-perceived uselessness as a dichotomous variable. Both sets of regression models produced very similar results. Similar to previous studies [15, 30], we pooled all four waves of the data together and adjusted for intrapersonal correlation across waves to obtain more robust and reliable results in that some respondents (both centenarians and non-centenarians) had more than two observations during the study period 2005–2014.

Two sets of analysis were designed: Period and cohort. The period analysis relied on the pooled dataset of the latest four waves from 26,624 respondents with 48,476 observations. Six nested models were analyzed for period analysis with different sets of control variables. Model I included demographic attributes (i.e., age, sex, urban-rural residence, ethnicity); Model II included resource factors (educational attainment, primary life occupation, economic independence, family economic condition, and access to healthcare services when in need) plus demographic attributes; Model III included social environmental factors (marital status, co-residence with children, primary caregivers) in addition to demographic attributes; Model IV included behavioral factors in terms of participation in leisure activities plus demographic attributes; Model V included health variables measured by ADL disability and cognitive impairment in addition to demographic attributes; and Model VI controlled for all covariates used in Models I to V. A variable reflecting the survey year was also included in all models to account for possible variations over time.

The same modeling strategy was applied to a cohort analysis that focused on those 2921 individuals who were born in 1906–1913. The cohort analysis compared two groups of people who were all born in the 1906–1913: one group survived to age 100 and the other group who reached age 90 yet died before age 100 in the study period 2005–2014. The reason that we selected these birth cohorts was because individuals who were born in 1906–1913 would all have passed age 100 in the 2014 wave if they were still alive so that we could identify for each respondent whether he or she lived to age 100 or not. An indicator variable capturing whether each respondent survived to age 100 or not was included in the model. This indicator variable had three categories: died at ages 91–94, died at ages 95–99, and died at age 100 or beyond. A variable of single year of birth cohort was included, while the variables of age and wave were dropped in all models of the cohort analysis.

Among those samples included in the analysis, the proportions of missing values for all study variables were less than 2%. To keep as many cases as possible in the analyses, we imputed these missing values using a regression-based approach by assuming that those respondents with missing values would have the same answer as those without missing values if their demographics, resources, social environments, behaviors, and health were the same. We also used other approaches (such as the mode for categorical variables and means for continuous variables) to impute the missing values and produced very similar results. In regression analyses, we did not apply the sampling weights because the weighted regression results could unnecessarily enlarge standard errors when the variables that are used for a construction of sampling weight are controlled for in the regression models [7, 8, 45]. All analyses were performed using Stata version 15.

Results

Table 1 presents the percentage distribution of study variables by the frequency of self-perceived perception of uselessness for 48,476 observations collected in 2005–2014 from 26,624 participants. A smaller proportion of the centenarians reported high frequency of self-perceived uselessness compared to non-centenarians, yet centenarians had a much higher proportion of "unable to answer". Among the 2921 individuals who were born in 1906–1913 included in the cohort analysis, those who became centenarians in 2005–2014 had a higher proportion of the low frequency of self-perceived uselessness compared to those who died between ages 91 and 99 in 2005–2014.

Table 2 presents the relative risk ratios (RRRs) of reporting high and moderate frequencies versus the low frequency of self-perceived uselessness for centenarians as compared to older adults in other age groups from the period analysis. Model I reveals that although centenarians had no difference in self-perceived uselessness compared to octogenarians and nonagenarians when only demographics were controlled for, they were respectively associated with 84% (RRR = 1.84, 95% CI: 1.69–2.01) and 35% (RRR = 1.35, 95% CI: 1.25–1.46) higher risk of reporting the high and the moderate frequencies of self-perceived uselessness relative to the low frequency in comparison with older adults aged 65–79. Model II shows that the elevated RRRs were mildly attenuated to 52% (RRR = 1.52, 95% CI: 1.39–1.67) and 23% (RRR = 1.23, 95% CI: 1.13–1.33), respectively, when resources were added to Model I; and Model III shows that these RRRs were 56% (RRR = 1.56, 95% CI: 1.42–1.72) and 21% (RRR = 1.21, 95% CI: 1.11–1.31), respectively, when social environmental factors were included in Model I. So far, modeling results reveal that centenarians were more likely to perceive themselves as useless

Table 1 Distribution of the pooled datasets: 2005, 2008, 2011, and 2014 waves of the CLHLS

Variables	Sample % [a]	Self-perceived uselessness (percentage)			
		Always/often	Sometimes	Seldom /never	Unable to answer
Total observations	48,476 (100%)	11,147 (23.0%) [b]	15,122 (31.2%) [b]	16,000 (33.0%)[b]	6207 (12.8%)[b]
Age groups					
Age 65–79	30.3	19.7	34.3	43.8	2.3
Age 80–89	26.7	26.4	33.3	32.7	7.6
Age 90–99	26.0	24.7	29.9	28.1	17.3
Age 100+	17.0	20.9	24.4	21.9	32.8
Other demographics					
Female	56.4	25.0	30.2	28.8	16.0
Male	43.6	20.4	32.5	38.4	8.7
Non-Han ethnicity	16.3	19.3	34.0	34.2	12.5
Han ethnicity	83.7	23.7	30.7	32.8	12.9
Resources					
Own education, 0 years of schooling	66.0	24.9	30.7	28.5	15.9
Own education, 1–6 years of schooling	25.1	20.8	32.9	38.7	7.6
Own education, 7+ years of schooling	8.9	15.0	29.9	50.2	4.9
Rural	56.4	24.7	31.4	30.2	13.8
Urban	43.6	20.9	30.9	36.7	11.6
Non-white collar occupation	92.3	23.7	31.3	31.7	13.3
White collar occupation	7.7	14.2	29.7	49.2	6.9
Economic dependence	72.2	25.2	30.7	28.4	15.7
Economic independence	27.8	17.3	32.5	45.0	5.2
Fair or poor family economic condition	84.8	24.1	31.5	31.0	13.4
Rich family economic condition	15.2	16.8	29.3	44.5	9.3
Not covered by state medical insurance scheme	8.5	35.7	27.7	15.5	21.1
Covered by state medical insurance scheme	91.5	21.8	31.5	34.7	12.0
Family/social support					
Currently not married	66.0	24.5	30.2	28.2	17.1
Currently married	34.0	20.1	33.1	42.3	4.5
Coresidence with children - no	39.3	24.3	32.5	35.6	7.6
Coresidence with children - yes	60.7	22.2	30.4	31.3	16.2
Receiving money/food from children - no	20.0	21.5	28.5	33.5	16.6
Receiving money/food from children - yes	80.0	23.4	31.9	32.9	11.9
Giving money/food to children - yes	77.0	24.5	30.2	30.2	15.1
Giving money/food to children - no	23.0	18.1	34.5	42.5	5.0
Behaviors					
Frequency of leisure activities-low level	75.6	25.2	30.6	28.5	15.7
Frequency of leisure activities- medium level	11.0	16.7	34.6	43.4	5.4
Frequency of leisure activities -high level	13.6	15.8	31.6	49.8	2.8
Health conditions					
ADL independent	74.6	21.8	33.7	38.1	6.5
ADL dependent	25.4	26.4	24.0	18.2	31.5
Cognitively unimpaired	60.1	21.1	35.7	41.7	1.4

Table 1 Distribution of the pooled datasets: 2005, 2008, 2011, and 2014 waves of the CLHLS *(Continued)*

Variables	Sample % [a]	Self-perceived uselessness (percentage)			
		Always/often	Sometimes	Seldom /never	Unable to answer
Cognitively impaired	39.9	25.8	24.4	19.9	30.0
Survey years					
Wave 2005	31.6	23.2	32.2	33.4	11.3
Wave 2008	33.7	23.9	29.1	31.9	15.1
Wave 2011	20.0	22.1	31.9	34.4	11.6
Wave 2014	14.7	21.7	33.0	33.0	12.3
Cohorts born in 1906–1913 (2921) [c]					
Died at ages 91–94	10.2	29.4	33.1	21.7	15.7
Died at ages 95–99	58.8	23.5	28.0	27.1	21.4
Died at ages 100+	31.0	25.3	29.3	29.3	16.1

Note: (1) Except for the total number of observations in the top line, all numbers were percentages unless otherwise stated. (2) a, this column referred to percentage distribution of each category of the study variables among 48,476 observations from 26,624 individuals who were interviewed from 2005 to 2014. The distributions by 26,624 individuals at their baseline were similar to what were presented in the Table 3b, percentages of self-perceived uselessness were calculated by row. The row sum of percentage of self-perceived uselessness may not be equal to 100% due to roundness. (4) c, Distribution for cohorts born in 1906–1913 was based on 2972 individuals who were followed-up till the 2014 wave or died before 2014. Those who were lost to follow-up between 2005 and 2014 were excluded. (5) All distributions were unweighted

compared to the youngest older adults aged 65–79 and had no difference in self-perceived uselessness as compared to older adults aged 80–99.

However, when behavioral factors were controlled in addition to demographics (Model IV), centenarians had 25% (RRR = 0.75, 95% CI: 0.69–0.82) and 15% (RRR = 0.85, 95% CI: 0.78–0.93) lower risk ratios of having the high frequency of self-perceived uselessness relative to the low frequency compared to octogenarians and

nonagenarians, respectively, although they still had a 11% higher risk ratio of having the moderate frequency relative to low frequency of self-perception of uselessness than older adults aged 65–79. When ADL disability and cognitive impairment were controlled for in addition to demographics (Model V), the centenarians were 34% (RRR = 0.66, 95% CI: 0.60–0.72) and 22% (RRR = 0.78, 95% CI: 0.71–0.85) less likely than octogenarians and nonagenarians to have the high frequency of

Table 2 Relative risk ratios of the high and the moderate frequencies relative to the low frequency of self-perceived uselessness among centenarians in comparison with non-centenarians, CLHLS 2005–2014

Ages at survey	Model I	Model II	Model III	Model IV	Model V	Model VI
High frequency relative to low frequency						
Ages 100+ vs. ages 65–79	1.84[***] (1.69–2.01)	1.52[***] (1.39–1.67)	1.56[***] (1.42–1.71)	1.08 (0.98–1.18)	0.97 (0.89–1.07)	0.69[**] (0.54–0.88)
Ages 100+ vs. ages 80–89	1.04 (0.95–1.13)	0.99 (0.91–1.08)	0.99 (0.91–1.08)	0.75[***] (0.69–0.82)	0.66[***] (0.60–0.72)	0.57[***] (0.49–0.68)
Ages 100+ vs. ages 90–99	0.98 (0.90–1.07)	0.96 (0.88–1.04)	0.98 (0.90–1.07)	0.85[*] (0.78–0.93)	0.78[***] (0.71–0.85)	0.75[***] (0.67–0.83)
Moderate frequency relative to low frequency						
Ages 100+ vs. ages 65–79	1.35[***] (1.25–1.46)	1.23[***] (1.13–1.33)	1.21[***] (1.11–1.31)	1.11[*] (1.02–1.21)	1.09[*] (1.00–1.19)	0.82+ (0.66–1.02)
Ages 100+ vs. ages 80–89	1.04 (0.96–1.13)	1.01 (0.93–1.10)	1.00 (0.92–1.08)	0.93+ (0.85–1.00)	0.89[**] (0.82–0.96)	0.78[**] (0.67–0.90)
Ages 100+ vs. ages 90–99	1.00 (0.92–1.09)	0.99 (0.91–1.07)	0.99 (0.92–1.08)	0.95 (0.88–1.03)	0.91[*] (0.85–0.99)	0.87[**] (0.79–0.96)

Note: (1) Figures in the table were relative risk ratios based on unweighted multinomial logistic regression models adjusting for intrapersonal correlation from 26,624 respondents consisting of 48,476 observations. (2) The high frequency of feelings of useless referred to always/often; the moderate frequency referred to sometimes; and the low frequency referred to seldom/never. The category of "unable to answer" of the self-perceived uselessness was included in the analyses, but their results were not presented because they are not our focuses. (3) Model I controlled for demographic attributes (sex, urban-rural residence, ethnicity), and the years of survey; Model II added resource factors (educational attainment, primary life occupation, economic independence, family economic condition, and adequate access to healthcare services when in need) in Model I; Model III controlled for social environmental factors (marital status, coresidence with children, primary caregivers) in addition to covariates in Model I; Model IV controlled for behavioral factors (leisure activities) in addition to covariates in Model I; Model V controlled for health-related factors (disability in activities of daily living and cognitive impairment) in addition to covariates in Model I; and Model VI controlled for all covariates in Models I to V. (4) + $p < 0.1$, [*] $p < 0.05$, [**] $p < 0.01$, [***] $p < 0.001$

self-perceived uselessness relative to the low frequency. The corresponding figures for the moderate relative to the low frequency of self-perception were 11% (RRR = 0.89, 95% CI: 0.82–0.96) and 9% (RRR = 0.91, 95% CI: 0.85–0.99).

When all covariates were taken into consideration, centenarians had 31% (RRR = 0.69, 95% CI: 0.54–0.88), 43% (RRR = 0.57, 95%CI: 0.49–0.68), and 25% (RRR = 0.75, 95%CI: 0.67–0.83) respectively lower risk ratios of having the high frequency relative to the low frequency of self-perceived uselessness compared to older adults aged 65–79, 80–89, and 90–99. In the case of the moderate frequency relative to the low frequency, these reduced risk ratios were 18% (RRR = 0.82, 95% CI: 0.66–1.02), 22% (RRR = 0.78, 95% CI: 0.67–0.90), and 13% (RRR = 0.87, 95% CI: 0.79–0.96), respectively. These results of the sequential models indicate that all sets of factors played a certain role in distinguishing the self-perception of uselessness between centenarians and older adults at other age groups, but health practice and health conditions played a greater role than other factors.

In the case of the cohort analysis among those who were born in 1906–1913 and survived to age 91 or above, Table 3 shows that compared with those who died at ages 91–94, those who became centenarians were 36–39% less like to have the high and the moderate frequencies of self-perceived uselessness versus the low frequency when demographic factors plus either resources factors or social environmental factors were taken into account. When the participation in leisure activities or the health condition was taken into consideration, the relative risk of the high frequency versus the low

frequency of self-perceived uselessness among centenarians was not statistically significant compared with those who died at age 91–94, although the RRR was significant in the case of the moderate frequency versus the low frequency controlling for health behaviors and demographics (Model IV). In other words, when participation in leisure activities and health condition of those who died at age 100 or beyond was the same as those who died at ages 91–94, there would have no difference in self-perceived uselessness between these two groups. In our sample, those who died at age 100 or beyond were in better health and were more likely to participation in leisure activities (not shown). When all factors were controlled for, there was only a very slight change in RRRs (Model VI) compared to the model that controlled for health (Model V). These results suggest that all factors under study other than participation in leisure activities and health conditions had a little impact on differentiating self-perception of uselessness between centenarians and those died at ages 91–94. This implies that participation in leisure activities and health condition played a greater role than other factors in differing those who lived to age 100 from those from the same birth cohort who died earlier in 2005–2014. No significant difference was found between those who died at age 100 or older and those who died at ages 95–99.

Discussion

Based on the 2005, 2008, 2011, and 2014 four waves of the Chinese Longitudinal Healthy Longevity Survey, the largest nationally representative survey of older adults in China, we examined whether centenarians were less

Table 3 Relative risk ratios of high and moderate frequencies relative to low frequency of self-perceived uselessness for those lived to age 100 and above in comparison with those lived to age 91 yet died before age 100 among those born in 1906–1913, CLHLS 2005–2014

Age at death	Model I	Model II	Model III	Model IV	Model V	Model VI
High frequency relative to low frequency						
Survived to age 100 vs. died at ages 91–94	0.62* (0.41–0.91)	0.64* (0.42–0.97)	0.62* (0.41–0.84)	0.74 (0.48–1.12)	0.80 (0.52–1.22)	0.85 (0.55–1.32)
Survived to age 100 vs. died at ages 95–99	0.98 (0.77–1.24)	1.02 (0.80–1.29)	0.98 (0.78–1.24)	1.11 (0.88–1.43)	1.16 (0.91–1.47)	1.25 (0.97–1.60)
Moderate frequency relative to low frequency						
Survived to age 100 vs. died at ages 91–94	0.61* (0.41–0.91)	0.62* (0.42–0.93)	0.61* (0.41–0.91)	0.64* (0.43–0.97)	0.69+ (0.47–1.04)	0.71+ (0.48–1.06)
Survived to age 100 vs. died at ages 95–99	0.93 (0.75–1.17)	0.95 (0.76–1.19)	0.94 (0.75–1.17)	0.98 (0.78–1.23)	1.02 (0.81–1.28)	1.04 (0.82–1.31)

Note: (1) Figures in the table were relative risk ratios based on unweighted multinomial logistic regression models from 2921 respondents who were born between January 1, 1906 and December 31, 1913. (2) The high frequency of feelings of useless referred to always/often; the moderate frequency referred to sometimes; and the low frequency referred to seldom/never. The category of "unable to answer" of the self-perceived uselessness was included in the analyses, but their results were not presented because they are not our focuses. (3) Model I controlled for demographic attributes (sex, urban-rural residence, ethnicity), and the years of survey; Model II added resource factors (educational attainment, primary life occupation, economic independence, family economic condition, and adequate access to healthcare services when in need) in Model I; Model III controlled for social environmental factors (marital status, coresidence with children, primary caregivers) in addition to covariates in Model I; Model IV controlled for behavioral factors (leisure activities) in addition to covariates in Model I; Model V controlled for health-related factors (disability in activities of daily living and cognitive impairment) in addition to covariates in Model I; and Model VI controlled for all covariates in Models I to V. (4) + p < 0.1, *p < 0.05, **p < 0.01, ***p < 0.001

likely to perceive themselves as useless compared to younger cohorts. In general, we found that when only demographic attributes, socioeconomic resources, and social environmental factors were taken into consideration, centenarians had a higher proportion of having a negative self-perception about their own usefulness than younger generations aged 65–79, although the centenarians had a similar proportion compared to octogenarians and nonagenarians. However, when behavioral factors or heath conditions were taken into account, centenarians were less likely to have a perception of self-perceived uselessness than octogenarians and nonagenarians; and when all factors under study were controlled for, centenarian were also less likely to have a negative perception about their usefulness compared to all four younger age groups under study. More importantly, we further found from the cohort analysis of those born in 1906–1913 that in comparison with those who were from the same cohort but died at ages 91–94, those who became centenarians were less likely to perceive themselves as useless when demographic attributes, resource factors, and social environmental factors were controlled for. Overall, these results convey a clear message that centenarians hold more positive attitudes and views about their aging than non-centenarians, and that these positive views may attribute to better chances for survival.

One important finding of the present study is that health in terms of physical and cognitive functions and behaviors played a more important role than other factors in distinguishing the self-perceive uselessness between centenarians and non-centenarian older adults. Health behaviors were measured by leisure activities, which is closely related physical function. This finding provides additional evidence to support the contribution of health and active lifestyle to self-perception about one's views and attitudes toward aging or usefulness. Studies have shown that a good health condition is associated with a better self-perception about one's usefulness to family and others [30]. Our findings also enrich the existing literature on factors associated with self-perceived usefulness and self-perception of aging [15] and the literature on centenarians' positive psychological attributes [26].

Research has indicated that perceptions of usefulness or uselessness may impact one's health psychologically, behaviorally, and physiologically [7, 14, 15]. Physiologically, having a strong feeling of usefulness could avoid a dysregulation of the central nervous system, neurotransmitters, and/or immune system for the onset and progression of disease, disability, and other manifestations of aging [46, 47]. Behaviorally, positive views and attitudes about one's aging could maintain healthy lifestyles that promote health [5]. Psychologically, a strong sense or perception about own usefulness to others could avoid diminishment of beliefs about self-control and

self-efficacy, help prevent social isolation, and improve resilience capacity to deal with negative views/thoughts and difficulties in daily life [5, 15, 48].

It is possible that with increasing age, some very old adults, especially centenarians have developed strategies to cope with challenges and changes in their environments so that the sense of perceived usefulness to family, others, and society is maintained [6, 32, 49–52]. Some previous studies have shown that a fairly large portion of centenarians are still in a good function [35], that vast majority of centenarians are quite independent in performing daily activities when they were at early 90s [38], and that they are more psychologically resilient than younger peers of the same birth cohort, or even as resilient as those younger birth cohorts [32, 50]. Overall, our findings are generally in accordance with previous findings that centenarians were more physically and psychologically robust than nonagenarians of their same birth cohorts in handling stress, depression, or other unfavorable conditions than their cohort peers [32, 36–38, 50]. The lower levels of self-perceived uselessness among the centenarians imply that positive attitudes and views about aging may be an important pathway to reach age 100.

Our finding that centenarians are less likely to feel useless to family and others compared to their cohort peers underscores the importance of maintaining positive self-perceptions with age at an individual level and suggests that it may never be too late to promote positive perspectives of aging [30]. In order to achieve exceptional longevity, it is thus recommended to promote positive views and attitudes among older people by building and maintaining adequate emotional capacity, neutralizing negative emotionality, developing resistance to counteract negative age-associated stressors, and nurturing positive views of health and life [53, 54]. Given recent evidence on the negative perceptions of aging among older adults in China [55], and eroding practice of filial piety and respecting for older adults due to rapid social and economic changes [7, 56, 57], promoting positive views about one's own aging and creation of age-friendly environments are especially timely and needed so as to achieving successful aging [58].

While highlighting the strengths, we acknowledge the following limitations. First, the CLHLS only used a single item to collect data on self-perceived uselessness, which may not capture the multidimensionality of the concept of uselessness [15, 28]. Second, because the CLHLS is not designed to be a cohort study, the sample size at each individual age only consists of a couple of hundred participants, which may be not sufficient in follow-up wave due to high mortality among these participants, although the total sample size is relatively large. Furthermore, the follow-up length only lasted for

10 years in the present study, which is a relatively short follow-up period. In addition, in our cohort analysis, more than 60% of the samples were aged 95–99 at the time of their initial interview and more than 85% of those who did not live to age 100 died at age 95–99. In other words, our cohort results mainly refer to a comparison between those aged to 95–99 years old and those who became centenarians. Overall, larger sample size and longer follow-up period are warranted to have more robust results. Third, although we examined factors associated with self-perceived uselessness for centenarians in comparison with non-centenarians and found that centenarians were more likely to have a low frequency of self-perceived uselessness compared with their same birth cohort peers who did not become centenarians. However, the casual mechanism responsible for how such positive attitudes or perceptions have enhanced their healthy longevity deserves further investigations. Studies combining phenotypic and genotypic data and adopting an interdisciplinary perspective may be a promising area for further explorations. Fourth, studies have shown that people may change their perception of age over time [59]. It is thus possible that the sense of longevity may influence their perceived usefulness, either negatively or positively, when they live longer and longer. Yet it is unknown whether, how, and to what extent aging itself or longevity can improve positive perception about own usefulness. We welcome more studies to shed light onto better understanding of the underlying mechanism of positive perception and longevity. Finally, although to our knowledge the present study is the first to investigate centenarians' own perceptions about their usefulness in comparison with those of non-centenarians, many factors that moderate or mediate the association between self-perception of usefulness, and other factors such as psychosocial and biological traits that are important factors in linking self-perceptions of aging with longevity were not included in the analyses [60]. We hope that in the future more studies will investigate the underlying mechanism between self-perceptions of own aging and longevity.

Conclusions

Based on a large nationally representative multi-wave survey of older adults in China from 2005 to 2014, we found that centenarians were less likely to have a negative perception about their own usefulness compared with younger elders when holding other personal characteristics and conditions equal and compared with those non-centenarian peers of their own birth cohorts. Our findings provided additional evidence to support the notion that centenarians are more positive about their aging. The results from this study could broaden our understanding of how internalized perceptions of aging could have significant consequences for the survival and longevity of older adults in a rapidly aging society.

Abbreviations
ADL: Activities of daily living; CLHLS: Chinese Longitudinal Healthy Longevity Survey; MMSE: Mini-mental status examination; RRR: Relative Risk Ratio

Acknowledgements
Not applicable.

Funding
The authors declare that they have no financial support for this study.

Authors' contributions
DG designed, drafted, and revised the text. DG also supervised the data analysis. YZ, HF, and AG drafted the paper. LQ prepared the data and performed the analyses. KSLC, BW, and DJ revised the paper. All authors read and approved the final version of the manuscript. Views expressed in this paper are solely those of authors, and do not necessarily reflect the views of Nanjing Normal University (China), Mindlink Institute (Hong Kong), New York University, University of Lausanne, or the United Nations.

Competing interests
DG is a section editor of the Journal. and DJ are Associate Editors of the Journal.

Author details
[1]Ginling College, School of Geographical Science, Nanjing Normal University, Nanjing, China. [2]Jiangsu Center for Collaborative Innovation in Geographical Information Resource Development and Application, Nanjing, China. [3]School of Psychology, Nanjing Normal University, Nanjing, China. [4]Ginling College, International Center for Aging Studies, Nanjing Normal University, Nanjing, China. [5]Independent Researcher, New York, USA. [6]Mindlink Institute, Hong Kong, Hong Kong. [7]Rory Meyers College of Nursing and NYU Aging Incubator, New York University, New York, USA. [8]Department of Psychology and National Centre for Research LIVES, University of Lausanne, Lausanne, Switzerland. [9]United Nations Population Division, Two UN Plaza, DC2-1910, New York, NY 10017, USA.

References
1. Allen PM, Mejía ST, Hooker K. Personality, self-perceptions, and daily variability in perceived usefulness among older adults. Psychol Aging. 2015;30(3):534–43.
2. Bryant C, Bei B, Gilson K, Komiti A, Jackson H, Judd F. The relationship between attitudes to aging and physical and mental health in older adults. Int Psychogeriatr. 2012;24(10):1674–83.
3. Chan KW, Hubbard RE. Attitudes to ageing and to geriatric medicine. Turkish J Geriatr. 2014;17(1):90–4.
4. Coleman PG, Ivani-Chalian C, Robinson M. Self and meaning in the lives of older people: Case studies over twenty years. Cambridge: Cambridge University Press; 2015.
5. Gruenewald TL, Karlamangla AS, Greendale GA, Singer BH, Seeman TE. Feelings of usefulness to others, disability, and mortality in older adults: the MacArthur study of successful aging. J Gerontol B Psychol Sci Soc Sci. 2007;62(1):28–37.
6. Gruenewald TL, Karlamangla AS, Greendale GA, Singer BH, Seeman TE. Increased mortality risk in older adults with persistently low or declining feelings of usefulness to others. J Aging Health. 2009;21(2):398–425.
7. Gu D, Brown BL, Qiu L. Self-perceived uselessness is associated with lower likelihood of successful aging among older adults in China. BMC Geriatr. 2016;16(1):172. https://doi.org/10.1186/s12877-016-0348-5.
8. Gu D, Dupre ME, Qiu L. Self-perception of uselessness and mortality among older adults in China. Arch Gerontol Geriatr. 2017;68:186–94.

9. Lakra DC, Ng R, Levy BR. Increased longevity from viewing retirement positively. Ageing Soc. 2012;32(8):1418–27.

10. Levy BR, Myers LM. Relationship between respiratory mortality and self-perceptions of aging. Psychol Health. 2005;20(5):553–64.

11. Levy BR, Slade MD, Kasl SV. Longitudinal benefit of positive self-perceptions of aging on functional health. J Gerontol B Psychol Sci Soc Sci. 2002;57(5):409–17.

12. Moser C, Spagnoli J, Santos-Eggimann B. Self-perception of aging and vulnerability to adverse outcomes at the age of 65-70 years. J Gerontology. 2011;66(6):675–80. https://doi.org/10.1093/geronb/gbr052.

13. Sargent-Cox KA, Anstey KJ, Luszcz MA. The relationship between change in self-perceptions of aging and physical functioning in older adults. Psychol Aging. 2012;27(3):750–60.

14. Wolff JK, Warner LM, Ziegelmann JP, Wurm S. What do targeting positive views on ageing add to a physical activity intervention in older adults? Results from a randomised controlled trial. Psychol Health. 2014; 29(8):915–32.

15. Zhao Y, Dupre ME, Qiu L, Gu D. Changes in perceived uselessness and risks for mortality: evidence from a national sample of older adults in China. BMC Public Health. 2017;17(561):1–9.

16. Levy BR, Zonderman AB, Slade MD, Ferrucci L. Age stereotypes held earlier in life predict cardiovascular events in later life. Psychol Sci. 2009;20(3):296–8.

17. Wurm S, Tesch-Römer C, Tomasik MJ. Longitudinal findings on aging related cognitions, control beliefs and health in later life. J Gerontol B Psychol Sci Soc Sci. 2007;62:156–P164.

18. Law J, Laidlaw K, Peck D. Is depression viewed as an inevitable consequence of age? The "understandability phenomenon" in older people. Clin Gerontol. 2010;33(3):194–209.

19. Levy BR, Banaji MR. Implicit ageism. In: Nelson TD, editor. Ageism: Stereotyping and prejudice against older persons, vol. 2004. Cambridge: MIT Press. p. 49–75.

20. Quinn KM, Laidlaw K, Murray LK. Older peoples' attitudes to mental illness. Clin Psychol Psychother. 2009;16(1):33–45.

21. Bodner E, Cohen-Fridel S. Relations between attachment styles, ageism and quality of life in late life. Int Psychogeriatr. 2010;22(8):1353–61.

22. Bodner E, Cohen-Fridel S, Yaretzky A. Sheltered housing or community dwelling: quality of life and ageism among elderly people. Int Psychogeriatr. 2011;23(8):1197–204.

23. Coudin G, Alexopoulos T. Help me! I'm old!' how negative aging stereotypes create dependency among older adults. Aging Ment Health. 2010;14(5):516–23.

24. Hausdorff JM, Levy BR, Wei JY. The power of ageism on physical function of older persons: reversibility of age-related gait changes. J Am Geriatr Soc. 1999;47(11):1346–9.

25. Levy BR. Mind matters: cognitive and physical effects of aging self-stereotypes. J Gerontol B Psychol Sci Soc Sci. 2003;58(4):203–11.

26. Allen JO. Ageism as a risk factor for chronic disease. The Gerontologist. 2016;56(4):610–4.

27. Levy BR, Slade MD, Kunkel SR, Kasl SV. Longevity increased by positive self-perceptions of aging. J Pers Soc Psychol. 2002;83(2):261–70.

28. Okamoto K, Tanaka Y. Subjective usefulness and 6-year mortality risks among elderly persons in Japan. J Gerontol Psychol Sci. 2004;59(5):246–9.

29. Stewart TL, Chipperfield JG, Perry RP, Weiner B. Attributing illness to 'old age:' consequences of a self-directed stereotype for health and mortality. Psychol Health. 2012;27(8):881–97.

30. Zhao Y, Sautter JM, Qiu L, Gu D. Self-perceived uselessness and associated factors among older adults in China. BMC Geriatr. 2017;17(12):1–19.

31. Andersen-Ranberg K, Chroll M, Jeune B. Healthy centenarians do not exist, but autonomous centenarians do: a population-based study of morbidity among Danish centenarians. J Am Geriatr Soc. 2001;49:900–8.

32. Gu D, Feng Q. Psychological resilience of Chinese centenarians and its associations with survival and health: A fuzzy set analysis. J Gerontolo. 2016; Online first. https://doi.org/10.1093/geronb/gbw071.

33. Kwan JSK, Lau BHP, Cheung KSL. Toward a comparehensive model of frailty: an emerging concept from the Hong Kong centenarian study. JAMDA. 2015;15:536e1–7.

34. Durate N, Teixeira L, Riberio O, Paul C. Frailty phenotype criteria in centenarians: findings from the Oporto centenarian study. Eur Geriatr Med. 2014;5(6):371–6.

35. Evert J, Lawler E, Bogan H, Perls TT. Morbidity profiles of centenarians:

survivors, delayers, escapers. J Gerontol. 2003;58:232–7. https://doi.org/10.1093/gerona/58.3.M232.

36. Jopp DS, Rott C. Adaptation in very old age: exploring the role of resources, beliefs, and attitudes for centenarians' happiness. Psychol Aging. 2006;21(2): 266–80.

37. Gondo Y, Hirose N, Arai Y, et al. Functional status of centenarians in Tokyo, Japan: developing better phenotypes of exceptional longevity. J Gerontol Ser A Biol Sci Med Sci. 2006;61(3):305–10.

38. Perls TT. The different paths to 100. Am J Clin Nutr. 2006;83:484S–7S.

39. Zeng Y, Poston DL Jr, Vlosky DA, Gu D. Healthy longevity in China: demographic, socioeconomic, and psychological dimensions. Dordrecht: Springer Publishing; 2008.

40. Xu Q. Accuracy and validation of age-reporting among the oldest-old in the CLHLS. Market Demogr Anal. 2001;2:1–9 [in Chinese].

41. Zhang X, Dupre ME, Qiu L, Zhou W, Zhao Y, Gu D. Urban-rural differences in the association between access to healthcare and health outcomes among older adults in China. BMC Geriatr. 2017;17(151):1–11.

42. Lee KH, Wu B, Plassman B. Cognitive function and oral health-related quality of life in older adults. J Am Geriatr Soc. 2013;61(9):1602–7. https://doi.org/10.1111/jgs.12402.

43. Wen M, Gu D. The effects of childhood, adult, and community socioeconomic conditions on health and mortality among older adults in China. Demography. 2011;48(1):153–81.

44. Xiang Y, Hao L, Qiu L, Zhao Y, Gu D. Greater financial resources are associated with lower self-perceived uselessness among older adults in China: the urban and rural difference. Arch Gerontol Geriatr. 2018;75:171–80.

45. Winship C, Radbill L. Sampling weights and regression analysis. Sociol Methods Res. 1994;23:230–57.

46. Grippo AJ, Johnson AK. Stress, depression, and cardiovascular dysregulation: a review of neurobiological mechanisms and the integration of research from preclinical disease models. Stress. 2009;12(1):1–21. https://doi.org/10.1080/10253890802046281.

47. Levy BR. Stereotype embodiment: a psychosocial approach to aging. Curr Dir Psychol Sci. 2009;18(6):332–6.

48. von Humboldt S. Conceptual and methodological issues on the adjustment to aging: perspectives on aging well. Lisbon: Springer Publisher; 2016.

49. Baltes PB, Baltes MM. Psychological perspectives on successful aging: the model of selective optimization with compensation. In: Baltes PB, Baltes MM, editors. Successful aging: perspectives from the behavioral sciences. New York: Cambridge University Press; 1990. p. 1–4.

50. Gu D, Feng Q, Zeng Y. Chinese Longitudinal Healthy Longevity Study. In: Pachana N, editor. Encyclopedia of Geropsychology. Singapore: Springer; 2017. p. 469–82. https://doi.org/10.1007/978-981-287-080-3_76-1.

51. Zeng Y, Shen K. Resilience significantly contributes to exceptional longevity. Current Gerontology and Geriatrics Research, 2010, Article ID 525693.

52. Poon LW, Cheung SLK. Centenarian research in the past two decades. Asian J Gerontol Geriatr. 2012;7(1):8–13.

53. Lucas RE. Adaptation and the set-point model of subjective well-being: does happiness change after major life events? Curr Dir Psychol Sci. 2007;16:75–9.

54. Poon LW, Martin P, Bishop A, et al. Understanding centenarians' psychosocial dynamics and their contributions to health and quality of life. Current Gerontology and Geriatrics Research, 2010, Article ID 680657.

55. Dong X, Simon MA, Gorbien M, Percak J, Golden R. Loneliness in older Chinese adults: a risk factor for elder mistreatment. J Am Geriatr Soc. 2007; 55(11):1831–5.

56. Bai X, Lai DWL, Guo A. Ageism and depression: perceptions of older people as a burden in China. J Soc Issues. 2016;72(1):26–46. https://doi.org/10.1111/josi.12154.

57. Qi X. Filial obligation in contemporary China: evolution of the culture system. J Theory Soc Behav. 2015;45(1):141–6.

58. Cheung KSL, Lau BH-P. Successful aging among Chinese near-centenarians and centenarians in Hong Kong: a multidimensional and interdisciplinary approach. Aging Ment Health. 2016;20(12):1314–26.

59. Chopik WJ, Bremner RH, Johnson DJ, Giasson HL. Age differences in age perceptions and developmental transitions. Front Psychol. 9:67. https://doi.org/10.3389/fpsyg.2018.00067.

60. Poon LW, Perls TT. The trails and tribulations of studying the oldest old. In: Poon LW, Perls TT, editors. Annual review of gerontology and geriatrics: biopsychosocial approaches to longevity. New York: Springer; 2007. p. 1–7.

23

Mixed methods developmental evaluation of the CHOICE program: a relationship-centred mealtime intervention for long-term care

Sarah Wu[1], Jill M. Morrison[1], Hilary Dunn-Ridgeway[2], Vanessa Vucea[1], Sabrina Iuglio[1] and Heather Keller[1,2*] (iD)

Abstract

Background: Mealtimes are important to quality of life for residents in long-term care (LTC). CHOICE (which stands for Connecting, Honouring dignity, Offering support, supporting Identity, Creating opportunities, and Enjoyment) is a multi-component intervention to improve relationship-centred care (RCC) and overall mealtime experience for residents. The objective of this developmental evaluation was to determine: a) if the dining experience (e.g. physical, social and RCC practices) could be modified with the CHOICE Program, and b) how program components needed to be adapted and/or if new components were required.

Methods: A mixed methods study conducted between April–November 2016 included two home areas (64 residents; 25 care staff/home management) within a single LTC home in Ontario. Mealtime Scan (MTS), which measures mealtime experience at the level of the dining room, was used to evaluate the effectiveness of CHOICE implementation at four time points. Change in physical, social, RCC dining environment ratings and overall quality of the mealtime experience over time was determined with linear mixed-effects analyses (i.e., repeated measures). Semi-structured interviews ($n = 9$) were conducted with home staff to identify what components of the intervention worked well and what improvements could be made.

Results: Physical and overall mealtime environment ratings showed improvement over time in both areas; one home area also improved social ratings ($p < 0.05$). Interviews revealed in-depth insights into the program and implementation process: i) Knowing the context and culture to meet staff and resident needs; ii) Getting everyone on board, including management; iii) Keeping communication lines open throughout the process; iv) Sharing responsibility and accountability for mealtime goals and challenges; v) Empowering and supporting staff's creative mealtime initiatives.

Conclusions: This developmental evaluation demonstrated the potential value of CHOICE. Findings suggest a need to: extend the time to tailor program components; empower home staff in change management; and provide increased coaching.

Keywords: Dining, Complex intervention implementation, Evaluation, Program development, Implementation science, Mealtimes, Long-term care, Residential care, Relationship-centred care, Personal support workers

* Correspondence: hkeller@uwaterloo.ca
[1]University of Waterloo, 200 University Avenue West, Waterloo, Ontario N2L 3G1, Canada
[2]Research Institute for Aging, 250 Laurelwood Drive, Waterloo, Ontario N2J 0E2, Canada

Background

Mealtimes have the potential to foster and support important and meaningful social relationships over the life course [1, 2]. Consequently, food and mealtimes are considered key aspects of quality of life and satisfaction for residents living in long-term care (LTC) homes [3–5]. Specifically, mealtimes in LTC have the capacity to act as a starting point for creating and sustaining social relationships [6]. The concept of reciprocity is strongly associated with meals [1, 7]; to extend this idea to LTC environments is to arrive at what many refer to as relationship-centred care (RCC), a social model that reflects the "importance of interactions amongst people as the foundation of any therapeutic or healing activity" [8]. The RCC model was purposefully selected for this intervention over the more commonly used philosophy of person-centred care, as it actively situates the resident within their social networks instead of viewing the resident as an unassociated, independent being [9]. Further, we may more effectively position the resident within the context of important and significant relationships (i.e., care staff, dietary aids, home management, etc.) during mealtimes in LTC through the adoption of an RCC model of care [9, 10].

A recent study identifying the determinants of poor food intake among LTC residents found that the mealtime experience and the way care is provided at meals plays a critical role in supporting food intake [11]. Yet, only a handful of intervention studies have attempted to improve the mealtime experience in LTC by intentionally or unintentionally including a psychosocial component in their design [12, 13]. Interventions developed to improve social interaction among residents have focused on the built dining environment, such as smaller dining spaces [14] while others have created meaningful mealtime opportunities for residents through involving them in meal preparation activities, such as making breakfast [15]. Rather than emphasizing the social aspects of routine meals, care staff or volunteer training interventions focus on tasks to promote food intake [12, 13], and no program identified to date has explicitly promoted dignity, honouring of individual identity, or the supporting of social connections between residents and staff at meals. Specifically, no training described in prior research has adopted an RCC model of care as a basis from which to enhance team member (i.e., care staff) capabilities or attempt to change behaviour to enhance reciprocal dining experiences for LTC residents.

Development of the CHOICE program

The concept of the CHOICE Program was developed over several years of research that identified the potential for dining in LTC to be more relationship-focused. Early research by this team identified the role meals played in the family home for persons living with dementia and their family care partners [16]. As families moved into residential environments, the understanding that these meals did not live up to expectations was identified [17]. Observations in a variety of residential environments demonstrated the social engagement and potential for building of relationships for residents and staff [6] and finally the concept of relational dining which encapsulates RCC and person-centred care practices was formed [18]. It was believed that the overall experience of a mealtime that captured physical, social and relationship-centred components could be measured and thus the Mealtime Scan (MTS) was developed and used in a large multi-site study [19]. The way that care was provided, and specifically more person- and relationship-centred was found to be associated with improved food intake [19]. This team then embarked on a journey to develop the CHOICE Program based on this acquired knowledge and experience with mealtimes in LTC settings.

The first step in development of the training program was to articulate more fully what relationship-centred and relational care could look like in the dining room and draw upon important principles from a substantive theory developed in a previous study with persons living with dementia and their care partners on the meaning of mealtimes [17]. This lead to the development of the CHOICE Principles which stand for Connecting, Honouring dignity, Offering support, supporting Identity, Creating opportunities and Enjoyment (Table 1). These principles were discussed at a variety of provider conferences and decision-maker discussion groups to see whether they resonated with those outside of the research program. In line with RCC, the program needed to enhance the mealtime experiences for residents and team members (i.e., Personal Support Workers and Dietary Aids) by changing team member attitudes, knowledge, and behaviour in order to promote and re-emphasize the importance of meaningful social interactions with residents. To be effective and responsive to the changing needs of residents and team members, the CHOICE Program needed to be tailored to the individual home area based on the priorities identified by the team members. Thus, the focus of training was on the principles and how they could be enacted within a specific care setting. Training materials for the CHOICE Program were developed based on models typically utilized by LTC home chains, and where this developmental evaluation was to be conducted. This included: a) a presentation that described each CHOICE Principle, b) scenarios on each principle for staff huddles (i.e., brief direct care staff meetings), c) brainstorming ideas for making specific improvements in physical, social and relationship-centred care, and d) verbal and visual reminders to enact identified ideas for mealtime improvements. The physical dining room and the team members within it were the targets for the intervention.

Table 1 The Six Principles of CHOICE

Connecting	Feeling a sense of togetherness and belonging with others. It is important to get to know who the resident is and how they like to connect with others at mealtimes.
Honouring Dignity	Respecting a resident's decisions, choices, and actions at mealtimes.
Offering Support	Adapting to what a resident needs in the moment. The amount and type of support may change from meal to meal. It is best to ask a resident what they need or want instead of making assumptions.
Supporting Identity	Accepting and acknowledging a resident for who they are today, while working to understand their life story that includes significant events, roles, and important relationships. Who they are will impact how they experience mealtimes.
Creating Opportunities	Engaging in meaningful mealtime roles is important to all of us. Involve residents in familiar or new meal related activities to make them feel a part of a familiar routine.
Enjoyment	Creating a welcoming, relaxed, and friendly dining environment can lead to more enjoyment at mealtimes. Create mealtime events for special occasions, such as birthdays or cultural holidays.

Methods

Study aim

This study describes the developmental evaluation of the CHOICE Program for LTC staff delivered in a single pilot site. The aim of this study is to determine: a) if the mealtime experience (e.g. physical, social and RCC practices) could be modified with the CHOICE Program, and b) how program components needed to be adapted and/or if new components were required.

Research design

Developmental evaluation is used in the early stages of an intervention or program to understand what works and what does not, especially in multi-component programs designed for complex environments [20]. A key purpose of such an evaluation is to learn and adapt the intervention as it is being delivered, and thus a 'bottom-up' approach is needed [20]. This form of evaluation is especially relevant for complex interventions that involve coordination of diverse staff and attempts to change their social interactions with others. As a result, components of CHOICE were revised or discarded and new components developed during the course of this evaluation. An explanatory sequential mixed methods (QUANTITATIVE → qualitative) pre-test post-test time series design was used to evaluate the CHOICE Program. This evaluation began with the collection of quantitative data using the observational tool, the Mealtime Scan for Long-Term Care (MTS), at four time points during a 24-week period. Quantitative results informed the subsequent qualitative data collection using semi-structured interviews [21]. Findings were merged to address study objectives. Ethical clearance was obtained from the University of Waterloo Office of Research Ethics (#21413).

Intervention participants and setting

It was anticipated that learnings would be enhanced and strengthened if two home areas (sometimes referred to as "care units") - Parker and Wellesley (pseudonyms) - in a single LTC were included, as resident differences with respect to eating capacity would likely influence types of team member activities undertaken to make improvements. The LTC home was located in Southern Ontario, Canada, and is part of an Ontario chain of for-profit homes. The Schlegel-University of Waterloo Research Institute for Aging (RIA) facilitated the incubation of this innovation in a research-friendly home so that the learnings from this work could contribute to the acceleration and eventual mobilization of the innovation to the broader LTC sector. The participating home has a total of 192 beds within 6 home areas and was also selected based on a self-identified need to refocus team member efforts on resident mealtimes. As well, this home had minimal prior exposure to external mealtime-focused research initiatives. As the quantitative data collection procedure was based on dining room-level observations, written consent was not required as per the University of Waterloo Office of Research Ethics from individual team members and residents, as only global aspects of the mealtime experience were being assessed. Informational posters and newsletters were provided to residents, families, and team members prior to the start of implementation to ensure that everyone who lived and worked in this home area was aware of the initiative and the use of observations to measure potential changes. Signs were posted advising the home areas when meal observations were to occur. Those care team members and home management who played critical roles in the implementation of the CHOICE Program were invited to participate in interviews in the qualitative phase; informed written consent was provided.

Implementation overview

Prior to pilot implementation, the research team (i.e., Principal Investigator HK, HD Study Coordinator, and doctoral student, SW) met with the home's administrators to discuss program components, implementation process, and potential barriers and facilitators of care team behaviour change during mealtimes (Table 2). A mutual agreement was reached on study timeline (i.e., 8-month involvement of care staff implementation process and evaluation), time commitments (i.e., time dedicated to staff huddles and coaching phone calls), support resources

Table 2 CHOICE Intervention Components and Functions

Intervention Components	Description	Dosage	Frequency over 8 months
Education Session and Training Modules	Overview of program components and best-practices to enhance mealtime experience for residents using relationship-centred approaches. Education session was developed into training module to ensure all staff received education sessions.	45 min./home area	1 per home area or as needed for new hires/refresher for current team members
Staff Huddles and Huddle Diary	Mealtime-focused huddles scheduled during shift changeover to promote CHOICE Principles, problem-solve, record progress in huddle diaries, and facilitate communication between care staff.	5–10 min./huddle	1 x week or as needed
Visual Reminders	Posters provided weekly reminders of each CHOICE Principle for care staff and posted strategically around dining room and servery.	1 poster/week	2–3 posters per dining room or as needed
Reference Binder	CHOICE reference binder provided resources staff would need to carry out program, including program overview, huddle schedule, huddle diary sheets, and reminder posters.	1 binder/home area	As needed by care staff and leadership
MT Champion Meetings	Teleconference meetings held when CHOICE Coach not on site in order to discuss progress, identify areas for improvement, problem-solve, and identify ways to respond to MTS feedback. In-person meetings held when Coach on site.	10–20 min/home area	1 per week
Continuous Feedback	Progress reports were generated based on MTS data collected by external auditors. Reports were reviewed by the MT Champions, DFS, project coordinator, with the research team prior to being shared with the care staff and other home administrators. Reports assisted in identifying areas that had improved and/or needed improvement	Comprehensive report based on MTS Data.	Baseline, 8 weeks, 16 weeks, 28 weeks for each home area (missing 5th meal audit because of outbreak)
CHOICE Coach	CHOICE Coach worked closely with MT Champions and DFS to facilitate and support each component of CHOICE program and assist in tailoring components when needed. Coach provided feedback on barriers and facilitators of program components, implementation process, and important contextual factors, such as organizational climate.	In-person visit: 5–7 h per home area. MT Champion Meetings 10–20 min.	In-person visit 2 per month for 5 months for each home area. Teleconference 1 per week for 3 months.

Abbreviations: *MT* mealtime, *MTS* Mealtime Scan, *DFS* director of food service

(i.e., informational resources on care delivery, program print materials), and outcome goals (i.e., what was feasible for each home area to achieve in this program). The home's administrators identified two Mealtime Champions (MT Champions) per home area to act as leaders to guide fellow team members through the implementation process. MT Champions play a critical role as point of contact for the interventionists as a way to give and receive feedback during implementation. The MT Champions were selected based on: a) their interest and dedication to care improvement, b) their positive social influence among their colleagues and reciprocated respect they received, and c) full-time employment to ensure their knowledge of the home area. Each home area attempted to work on one CHOICE Principle at a time to raise awareness and identify areas for improvement. Flexibility in the program allowed home areas to spend as much time as needed on a principle. The Director of Food

Services (DFS), acted as both an internal resource and CHOICE advocate to hold the team members within each home area accountable to their goals each week. It became apparent immediately that the MT Champions and DFS needed further support post training to stimulate change among the care team. The research team took on this role collectively; the PI provided support on techniques and theory to make change; the study coordinator who was an employee of the RIA facilitated communications among home management, the dining team and the researchers, while the doctoral student visited the site, initially with the study coordinator, and took on the role of 'CHOICE Coach' on-site as the implementation progressed. The Coach visited the study site twice per month for 5 months, spending 1 day in each home area to attend team member huddles, support the completion of the huddle diary, observe mealtimes, gain feedback from team members and residents, and strategize and problem-solve with the MT Champions. She also took this time to meet with the DFS to review progress reports generated by the research team using MTS results in order to strategize on ways to support team members in areas identified as needing improvement. Over the last 3 months of implementation, the Coach reduced in-person presence in order to promote capacity and independence among the MT Champions and team members; however, bi-weekly coaching teleconference meetings continued with the research team.

As the MT Champions and the DFS started to consider how to make improvements, it was recognized that they needed coaching on change management. The Theoretical Domains Framework was chosen as a basis for coaching on strategies to make change [22, 23]. In this framework, fourteen domains (i.e., knowledge, skill, beliefs about capabilities, intentions, goals, etc.) can be condensed into three core components in relation to behaviour change: capability, opportunity, and motivation (e.g. COM-B; [24]). The COM-B model was selected specifically for this LTC intervention as it places emphasis on the importance of context (i.e., opportunity) when looking to change behaviour, which is critical when designing feasible and acceptable interventions for health care environments. Without explicitly educating team members on this framework, coaching was provided by the research team to support the adoption, uptake and execution of the program components. For example, celebrating success was an incentive to further motivate team members to complete a specific care activity.

The intervention evolved over the course of the pilot, as is typical of developmental evaluation [20]. It ultimately included 8 components that supported team members in their change efforts, as outlined in Table 2. Team members and the research team worked to tailor these components over the course of the implementation process to meet specific needs of the individual home areas. For example, the in-person educational session on CHOICE Principles was translated into an online education module and made available on the home's intranet training platform for those team members and administrators who were not present for the in-person sessions, as well as new team member hires.

Quantitative phase
Data collection
To understand impact of CHOICE on mealtime processes and interactions among residents and team members, several mealtime observations were conducted every two months using a standardized tool. Mealtime audits were completed with the Mealtime Scan [MTS] [25]. This observational tool is a construct valid and reliable assessment that measures the psychosocial environment, as well

as physical aspects of a dining environment that impact the mealtime experience [25, 26]. Observations are conducted at the dining room level, and not at the individual resident level, to attain an overall impression and summary of key aspects of the observed meal. As part of this developmental evaluation, a modified version of MTS was trialed to determine its responsiveness to the intervention. Modifications as recommended after extensive use [11, 25] included more detailed tracking of social interactions and improved scaling of items (i.e. dichotomous items changed to a 0–4 scale) that are intended to promote responsiveness to change over time. The physical environment meter (e.g. temperature, sound, humidity, and illumination) was removed from the original tool, as the protocol to collect these data was potentially disruptive to mealtimes [25]. In addition to the physical, social and person/relationship-centred summative scales included on the original MTS, a summative scale was also created to capture the overall quality of the dining environment; preliminary data demonstrated good inter-rater reliability of this summative scale (intraclass correlation coefficient = 0.76; unpublished). Maximum score for these four MTS summative scales was 8. Further details on the MTS are described in Keller et al., 2018 [25].

Two trained assessors arrived in their respective dining room several minutes before the scheduled meal start time, before residents entered, and continued observation until the end of the meal when most residents had left the dining room. Data collection was originally planned to be carried out at baseline, 8 weeks, 16 weeks, 24 weeks, and 32 weeks, however, due to concerns about illness outbreak and other home events (i.e., special events, accreditation, etc.), data collection could not be carried out at Week 32. At each of the four time points, the MTS was completed at 5 meals (1 breakfast, 2 lunches, 2 dinners) over a two-day period. Five meals had been previously used to assess the mealtime environment [25] in a large multi-site study and found to represent the meal context. The same assessor completed all assessments ($n = 20$) in the same assigned home area throughout the study to promote consistency.

Resident-level data were collected from the inter-RAI Minimum Data Set (MDS) to characterize those living in each area. Data included residents' age, sex, Cognitive Performance Score (CPS), and Activities of Daily Life – Long Form (ADL-LF). CPS is an ordinal scale from 0 to 6 that rates residents on their cognitive capacity, where 0 = intact condition and 6 = high cognitive impairment [27]. For this analysis, CPS score was dichotomized into two groups: CPS < 3 and CPS ≥ 3 to differentiate between distinct levels of cognitive capacity. The ADL-LF is a 7-item summary scale that measures a resident's capacity to perform activities of daily living (i.e., transfers, toilet use, and eating). Higher values on the continuous score (maximum = 28) indicate more impairment on ADLs [28].

Data analysis

To provide context, descriptive comparisons were made between home areas based on resident data and mealtime characteristics that were not expected to change with the intervention (e.g., number of residents, staff) using chi-square or two-sample t-tests (or non-parametric equivalent, e.g., Wilcoxon signed rank test). Each of the four MTS summative scales and subscales (e.g. Mealtime Relational Care Checklist) were tested for normality and described (mean, standard deviation [SD]) by time point and dining room. Linear mixed models (Proc MIXED) with repeated measures over time within dining room were used to analyze each of the four MTS summative scales as outcomes. Dining room, time point (categorical with time 0 as referent), and the interaction between dining room and time point were included in the model as independent variables tested as fixed effects. As both home areas received the CHOICE program, there was no control. The time effect demonstrated the potential for the MTS scales to change over time with implementation of the program, while time-home area interactions demonstrate differences by home area in this effect. Data were analyzed using SAS® Studio Statistical Software (SAS Institute Inc., Cary, North Carolina). Statistical significance was determined at $p < 0.05$ unless otherwise specified.

Qualitative phase
Data collection

Semi-structured interviews were used to explain quantitative results rather than confirm. Specifically, interviews identified what program components worked well (e.g. using data to stimulate change, educational activities), the implementation process (e.g. use of champions to lead effort), especially as it varied among home areas. Key informants were recruited based on their involvement with the implementation of the CHOICE Program (i.e., MT Champions, management, highly involved team members) at the completion of the study. Interview guides for team members and home management were developed based on key findings from the progress reports generated for each home area (i.e., MTS data over time). In particular, the following areas were addressed during the interviews:

- *Team members:* their perceptions of the impact of the intervention on resident mealtime experience; their experiences adopting and carrying out intervention components; their opinions on how the program could be improved and sustained; what mealtime changes were noticed
- *Home Management:* their perceptions of the program components and how they were received

by team members; their experiences with the implementation process; how better to support team members to sustain the program; what mealtime changes were noticed.

In addition, brief qualitative comments were recorded by each of the auditors on each MTS audit form to account for and contextualize unusual events that may have impacted a particular meal's score during MTS observations. These were reviewed and used to support the linkage between quantitative and qualitative findings. Interviews were conducted by the CHOICE Coach (SW) over one month following the end of the intervention in November 2016.

Data analysis

Data analyses were conducted concurrently with data collection conducted by SW until informational redundancy was reached [29]. Interviews were transcribed verbatim and were then analyzed using a generalized inductive approach, whereby codes were applied to small segments of data and individual codes collapsed into larger categories that were interpreted into themes [30]. Emergent codes and the formation of categories and overarching themes were reviewed and discussed with co-authors HK, VV, and SI throughout analysis. The analytical process focused on the intervention implementation, the intervention components, and the changes that occurred during mealtimes on each home area. MTS text data was coded deductively and incorporated into the main interview themes in order to contextualize findings to the dining areas [31].

Results

A total of 64 residents resided in the two home areas that participated in the study (Wellesley $n = 32$; Parker $n = 32$). Descriptive characteristics of residents are presented in Table 3. The average age of residents from both home areas was 85 years, with the majority of residents being female (70%). Data from the Minimum Data

Table 3 Resident Characteristics of Two Home Areas ($N = 64$)

Characteristic	Both Home Areas ($N = 64$)	Wellesley ($n = 32$)	Parker ($n = 32$)
Age, mean (SD)	85 (11.7)	84 (13.3)	85 (10.0)
Male (n)	30.4% (4)	26.1% (6)	34.8% (8)
CPS Score,[a] mean (SD)	2.6 (1.7)	3.1 (1.5)	2.0 (1.7)
Moderate/severe impairment (n)	52.2% (24)	65.2% (15)	39.1% (9)
ADL-LF[b] Score, mean (SD)	16.4 (8.7)	16.9 (9.3)	16.0 (8.3)

[a]*CPS* Cognitive Performance Scale, scoring 0–6; scores ≥3 indicate moderate/severe cognitive impairment

[b]*ADL-LF* Activities of Daily Living Long Form Scale, scoring 0–28 with higher scores indicating more impairment of ADL independence performance

Note: Home areas were not significantly different on any of the resident characteristics, $p < 0.05$

Set (MDS, [28]) collected during the baseline period indicates that 65% of residents living in Wellesley had a Cognitive Performance Scale (CPS) Score of 3 or greater, as compared to Parker where less than half of residents showed signs of significant cognitive impairment (CPS ≥ 3); this difference was not statistically significant. Residents in the two home areas did not differ on mean ADL-LF scores. However, the observations from the MTS indicated that Wellesley had a significantly greater number of residents who required assistance with tasks related to eating (mean = 4.8 ± 0.9 persons/meal) than Parker (mean = 3.8 ± 1.2; $p < 0.01$).

A total of 16 team members (10 Personal Support Workers (PSW), 3 Dietary Aids (DA), 2 Registered Practical Nurse (RPN), 1 Recreational Therapist) and 5 members of home management (2 home area coordinators, 1 DFS, 1 Assistant DFS, 1 Director of Care, 1 quality indicators manager) received CHOICE training. Four PSWs, two from each home area, were selected as MT Champions by home management. However, half way through the implementation process only one Champion remained on each unit due to staff scheduling changes.

Quantitative phase
Descriptive characteristics of two dining areas assessed by MTS
The two dining areas were statistically different in key physical characteristics over the course of the intervention (Table 4); Parker had more residents eating in the dining room than Wellesley ($t = -5.86$, $p < 0.0001$). The total number of team members in either dining room did not significantly differ. However, in terms of team members' mealtime activities, a statistical significant difference was found between the number of team members passing food (Wilcoxon; z = − 4.68, $p < 0.0001$) as well as the number of team members assisting residents with their meals (Wilcoxon; z = 4.06, $p < 0.0001$) with Wellesley having fewer food servers, but more team members assisting with eating. There was no observed difference between the number of family/volunteers present during meals, nor the number of residents eating outside the main dining area.

MTS changes over time by home area
Five meals were observed at each of four time-points in each dining room, for a total of 20 mealtime observations per home area. Linear mixed models were used to determine change in MTS summative scales (i.e., physical environment, social environment, and overall quality of mealtime environment) over time for both home areas. Table 5 presents the descriptive data for each of the summative scales at each time point by home area. After adjusting for repeated measures across time within each dining room, the physical ($p < 0.01$), social ($p = 0.02$), and overall quality ($p = 0.02$) of the dining environment were significantly different, with improvements in Parker for all three scales, while Wellesley did not experience an improvement in the social summative scale. Of the MTS subscales there were several differences between dining rooms, however, only the Mealtime Relational Care Checklist score showed a significant improvement over time ($p < 0.01$) (Additional file 1: Table S1) [26].

Models of the social environment and overall quality scores demonstrated significant interactions between home area and time. Significant interactions indicate that changes in these MTS scores across the time points varied by dining room; the intervention's effect was not consistent over time for the two home areas. Figures 1 and 2 display the difference in change from baseline of social environment score and the overall mealtime environment rating between Wellesley and Parker. The social environment scores slightly decreased in Wellesley over the four observation points, whereas Parker's social environment improved (Figure 1; Table 5). Overall quality of dining environment improved for Parker, however, Wellesley had a more modest improvement maintained for this scale from baseline (Figure 2; Table 5).

Qualitative phase
Nine interviews were conducted with four PSWs (two of whom were MT Champions), two DAs, two home management members (HM), and one registered nurse (RN). Six themes emerged from the analysis. In addition, we provide key learnings and/or materials developed in response to the

Table 4 Descriptive Characteristics of Two Dining Areas Assessed by MTS Over All Observed Meals ($n = 40$)

Variable	Both Home Areas	Wellesley	Parker
Residents in dining room, mean (SD)	24.3 (2.90)	22.4 (1.98)	26.3 (2.27)*
Any staff who entered dining room during meal observation, mean (SD)	6.7 (1.38)	7.2 (1.42)	6.3 (1.23)
Staff serving food[a], mean (SD)	2.1 (0.94)	1.4 (0.51)	2.8 (0.77)*
Staff assisting residents to eat[a], mean (SD)	2.6 (0.98)	3.2 (0.70)	2.0 (0.82)*
Family/Volunteers, mean (SD)	0.6 (0.89)	0.4 (0.59)	1.0 (1.05)
% of meals where at least 1 resident eating meal in adjacent area, % (freq.)	55.0 (22)	63.6 (14)	36.4 (8)

*Difference between home areas is statistically significant, $p < 0.001$
[a]Staff involved in meal service included full-time and part-time staff, LPN, and DA
Abbreviations: *MTS* Mealtime scan, *SD* Standard Deviation

Table 5 Descriptive and Linear Mixed Model Analysis of MTS Summative Global Scores At Each Time Point By Home Area

Time Point (weeks)	Descriptives by dining room		Mixed model analysis with interaction	
	Summative Scale Scores, Mean (SD)[a]		Effect	p-value[b]
	Wellesley	Parker		
	Physical Environment		Physical Environment	
0	5.2 (0.84)	4.8 (0.45)	Dining Room	0.37
8	5.6 (0.89)	4.6 (0.89)	Time	< 0.01
16	4.6 (0.55)	5.2 (0.45)	Dining Room x Time	0.09
24	6.2 (0.84)	6.2 (0.45)		
	Social Environment		Social Environment	
0	5.4 (1.14)	4.4 (0.55)	Dining Room	0.04
8	4.4 (0.55)	4.6 (0.89)	Time	0.02
16	3.0 (1.00)	5.6 (1.14)	Dining Room x Time	< 0.01
24	5.2 (1.30)	6.0 (0.71)		
	Relationship-Centred Care		Relationship-Centred Care	
0	4.4 (1.14)	4.2 (0.45)	Dining Room	0.15
8	5.0 (0.71)	4.8 (0.84)	Time	0.40
16	3.8 (1.30)	5.6 (0.55)	Dining Room x Time	0.09
24	4.8 (1.30)	5.2 (1.10)		
	Overall Quality of Dining Environment		Overall Quality of Dining Environment	
0	4.8 (0.84)	4.2 (0.45)	Dining Room	0.41
8	5.0 (0.71)	4.6 (0.89)	Time	0.02
16	4.2 (0.84)	5.6 (0.55)	Dining Room x Time	0.02
24	5.4 (0.89)	5.8 (0.84)		

[a] $n = 5$ observations per time point per dining room
[b] P-values from type 3 test of fixed effects

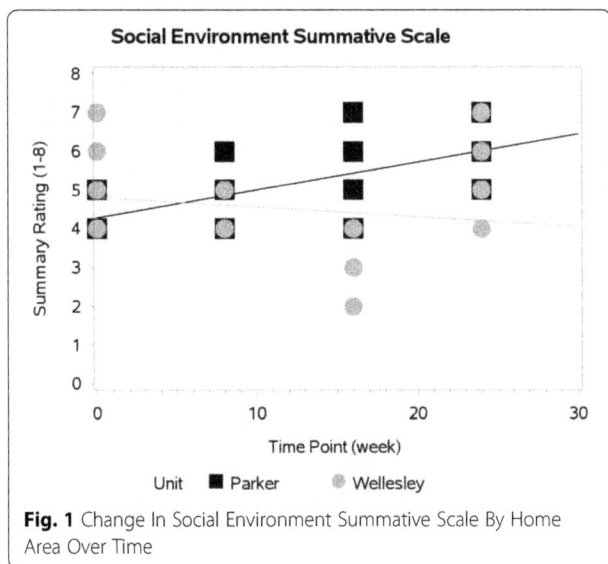

Fig. 1 Change In Social Environment Summative Scale By Home Area Over Time

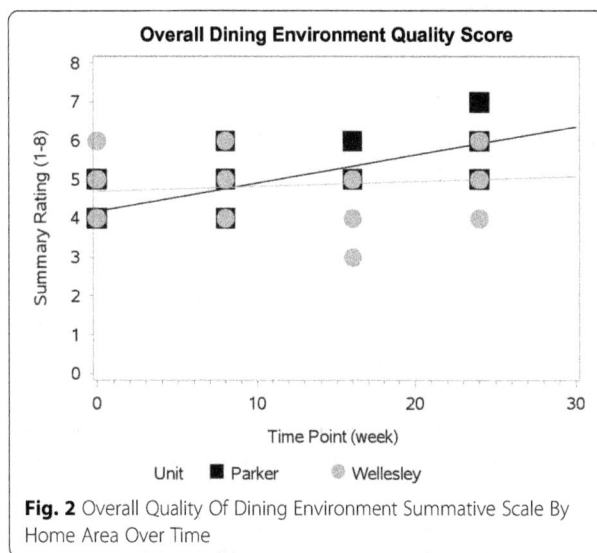

Fig. 2 Overall Quality Of Dining Environment Summative Scale By Home Area Over Time

needs of each dining room identified during the implementation process for each theme (Table 6).

New appreciation for mealtimes: "It's not about us, it's about them"

After implementation of the CHOICE Program, all participants expressed a new appreciation and greater understanding of the importance of the mealtime experience for residents in their home areas, *"I'm going to be honest, we forget that we are in their dining room"* (PSW 2). Leadership saw CHOICE as *"a great opportunity for [them] to take a look at [the dining experience] more in-depth."* (MG 2), but as demonstrated in both qualitative and quantitative data, this was only a start to making change within each of the home areas. The program also served as a way to reflect on how team members' behaviours impacted residents' mealtimes, *"I feel like it was a really big eye-opener about things we could change and how me and [the other team members] were acting in the dining room. These are human beings – they're not robots. This is their home and we should be engaging with them"* (PSW 3).

Knowing the context and culture

Dining rooms in Wellesley and Parker differed in terms of context and subculture, which meant that strategies to make change that worked well in one home area did not necessarily work well in the other. Gaining an understanding and appreciation for these differences meant tailoring how the CHOICE Principles were enacted to meet the mealtime needs of team members and residents. Characteristics of each home area (e.g., differences in the number of residents needing eating assistance) influenced which improvements could be easily adopted, and why others were not as acceptable; context drove what was done to improve dining and how it was implemented. As one RN explained, *"Wellesley is one of our heavier care units where we do struggle with team members a lot. I think that was a barrier in the research"* (RN). As there were more residents who required eating assistance on Wellesley, less team members were available to partake in mealtime processes such as serving food and socializing with residents.

Getting everyone on board

Interviews identified the importance of ensuring that care team members and management were aware of what would be involved in implementing the CHOICE Program from the outset. For example, team members felt that reassurance was needed in order to spend additional time socializing with residents without being penalized, *"You can't sit down [at the dining table with residents], you're going to get in trouble if the general manager walks on the floor and you're sitting down"* (PSW 1). Team members believed that CHOICE would

give them the opportunity to dedicate their time and efforts to meals, *"I hear that a lot, 'we don't have time to get to talk with them or help them more than we want to'. So, this was actually the time when you can do it."* (DA 2). However, dedicated time to the implementation process was identified by some leadership as difficult to achieve, *"I would have loved to have been more involved in it, but I found myself at times... I get pulled in every direction"* (HM 1). Restrictions in leadership's ability to both dedicate time to the implementation process, as well as being aware of the additional time that team members require to execute CHOICE meal practices, may help to explain the lack of change in some aspects of the mealtime experience, such as a more relaxed dining environment, *"knowing that management is well aware that mealtime is going to take a bit longer"* (PSW 3).

Keeping communication lines open

Communication between the research team, team members, and leadership was needed in order to problem-solve and overcome barriers throughout the implementation process. In-person contact was made by the CHOICE Coach, MT Champion, and leadership on a bi-weekly basis; however, mechanisms that supported more frequent communication were needed between the two home areas. In response, the research team began teleconferences with MT Champions and leadership during those weeks where the CHOICE Coach was not on site. Selecting MT Champions who possessed effective communication skills and were respected by their co-workers was also vital to spreading the CHOICE Principles and components, *"to be honest, you picked a really good communicator... Communication, I think, is the biggest thing"* (DA1).

Sharing responsibilities and accountability

Team members and leadership expressed the need for accountability as a source of motivation for themselves to both critically evaluate current mealtime practices and to re-consider ways to improve mealtime experience for residents, *"With having you guys there, I noticed a lot of things that are wrong with our dining room service. The first time when you came, I thought, 'Oh, we do everything great'. Well, these past couple of days I've noticed so many things that are wrong."* (DA2). Self-reflection and accountability to the research team and CHOICE Coach served as motivation for team members and leadership to focus on their weekly mealtime goals. Feeding back results from the mealtime audits specifically to champions and leadership also supported this accountability. Leadership recognized the need to be present in the home areas if the program was to be sustainable, *"We really need to make our spot checks, we need to ensure that what we're saying is actually happening. Follow through and follow-up – that's a huge component"* (HM 2).

Table 6 Learnings and Improvements to the CHOICE Program

Findings	Learnings	Planned Improvements to Program
New Appreciation for Mealtimes: "It's not about us; it's about them."	• CHOICE provided dedicated time for care staff and management to reflect and reconsider the meaning of mealtimes within their home area. • Care staff took advantage of this opportunity to share insights, learnings, and revelations amongst care teams as another way to reinforce the importance of what they are undertaking. • Staff huddles and meetings serve as a great opportunity to engage in self-reflection.	• Staff huddles and meetings proved to be more beneficial to staff to communicate with one another than using Huddle Diaries. The use of diaries ceased, which left additional time for staff to consider what aspect of mealtimes were improving, and what needed more attention. • Self-reflection based on checklists of relationship-centred care practices at mealtimes. • Adapting training on CHOICE Principles to video to allow for individual review and goal setting.
Knowing context and culture	• Additional time is needed prior to implementation to tailor the intervention components to each home area, support communication across all stakeholders and build consensus on what needs to be improved. • Changes to both the physical and social environment can improve the mealtime experience. Taking time to reflect on both environments and how they interact with one another is important. • Spending time with staff discussing how each CHOICE Principle would be enacted during their mealtimes and collectively identifying specific approaches to make change as opposed to offering vague recommendations that are not relevant to their context.	• Program extended to 52 weeks to allow for a preparatory phase where a CHOICE Dining Team is developed and trained on change management techniques. • Engagement of the residents, family and greater team with baseline findings and what areas need to be improved and identification of priority areas for change based on the perspectives of all stakeholders • Self-assessment checklist for mealtime practices as well as physical aspects of dining. • CHOICE Dining Team takes priority areas identified by family, residents and the greater care team and develops concrete action plans that are negotiated and communicated with all stakeholders in the area.
Getting everyone on board	• Additional time spent at the early stages of implementation to ensure that everyone understands what changes need to be made is critical to buy-in from care staff and management. • The development of a dining team that includes members from home management would assist in tailoring implementation components that were acceptable and feasible for a specific home area • Basic change management principles should become part of educational component for Mealtime Champions (and a dining team) so that home areas can utilize implementation methods and tools that work best for their home area.	• Greater team engagement and self-reflection checklists mentioned above to bring awareness as to what aspects of mealtimes could be improved. • CHOICE Dining Team to include residents, family, care team champions, management and CHOICE Coach; ownership and leadership transferred from Coach to home members over the course of the implementation. • Training components for the CHOICE Dining Team on change management; mentorship by Coach on change management principles.
Keeping communication lines open	• More frequent communication was needed between the CHOICE Coach, the Mealtime Champions, and the home area for guidance and support in determining what aspects of mealtimes to target and how to go about it. • Once implementation is underway, clear and consistent methods of communication are needed to understand how the intervention is progressing and what support is needed in the home area.	• Establish communication processes with Choice Dining Team and greater team, including residents and family. • Use a variety of communication formats to reach diverse audiences and once established use consistently.
Sharing responsibilities and accountability	• The CHOICE Program gave the home areas the opportunity and space to reflect on how mealtimes could be improved and what their roles were to make changes. • Mealtime Champions expressed additional pressure associated with the responsibility of leading the change efforts in their home areas. • The development of a Dining Team would assist in sharing some of the change management tasks that were originally given to the Mealtime Champions.	• Development of a CHOICE Dining Team to share responsibility and promote accountability. • Use of informal audit of new practices to promote accountability and embedding.

Table 6 Learnings and Improvements to the CHOICE Program *(Continued)*

Findings	Learnings	Planned Improvements to Program
Empowering and supporting creativity	• From the outset of implementation, care staff and management need to collaborate to identify feasible mealtime improvements and change management strategies that work best for their home area. • Care staff have creative ideas and solutions to improve the mealtime experience for residents, however, they require time, resources, and support to make them a reality.	• CHOICE Dining Team needs to include a management representative to facilitate some changes considered a priority. • To ensure that care staff do not feel overwhelmed with change efforts, 1–2 CHOICE Principles could be prioritized. • Provide opportunities for engaging staff in identifying solutions; potentially post review of evaluation data to stimulate priority setting and motivation for change.

Empowering and supporting creativity

Leadership and team members were the experts in knowing how CHOICE Principles could be enacted, what would be feasible and acceptable within the subculture and context of their home area. Part way through implementation and with the help of the CHOICE Coach they felt empowered to make the CHOICE Principles their own. Several team members took the initiative to implement creative ways to enhance the mealtime experience for residents, *"Having the ideas and trying them, and then once you've tried them it gives you the motivation to think of other things" (PSW 4)*. For instance, team members took it upon themselves to bake bread in the living room so as to entice residents' appetites, which may have contributed to the significant improvement in the overall MTS physical environment score. Other team members held weekly Supper Clubs that involved a theme dinner with costumes, decorations, and music. These efforts were reflected in the MTS analysis where both the physical environment and overall mealtime ambiance scores improved over time. Ensuring that all team members felt that they had the capacity and opportunity to implement CHOICE was identified by team members as an area for improvement, in particular, the need for more reflection and hands-on approaches beyond education. In addition, targeting casual and part-time team members was identified as a priority to *"get them more comfortable with serving in the dining room, so that it's not always the same people, so that they all get those skills and they're more well-rounded" (DA 1)*.

Discussion

Mealtimes are often the most anticipated daily event for residents living in LTC homes. However, opportunities for meaningful social engagement are oftentimes missed within these settings, where the communal dining room can result in the pleasurable aspects of a mealtime coming second to concerns surrounding efficiency and sufficient food intake [4, 32]. It is the authors' contention that if mealtime experiences support relationships and positive social connections (a necessary aspect of quality of life), that improvements in nutritional intake will follow [11]. Team members and home management have an important role in assisting in defining and promoting a culture of care that centers around relationships, as it is this culture that ultimately impacts how residents experience their mealtimes [33].

This mixed methods developmental evaluation looked to determine whether the CHOICE Program was an intervention that was worthy of further development and testing. Despite each home identifying different areas for improvement, meta-inferences from both the quantitative and qualitative phases showed that the CHOICE Principles resonated with team members and were seen as a goal for dining. Those who were involved believed that the program was useful for addressing some of the challenges associated with mealtimes in their home areas [34]. Team members and management expressed a re-kindled appreciation for mealtimes and noted visible improvements in mealtime experiences in both home areas.

While the CHOICE Principles resonated with team members as a way to improve mealtimes, the feasibility of implementing and carrying out ways in which the principles could be enacted proved to be more challenging than initially anticipated. For example, as residents on Wellesley needed more one-on-one assistance with eating, there were fewer team members available to walk around the dining room to encourage conversation amongst residents and thus reach the goal of Connecting (refer to Table 1 for CHOICE Principles definitions). In this case, the motivation to perform certain aspects of the CHOICE Program on Wellesley was not the issue; it was a matter of addressing the feasibility of how that principle could be enacted within the context in order to create the opportunity for team members to engage in more socialization with residents. One strategy was inclusion of a recreation therapist at meals to support the care team. Contextual differences between home areas, played an important role in shaping how the CHOICE Principles were interpreted and enacted during meals; this confirms that linear, structured approaches to care within the LTC setting [4, 35] is a barrier to improvements that are contextually driven. When looking to build upon this developmental evaluation, there is a need to be responsive to influencing factors at the management and home levels that may hinder or promote the uptake of change initiatives early on in the implementation process [36, 37].

In addition, differences in improvements between the two home areas and feedback from interview participants reveal that more time with the Coach would have been beneficial to build capacity for both teamwork and change management techniques before change efforts were undertaken. No doubt, the large geographic distance (280 km) between the research team and the LTC resulted in less face-to-face time than what may have been needed with the home. This made it difficult to meet the needs of some team members and MT Champions during especially challenging times in the implementation process. Modifications to the CHOICE Program should acknowledge the face-time needed by the Coach [38] in order to empower team members, specifically MT Champions [39], so that they feel confident in applying change management approaches when tailoring principles in their home areas [40, 41]. Table 6 outlines key learnings and outcomes based on findings from this study, in addition to planned improvements for the future development of the CHOICE Program.

Working to make mealtimes more relationship-centred

Results from this developmental evaluation demonstrate the potential for the CHOICE Program to improve some aspects of the mealtime experience, namely physical and overall quality of the dining environment. It is important to note however, that these changes were not necessarily experienced in both home areas to the same extent. For example, although there was a significant time by dining room change noted in the social summative scale, there was a decrease in performance for one area (Wellesley = 5.4 to 5.2) over time. From baseline, one home area improved the overall quality of the environment significantly more than the other, demonstrating that comparisons across neighbourhoods can be challenging, as they are not equivalent with respect to their capacity for improvement. In areas where residents have significant dementia, social interactions are likely to never be high due to their limited verbal capacity. Relationship-centred care may also be challenging due to the higher demands for hands-on care. The physical and overall quality of the mealtime experience, which significantly improved in both areas included in this pilot, appear to be more readily changeable with the CHOICE program. These findings not only reinforce the need to account for contextual differences between environments, but also to temper expectations as to what can realistically be achieved within a short-period of time based on staffing and team member skills as well as the capacity of residents. Making improvements to an organization's care culture and social environment has been noted to be a challenging task [42] that requires additional time and effort when compared to making improvements to the physical dining environment [11]. Often such cultural changes require targeting roles and responsibilities with added quality supervision on the part of home leadership [36]. Thus, it is recommended that the feasible changes to the built environment be targeted in the initial stages of the implementation process, as altering the physical dining environment (i.e., clock on wall, decorations on table, music playing) provides visible improvements that change-making is underway.

Study limitations

Future evaluation of CHOICE should consider the use of a wait list control through a stepped-wedge design rather than a randomized control trial, as this pilot clearly demonstrated that the context of units greatly influences uptake and discernible change. Methodological limitations of this study include the MTS potentially being too insensitive, with too few observations, to capture the gradual improvements that team members and leadership referred to during interviews [25]. The issue of social desirability from interview participants may have led to responses, which may not have been entirely reflective of their experiences implementing the program. As well, there is the potential for confirmation bias, as the interventionist was the interviewer. Other forms of quantitative assessment to capture improvements should include team members' perspectives on mealtimes and dyads of the resident and family members. Furthermore, it should be noted that because of an illness outbreak at the LTC home, we were unable to capture the last point of data collection at 32 weeks, which may have indicated further improvements in the dining environment. Staff turnover was a barrier to continuity with initial study participants; most notably, a key individual from the home's management team was unable to participate in the interview process due to extenuating circumstances, which would have undoubtedly revealed critical insights into the feasibility and acceptability of the program. The research team appreciates the importance of the inclusion of family and residents in a relationship-centred intervention, however, these perspectives were not attained in this evaluation. Future development of the CHOICE Program will extend qualitative data collection to family and residents as well.

Conclusions

The CHOICE Program demonstrated that it was possible to improve some aspects of the mealtime experience in two home areas within a relatively short period of time. Capacity for improvements in relationship-centred and social interactions appear to be more challenging and less consistent, as they are likely influenced by resident care needs (e.g. need for eating assistance). CHOICE gave team members and home management the opportunity to (re)-consider the importance of mealtimes for residents living in LTC homes. Tailoring program components and implementation methods is absolutely critical for initial uptake and sustainability of change efforts. This involves including not only team members in the implementation of CHOICE, but also a vested interest and support from home management. Future directions for CHOICE development include a more collaborative approach to tailoring, implementation and evaluation, including the involvement of residents, family members, and volunteers, as they have the capacity to enhance and support relationship-centred dining.

Abbreviations
ADL-LF: Minimum Data Set Activities of Daily Living-Long Form; CPS: Cognitive Performance Scale; DA: Dietary Aid; DFS: Director of Food Service; HM: Home Management; LTC: Long-Term Care; MDS: Minimum Data Set; M-RCC: Mealtime Relational Care Checklist; MT Champions: Mealtime Champions; MTS: Mealtime Scan for Long-Term Care; PSW: Personal Support Worker; RCC: Relationship-Centred Care; RIA: Research Institute for Aging; RN: Registered Nurse; RPN: Registered Practical Nurse

Acknowledgements
The authors wish to acknowledge and thank the long-term care home, team members, and residents for contributions and involvement in this developmental evaluation study.

Funding
This work was supported by the Seed Catalyst Grant from the Network on Aging Research at the University of Waterloo. Research Institute on Aging provided project management and facilitation.

Author's contributions
The Primary Investigator, SW, assisted in the development of the CHOICE Program and acted as the CHOICE Coach. SW conducted and analyzed participant interviews, integrated quantitative and qualitative datasets, and developed the initial draft of this manuscript. Principal investigator HK conceived and developed the CHOICE Program and created the validated measurement tool used throughout the study (MTS). HK made substantial intellectual contributions to the analysis and co-wrote the manuscript. Co-Investigator HD aided in the development of the CHOICE Program and was the main point of contact for the study site. Co-Investigator JMM made substantial intellectual contributions in the form of analysis and presentation of data and critically reviewed early and final drafts of the manuscript. VV and SI were site leads for the acquisition of data collection at the study site. All authors reviewed and provided final approval of this manuscript. All authors agree to be accountable for all aspects of the work.

Competing interests
All authors declare they have no competing interests.

References

1. Devine CM. A life course perspective: understanding food choices in time, social location, and history. J Nutr Educ Behav. 2005;37(3):121–8.
2. Evans BC, Crogan NL, Shultz JA. The meaning of mealtimes: connection to the social world of the nursing home. J Gerontol Nurs. 2005;31(2):11–7.
3. Cranley LA, Norton PG, Cummings GG, Barnard D, Batra-Garga N, Estabrooks CA. Identifying resident care areas for a quality improvement intervention in long-term care: a collaborative approach. BMC Geriatr. 2012;12(1):59.
4. Lowndes R, Daly T, Armstrong P. "Leisurely dining": exploring how work organization, informal care, and dining spaces shape residents' experiences of eating in long-term residential care. Qual Health Res. 2018;28(1):126–44.
5. Watkins R, Goodwin VA, Abbott RA, Backhouse A, Moore D, Tarrant M. Attitudes, perceptions and experiences of mealtimes among residents and staff in care homes for older adults: a systematic review of the qualitative literature. Geriatr Nurs. 2017;38(4):325–33.
6. Curle L, Keller H. Resident interactions at mealtime: an exploratory study. Eur J Ageing. 2010;7(3):189–200.
7. Kaplan H, Gurven M, Hill K, Hurtado AM. The natural history of human food sharing and cooperation: a review and a new multi-individual approach to the negotiation of norms. Moral sentiments and material interests: the foundations of cooperation in economic life 2005;6:75–113.
8. Tresolini CP, Force PF. Health professions education and relationship-centered care, vol. 8. San Francisco: Pew Health Professions Commission; 1994.
9. Nolan MR, Davies S, Brown J, Keady J, Nolan J. Beyond 'person-centred'care: a new vision for gerontological nursing. J Clin Nurs. 2004;13:45–53.
10. Sheard D. Bringing relationships into the heart of dementia care. J of Dementia Care. 2004;12(4):22–4.
11. Keller HH, Carrier N, Slaughter SE, Lengyel C, Steele CM, Duizer L, et al. Prevalence and determinants of poor food intake of residents living in long-term care. J Am Med Dir Assoc. 2017;18(11):941–7.
12. Abbott RA, Whear R, Thompson-Coon J, Ukoumunne OC, Rogers M, Bethel A, et al. Effectiveness of mealtime interventions on nutritional outcomes for the elderly living in residential care: a systematic review and meta-analysis. Ageing Res Rev. 2013;12(4):967–81.
13. Vucea V, Keller HH, Ducak K. Interventions for improving mealtime experiences in long-term care. J Nutr Gerontol Geriatr. 2014;33(4):249–324.
14. Chaudhury H, Hung L, Badger M. The role of physical environment in supporting person-centered dining in long-term care: a review of the literature. Am J Alzheimers Dis Other Demen. 2013;28(5):491–500.
15. Perivolaris A, Leclerc CM, Wilkinson K, Buchanan S. An enhanced dining program for persons with dementia. Alzheimer's care today. 2006;7(4):258–67.
16. Genoe R, Dupuis SL, Keller HH, Martin LS, Cassolato C, Edward HG. Honouring identity through mealtimes in families living with dementia. J Aging Stud. 2010;24(3):181–93.
17. Henkusens C, Keller HH, Dupuis S, Schindel Martin L. Transitions to long-term care: how do families living with dementia experience mealtimes after relocating? J Appl Gerontol. 2014;33(5):541–63.
18. Ducak K, Sweatman G, Keller H. Dining culture change in long-term care homes: transitioning to resident-centered and relational meals. Ann Longterm Care. 2015;23(6):28–36.
19. Keller HH, Carrier N, Slaughter S, Lengyel C, Steele CM, Duizer L, et al. Making the Most of mealtimes (M3): protocol of a multi-Centre cross-sectional study of food intake and its determinants in older adults living in long term care homes. BMC Geriatr. 2017;17(1):15.
20. Patton MQ. Developmental evaluation: applying complexity concepts to enhance innovation and use. New York: Guilford Press; 2010.
21. Creswell JW, Clark VL. Designing and conducting mixed methods research. California: Sage publications; 2017.
22. Cane J, O'Connor D, Michie S. Validation of the theoretical domains framework for use in behaviour change and implementation research. Implement Sci. 2012;7(1):37.
23. Michie S, Johnston M, Abraham C, Lawton R, Parker D, Walker A. Making psychological theory useful for implementing evidence based practice: a consensus approach. BMJ Qual Saf. 2005;14(1):26–33.
24. Michie S, Atkins L, West R. The behavior change wheel: a guide to designing interventions. Great Britain: Silverback Publishing; 2014.
25. Keller HH, Chaudhury H, Pfisterer KJ, Slaughter SE. Development and inter-rater reliability of the mealtime scan for long-term care. Gerontologist. 2018; 58(3):e160-167. https://doi.org/10.1093/geront/gnw264.
26. Iuglio S, Keller H, Chaudhury H, Slaughter SE, Lengyel C, Morrison J, et al.

Construct validity of the mealtime scan: a secondary data analysis of the making Most of mealtimes (M3) study. J Nutr Gerontol Geriatr. 2018;18:1–23.

27. Hirdes JP, Ljunggren G, Morris JN, Frijters DH, Soveri HF, Gray L, Björkgren M, et al. Reliability of the interRAI suite of assessment instruments: a 12-country study of an integrated health information system. BMC Health Serv Res. 2008;8(1):277.

28. Morris JN, Fries BE, Morris SA. Scaling ADLs within the MDS. J Gerontol A Biol Sci Med Sci. 1999;54(11):M546–53.

29. Sandelowski M. Sample size in qualitative research. Res Nurs Health. 1995;18(2):179–83.

30. Thomas DR. A general inductive approach for analyzing qualitative evaluation data. Am J Eval. 2006;27(2):237–46.

31. Pope C, Ziedland S, Mays N. Qualitative research in health care: Analysing qualitative data. 320.

32. Milte R, Shulver W, Killington M, Bradley C, Miller M, Crotty M. Struggling to maintain individuality–describing the experience of food in nursing homes for people with dementia. Arch Gerontol Geriatr. 2017;72:52–8.

33. Harnett T, Jönson H. Shaping nursing home mealtimes. Ageing Soc. 2017;37(4):823–44.

34. Sidani S, Braden CJ. Design, evaluation, and translation of nursing interventions. United Kingdom: Wiley; 2011.

35. Keller H, Carrier N, Duizer L, Lengyel C, Slaughter S, Steele C. Making the Most of mealtimes (M3): grounding mealtime interventions with a conceptual model. J Am Med Dir Assoc. 2014;15(3):158–61.

36. Coleman CK, Medvene LJ. A person-centered care intervention for geriatric certified nursing assistants. Gerontologist. 2012;53(4):687–98.

37. Estabrooks CA, Squires JE, Hayduk L, Morgan D, Cummings GG, Ginsburg L, et al. The influence of organizational context on best practice use by care aides in residential long-term care settings. J Am Med Dir Assoc. 2015;16(6): 537–e1.

38. Cummings GG, Hewko SJ, Wang M, Wong CA, Laschinger HK, Estabrooks CA. Impact of managers' coaching conversations on staff knowledge use and performance in long-term care settings. Worldviews Evid-Based Nurs. 2018;15(1):62–71.

39. Woo K, Milworm G, Dowding D. Characteristics of quality improvement champions in nursing homes: a systematic review with implications for evidence-based practice. Worldviews Evid-Based Nurs. 2017;14(6):440–6.

40. McNally M, Martin-Misener R, McNeil K, Brillant M, Moorhouse P, Crowell S, et al. Implementing oral care practices and policy into long-term care: the brushing up on mouth care project. J Am Med Dir Assoc. 2015;16(3):200–7.

41. Rahman AN, Simmons SF, Applebaum R, Lindabury K, Schnelle JF. The coach is in: improving nutritional care in nursing homes. Gerontologist. 2011;52(4):571–80.

42. Viau-Guay A, Bellemare M, Feillou I, Trudel L, Desrosiers J, Robitaille MJ. Person-centered care training in long-term care settings: usefulness and facility of transfer into practice. Can J Aging. 2013;32(1):57–72.

24

Handgrip strength in old and oldest old Swiss adults

Julia Wearing[1,2], Peter Konings[3], Maria Stokes[4] and Eling D. de Bruin[5,6*] iD

Abstract

Background: Handgrip strength is indicative of overall physical health and mobility in the elderly. A reduction in strength below a certain threshold severely increases the risk of mobility limitations and is predictive for adverse outcomes such as dependence in daily activities and mortality. An overview of age- and geography- specific handgrip strength values in older adults provide a reference for further investigations and measures in clinical practice to identify people at risk for clinically meaningful weakness. The aim of this study was to evaluate handgrip strength in the Swiss-German population aged 75 and over.

Methods: In a cross-sectional study, maximal isometric handgrip strength of the dominant hand was evaluated in 244 Swiss people aged 75 years and over (62.7% women), with mean age (SD) of 84.5 (5.6) years in men and 83.1 (5.9) years in women. Demographic data and information about comorbidities, medication, fall history, global cognitive function, self-reported physical activity and dependence in activities of daily living were collected, and correlated with grip strength measures. Age- and gender specific grip strength values are reported as means, standard deviations and standard error of mean.

Results: Sex-stratified handgrip strength was significantly lower with advancing age in men ($p < .01$), from 37.7 (6.5) kg to 25.6 (7.6) kg and in women ($p < .01$) from 22.2 (4.0) kg to 16.5 (4.7) kg. Handgrip strength in our sample was significantly higher than in Southern European countries. Handgrip strength was independently associated with age, height and ADL dependence in men and women. Overall, 44% of men and 53% of women had handgrip strength measures that were below the clinically relevant threshold for mobility limitations.

Conclusion: This study reports the age- and sex-stratified reference values for handgrip strength in a representative sample of the Swiss population, aged 75–99 years. Although grip strength decreased with advancing age in both sexes; the relative decline was greater in men than women. Nonetheless men had significantly higher grip strength in all age groups. While the Swiss population sampled had greater grip strength than that reported in other European countries, about 50% were still classified as at risk of mobility limitations.

Keywords: Grip strength, Aged, Geriatric assessment

Background

Muscle strength is an important determinant of healthy aging [1]. A reduction in muscle mass and strength is known to impair body function and can have substantial consequences directly for the individual but also for economic costs [2]. Impairment in body function initially results in difficulties in performing common daily activities such as carrying household items; however, once body strength drops below a clinically relevant threshold, mobility limitations increase and can affect independence in basic daily life activities [3, 4]. Loss of independence requires the support of care-givers and often leads to social withdrawal and negatively effects on wellbeing and quality of life [2]. Early detection of low muscle strength in the elderly may help identify those at risk of mobility limitations and apply interventions to avoid or slow down the spiral of negative outcomes.

* Correspondence: eling.debruin@hest.ethz.ch
[5]Insitute of Human Movement Sciences and Sport (IBWS) ETH, Department of Health Sciences and Technology, HCP H 25.1, Leopold-Ruzicka-Weg 4, 8093 Zürich, ETH, Zurich, Switzerland
[6]Division of Physiotherapy, Department of Neurobiology, Care Sciences and Society, Karolinska Institutet, Stockholm, Sweden
Full list of author information is available at the end of the article

Muscle deterioration in old age is primarily explained by neural and muscular decline due to the aging process and concomitant physical inactivity and malnutrition [1]. However, mobility-limiting muscle weakness can potentially be counteracted or improved through preventive exercise and rehabilitation respectively [1, 5]. Increased physical activity and resistance exercise have been shown to improve muscle strength and -function even in older people with severe disability [6].

An easily applicable measure of muscle strength is a handgrip strength test. Maximal isometric handgrip strength, measured with a dynamometer in a standard procedure, has high to excellent inter-tester and test-retest reliability [7]. Low handgrip strength is indicative for decline of upper extremity strength [8] and lower extremity function [9] with high predictive value of adverse outcomes [10]. In clinical research, grip strength is often used in detection of age-related changes of muscle strength, associated with sarcopenia [11] and frailty [12]. Low grip strength is related to poor mobility of the elderly [13] and dependence in activities of daily living [14], and even predicts decline in body function and mortality [10].

Moreover, measurement of grip strength alone has been proposed to be a reliable marker of frailty [15] and has, in combination with gait speed, a positive predictive value of 87.5% to identify frailty [16]. Handgrip strength in older adults is considered a meaningful measure of current physical decline and future outcome by the World Health Organization [17].

Theoretical models of demographic trends show an increasing average life expectancy in industrial countries [18]. Particularly the percentage of older adults over 65 years will expand, in Switzerland from 18% in 2015 to 26% in 2045, whereas the old and oldest old age group (75 years and over) will increase the most. 60% of the over 80 year olds in Switzerland seek private help or live in old peoples- or nursing- homes because of limitations in basic and/or complex activities in daily living [19, 20].

The severity of consequences of age-associated muscle weakness provides significance to determine strength across all ages, particularly in the 75 years and over group. In this context, "hand-grip dynamometry can be considered a fundamental element of the physical examination of patients, particularly if they are older adults" [21].

Although many studies have collected grip strength data in the elderly, only few have systematically assessed grip strength in the most advanced age groups spanning the range from 90 up to 100 years and over [22, 23]. To the best of our knowledge, so far only one study evaluated grip strength in the Swiss population [24]. Since average grip strength differs depending on geographic regions [25, 26], an extension of Swiss reference values

is important for interpreting region-specific handgrip strength measures in clinical practice.

This study aimed to assess handgrip strength in the Swiss population aged 75 years and above to provide reference values for further investigations and measures in clinical practice.

Methods
Study design
A cross-sectional study of handgrip strength involving older people living in two different urban regions (Basel and St Gallen) of the German-speaking part of Switzerland was undertaken. Recruitment targeted community-living elderly, as well as those dwelling in assisted living apartments, and residential aged-care/nursing homes to ensure a broad representative sample of the general older population. Participants meeting the following inclusion criteria were eligible for the study: male and female adults aged 75 years or older, able to follow verbal instructions in German, able and willing to sign informed consent. Participants were excluded from the study based on the following criteria: self-reported upper extremity pain, aching or stiffness of the upper extremity on most days (over 50%) of the past month, injury or surgery or acute diseases of upper extremity within the past 6 months, and inability to follow the procedures of the study.

Sample size
Participant numbers ($n = 240$) were estimated a priori based on previously published grip strength data for Swiss older adults. The number would be sufficient to detect a 30% difference in grip strength for each 10-years age group cluster at an alpha (α) level of .05 and with 80% power ($\beta = .20$).

Data collection and methods
Prior to data collection, research assistants at both study sites were trained in conducting the interview of the participants and in using the study equipment for measuring handgrip strength according to the study protocol. Factors previously shown to influence handgrip strength including demographic characteristics, medication and fall history, osteoarthritis of the hands, global cognitive function, physical activity and dependence in activities of daily living were also collected.

Information about the intake of sedative medication, fall history and osteoarthritis of the hands were self-reported by the participants.

Measurements of body height were made to the nearest centimeter with a stadiometer and body weight was measured to the nearest kilogram on a digital weigh scale.

Global cognitive function was evaluated with the Mini Mental State Exam (MMSE) [27] and expressed as a score out of 30. The MMSE has a reported sensitivity of 77% and specificity of 91% in detecting cognitive impairment in older, community dwelling, hospitalized and institutionalized adults [28].

Independence in daily activities was assed via two questionnaires; the Barthel Index, which assesses basic activities of daily living (ADL) [29], and the Lawton Scale which evaluates instrumental activities of daily living (IADL) such as telephone use, shopping and food preparation [30]. Both self-rated assessments are widely used in elderly cohorts and have been shown to have high levels of reliability (intraclass correlation coefficient and Cronbach's alpha 0.9) [31, 32]. The questionnaires were conducted as interviews and categorized participants as independent (when all activities were scored highest), dependent in IADL (when at least one complex activity was rated with 0 points) or dependent in ADL (when at least one basic activity was rated with less than maximum score).

Physical activity was assessed with the Freiburg Questionnaire of Physical Activity; a self-reported questionnaire comprised of 8 items evaluating occupational, household, and leisure activities during the previous 7-day/30-day period [33]. Energy cost per week was quantified using a specific coding scheme that classifies physical activity by rate of energy expenditure [34, 35].

Handgrip strength was assessed using a hydraulic hand dynamometer (Jamar®) according to the standardized protocol recommended by the American Society of hand therapists [36]. The participant was seated in a chair without arm support, and with their hips flexed at 90° and feet resting on the floor. The elbow of the test arm was flexed to 90°, the forearm in neutral, and the wrist positioned at 15–30° of extension (dorsiflexion) and 0–15° of ulnar deviation. The examiner supported the base of the dynamometer for testing and the second smallest dynamometer handle position was used. Following a demonstration of the protocol, the participant was asked to squeeze the handle with as much force as possible for three seconds. Three repeated trials were recorded for both hands with a rest period of at least 15 s between trials. The maximum value of the three trials was used for analysis and data presentation. To enable comparison of results with those of other authors, the mean value of three trials was also reported. Hand dominance was self-reported by the participant based on their preferred hand use in activities including writing and brushing teeth, according to the Edinburgh Handedness Inventory [37].

IBM SPSS Statistics, Version 23 was used for statistical analysis. Descriptive statistics for categorical variables were expressed in percentage frequency distribution, for continuous variables mean and standard deviation was used. Grip strength of the dominant hand (mean and maximum value of three trials) was reported as means and standard deviations (SD) and standard error of mean (SEM) for men and women by age group. Measures of handgrip strength controlled for height were also presented. Spearman's correlation coefficient and multiple regression analysis was used to calculate relationships of grip strength with demographic data and information about comorbidities, medication, fall history, global cognitive function, self-reported physical activity and dependence in activities of daily living. Multivariate analysis of variance with Bonferroni-adjusted post-hoc analysis was used to detect strength differences between age groups and sexes.

This manuscript adheres to reporting guidelines for cross-sectional studies [38].

Results

A total of 244 participants were recruited in the period from June 2016 to march 2017, including 164 people from the canton Basel and 80 from the canton St Gallen. There was no statistically significant difference in mean age- and sex-stratified grip strength between the two sites ($p = .24$).

Characteristics of participants (62.7% female) and mean grip strength are shown in Table 1. There were no differences between sexes for age, global cognitive function, dependence in activities in daily living, amount of people living in assisted-living facilities, taking sedative medication or experiencing a fall but males were significantly taller, heavier, stronger, more physically active and had less hand osteoarthritis than females.

Handgrip strength in men significantly correlated with age ($\rho = -.41$, $p < .01$), height ($\rho = .31$, $p < .01$) and ADL dependence ($\rho = -.42$, $p < .01$). After multiple regression analysis, all three variables showed independent association with grip strength, with a regression coefficient of $-.4$ for age in years and $.3$ for height in m and -7.5 for ADL dependence. In women, handgrip strength significantly correlated with age ($\rho = -.49$, $p < .01$), weight ($\rho = .20$, $p < .02$), height ($\rho = .30$, $p < .01$) and ADL dependence ($\rho = -.49$, $p < .01$). After multiple regression analysis, only age, height and ADL dependence were independently associated with grip strength, with a regression coefficient of $-.2$ for age in years and $.1$ for height in m and -2.8 for ADL dependence.

For presentation of handgrip strength results as reference values and to aid comparisons with previous research, mean as well as maximum values of three trials were given for participants categorized into age groups, with each group including at least 20 individuals: age groups 75–79 years, 80–84 years, 85–89 years and 90–

Table 1 Participants characteristics

Characteristic	men mean (SD) or %	women mean (SD) or %
age (years)	83.1 (5.6)	84.5 (5.9)
height (m)	1.73 (0.7)	1.59 (0.7)*
weight (kg)	75.2 (10.4)	63.3 (13.2)*
handgrip strength (kg)	32.0 (8.2)	19.4 (4.3)*
Global cognitive function (points)	27.6 (2.4)	26.9 (3.1)
Physical activity (kcal/week)	1467.4 (1435.9)	828.2 (1005.1)*
ADL dependence		
in instrumental activities of daily living	18.2	16.0
in instrumental and basic activities of daily living	17.0	23.7
Living in assisted-living facilities/nursing homes	6.8	9.6
Medication	23.9	34.0
Osteoarthritis in hands	11.4	27.6*
Fall history	52.3	64.7

*significant difference between values of men and women with $p < .05$

99 years for women and age groups 75–79 years, 80–84 years, 85–99 years for men. Age distribution is presented in Tables 2 and 3. Handgrip strength was calculated for men and women separately. Handgrip strength results in kg of male and female participants are presented with and without controlling the values for height (assuming all males and females had the same height within their respective groups) in Tables 4, 5, 6 and 7, respectively. Unadjusted maximum handgrip strength is graphically shown in Fig. 1.

Analysis of variance for maximum handgrip strength in men showed that age group 75–79 was significantly stronger than age group 80–84 ($p < .01$, 95% CI 4.3–13.5) and 85–99 ($p < .01$, 95% CI 3.9–13.0). Handgrip strength between age group 80–84 and 85–99 did not differ significantly ($p = 1.0$, 95% CI -5.1 - 4.1).

Difference in mean handgrip strength between the youngest two age groups (75–79 and 80–84) was 8.9 ± 1.8 kg (23.6 ± 4.7%), and 8.4 ± 1.8 kg (22.3 ± 4.7%) between age groups 75–79 and 85–99.

In women, analysis of variance for handgrip strength was significantly higher in age group 75–79 than in the other three groups (80–84, $p = .02$, 95% CI 0.2–4.8, 85–89, $p < .01$, 95% CI 0.8–5.6; and 90–99, $p < .01$, 95% CI 3.4–8.2). Handgrip strength of age group 80–84 and 85–89 were significantly stronger than age

group 90–99 ($p < .01$, 95% CI 0.9–5.5; $p = .03$, 95% CI 0.1–5.0), but did not differ from each other ($p = 1.0$).

Difference in mean handgrip strength between the youngest two age groups (75–79 and 80–84) was 2.5 kg ± 0.9 (11.3 ± 4.1%), and 5.8 ± 0.9 kg (26.1 ± 4.1%) between the youngest and the oldest (75–79 and 90–99).

For identification of participants with clinically meaningful weakness, handgrip strength was classified in three categories: weak, intermediate and normal, according to cut-off values published by Alley et al. [3]. Allocation of participants to individual categories is presented in Table 8. Men and women show equal percentage distribution for each category except for intermediate strength, where women were significantly higher. About 50% of both sexes have normal strength and 50% were categorised as having reduced strength (category weak and intermediate). The percentage distribution of participants living in assisted-living facilities did not differ between sexes but significantly differed between categories. In men and women, more people categorised as weak lived in assisted-living facilities than people with intermediate or normal strength.

Discussion

The present study evaluated handgrip strength in a sample of Swiss individuals aged 75 years and over to

Table 2 Number of male participants per age group in absolute (n) and percentage values (%)

Age (years)	75–79	80–84	85–99
Men			
Absolute n	30	28	30
percentage %	34.1	31.8	34.1

Table 3 Number of female participants per age group in absolute (n) and percentage values (%)

Age (years)	75–79	80–84	85–89	90–99
Women				
absolute n	37	45	37	37
percentage %	23.7	28.8	23.7	23.7

Table 4 Height-adjusted handgrip strength (kg) of the dominant hand in men, categorized in age groups

Age (years)	75–79	80–84	85–99
Men			
mean of 3 trials	35.9 ± 6.3	27.5 ± 7.7	28.1 ± 7.1
max of 3 trials	37.7 ± 6.5	28.8 ± 7.7	29.6 ± 7.2

Handgrip strength is presented as maximum value of three trials and mean value of three trials ± SD

Table 6 Handgrip strength (kg), unadjusted to height, of the dominant hand in men, categorized in age groups

Age (years)	75–79	80–84	85–99
Men			
mean of 3 trials	35.9 ± 6.3 (1.2)	27.5 ± 7.7 (1.5)	27.8 ± 7.3 (1.3)
max of 3 trials	37.7 ± 6.5 (1.2)	28.8 ± 7.7 (1.5)	29.3 ± 7.3 (1.3)

Handgrip strength is presented as maximum value of three trials and mean value of three trials ± SD (SEM – standard error of mean)

provide reference values for further investigations and measures in clinical practice. Our study results showed handgrip strength values confirm and equal previously published data in the Swiss population 75–85 years [24] and confirmed the validity of provided reference values for this geographic region. For the first time, additional reference values for women specifically for the age groups 85–90 and 90–99 years of the Swiss population are presented. There is a need to provide reference values for screening tests, such as handgrip strength, particularly for this age group 85 and over, as with increased life expectancy, the risk of poor health increases. The old and oldest age groups are expected to increase the most; age-specific handgrip strength helps to identify individuals with low strength and to plan specific preventive health services to lower the risk of mobility limitations and dependence in activities of daily living.

Compared to grip strength data of a previously published Swiss sample (up to 85 years of age) [24], the older people in our study presented with comparable strength values (mean of three trials) in all age groups, except from women aged 75–79 years who were significantly weaker in the present study. Where Werle et al. included community-living older adults and elderly living in senior residences, our sample included nursing home dwellers as well. It is possible, therefore, that our sample had a lower level of physical condition than participants in the Werle et al. study. Therefore, handgrip strength could be expected to be lower in our sample as seen in women aged 75–79 years. The age group 85+ reported in the study of Werle et al. could not be compared to our sample since information on average age of their 85+ cohort was not provided.

In comparison to handgrip strength values published by other authors who included a random sample of the general nonagenarian population [22, 23], mean

handgrip strength of the 90–99-year-old participants were significantly higher than in Southern France and Italy. These findings are consistent with previous comparisons among different European countries showing a North-South slope [22, 25]. Contrasting our results of the oldest women with studies of two cohorts from Denmark (women mean age 100 years, 92–92 years respectively) who included volunteers of oldest old people registered in the national civil registration system [22, 23], women of our Swiss sample were significantly stronger. The difference could be due to variances in mean age, with women of one Danish cohort being 7 years older on average, as well as due to higher percentage of the participants living in assisted living facilities/nursing homes in both Danish samples (30.6% [22] and 47.6% [23] versus 8.4% in our sample).

The differences in age- and gender-specific grip strength among different countries likely vary due to e.g. birth weight, lifestyle and health care in the elderly [25]. In the Swiss population, these factors are above average on international comparison, which might contribute to the higher grip strength observed in the elderly Swiss. More specifically, the average birth weight (3.3 kg) of Swiss newborns in 2016 [39] corresponds with the average value of international standards for newborns [40]. However, at 83.3 years, the Swiss population had the second highest life expectancy at birth in 2016 [41]. Moreover, 56% of the population aged 75 years and over met the WHO-recommendations for physical activity in 2016, and therefore were within the highest quartile of the prevalence range (20–60%) of physical activity in older adults [42]. Remarkably, Switzerland has the highest social and economic wellbeing of older people worldwide, considering income and health status, education and employment, and enabling environment [43], which may be important preconditions for remaining active in old age.

Another finding of our study, consistent with previous research in the elderly [14, 25], was that handgrip strength in men and women was independently associated with age, height and ADL dependence. Handgrip strength did not correlate with Body Mass Index (BMI), probably owing to homogenous BMI values across sexes and age groups. Since percentage of muscle and fat mass was not specified in the study participants, no conclusion about association between

Table 5 Height-adjusted handgrip strength (kg) of the dominant hand in women, categorized in age groups

Age (years)	75–79	80–84	85–89	90–99
Women				
mean of 3 trials	21.0 ± 3.9	18.2 ± 3.0	18.0 ± 3.7	15.4 ± 4.6
max of 3 trials	22.2 ± 4.0	19.7 ± 3.0	19.0 ± 3.8	16.5 ± 4.7

Handgrip strength is presented as maximum value of three trials and mean value of three trials ± SD

Table 7 Handgrip strength (kg), unadjusted to height, of the dominant hand in women, categorized in age groups

Age (years)	75–79	80–84	85–89	90–99
Women				
mean of 3 trials	21.0 ± 3.9 (0.6)	18.2 ± 3.0 (0.4)	18.1 ± 3.7 (0.6)	15.3 ± 4.6 (0.8)
max of 3 trials	22.2 ± 4.0 (0.7)	19.7 ± 3.0 (0.4)	19.0 ± 3.8 (0.6)	16.5 ± 4.7 (0.8)

Handgrip strength is presented as maximum value of three trials and mean value of three trials ± SD (SEM – standard error of mean)

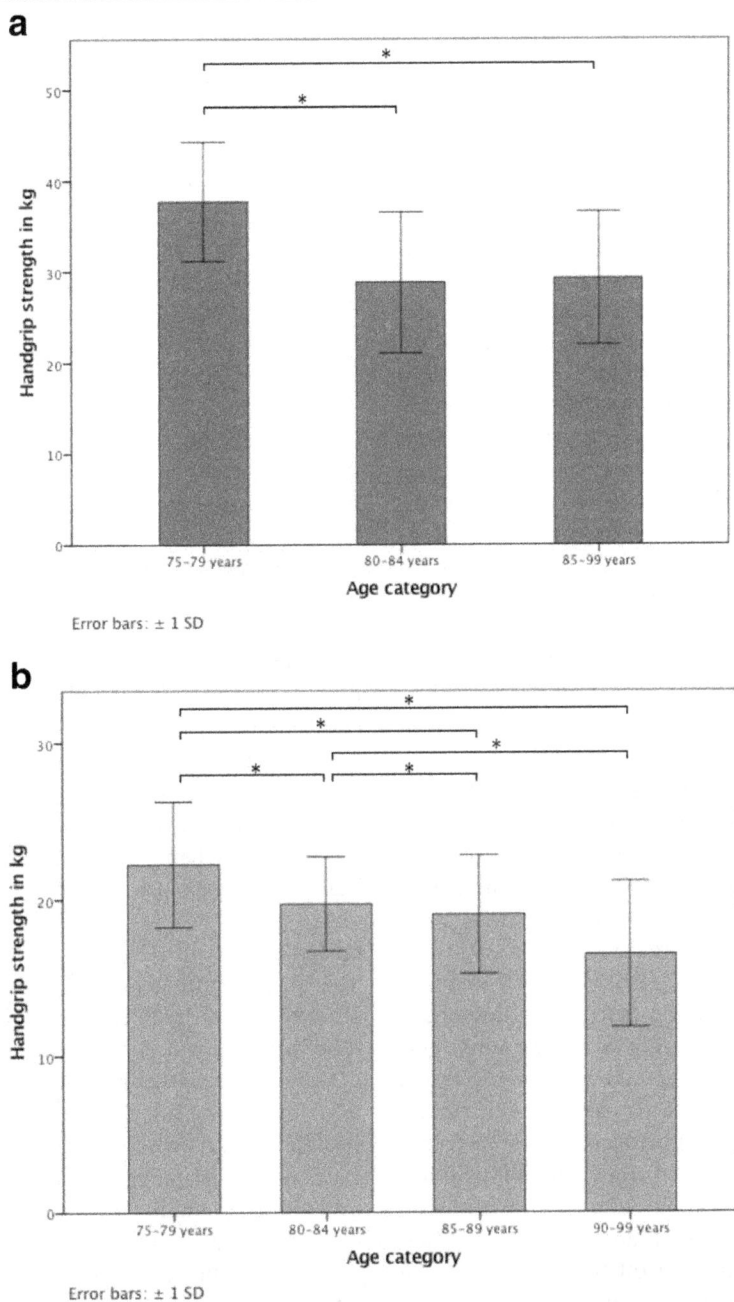

Fig. 1 a Maximum handgrip strength (kg) in men of the Swiss population 75 years and over. * Significant difference in grip strength ($p < .05$). **b** Maximum handgrip strength (kg) in women of the Swiss population 75 years and over. * Significant difference in grip strength ($p < .05$)

Table 8 Classification of participants (%) into three handgrip strength categories

	men (%)	women (%)
Weak (men < 26 kg, women < 16 kg)	22.7	18
assisted-living	20˚	21˚
community-living	80	79
Intermediate (men ≥26 < 32 kg, women ≥16 < 20 kg	21.6	35.3*
assisted-living	7	10
community-living	93	90
Normal (men ≥32 kg, women ≥20 kg)	55.7	46.7
assisted-living	4	5
community-living	96	95

Three groups for handgrip strength: weak, intermediate and normal. Percentage of people living in assisted-living facilities per group is presented in %
*Significant difference between men and women, p < .05
˚Significant difference of people living assisted (%) between strength categories, p < .05

grip strength and body composition could be drawn. Therefore, age-specific grip strength values were demonstrated only with and without adjustment to height and not BMI. Handgrip strength decreased significantly with age in men and women. Between 75 and 99 years, men demonstrated a greater decrease in strength than women but had still higher overall values even in the oldest age group. When considering the entire age range (75–99 years), the largest reduction in grip strength occurred in men in their early 80's while the biggest difference in women's strength appeared in their early 90's. The finding is consistent with a longitudinal study of Danish older adults, in which males lost handgrip strength more rapidly than females but were still stronger in absolute values [44] and less dependent in daily living [23]. As more women of the oldest age group in the current study were dependent in daily activities than men (51% of women, 10% men), it would appear that absolute strength rather than relative grip strength reduction may be more important for remaining independent in daily living in the elderly.

To identify people with a clinically meaningful reduction in handgrip strength in our sample of Swiss older adults, we applied cut-off values for detection of people at risk for mobility limitations, associated with sarcopenia/ dynapenia [2, 3]. According to cut off values published by Alley et al. [3] classifying people as weak (grip strength less than 26 kg for men and 16 kg for women), 22.7% male and 18% female participants in our sample were in this category. These individuals have a 7.6 (men) and 4.4 (women) times increased risk for mobility limitations, compared to older people with normal strength. In addition, 35.3% of the women and 21.6% of the men had "intermediate strength" (cut-off thresholds of 32 kg in men and 20 kg in women), with concomitant 3.6 (men) and 2.4 (women) times higher risk of impairment compared to older adults with normal strength values.

In total, the percentage of participants with reduced strength according the proposed thresholds is 44% in men and 53% in women. Comparing the men and women with normal strength to the at risk of mobility limitation groups regarding dependency in daily living, those with normal strength were more than 2–5 times less likely living in a care home facility.

Even though cut-off values are not confirmed to be valid in detecting mobility limitations in the Swiss population yet, these results might give insight into current physical health and might indicate future need for help and care in the Swiss population.

In this study, handgrip strength was evaluated in two urban regions of German-speaking Switzerland with comparable handgrip strength observed at both sites. The age- and gender- distribution, as well as the percentage of people dependent in daily activities, were comparable with the Swiss population of the same geographic region [19, 20]. Hence, grip strength values reported in this study are likely representative of the urban, German-Swiss population. We cannot rule out, however, that handgrip strength may differ in French-, Italian- and Romansh-speaking areas of Switzerland.

Limitations

This study recruited people from urban rather than rural areas of Switzerland. As people from rural backgrounds have been shown to have greater grip strength than those from urban environments [45], reference values in this study may be viewed as lower estimates of grip strength in the Swiss population. It is noteworthy, however, that our data are comparable with previously published grip strength in Swiss adults (aged 75–85) which included urban, suburban and rural populations.

Secondly, our study included people of various health status. Grip strength differences between men and women might therefore be different to results of other authors that included only healthy people [24, 46], since reduced wellbeing could influence the range of handgrip strength values and change the sex differences.

Conclusion

This study reports the age- and sex-stratified reference values for handgrip strength in a representative sample of the Swiss population, aged 75–99 years. Grip strength decreased with age in both sexes with the relative decline being greater in men than in women. Nonetheless, men had significantly higher grip strength values in all age groups. While the Swiss population sample had a greater grip strength than that reported in other European countries, 44% (men) and 53% (women) were still classified as being at risk of developing mobility limitations.

Abbreviations

ADL: Activities of daily living; CI: Confidence interval; IADL: Instrumental activities of daily living; MMSE: Mini Mental State Exam; SD: Standard deviation; SEM: Standard error of the mean

Acknowledgements

The authors acknowledge the assistance of Adullam Spital und Pflegezentren Basel and Geriatrische Klinik St Gallen in providing equipment and participant recruitment.

Funding

No funding.

Authors' contributions

JW, EdB, MS and PK designed the study, PK and JW contributed to participant recruitment and data collection. JW conducted the statistical analysis. All authors contributed to drafting and revision of the manuscript and approved the final version for submission.

Competing interests

The authors declare that they have no competing interests.

Author details

[1]Faculty of Health, Medicine and Sciences, School for Public Health and Primary Care, University Maastricht, Minderbroedersberg 4-6, Maastricht, LK 6211, The Netherlands. [2]Adullam Stiftung, Mittlere Strasse 15, 4056 Basel, Switzerland. [3]Geriatrische Klinik St. Gallen, Rorschacher Strasse 94, 9000 St. Gallen, Switzerland. [4]Faculty of Health Sciences, University of Southampton, Building 45, Highfield Campus, Southampton SO17 1BJ, UK. [5]Insitute of Human Movement Sciences and Sport (IBWS) ETH, Department of Health Sciences and Technology, HCP H 25.1, Leopold-Ruzicka-Weg 4, 8093 Zürich, ETH, Zurich, Switzerland. [6]Division of Physiotherapy, Department of Neurobiology, Care Sciences and Society, Karolinska Institutet, Stockholm, Sweden.

References

1. McLeod M, Breen L, Hamilton DL, Philp A. Live strong and prosper: the importance of skeletal muscle strength for healthy ageing. Biogerontology. 2016;17(3):497–510.
2. Clark BC, Manini TM. Functional consequences of sarcopenia and dynapenia in the elderly. Curr Opin Clin Nutr Metab Care. 2010;13(3):271–6.
3. Alley DE, Shardell MD, Peters KW, McLean RR, Dam TT, Kenny AM, et al. Grip strength cutpoints for the identification of clinically relevant weakness. J Gerontol A Biol Sci Med Sci. 2014;69(5):559–66.
4. Hasegawa R, Islam MM, Lee SC, Koizumi D, Rogers ME, Takeshima N. Threshold of lower body muscular strength necessary to perform ADL independently in community-dwelling older adults. Clin Rehabil. 2008; 22(10–11):902–10.
5. Manini TM, Clark BC. Dynapenia and aging: an update. J Gerontol A Biol Sci Med Sci. 2012;67(1):28–40.
6. de Souto BP, Morley JE, Chodzko-Zajko W, Pitkala KH, Weening-Djiksterhuis E, Rodriguez-Manas L, et al. Recommendations on physical activity and exercise for older adults living in long-term care facilities: a taskforce report. J Am Med Dir Assoc. 2016;17(5):381–92.
7. Mathiowetz V, Weber K, Volland G, Kashman N. Reliability and validity of grip and pinch strength evaluations. J Hand Surg Am. 1984;9(2):222–6.
8. Bohannon RW. Hand-grip dynamometry provides a valid indication of upper extremity strength impairment in home care patients. J Hand Ther. 1998;11(4):258–60.
9. Fragala MS, Alley DE, Shardell MD, Harris TB, McLean RR, Kiel DP, et al. Comparison of handgrip and leg extension strength in predicting slow gait speed in older adults. J Am Geriatr Soc. 2016;64(1):144–50.
10. Rijk JM, Roos PR, Deckx L, van den Akker M, Buntinx F. Prognostic value of handgrip strength in people aged 60 years and older: a systematic review and meta-analysis. Geriatr Gerontol Int. 2016;16(1):5–20.
11. Cruz-Jentoft AJ, Baeyens JP, Bauer JM, Boirie Y, Cederholm T, Landi F, et al. Sarcopenia: European consensus on definition and diagnosis: report of the European working group on sarcopenia in older people. Age Ageing. 2010; 39(4):412–23.
12. Fried LP, Tangen CM, Walston J, Newman AB, Hirsch C, Gottdiener J, et al. Frailty in older adults: evidence for a phenotype. J Gerontol A Biol Sci Med Sci. 2001;56(3):M146–56.
13. Lauretani F, Russo CR, Bandinelli S, Bartali B, Cavazzini C, Di Iorio A, et al. Age-associated changes in skeletal muscles and their effect on mobility: an operational diagnosis of sarcopenia. J Appl Physiol. 2003;95(5):1851–60.
14. Matsui Y, Fujita R, Harada A, Sakurai T, Nemoto T, Noda N, et al. Association of grip strength and related indices with independence of activities of daily living in older adults, investigated by a newly-developed grip strength measuring device. Geriatr Gerontol Int. 2014;14(Suppl 2):77–86.
15. Syddall H, Cooper C, Martin F, Briggs R, Aihie SA. Is grip strength a useful single marker of frailty? Age Ageing. 2003;32(6):650–6.
16. Lee L, Patel T, Costa A, Bryce E, Hillier LM, Slonim K, et al. Screening for frailty in primary care: accuracy of gait speed and hand-grip strength. Can Fam Physician. 2017;63(1):e51–e7.
17. World Health Organisation. Guidelines on Integrated Care for Older People (ICOPE). http://www.who.int/ageing/publications/guidelines-icope/en/; 2017.
18. Kontis V, Bennett JE, Mathers CD, Li G, Foreman K, Ezzati M. Future life expectancy in 35 industrialised countries: projections with a Bayesian model ensemble. Lancet. 2017;389(10076):1323–35.
19. Bundesamt für Statistik. Betagte Personen in Institutionen [web page]. https://www.bfs.admin.ch/bfs/en/home/news/whats-new.assetdetail.348174. html: BFS; 2011.
20. Bundesamt für Statistik. Functional health of older, community-living people [web page].https://www.bfs.admin.ch/bfs/de/home/statistiken/gesundheit/ gesundheitszustand/alter.assetdetail.349311.html: BFS; 2014.
21. Bohannon RW. Muscle strength: clinical and prognostic value of hand-grip dynamometry. Curr Opin Clin Nutr Metab Care. 2015;18(5):465–70.
22. Jeune B, Skytthe A, Cournil A, Greco V, Gampe J, Berardelli M, et al. Handgrip strength among nonagenarians and centenarians in three European regions. J Gerontol A Biol Sci Med Sci. 2006;61(7):707–12.
23. Nybo H, Gaist D, Jeune B, McGue M, Vaupel JW, Christensen K. Functional status and self-rated health in 2,262 nonagenarians: the Danish 1905 cohort survey. J Am Geriatr Soc. 2001;49(5):601–9.

24. Werle S, Goldhahn J, Drerup S, Simmen BR, Sprott H, Herren DB. Age- and gender-specific normative data of grip and pinch strength in a healthy adult Swiss population. J Hand Surg Eur Vol. 2009;34(1):76–84.

25. Andersen-Ranberg K, Petersen I, Frederiksen H, Mackenbach JP, Christensen K. Cross-national differences in grip strength among 50+ year-old Europeans: results from the SHARE study. Eur J Ageing. 2009;6(3):227–36.

26. Leong DP, Teo KK, Rangarajan S, Kutty VR, Lanas F, Hui C, et al. Reference ranges of handgrip strength from 125,462 healthy adults in 21 countries: a prospective urban rural epidemiologic (PURE) study. J Cachexia Sarcopenia Muscle. 2016;7(5):535–46.

27. Folstein MF, Folstein SE, McHugh PR. "Mini-mental state". A practical method for grading the cognitive state of patients for the clinician. J Psychiatr Res. 1975;12(3):189–98.

28. Thalmann B, Spiegel R, Stähelin HB, Brubacher D, Ermini-Fünfschilling D, Bläsi S, et al. Dementia screening in general practice: optimised scoring for the clock drawing test. Brain Aging. 2002;2(2):36–43.

29. Mahoney FI, Barthel DW. Functional evaluation: the Barthel index. Md State Med J. 1965;14:61–5.

30. Lawton MP, Brody EM. Assessment of older people: self-maintaining and instrumental activities of daily living. Gerontologist. 1969;9(3):179–86.

31. Hokoishi K, Ikeda M, Maki N, Nomura M, Torikawa S, Fujimoto N, et al. Interrater reliability of the physical self-maintenance scale and the instrumental activities of daily living scale in a variety of health professional representatives. Aging Ment Health. 2001;5(1):38–40.

32. Minosso JSM, Amendola F, Alvarenga MRM, de Campos Oliveira MA. Validation of the Barthel index in elderly patients attended in outpatient clinics, in Brazil. Acta Paul Enferm. 2010;23(2):218–23.

33. Frey I, Berg A, Grathwohl D, Keul J. Freiburg questionnaire of physical activity--development, evaluation and application. Soz Praventivmed. 1999; 44(2):55–64.

34. Ainsworth BE, Haskell WL, Leon AS, Jacobs DR Jr, Montoye HJ, Sallis JF, et al. Compendium of physical activities: classification of energy costs of human physical activities. Med Sci Sports Exerc. 1993;25(1):71–80.

35. Ainsworth BE, Haskell WL, Whitt MC, Irwin ML, Swartz AM, Strath SJ, et al. Compendium of physical activities: an update of activity codes and MET intensities. Med Sci Sports Exerc. 2000;32(9 Suppl):S498–504.

36. Shechtman O, Sindhu BS. Grip Strength. In: ASTH, editor. Clinical Assessment Recommendations. 3rd ed; 2013.

37. Oldfield RC. The assessment and analysis of handedness: the Edinburgh inventory. Neuropsychologia. 1971;9(1):97–113.

38. von Elm E, Altman DG, Egger M, Pocock SJ, Gotzsche PC, Vandenbroucke JP, et al. The strengthening the reporting of observational studies in epidemiology (STROBE) statement: guidelines for reporting observational studies. Int J Surg. 2014;12(12):1495–9.

39. BFS BfS. Health of newborns [web page]. https://www.bfs.admin.ch/bfs/de/home/statistiken/gesundheit/gesundheitszustand/gesundheit-neugeborenen.html: Bundesamt für Statistik BFS; 2016.

40. Villar J, Cheikh Ismail L, Victora CG, Ohuma EO, Bertino E, Altman DG, et al. International standards for newborn weight, length, and head circumference by gestational age and sex: the newborn cross-sectional study of the INTERGROWTH-21st project. Lancet. 2014;384(9946):857–68.

41. World Health Organisation. Life expectancy at birth [web page]. http://apps.who.int/gho/data/node.main.688 /gho/mortality_burden_disease/life_tables/situation_trends/en/: who.int; 2015.

42. Sun F, Norman IJ, While AE. Physical activity in older people: a systematic review. BMC Public Health. 2013;13:449.

43. helpage. Global AgeWatch Index 2015 [web page]. http://www.helpage.org/global-agewatch/population-ageing-data/global-rankings-table/: helpage.org; 2015.

44. Oksuzyan A, Maier H, McGue M, Vaupel JW, Christensen K. Sex differences in the level and rate of change of physical function and grip strength in the Danish 1905-cohort study. J Aging Health. 2010;22(5):589–610.

45. Carvalho Sampaio RA, Sewo Sampaio PY, Yamada M, Ogita M, Arai H. Urban-rural differences in physical performance and health status among older Japanese community-dwelling women. J Clin Gerontol Geriatr. 2012; 3(4):127–31.

46. Malhotra R, Ang S, Allen JC, Tan NC, Ostbye T, Saito Y, et al. Normative Values of Hand Grip Strength for Elderly Singaporeans Aged 60 to 89 Years: A Cross-Sectional Study. J Am Med Dir Assoc. 2016;17(9):864–e1–7.

25

The pace and prognosis of peripheral sensory loss in advanced age: association with gait speed and falls

Lewis A. Lipsitz[1,2,3*], Brad Manor[1,2,3], Daniel Habtemariam[1], Ikechukwu Iloputaife[1], Junhong Zhou[1,2,3] and Thomas G. Travison[1,2,3]

Abstract

Background: Peripheral sensory loss is considered one of many risk factors for gait impairments and falls in older adults, yet no prospective studies have examined changes in touch sensation in the foot over time and their relationship to mobility and falls. Therefore, we aimed to determine the prevalence and progression of peripheral sensory deficits in the feet of older adults, and whether sensory changes are associated with the slowing of gait and development of falls over 5 years.

Methods: Using baseline, and 18 and 60 month followup data from the Maintenance Of Balance, Independent Living, Intellect, and Zest in the Elderly (MOBILIZE) Study in Boston, MA, we determined changes in the ability to detect stimulation of the great toe with Semmes Weinstein monofilaments in 351 older adults. We used covariate-adjusted repeated measures analysis of variance to determine relationships between sensory changes and gait speed or fall rates.

Results: Subjects whose sensory function was consistently impaired over 5 years had a significantly steeper decline in gait speed (− 0.23 m/s; 95% CI: -0.28 to − 0.18) compared to those with consistently intact sensory function (− 0.12 m/s; 95% CI: -0.15 to − 0.08) and those progressing from intact to impaired sensory function (− 0.13 m/s; − 0.16 to − 0.10). Compared to subjects with consistently intact sensation, those whose sensory function progressed to impairment during followup had the greatest risk of falls (adjusted risk ratio = 1.57 (95% confidence interval = 1.12 to 2.22).

Conclusions: Our longitudinal results indicate that a progressive decline in peripheral touch sensation is a risk factor for mobility impairment and falls in older adults.

Keywords: Neuropathy, Elderly, Mobility, Longitudinal, Feet

Background

Falls are a leading cause of morbidity and mortality among older adults, occurring in approximately one-third of community-dwelling persons over age 65 and costing over $31 billion in related injuries annually [1–3]. The presence of peripheral sensory loss is considered to be one of many different risk factors for falls [3–8]. A few previous studies demonstrated that older adults with peripheral sensory loss at the outset had an increased risk of subsequent falls [5–9]. However, these studies relied on single baseline measures of sensory function and did not examine the effect of changes over time [7, 8]. The longitudinal relationship between changes in peripheral sensory function and the development of falls is not known.

Peripheral neuropathy is common among older adults, [10] especially in those with diabetes [11, 12]. The prevalence of peripheral neuropathy has been reported to be approximately 7% in older adult populations worldwide [11, 13]. While there are many causes, including alcohol ingestion, vitamin B_{12} deficiency, cancer, chemotherapy, chronic kidney disease, and paraproteinemias, diabetes is the most frequent, accounting for 32–44% of patients with polyneuropathy [14, 15].

* Correspondence: Lipsitz@hsl.harvard.edu
[1]Hebrew SeniorLife Institute for Aging Research, 1200 Centre Street, Boston Roslindale, MA 02131, USA
[2]Division of Gerontology, Beth Israel Deaconess Medical Center, Boston, MA, USA
Full list of author information is available at the end of the article

Many factors associated with peripheral neuropathy may increase the risk of falls, including impaired balance, muscle weakness, nutritional deficiencies, and medications [2, 16]. One mechanism by which the progression of sensory neuropathy may predispose people to falls is through alterations in gait. While slow gait speed has been reported to be cross-sectionally associated with distal sensory neuropathy [17], this could be either a cause of falls or protective mechanism to prevent falls. The present study takes advantage of longitudinal data from the Maintenance Of Balance, Independent Living, Intellect, and Zest in the Elderly (MOBILIZE) Study in Boston, MA, to assess the prevalence and progression of peripheral sensory deficits in the feet, and whether they are associated with slowing of gait and falls over a 5-year period.

Methods

Participants

The MOBILIZE Boston Study (MBS) is a prospective cohort study of a unique set of risk factors for falls in community-dwelling seniors living in the Boston area. The design and methodology for this study have been previously described in detail [18, 19]. In brief, 765 persons eligible for the MBS were enrolled using door-to-door population based recruitment. To be included, individuals had to be: > 70 years of age (or > 65 years if living with a participant), able to understand and communicate in English, able to walk 20 ft without personal assistance (walking aids permitted), expecting to live in the area for at least 2 years, and able to provide written informed consent. Exclusion criteria included terminal disease, severe vision or hearing deficits, and a Mini-Mental State Examination score < 18 [20, 21].

All subjects underwent a complete home and laboratory assessment of demographic characteristics, medical conditions, medications, functional status, gait speed, smoking status, alcohol use, blood pressure, and cerebral hemodynamics, then were followed prospectively for falls using a monthly postcard calendar (see below). These assessments were repeated at 18 months and 5 years, while monthly falls data were collected continuously.

The analysis described here utilized longitudinal data from three waves of MBS data collection over approximately five years. Of the original 765 MOBILIZE Boston participants, data from only 351 subjects were available for the current study because of death, institutionalization, or loss to followup. As expected, the study sample that survived the 5 year followup was healthier that the original cohort, with better scores on the Mini-mental State Examination [20], Trail-making Test [22], Short Physical Performance Battery [23], and Berg Balance Scale [24], and a lower prevalence of diabetes, less use of a walking aid, and faster gait speed.

Clinical measures

Sensory function

We used an abbreviated Semmes-Weinstein monofilament test (SWMT) to assess the threshold for light touch sensation on the dorsum of each great toe, which uses a buckling monofilament to impart a known force to the skin, following the procotol suggested by Perkins et al. [25] The dorsum of the toe was used to avoid callouses on the plantar surface, which interfere with the sensory stimulus. The SWMT is a diagnostic tool to evaluate loss of protective sensation that often leads to ulcer formation. We employed two of the most-widely used monofilaments: the 5.07 monofilament (providing a standardized 10 g buckling force) and the 4.17 monofilament (providing a standardized force of 1.4 g). Failure to feel the 5.07 monofilament represents a loss of protective sensation [26, 27]. The 4.17 monofilament is used to determine whether the participant has normal light touch sensation. Inability to detect the 4.17 may indicate early neuropathy. The protocol began with the 4.17 monofilament, and if the participant could not feel it, he or she was tested with the 5.07 monofilament.

Monofilament testing was conducted while the participant was lying on an exam table, without shoes or socks. The procedure was demonstrated on the participant's hand or arm before foot measurements were taken. Touch sensation was assessed at a single site on the dorsum of the great toe, 1 cm proximal to the nail bed (distal to the knuckle). The participant covered or closed their eyes throughout the test.

The test results were categorized into sensory loss groupings of intact, mild-to-moderate, and severe deficits, as defined in Table 1. The prevalence of each group is also shown. Changes in sensation over 5 years were grouped into 4 categories as shown in Table 2; including intact to intact, intact to mild-to-moderate impairment, mild-to-moderate impairment to severe, or severe to severe. Nine subjects who exhibited improved sensation were excluded from the longitudinal analysis.

Gait speed

Gait speed was assessed with a stopwatch as participants walked at their preferred pace over a four meter course. Timing started with a signal while subjects were standing still and ended when they traversed 4 m. To prevent terminal slowing, they were not told where the course ended. They were asked to walk at their comfortable speed as if taking a purposeful walk on the street, going to a store. They were allowed to use an assistive device if they used it at home or outdoors. The fastest time of two separate trials was used for analysis. The time to walk 4 m is a component of the Short Physical Performance Battery (SPPB), described below.

Table 1 The definition and prevalence of each category of somatosensory impairment

	Definition	Prevalence at baseline, n (%)
Intact	Able to feel *at least* 3 monofilament touches out of 4 attempts for a 4.17 g monofilament in the left *and* right great toes	292 (83%)
Mild-moderate impairment	Able to feel *fewer* than 3 monofilament touches out of 4 attempts for a 4.17 g monofilament in the left *or* right great toe *and* able to feel *at least* 3 monofilament touches out of 4 attempts for a 5.07 g monofilament in the left *and* right great toes	22 (6%)
Severe impairment	Able to feel *fewer* than 3 monofilament touches out of 4 attempts for *both* 4.17 *and* 5.07 g monofilaments in the left *or* right great toe	37 (11%)

Berg balance scale

The Berg Balance Scale is a multi-component assessment of standing balance, consisting of 14 balance tasks with each task scored from 0 to 4, for a summed score of 0 to 56 [24]. The scale has been well-validated and shown to predict risk of falls in community dwelling elders [28]. Only baseline data were available.

Physical performance

The Short Physical Performance Battery (SPPB) was used to measure lower extremity mobility performance [23]. The SPPB includes measures of standing balance, 4-m usual-paced walking speed, and ability and time to rise from a chair 5 times. The validity of this scale has been demonstrated by showing a gradient of risk for admission to a nursing home and mortality along the full range of the scale from 0 to 12 [29, 30].

Falls detection

During a five-year follow-up period, a fall was defined as unintentionally coming to rest on the ground or other lower level, not as a result of a major intrinsic event (e.g., myocardial infarction, stroke, or seizure) or an overwhelming external hazard (e.g., hit by a vehicle) [18, 31]. Participants were instructed to complete and return monthly falls calendar postcards designed to be posted on a refrigerator. On the postcards, participants were to record an "F" for each fall on the day it occurred and an "N" on days when no falls occurred. If the postcard was not returned, a research assistant called the participant to determine whether a fall occurred during the preceeding month and to remind them to complete and return future cards. This approach has been well-validated for use in epidemiological cohort studies and described in

Table 2 Categories of change in sensory function over 5 years of followup; count and row percentages shown

Baseline	Follow-up	
	Intact	Impaired
Intact	150 (51%)	142 (49%)
Impaired	9 (15%)[a]	50 (85%)

[a]Not included in longitudinal analyses due to small cell size

previous studies [32]. All subjects who reported falls were also called to determine the circumstances of the fall and clinical outcomes, including whether any injuries (e.g. fractures) and hospital visits occurred.

Other variables

Sociodemographic characteristics assessed at baseline in the home interview included age, sex, race (self-identified), and years of education. At each wave we used the validated Physical Activity Scale for the Elderly (PASE) to measure self-assessed physical activity in the previous week [33]. Participants were asked about physician-diagnosed major medical conditions.

Diabetes was defined using an algorithm based on self-reported diabetes, use of antidiabetic medications, and laboratory measures from the baseline clinic visit, including random glucose (> 200 mg/dL) and hemoglobin A1C ($> 7\%$). Body mass index (BMI, calculated as weight in kilograms divided by height in meters squared) was calculated from measured height and weight. Comorbidity was measured using a count of relevant self-reported medical conditions, including: coronary heart disease, high blood pressure, ulcer or other stomach disease, kidney disease, liver disease, anemia, cancer, depression, osteoarthritis and degenerative arthritis, and rheumatoid arthritis [34]. Baseline subject characteristics also included the Center for Epidemiologic Studies Depression Scale – revised [35], Mini-Mental State Examination and Trail-making Test.

Data analysis

We summarized baseline characteristics of groups of participants with and without sensory loss using means and standard deviations or frequency distributions and compared groups of participants using t-tests for continuous variables, chi-square tests for categorical variables, and negative binomial regression for count variables.

Participants were grouped into 4 peripheral sensory loss categories based on their changes from baseline to 60 months: those with intact sensory function both at baseline and 60 months of follow-up (hereafter called **consistently intact**), those with intact sensory function at baseline and loss of function to at least mild impairment by 60 months (**progressing to impairment**), those with at least mildy impaired sensory function at both baseline and 60 months (**consistently impaired**), and those with impaired sensory function at baseline but intact function at 60 months. (**improved**) (Table 2). Those with mild-to-moderate and severe sensory loss were grouped together into the impaired category for the derivation of these sensory loss trajectories. Due to the small number of participants (9) in the improved category, this group was excluded from consideration in longitudinal analyses, leaving 342 participants for the analyses of change over time.

Analysis of the relationship between sensory loss categories and change in gait speed was done using repeated measures analysis of variance models. Gait speeds measured at baseline, 18 months, and 60 months were used as dependent variables, and tests of global mean differences across all time points as well as pairwise tests comparing mean gait speeds at each time point were conducted. The relationship to the falls rate outcome was analyzed using negative binomial regression, as falls rates exhibited a high degree of variance between participants through the course of study follow-up. Since falls were recorded as present or absent on each day of the 5-year followup period, there were no missing falls data.

Adjusted analyses for gait speed included age, sex, comorbidity count, use of a walking aid, baseline Berg balance score, and diabetes as covariates. Adjusted analyses for falls included age, sex, average weekly physical activity (PASE), baseline Berg balance score, diabetes, comorbidity count, and the SPPB score. For hypothesis testing, a two-sided type-I error probability of 0.05 was allowed. Models were estimated using Stata/MP version 13.1 (Statacorp, College Station, Tx).

Results

The characteristics of the full study cohort and those with (mild, moderate, or severe) and without (intact) baseline sensory impairment are shown in Table 3. At baseline, participants with any sensory impairment were four years older on average than their intact counterparts, were more likely to be male, and had diminished executive function (as indicated by 20s longer Trails B time on average). They also exhibited more multimorbidity and diminished physical functioning than their intact counterparts, reporting a greater prevalence of diabetes and peripheral neuropathy, and 0.3 greater mean comorbidity count on average. They were twice as likely to report use of a walking aid and exhibited diminished physical function, scoring an average of 1.4 points lower on the SPPB and 0.1 m/s slower gait speed, both differences well above established thresholds of clinical significance. Despite these differences, however, a history of one or more falls was similar in the two groups.

The relationship between changes in peripheral sensory function and change in gait speed over 18 and 60 months is illustrated in Fig. 1. After model adjustment, participants in the three groups had comparable mean baseline gait speed. The group of subjects with consistently intact sensory function over this time period had the smallest declines in gait speed over 60 months (– 0.12 m/s; 95% CI: -0.15 to – 0.08). This decline in gait speed was of similar magnitude to the decline observed in subjects whose sensory function progressed to impairment (– 0.13 m/s; – 0.16 to – 0.10).Those whose sensory function was consistently impaired had a steeper decline in gait speed (– 0.23 m/s; 95% CI: -0.28 to – 0.18). The difference between the consistently impaired group and the others was statistically significant and consistent with a 'substantially' meaningful difference for gait speed metrics in older populations [36].

Declines in peripheral sensory function were also associated with fall risk. Table 4 shows the absolute and relative risk of falls by temporal pattern of impairment. Those whose sensory function progressed to impairment during followup had a greater risk of falls than those whose sensory function was consistently intact (adjusted risk ratio = 1.57 (95% confidence interval = 1.12 to 2.22). The group that remained consistently impaired over the 5 years had an elevated fall rate, but it was not statistically significantly different from that of the consistently intact group (adjusted risk ratio = 1.47, 95% confidence interval = 0.89 to 2.45).

Discussion

The results of this study demonstrate the course of tactile sensory loss in the feet of older community-dwelling people over 5 years, and relationships between peripheral sensory loss and the concurrent slowing of gait and development of falls. Over the 5-year course of the study, older adults with consistently impaired peripheral sensory function had a significantly greater decline in gait speed compared to those with consistently intact or progressive impairment over 5 years. Compared to those with consistently intact sensory function, older adults who developed sensory impairments had a greater risk of falls. These results indicate that the loss of peripheral sensory function is a significant contributor to slowing of gait and an increased risk of falls in a community-dwelling older adult population.

The absolute number (59) and percent (17%) of participants with sensory impairment were relatively low in the MOBILIZE Boston population, but higher than the 7% reported in other older populations [11, 13]. Most of our participants had intact sensation at baseline, but this enabled us to observe the development of impairments over time. Nearly half (49%) of those initially intact developed sensory impairment over 5 years of followup.

Table 3 Baseline characteristics and descriptive statistics of the study sample (N = 351); mean (standard deviation) or count (percent) is shown

	Full cohort (n = 351)	Baseline somatosensory function	
		Intact (n = 292)	Impaired (n = 59)
Age, years	78 (5)	77 (5)	81 (5)
Female	230 (66%)	203 (70%)	27 (46%)
White	283 (81%)	230 (79%)	53 (90%)
Education			
Less than high school	19 (5%)	15 (5%)	4 (7%)
High school	68 (19%)	53 (18%)	15 (25%)
Some college/college	136 (39%)	119 (41%)	17 (29%)
Graduate/professional education	127 (36%)	104 (36%)	23 (39%)
Body mass index, kg/m^2	27.2 (4.9)	27.0 (4.9)	27.9 (5.0)
Current smoker	11 (3%)	10 (3%)	1 (2%)
Daily alcohol use (percent yes)	34 (10%)	28 (10%)	6 (10%)
Comorbidity count[a]	2.4 (1.5)	2.4 (1.5)	2.7 (1.5)
CES-D score	9.9 (10.2)	9.8 (10.0)	10.3 (11.0)
Medication use			
Antihypertensive medication	237 (68%)	194 (66%)	43 (73%)
Antidepressants	35 (10%)	29 (10%)	6 (10%)
Anti-seizure medications	12 (3%)	10 (3%)	2 (4%)
Statins	160 (46%)	131 (45%)	29 (49%)
Anxiolytics	42 (12%)	33 (11%)	9 (15%)
Antihistamines	35 (10%)	29 (10%)	6 (10%)
Opioids	14 (4%)	10 (3%)	4 (7%)
Nonsteroidal anti-inflammatory drugs	65 (19%)	51 (18%)	14 (24%)
Analgesics/antipyretics	82 (24%)	71 (25%)	11 (19%)
Cognitive function			
Mini-Mental State Examination	27.7 (2.3)	27.8 (2.3)	27.5 (2.3)
Trail Making Test, seconds			
Part A	52 (33)	51 (33)	56 (33)
Part B	123 (68)	120 (66)	140 (72)
Part B less A	74 (55)	72 (55)	84 (55)
Medical conditions (self-report)			
Stroke	32 (9%)	26 (9%)	6 (10%)
Diabetes mellitus	47 (13%)	33 (11%)	14 (24%)
Hyperlipidemia	179 (51%)	148 (51%)	31 (53%)
Hypertension	259 (75%)	214 (74%)	45 (78%)
Peripheral artery disease	29 (8%)	22 (8%)	7 (12%)
History of back pain or spinal stenosis	138 (39%)	116 (40%)	22 (37%)
History of falls	129 (37%)	106 (36%)	23 (40%)
Parkinson's disease	6 (2%)	5 (2%)	1 (2%)
Peripheral neuropathy	69 (21%)	35 (13%)	34 (63%)
Cancer, excluding skin cancer	81 (23%)	63 (22%)	18 (31%)

Table 3 Baseline characteristics and descriptive statistics of the study sample ($N = 351$); mean (standard deviation) or count (percent) is shown *(Continued)*

	Full cohort ($n = 351$)	Baseline somatosensory function	
		Intact ($n = 292$)	Impaired ($n = 59$)
Physical function			
Uses walking aid	36 (10%)	24 (8%)	12 (20%)
Physical Activity Scale for the Elderly	111 (69)	114 (70)	97 (61)
Short Physical Performance Battery	9.8 (2.2)	10.0 (2.0)	8.6 (2.8)
Gait speed at baseline, m/s	1.00 (0.25)	1.02 (0.24)	0.92 (0.29)
Falls during first year of follow-up	1.1 (1.7)	1.1 (1.8)	1.0 (1.4)
Berg Balance score	51 (5)	52 (5)	48 (8)

[a]*Comorbidity count includes coronary heart disease, high blood pressure, diabetes, ulcer or other stomach disease, kidney disease, liver disease, anemia, cancer, depression, osteoarthritis and degenerative arthritis, rheumatoid arthritis, and other unlisted medical problem* [34]

This high incidence of sensory loss has not been fully appreciated in other studies nor in clinical practice.

To our knowledge previous studies have not examined changes in peripheral sensory function over time nor their relationship to mobility outcomes. However, several cross-sectional and longitudinal studies have examined relationships between baseline abnormalities in foot sensation (including sense of vibration and touch), functional impairments, and fall risk. Most of these studies demonstrated that the loss of vibratory sensation was

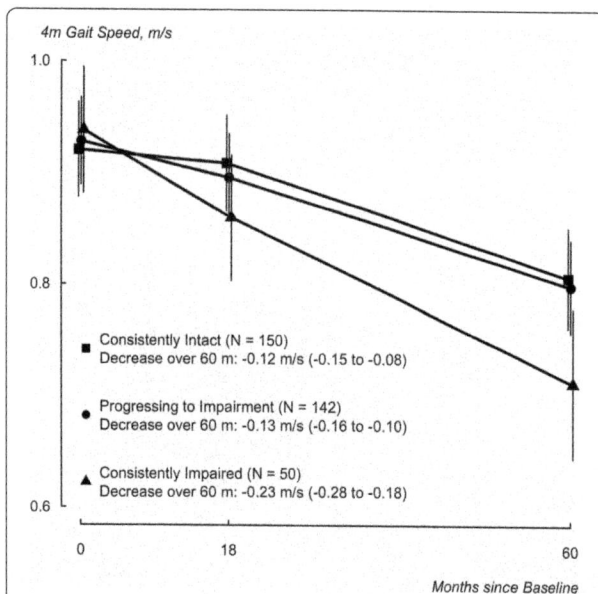

Fig. 1 Model-generated mean and 95% confidence interval estimates of 60-month decrease in 4 m gait speed are provided for each temporal pattern of sensory functioning. Those 'consistently intact' displayed intact function at both baseline and follow-up measurements. Those 'progressing to impairment' exhibited intact perception at baseline but were impaired at follow-up. Those 'consistently impaired' had sensory impairment at both time points. Estimates and 95% confidence intervals were derived from repeated measures ANOVA adjusted for age, sex, comorbidity count, use of walking aids, baseline Berg balance score, and diabetes

associated with increased fall risk [5, 37, 38]. For example, Patel et al. [37] found among older women with diabetes that fallers had higher vibratory sensory thresholds than non-fallers, but both fallers and non-fallers had similar touch sensation. Using cross-sectional data from the 2003–2004 National Health and Nutrition Examination Survey (NHANES), Wilson et al. [38] found no association between sensory loss in the feet, as measured using 10 g SWMT, and a subjective report of "difficulty with falls during the past 12 months," assessed by questionnaire. However, after adjustments, participants who exhibited peripheral neuropathy had an increased risk of balance impairment compared to those without peripheral neuropathy. In a cross-sectional study exploring the effect of different sensory systems on postural stability, Lord and colleagues [5] found that poor tactile sensitivity to Semmes-Weinstein monofilaments at the lateral malleolus of the dominant ankle was associated with increased body sway. They also reported that peripheral sensation is the most important sensory system in the maintenance of static postural stability. Richardson et al. [39] found a cross-sectional relationship between peripheral neuropathy diagnosed by electromyography in a small referral population and a self-reported history of falls during the past year. Using longitudinal data from the Health, Aging and Body Composition study, Strotmeyer et al. [16] found that insensitivity to the 10 g Semmes Weinstein monofilament at the great toe was associated with lower quadriceps muscle strength. Thus, a number of neuromuscular deficits are associated with peripheral neuropathy and may lead to mobility impairments and falls.

Our longitudinal results are most consistent with those of Lord et al. [7] and Luukinen et al. [8] who found relationships between various modalities of sensory loss at the knees and recurrent falls in community-dwelling populations followed prospectively with fall questionnaires or diaries over 1 or 2 years, respectively. In Lord et al's study, touch sensation did not

Table 4 Risk of Falls According to temporal pattern in sensory function; point estimates and 95% confidence intervals shown

| | Absolute Risk of Fall | | [a]Relative Risk of Fall | |
	Events (py)	Rate per py	Unadjusted	[b]Adjusted
Consistently intact	384 (474)	0.81	Referent	Referent
Progressing to impairment	591 (454)	1.31	1.60 (1.16 to 2.22)	1.57 (1.12 to 2.22)
Consistently impaired	181 (161)	1.12	1.39 (0.89 to 2.18)	1.48 (0.89 to 2.45)

PY = patient year
[a]Estimates obtained using negative binomial regression
[b]Adjusted for age, sex, physical activity (PASE index), diabetes, comorbidity, Short Physical Performance Battery score

discriminate non-fallers from single or recurrent fallers. However, in another one-year prospective study of older adults living in an intermediate care facility, Lord and Clark [40] found that tactile sensitivity using a Semmes Weinstein Pressure Aesthesiometer did discriminate between fallers and non-fallers.

The subjects of our study who exhibited consistent sensory impairment at baseline and at follow-up were not more likely to fall than those who were consistently intact. The lack of a statistically significant difference between these groups could be due to the relatively small size of the consistently impaired group ($N = 50$) or adaptive behaviors learned by people with chronic sensory loss. Those with baseline sensory impairment were more likely to be using walking aids, which may have protected them from falls. There was also a trend towards lower physical activity as measured by PASE, suggesting that this group may have had less time at risk for falls.

The strength of the current study lies in its 5-year longitudinal design and rigorous detection of falls using state-of-the-art falls calendars and follow-up phone calls. There are several weaknesses to the current study. Participants did not receive a full neuropathic evaluation and the monofilament assessment of sensory function is only a quick screen that is specific, but not very sensitive to neuropathic sensory loss [41]. However, this simple, widely available, bed-side test of sensation on the dorsum of the great toe was sensitive to changes over time and predictive of a decrease in gait speed and increase in fall rate, even in the absence of more rigorous assessments of vibratory, proprioceptive, and motor nerve function. Although observed relationships could be confounded by underlying diseases such as diabetes, which affect sensation, gait and falls, the findings persisted after multivariate adjustments.

Our longitudinal results provide validation of the belief that peripheral sensory loss is a risk factor for mobility impairment. They also suggest that a decline in touch sensation at the great toe over time may be a more important predictor of slow gait speed and falls than a baseline sensory deficit. Therefore, simple, repeated clinical assessments of sensory function in the feet of older adults may be helpful in identifying and treating those at risk of falls to prevent their morbid consequences.

Abbreviations
BMI: Body mass index; MOBILIZE: Maintenance Of Balance, Independent Living, Intellect, and Zest in the Elderly; PASE: Physical Activity Scale for the Elderly; SPPB: Short Physical Performance Battery; SWMT: Semmes-Weinstein monofilament test

Acknowledgements
Not applicable.

Funding
This research was supported by grants P01 AG04390, R01 AG041785, and R01 AG025037 to Dr. Lipsitz from the National Institute on Aging. Dr. Manor was supported by grant K01 AG044543. This study was also supported by the infrastructural resources provided by the Boston Claude D. Pepper Older Americans Independence Center (P30-AG013679). Dr. Lipsitz holds the Irving and Edyth S. Usen and Family Chair in Geriatric Medicine at Hebrew SeniorLife, Boston, MA.

Authors' contributions
Conception and design of the work: LL, BM and TT; Acquisition, analysis, interpretation of data for the work: LL, BM, DH, II, JZ and TT; Drafting the work and revising it for important intellectual content: LL, BM, JZ and TT. All authors read and approved the final manuscript.

Competing interests
The authors declare that they have no competing interests.

Author details
[1]Hebrew SeniorLife Institute for Aging Research, 1200 Centre Street, Boston Roslindale, MA 02131, USA. [2]Division of Gerontology, Beth Israel Deaconess Medical Center, Boston, MA, USA. [3]Harvard Medical School, Boston, MA, USA.

References
1. Centers for Disease Control and Prevention. Falls are Leading Cause of Injury and Death in Older Americans. CDC Newsroom. 2016. https://www.cdc.gov/media/releases/2016/p0922-older-adult-falls.html. Accessed 22 Sept 2016.
2. Gu Y, Dennis SM. Are falls prevention programs effective at reducing the risk factors for falls in people with type-2 diabetes mellitus and peripheral neuropathy: a systematic review with narrative synthesis. J Diabetes Complicat. 2017;31:504–16.
3. Rubenstein LZ. Falls in older people: epidemiology, risk factors and strategies for prevention. Age Ageing. 2006;35:ii37–41.
4. Richardson JK, Hurvitz EA. Peripheral neuropathy: a true risk factor for falls. J Gerontol A Biol Sci Med Sci. 1995;50:M211–5.
5. Lord SR, Clark RD, Webster IW. Physiological factors associated with falls in an elderly population. J Am Geriatr Soc. 1991;39:1194–200.
6. Lord SR, Clark RD, Webster IW. Postural stability and associated physiological factors in a population of aged persons. J Gerontol. 1991;46:M69–76.
7. Lord SR, Ward JA, Williams P, Anstey K. Physiological factors associated with falls in older community-dwelling women. J Am Geriatr Soc. 1994;42:1110–7.

8. Luukinen H, Koski K, Laippala P, Kivela SL. Predictors for recurrent falls among the home-dwelling elderly. Scand J Prim Health. 1995;13:294–9.
9. Cavanagh PR, Derr JA, Ulbrecht JS, Maser RE, Orchard TJ. Problems with gait and posture in neuropathic patients with insulin-dependent diabetes mellitus. Diabetic Med. 1992;9:469–74.
10. Baldereschi M, Inzitari M, Di Carlo A, et al. Epidemiology of distal symmetrical neuropathies in the Italian elderly. Neurology. 2007;68:1460–7.
11. Chiles NS, Phillips CL, Volpato S, et al. Diabetes, peripheral neuropathy, and lower-extremity function. J Diabetes Complicat. 2014;28:91–5.
12. Katon JG, Reiber GE, Nelson KM. Peripheral neuropathy defined by monofilament insensitivity and diabetes status. Diabetes Care. 2013;36: 1604–6.
13. Hanewinckel R, Van Oijen M, Ikram MA, Van Doorn PA. The epidemiology and risk factors of chronic polyneuropathy. Eur J Epidemiol. 2016;31:5–20.
14. Callaghan B, Kerber K, Langa KM, et al. Longitudinal patient-oriented outcomes in neuropathy: importance of early detection and falls. Neurology. 2015;85:71–9.
15. Dyck PJ, Litchy WJ, Lehman KA, Hokanson JL, Low PA, O'Brien PC. Variables influencing neuropathic endpoints: the Rochester diabetic neuropathy study of healthy subjects. Neurology. 1995;45:1115–21.
16. Strotmeyer ES, De Rekeneire N, Schwartz AV, et al. Sensory and motor peripheral nerve function and lower-extremity quadriceps strength: the health, aging and body composition study. J Am Geriatr Soc. 2009;57:2004–10.
17. Wuehr M, Schniepp R, Schlick C, et al. Sensory loss and walking speed related factors for gait alterations in patients with peripheral neuropathy. Gait Posture. 2014;39:852–8.
18. Leveille SG, Kiel DP, Jones RN, et al. The MOBILIZE Boston study: design and methods of a prospective cohort study of novel risk factors for falls in an older population. BMC Geriatr. 2008;8:16.
19. Samelson EJ, Kelsey JL, Kiel DP, et al. Issues in conducting epidemiologic research among elders: lessons from the MOBILIZE Boston study. Am J Epidemiol. 2008;168:1444–51.
20. Folstein MF, Folstein SE, McHugh PR. "Mini-mental state". A practical method for grading the cognitive state of patients for the clinician. J Psychiatr Res. 1975;12:189–98.
21. Escobar JI, Burnam A, Karno M, Forsythe A, Landsverk J, Golding JM. Use of the mini-mental state examination (MMSE) in a community population of mixed ethnicity cultural and linguistic artifacts. J Nerv Ment Dis. 1986;174:607–14.
22. Tombaugh TN. Trail making test a and B: normative data stratified by age and education. Arch Clin Neuropsychol. 2004;19:203–14.
23. Guralnik JM, Simonsick EM, Ferrucci L, et al. A short physical performance battery assessing lower extremity function: association with self-reported disability and prediction of mortality and nursing home admission. J Gerontol. 1994;49:M85–94.
24. Berg KO, Maki BE, Williams JI, Holliday PJ, Wood-Dauphinee SL. Clinical and laboratory measures of postural balance in an elderly population. Arch Phys Med Rehabil. 1992;73:1073–80.
25. Perkins BA, Olaleye D, Zinman B, Bril V. Simple screening tests for peripheral neuropathy in the diabetes clinic. Diabetes Care. 2001;24(2):250–6.
26. Abbott CA, Carrington AL, Ashe H, et al. The north-west diabetes foot care study: incidence of, and risk factors for, new diabetic foot ulceration in a community-based patient cohort. Diabet Med. 2002;19:377–84.
27. Dros J, Wewerinke A, Bindels PJ, Van Weert HC. Accuracy of monofilament testing to diagnose peripheral neuropathy: a systematic review. Ann Fam Med. 2009;7:555–8.
28. Shumway-Cook A, Baldwin M, Polissar NL, Gruber W. Predicting the probability for falls in community-dwelling older adults. Phys Ther. 1997;77:812–9.
29. Guralnik JM, Ferrucci L, Simonsick EM, Salive ME, Wallace RB. Lower-extremity function in persons over the age of 70 years as a predictor of subsequent disability. N Engl J Med. 1995;332:556–61.
30. Guralnik JM, Ferrucci L, Pieper CF, et al. Lower extremity function and subsequent disability: consistency across studies, predictive models, and value of gait speed alone compared with the short physical performance battery. J Gerontol A Biol Sci Med Sci. 2000;55:M221–31.
31. Gibson MJ, Andres RO, Isaacs B, Radebaugh T, Wormpetersen J. The prevention of falls in later life - a report of the Kellogg-international-work-group on the prevention of falls by the elderly. Dan Med Bull. 1987;34:1–24.
32. Tinetti ME, Liu WL, Claus EB. Predictors and prognosis of inability to get up after falls among elderly persons. JAMA. 1993;269:65–70.
33. Washburn RA, Smith KW, Jette AM, Janney CA. The physical activity scale for the elderly (PASE): development and evaluation. J Clin Epidemiol. 1993;46: 153–62.
34. Sangha O, Stucki G, Liang MH, Fossel AH, Katz JN. The self-administered comorbidity questionnaire: a new method to assess comorbidity for clinical and health services research. Arthritis Rheum. 2003;49:156–63.
35. Eaton WW, Muntaner C, Smith C, Tien A, Ybarra M. Center for Epidemiologic Studies Depression Scale: review and revision (CESD and CESD-R). In: ME M, editor. The use of psychological testing for treatment planning and outcomes assessment. Mahwah: Lawrence Erlbaum Assoc Inc; 2004.
36. Perera S, Mody SH, Woodman RC, Studenski SA. Meaningful change and responsiveness in common physical performance measures in older adults. J Am Geriatr Soc. 2006;54:743–9.
37. Patel S, Hyer S, Tweed K, et al. Risk factors for fractures and falls in older women with type 2 diabetes mellitus. Calcified Tissue Int. 2008;82:87–91.
38. Wilson SJ, Garner JC, Loprinzi PD. The influence of multiple sensory impairments on functional balance and difficulty with falls among U.S. adults. Prev Med. 2016;87:41–6.
39. Richardson JK, Ching C, Hurvitz EA. The relationship between electromyographically documented peripheral neuropathy and falls. J Am Geriatr Soc. 1992;40:1008–12.
40. Lord SR, Clark RD. Simple physiological and clinical tests for the accurate prediction of falling in older people. Gerontology. 1996;42:199–203.
41. Feng Y, Schlösser FJ, Sumpio BE. The Semmes Weinstein monofilament examination as a screening tool for diabetic peripheral neuropathy. J Vasc Surg. 2009;50:675–82.

Permissions

All chapters in this book were first published in GERIATRICS, by BioMed Central; hereby published with permission under the Creative Commons Attribution License or equivalent. Every chapter published in this book has been scrutinized by our experts. Their significance has been extensively debated. The topics covered herein carry significant findings which will fuel the growth of the discipline. They may even be implemented as practical applications or may be referred to as a beginning point for another development.

The contributors of this book come from diverse backgrounds, making this book a truly international effort. This book will bring forth new frontiers with its revolutionizing research information and detailed analysis of the nascent developments around the world.

We would like to thank all the contributing authors for lending their expertise to make the book truly unique. They have played a crucial role in the development of this book. Without their invaluable contributions this book wouldn't have been possible. They have made vital efforts to compile up to date information on the varied aspects of this subject to make this book a valuable addition to the collection of many professionals and students.

This book was conceptualized with the vision of imparting up-to-date information and advanced data in this field. To ensure the same, a matchless editorial board was set up. Every individual on the board went through rigorous rounds of assessment to prove their worth. After which they invested a large part of their time researching and compiling the most relevant data for our readers.

The editorial board has been involved in producing this book since its inception. They have spent rigorous hours researching and exploring the diverse topics which have resulted in the successful publishing of this book. They have passed on their knowledge of decades through this book. To expedite this challenging task, the publisher supported the team at every step. A small team of assistant editors was also appointed to further simplify the editing procedure and attain best results for the readers.

Apart from the editorial board, the designing team has also invested a significant amount of their time in understanding the subject and creating the most relevant covers. They scrutinized every image to scout for the most suitable representation of the subject and create an appropriate cover for the book.

The publishing team has been an ardent support to the editorial, designing and production team. Their endless efforts to recruit the best for this project, has resulted in the accomplishment of this book. They are a veteran in the field of academics and their pool of knowledge is as vast as their experience in printing. Their expertise and guidance has proved useful at every step. Their uncompromising quality standards have made this book an exceptional effort. Their encouragement from time to time has been an inspiration for everyone.

The publisher and the editorial board hope that this book will prove to be a valuable piece of knowledge for researchers, students, practitioners and scholars across the globe.

List of Contributors

Jae Myeong Kang and Seong-Jin Cho
Department of Psychiatry, Gil Medical Center, Gachon University College of Medicine, Incheon, Republic of Korea

Bo Kyung Sohn
Department of Psychiatry, SMG-SNU Boramae Medical Center, Boramae-Ro 5-Gil, Shindaebang-dong, Dongjak-gu, Seoul, Republic of Korea

Young-Sung Cho, Jeong-Seok Choi, Hee Yeon Jeong and Jun-Young Lee
Department of Psychiatry, SMG-SNU Boramae Medical Center, Boramae-Ro 5-Gil, Shindaebang-dong, Dongjak-gu, Seoul, Republic of Korea
Department of Psychiatry and Behavioral Science, Seoul National University College of Medicine, Boramae-Ro 5-Gil, Shindaebang-dong, Dongjak-gu, Seoul, Republic of Korea

Chi Hyun Choi
Department of Psychiatry and Behavioral Science, Seoul National University College of Medicine, Boramae-Ro 5-Gil, Shindaebang-dong, Dongjak-gu, Seoul, Republic of Korea

Soowon Park
Department of Education, Sejong University, Seoul, Republic of Korea

Byung Ho Lee
Department of Psychology, Salisbury University, Salisbury, Maryland, USA

Jae-Hong Lee
Department of Neurology, Asan Medical Center, University of Ulsan College of Medicine, Seoul, Republic of Korea

Dafne Piersma, Anselm B. M. Fuermaier, Dick De Waard, Michelle J. A. Doumen and Oliver Tucha
Department of Clinical and Developmental Neuropsychology, University of Groningen, Groningen, The Netherlands

Wiebo H. Brouwer
Department of Clinical and Developmental Neuropsychology, University of Groningen, Groningen, The Netherlands

Department of Neurology and Alzheimer Research Center, University of Groningen and University Medical Center Groningen, Groningen, The Netherlands

Ragnhild J. Davidse and Jolieke De Groot
SWOV Institute for Road Safety Research, The Hague, The Netherlands

Rudolf W. H. M. Ponds
Department of Psychiatry and Neuropsychology, School of Mental Health and Neurosciences (MHeNS), Maastricht University, Maastricht, The Netherlands

Peter P. De Deyn
Department of Neurology and Alzheimer Research Center, University of Groningen and University Medical Center Groningen, Groningen, The Netherlands

Lloyd D. Hughes
GP Registrar, Primary Care Directorate, NHS Education for Scotland, Edinburgh, UK

Miles D. Witham
Ageing and Health, University of Dundee, Ninewells Hospital, Dundee, UK

Franziska Saxer, Marcel Jakob, Norbert Suhm, Werner Vach and Nicolas Bless
Department of Orthopaedics and Traumatology, University Hospital Basel, Spitalstrasse 21, 4031 Basel, Switzerland

Patrick Studer
Department of Orthopaedics and Traumatology, University Hospital Basel, Spitalstrasse 21, 4031 Basel, Switzerland
Clinic for Orthopaedics and Trauma Surgery Stephanshorn, Brauerstrasse 95, 9016 St. Gallen, Switzerland

Salome Dell-Kuster
Basel Institute for Clinical Epidemiology and Biostatistics, University Hospital Basel, Spitalstrasse 12, 4031 Basel, Switzerland
Department of Department of Anaesthesiology, Surgical Intensive Care, Prehospital Emergency Medicine and Pain Therapy, University Hospital Basel, Spitalstrasse 21, 4031 Basel, Switzerland

Rachel Rosenthal
Faculty of Medicine, University of Basel, Klingelbergstr. 61, 4056 Basel, Switzerland

Sang Yhun Ju
Department of Family Medicine, Yeouido St. Mary's Hospital, College of Medicine, The Catholic University of Korea, 10, 63-Ro, Yeongdeungpo-Gu, Seoul 07345, Republic of Korea
Hospice Palliative Medicine, Division of Spirituality, Yeouido St. Mary's Hospital, College of Medicine, The Catholic University of Korea, 10, 63-Ro, Yeongdeungpo-Gu, Seoul 07345, Republic of Korea

June Young Lee
Department of Biostatistics, Korea University College of Medicine, 145, Anam-Ro, Seongbuk-Gu, Seoul 02841, Republic of Korea

Do Hoon Kim
Department of Family Medicine, Korea University Ansan Hospital, 70-9, Darigan 2-gil, Danwon-Gu, Ansan-Si, Gyeonggi-Do 15459, Republic of Korea

Bram Tilburgs and Myrra Vernooij-Dassen
Department of IQ healthcare, Radboudumc, Nijmegen, The Netherlands

Raymond Koopmans
Department of Primary and Community Care, Radboudumc, Nijmegen, The Netherlands
Radboudumc Alzheimer Centre, Nijmegen, The Netherlands
Joachim en Anna, Centre for Specialized Geriatric Care, Nijmegen, The Netherlands

Marieke Perry
Department of Primary and Community Care, Radboudumc, Nijmegen, The Netherlands
Radboudumc Alzheimer Centre, Nijmegen, The Netherlands
Department of Geriatric Medicine, Radboudumc, Nijmegen, The Netherlands

Marije Weidema
Department of Medical Oncology, Radboudumc, Nijmegen, The Netherlands

Yvonne Engels
Department of Anesthesiology, Pain and Palliative Medicine, Radboudumc, Nijmegen, The Netherlands

H W Donkers, D J Van der Veen and M J Vernooij-Dassen
Radboud university medical center, Radboud Institute for Health Sciences, IQ healthcare, 6500, HB, Nijmegen, The Netherlands
Radboud university medical center, Donders Institute for Brain, Cognition and Behaviour, Radboudumc Alzheimer Center, Nijmegen, The Netherlands

M W G Nijhuis-vander Sanden
Radboud university medical center, Radboud Institute for Health Sciences, IQ healthcare, 6500, HB, Nijmegen, The Netherlands
Department of Rehabilitation, Radboud university medical center, Donders Institute for Brain, Cognition and Behaviour, Nijmegen, The Netherlands

M J L Graff
Radboud university medical center, Radboud Institute for Health Sciences, IQ healthcare, 6500, HB, Nijmegen, The Netherlands
Radboud university medical center, Donders Institute for Brain, Cognition and Behaviour, Radboudumc Alzheimer Center, Nijmegen, The Netherlands
Department of Rehabilitation, Radboud university medical center, Donders Institute for Brain, Cognition and Behaviour, Nijmegen, The Netherlands

S Teerenstra
Department for Health Evidence, section Biostatistics, Radboud university medical center, Radboud Institute for Health Sciences, Nijmegen, The Netherlands

Min Gao, Weijun Zhang, Donghua Tian, Shengfa Zhang and Linni Gu
School of Social Development and Public Policy, China Institute of Health, Beijing Normal University, Beijing 100875, China

Zhihong Sa
School of Sociology, Beijing Normal University, No.19, Xinjiekou wai Street, Beijing 100875, China

Yanyu Li
School of Humanities and Social Sciences, North China Electric Power University, Baoding 071000, China

Michael Van der Elst, Birgitte Schoenmakers and Jan De Lepeleire
Department of Public Health and Primary Care, University of Leuven, Kapucijnenvoer 33 bus 7001, B-3000 Leuven, Belgium

Bert Vaes
Department of Public Health and Primary Care, University of Leuven, Kapucijnenvoer 33 bus 7001, B-3000 Leuven, Belgium
Institute of Health and Society, Université Catholique de Louvain, Clos Chapelle-aux-champs 30, B-1200 Brussels, Belgium

Daan Duppen, Deborah Lambotte and Bram Fret
Department of Educational Sciences, Vrije Universiteit Brussel, Pleinlaan 2, B-1050 Brussels, Belgium

Martha Therese Gjestsen
Centre for age-related medicine (SESAM), Stavanger University Hospital, Stavanger, Norway
University of Stavanger, Faculty of Health Sciences, Centre for Resilience in Healthcare (SHARE), Stavanger, Norway

Ingelin Testad
Centre for age-related medicine (SESAM), Stavanger University Hospital, Stavanger, Norway
University of Exeter Medical School, Exeter, Devon, UK

Kolbjørn Brønnick
Centre for Clinical Research in Psychosis (TIPS), Stavanger University Hospital, Stavanger, Norway
University of Stavanger, Faculty of Health Sciences, Stavanger, Norway

Zafirah Banu, Kai Zhen Yap and Hui Ting Ang
Department of Pharmacy, Faculty of Science, National University of Singapore, Singapore, Republic of Singapore

Ka Keat Lim, Yu Heng Kwan and Truls Ostbye
Program in Health Services and Systems Research, Duke-NUS Medical School, Singapore, Republic of Singapore

Julian Thumboo
Program in Health Services and Systems Research, Duke-NUS Medical School, Singapore, Republic of Singapore
Department of Rheumatology and Immunology, Singapore General Hospital, Singapore, Republic of Singapore

Chuen Seng Tan
Saw Swee Hock School of Public Health, National University of Singapore and National University Health System, Singapore, Republic of Singapore

Kheng Hock Lee and Lian Leng Low
Department of Family Medicine and Continuing Care, Singapore General Hospital, Singapore, Republic of Singapore
Duke-NUS Medical School, Singapore, Republic of Singapore

Warren Fong
Department of Rheumatology and Immunology, Singapore General Hospital, Singapore, Republic of Singapore
Duke-NUS Medical School, Singapore, Republic of Singapore
Department of Medicine, Yong Loo Lin School of Medicine, National University of Singapore, Singapore, Republic of Singapore

Madushika Wishvanie Kodagoda Gamage
Department of Nursing, Faculty of Allied Health Sciences, University of Ruhuna, Galle, Sri Lanka

Chandana Hewage
Department of Physiology, Faculty of Medical Sciences, University of Sri Jayewardenepura, Gangodawila, Nugegoda, Sri Lanka

Kithsiri Dedduwa Pathirana
Department of Medicine, Faculty of Medicine, University of Ruhuna, Galle, Sri Lanka

Samuel Kwaku Essien, Cindy Xin Feng and Marwa Farag
School of Public Health, University of Saskatchewan, Health Sciences Building E-Wing, 104 Clinic Place, Saskatoon, SK S7N 2Z4, Canada

Wenjie Sun
Robert Stempel College of Public and Social Work, Florida international University, Miami, FL 33199, USA
School of Food Science, Guangdong Pharmaceutical University, Zhongshan 528458, China

Yongqing Gao
School of Food Science, Guangdong Pharmaceutical University, Zhongshan 528458, China

Longhai Li
Department of Mathematics and Statistics, University of Saskatchewan, Saskatoon, SK S7N 5E6, Canada

Eva Lindqvist, Annika PerssonVasiliou and Louise Nygård
Department of Neurobiology, Care Sciences and Society (NVS), Division of Occupational Therapy, Karolinska Institutet, Fack 23 200, SE-141 83 Huddinge, Sweden

Amy S. Hwang and Alex Mihailidis
University of Toronto and Toronto Rehab Institute-UHN, Toronto, Canada

Arlene Astelle
University of Sheffield, Sheffield, UK

Andrew Sixsmith
Simon Fraser University, Vancouver, Canada

Michael A. Steinman
University of California, 3333 California St, San Francisco, CA 94118, USA
San Francisco VA Health Care System, 4150 Clement St, San Francisco, CA 94121, USA Clalit Research Institute, Tel Aviv, Israel University of Haifa, Haifa, Israel

Ran D. Balicer
Clalit Research Institute, Tel Aviv, Israel

Marcelo Low and Efrat Shadmi
Clalit Research Institute, Tel Aviv, Israel
University of Haifa, Haifa, Israel

Sooyoung Kwon, Soyun Hong and Sangeun Lee
College of Nursing, Yonsei University, Seoul, South Korea

Heejung Kim
College of Nursing, Yonsei University, Seoul, South Korea
Mo-Im Kim Nursing Research Institute, Yonsei University, Seoul, South Korea

Live Bredholt Jørgensen and Berit Marie Thorleifsson
Department of Public Health and Nursing, Norwegian University of Science and Technology (NTNU), Trondheim, Norway

Geir Selbæk
Norwegian National Advisory Unit on Ageing and Health, Vestfold Hospital Trust, Tønsberg, Norway
Centre for Old Age Psychiatric Research, Innlandet Hospital Trust, Ottestad, Norway
Institute of Health and Society, Faculty of Medicine, University of Oslo, Oslo, Norway

Anne-Sofie Helvik
Norwegian National Advisory Unit on Ageing and Health, Vestfold Hospital Trust, Tønsberg, Norway
Department of Public Health and Nursing, Faculty of Medicine and Health Sciences, Norwegian University of Science and Technology (NTNU), Trondheim, Norway
St Olavs University Hospital, Trondheim, Norway

Jūratė Šaltytė Benth
Centre for Old Age Psychiatric Research, Innlandet Hospital Trust, Ottestad, Norway
Institute of Clinical Medicine, University of Oslo, Oslo, Norway
Health Services Research Unit, Akershus University Hospital, Lørenskog, Norway

Huan-Ji Dong, Britt Larsson and Björn Gerdle
Pain and Rehabilitation Medicine, Department of Medicine and Health Sciences (IMH), Faculty of Health Sciences, Linköping University, SE-581 85 Linköping, Sweden

Lars-Åke Levin and Lars Bernfort
Division of Health Care Analysis, Department of Medical and Health Sciences, Linköping University, SE-581 85 Linköping, Sweden

Maria Bjerk, Therese Brovold and Astrid Bergland
Department of Physiotherapy, OsloMet – Oslo Metropolitan University, St. Olavs plass, 0130 Oslo, Norway

Dawn A. Skelton
School of Health and Life Sciences, Glasgow Caledonian University, Glasgow, UK

Sergei Muratov
Department of Health Research Methods, Evidence, and Impact, McMaster University, Hamilton, ON, Canada
Programs for Assessment of Technology in Health (PATH), The Research Institute of St. Joe's Hamilton, St. Joseph's Healthcare, Hamilton, ON, Canada

Anne Holbrook
Department of Health Research Methods, Evidence, and Impact, McMaster University, Hamilton, ON, Canada
Division of Clinical Pharmacology and Toxicology, Department of Medicine, McMaster University, Hamilton, ON, Canada

Lawrence Mbuagbaw
Department of Health Research Methods, Evidence, and Impact, McMaster University, Hamilton, ON, Canada
Biostatistics Unit, Father Sean O'Sullivan Research Centre, St Joseph's Healthcare, Hamilton, ON, Canada

Jean-Eric Tarride
Department of Health Research Methods, Evidence, and Impact, McMaster University, Hamilton, ON, Canada
Programs for Assessment of Technology in Health (PATH), The Research Institute of St. Joe's Hamilton, St. Joseph's Healthcare, Hamilton, ON, Canada
Center for Health Economics and Policy Analysis (CHEPA), McMaster University, Hamilton, Canada

Andrew Costa
Department of Health Research Methods, Evidence, and Impact, McMaster University, Hamilton, ON, Canada
Institute for Clinical Evaluative Sciences (ICES), Toronto, ON, Canada
Center for Health Economics and Policy Analysis (CHEPA), McMaster University, Hamilton, Canada

Justin Lee
Department of Health Research Methods, Evidence, and Impact, McMaster University, Hamilton, ON, Canada
Division of Geriatric Medicine, Department of Medicine, McMaster University, Hamilton, ON, Canada
Division of Clinical Pharmacology and Toxicology, Department of Medicine, McMaster University, Hamilton, ON, Canada
Geriatric Education and Research in Aging Sciences Centre, Hamilton Health Sciences, Hamilton, ON, Canada

Wayne Khuu
Institute for Clinical Evaluative Sciences (ICES), Toronto, ON, Canada

J. Michael Paterson
Institute for Clinical Evaluative Sciences (ICES), Toronto, ON, Canada
Institute of Health Policy, Management and Evaluation, University of Toronto, Toronto, ON, Canada

Tara Gomes
Institute for Clinical Evaluative Sciences (ICES), Toronto, ON, Canada
Leslie Dan Faculty of Pharmacy, University of Toronto, Toronto, Canada
Li Ka Shing Knowledge Institute, St. Michael's Hospital, Toronto, ON, Canada

Jason R. Guertin
Département de Médecine Sociale et Préventive, Faculté de Médecine, Université Laval, Quebec City, QC, Canada
Centre de recherche du CHU de Québec, Université Laval, Axe Santé des Populations et Pratiques Optimales en Santé, Québec City, QC, Canada

Maria Magdalena Bujnowska-Fedak
Department of Family Medicine, Wrocław Medical University, ul. Syrokomli 1, 51-141 Wrocław, Poland

Donata Kurpas and Katarzyna Szwamel
Department of Family Medicine, Wrocław Medical University, ul. Syrokomli 1, 51-141 Wrocław, Poland
Opole Medical School, ul. Katowicka 68, 45-060 Opole, Poland

Carol A. Holland
Centre For Ageing Research, Lancaster University, Lancaster, UK

Holly Gwyther
Centre For Ageing Research, Lancaster University, Lancaster, UK
Psychology, School of Life and Health Sciences, Aston University, Birmingham, UK

Rachel L. Shaw
Psychology, School of Life and Health Sciences, Aston University, Birmingham, UK

Barbara D'Avanzo
Istituto di Ricerche Farmacologiche Mario Negri IRCCS, Milan, Italy

Yuan Zhao
Ginling College, School of Geographical Science, Nanjing Normal University, Nanjing, China
Jiangsu Center for Collaborative Innovation in Geographical Information Resource Development and Application, Nanjing, China

Hong Fu
School of Psychology, Nanjing Normal University, Nanjing, China

Aimei Guo
Ginling College, International Center for Aging Studies, Nanjing Normal University, Nanjing, China

Li Qiu
Independent Researcher, New York, USA

Karen S. L. Cheung
Mindlink Institute, Hong Kong, Hong Kong

Bei Wu
Rory Meyers College of Nursing and NYU Aging Incubator, New York University, New York, USA

Daniela Jopp
Department of Psychology and National Centre for Research LIVES, University of Lausanne, Lausanne, Switzerland

Danan Gu
United Nations Population Division, Two UN Plaza, DC2-1910, New York, NY 10017, USA

Sarah Wu, Jill M. Morrison, Vanessa Vucea and Sabrina Iuglio
University of Waterloo, 200 University Avenue West, Waterloo, Ontario N2L 3G1, Canada

Heather Keller
University of Waterloo, 200 University Avenue West, Waterloo, Ontario N2L 3G1, Canada
Research Institute for Aging, 250 Laurelwood Drive, Waterloo, Ontario N2J 0E2, Canada

Hilary Dunn-Ridgeway
Research Institute for Aging, 250 Laurelwood Drive, Waterloo, Ontario N2J 0E2, Canada

Julia Wearing
Faculty of Health, Medicine and Sciences, School for Public Health and Primary Care, University Maastricht, Minderbroedersberg 4-6, Maastricht, LK 6211, The Netherlands
Adullam Stiftung, Mittlere Strasse 15, 4056 Basel, Switzerland

Peter Konings
Geriatrische Klinik St. Gallen, Rorschacher Strasse 94, 9000 St. Gallen, Switzerland

Maria Stokes
Faculty of Health Sciences, University of Southampton, Building 45, Highfield Campus, Southampton SO17 1BJ, UK

Eling D. de Bruin
Insitute of Human Movement Sciences and Sport (IBWS) ETH, Department of Health Sciences and Technology, HCP H 25.1, Leopold-Ruzicka-Weg 4, 8093 Zürich, ETH, Zurich, Switzerland
Division of Physiotherapy, Department of Neurobiology, Care Sciences and Society, Karolinska Institutet, Stockholm, Sweden

Daniel Habtemariam and Ikechukwu Iloputaife
Hebrew SeniorLife Institute for Aging Research, 1200 Centre Street, Boston Roslindale, MA 02131, USA

Lewis A. Lipsitz, Brad Manor, Junhong Zhou and Thomas G. Travison
Hebrew SeniorLife Institute for Aging Research, 1200 Centre Street, Boston Roslindale, MA 02131, USA
Division of Gerontology, Beth Israel Deaconess Medical Center, Boston, MA, USA
Harvard Medical School, Boston, MA, USA

Index